PET and PET-CT in Oncology

P. Oehr · H.-J. Biersack · E. Coleman (Eds.)

Springer-Verlag Berlin Heidelberg GmbH

P. Oehr
H.-J. Biersack
E. Coleman

PET and PET-CT in Oncology

With 157 figures, some in color and 60 tables

Springer

Prof. Dr. Peter Oehr
University of Bonn, and
Bio-Med-Pharma Consulting
Am Buechel 53a
53173 Bonn, Germany

Prof. Dr. Hans-Jürgen Biersack
University of Bonn
Dept. Nuclear Medicine
Sigmund-Freud-Str. 25
53127 Bonn, Germany

Prof. Dr. R. Edward Coleman
Duke University
Medical Center
Erwin Road
Durham, NC 27710, USA

ISBN 978-3-642-62298-4 ISBN 978-3-642-18803-9 (eBook)
DOI 10.1007/978-3-642-18803-9

Library of Congress Cataloging-in-Publication Data
A catalog record for this book is available from Library of Congress.

Bibliographic information published by Die Deutsche Bibliothek.
Die Deutsche Bibliothek lists this publication in the Deutsche Nationalbibliografie; detailed bibliographic data is available in the Internet at <http:/dnb.ddb.de>.

http:/www.springeronline.com

Originally published by Springer-Verlag Berlin Heidelberg New York in 2004
Softcover reprint of the hardcover 1st edition 2004

Production: PRO EDIT GmbH, Heidelberg, Germany
Cover Design: Erich Kirchner, Heidelberg, Germany
Typesetting: medio Technologies AG, Berlin, Germany

Printed on acid-free paper 30/3111 5 4 3 SPIN 11586098

Preface

Structure and function are basic principles, and the relationship between them plays an important role in religion, science, and art. Modern diagnostic devices are often specialized only to find deviations either in structure or function, at the expense of biological or medical information. CT and PET are examples of such developments. Nevertheless, various attempts have been made to combine the results of these two imaging procedures, and PET-CT (or CT-PET) now seems to have become one useful potential solution.

CT and PET scans obtained from combined PET-CT systems in a single imaging setting allow optimal co-registration of image data, and the fusion images lead to highly accurate interpretation of both CT and PET studies, which can be integrated for optimal decision making in patient care. This new imaging technique paves the way for high-precision target volume planning in radiotherapy and opens unexpected avenues for minimal invasive treatment.

We, the editors, intend, with this volume, (a) to give an overview of the present technical state of the art of using data from PET, CT, MRI and PET-CT for scientific purposes and (b) to apply the current knowledge gained in this way to medical oncology, combining biological approaches with molecular medicine. This could only be achieved given the excellent professional support provided by our authors and given the freedom our conceptual framework was granted by Springer-Verlag as represented by Dr. Ute Heilmann and her international staff.

Peter Oehr
Hans Jürgen Biersack
R. Edward Coleman

Bonn, Durham
August 2003

Contents

Part III: Clinical Applications

List of Contributors

Peter Albers, MD
Department of Urology
University of Bonn, Sigmund-Freud-Str. 25
53105 Bonn, Germany
e-mail: *Peter.Albers.@ukb.uni-bonn.de*

Simon-Mensah Ametamey, PhD
Center for Radiopharmaceutical Science ETH-PSI-USZ
Paul Scherrer Institute
5323 Villigen, Switzerland
e-mail: *simon-mensah.ametamey@psi.ch*

Gerald Antoch
Department of Diagnostic and Interventional Radiology, Department of Nuclear Medicine
University Hospital Essen
Hufelandstr. 55, 45122 Essen, Germany
e-mail: *gerald.antoch@uni-essen.de*

Hans Bender, MD
Röntgeninstitut, Kaiserwertherstr. 89
40476 Düsseldorf, Germany

Thomas Beyer, PhD
Department of Diagnostic and Interventional Radiology and Department of Nuclear Medicine
University Hospital Essen
Hufelandstr. 55, 45122 Essen, Germany
e-mail: *thomas.Beyer@uni-essen.de*

Andreas Bockisch, MD, PhD
Department of Nuclear Medicine
University Hospital Essen
Hufelandstr. 55, 45122 Essen, Germany
e-mail: *Andreas.bockisch@uni-essen.de*

Matthias Bruehlmeier, MD
Nuclear Medicine Physician
Department of Nuclear Medicine, Kantonsspital Aarau
Buchserstr. 1, 5001 Aarau, Switzerland
e-mail: *matthias.bruehlmeier@ksa.ch*

Andreas K. Buck, MD
Department of Nuclear Medicine
University Hospital Ulm
Robert-Koch-Strasse 8, 89081 Ulm, Germany
e-mail: *andreas.buck@medizin.uni-ulm.de*

R. Edward Coleman, MD
Division of Nuclear Medicine
Department of Radiology, Room 1410
Duke Hospital North, Erwin Road
Duke University Medical Center
Durham NC 27710, USA
e-mail: *colem010@mc.duke.edu*

Luke B. Connelly, BA MEconSt PhD UQ
Centre of National Research on Disability and Rehabilitation Medicine (CONROD)
The University of Queensland
Mayne Medical Building
Herston Road, Herston Q 4006,Australia
e-mail: *l.connelly@uq.edu.au*

Dominique Delbeke, MD, PhD
Nuclear Medicine and PET, Department of Radiology and Radiological Sciences
Vanderbilt University
Medical Center
21st Avenue South and Garland
Nashville, Tennessee 37232–2675, USA
e-mail: *Dominique.delbeke@vanderbilt.edu*

Michaela Diehl, MD
Department of Nuclear Medicine
Hospital of the Johann W. Goethe University
Theodor-Stern-Kai 7, 60590 Frankfurt, Germany
e-mail: *m.diehl@em-uni-frankfurt.de*

Markus Dietlein, MD
Klinik und Poliklinik für Nuklearmedizin der Universität Köln
50924 Köln, Germany
e-mail: *markus.dietlein@uni-koeln.de*

Patrick Flamen, MD, PhD
Department of Nuclear Medicine
University Hospital Leuven
Herestraat 49, 3000 Leuven, Belgium
e-mail: *Patrick.Flamen@zu.kuleuven.ac.be*

Lutz Freudenberg, MD
Department of Nuclear Medicine
University Hospital Essen
Hufelandstr. 55, 45122 Essen, Germany
e-mail: *lutz.freudenberg@uni-essen.de*

Nadine Gilbert
Institut für Klinische Biochemie, University of Bonn
Sigmund-Freud-Str. 25, 53105 Bonn, Germany

Frank Grünwald, MD
Department of Nuclear Medicine
Hospital of the Johann W. Goethe University
Theodor-Stern-Kai 7, 60590 Frankfurt, Germany
e-mail: *gruenwald@em.uni-frankfurt.de*

W.-D. Heiß, MD
Department of Neurology, University of Cologne
Gleuelerstr. 50, 50931 Cologne, Germany
e-mail: *wdh@pet.mpin-koeln.mpg.de*

Michael Honer, PhD
Center for Radiopharmaceutical Science ETH-PSI-USZ
Paul Scherrer Institute, 5323 Villigen, Switzerland
e-mail: *michael.honer@psi.ch*

R. Hustinx, MD, PhD
Division of Nuclear Medicine, CHU Sart-Tilman
4000 Liège, Belgium
e-mail: *rhustinx@chu.ulg.ac.be*

Michiru Ide, MD
HIMEDIC Imaging Center at Lake Yamanaka
Hirano 562–12, Yamanakako-mura
Minamitsuru-gun, Yamanashi, 401–0502, Japan
e-mail: *mide@mfi.or.jp*

Andreas H. Jacobs, MD
Laboratory of Gene Therapy and Molecular Imaging
Department of Neurology, University of Cologne
MPI for Neurological Research
Gleuelerstr. 50, 50931 Cologne, Germany
e-mail: *Andreas.Jacobs@pet.mpin-koeln.mpg.de*

Siaki Kawada
HIMEDIC Imaging Center at Lake Yamanaka
Hirano 562–12, Yamanakako-mura
Minamitsuru-gun, Yamanashi, 401–0502, Japan
e-mail: *h-kawada@mc.kcom.ne.jp*

Mehmet T. Kitapci, MD
Department of Nuclear Medicine, Gazi University
School of Medicine, Ankara, Turkey

Helmut Lemmoch
Institut für Klinische Biochemie, University Bonn
Sigmund-Freud-Str. 25, 53105 Bonn, Germany
e-mail: *Helmut_Lemoch@web.de*

Val J. Lowe, MD
Department of Radiology, Mayo Clinic, CH1–285
200 First Street SW, Rochester, MN 55905, USA

M. Ludwig, PhD, PD
Institut für Klinische Biochemie, University of Bonn
Sigmund-Freud-Str. 25, 53105 Bonn, Germany
e-mail: *mludwig@uni-bonn.de*

Christian Menzel, MD
Department of Nuclear Medicine
Hospital of the Johann Goethe University
Theodor-Stern-Kai 7, 60590 Frankfurt, Germany
e-mail: *.Christian.menzel@em.uni-frankfurt.de*

Kenneth A. Miles, MD
Brighton & Sussex Medical School
Medical School Building, University of Sussex
Falmer, Brighton BN1 9RH, United Kingdom

Luc Mortelmans, MD, PhD
Department of Nuclear Medicine
University Hospital Leuven
Herestraat 49, 3000 Leuven, Belgium
e-mail: *Luc.Mortelmans@zu.kuleuven.ac.be*

Stefan P. Müller, MD
Department of Nuclear Medicine
University Hospital Essen
Hufelandstr. 55, 45122 Essen, Germany
e-mail: *stefan.mueller@uni-essen.de*

Katsuhiko Nakai
(HIMEDIC Imaging Center at Lake Yamanaka)
Matsuda Hospital, Irino-cho 753, Hamamatsu-shi
Shizuoka, 432–8061, Japan
e-mail: *nakai@matsuda-hp.or.jp*

Ilse Novak-Hofer, PhD
Center for Radiopharmaceutical Science ETH-PSI-USZ
Paul Scherrer Institute, 5323 Villigen, Switzerland
e-mail: *ilse.novak@psi.ch*

Peter Oehr, PhD
University of Bonn, and Bio-Med-Pharma Consulting,
Am Buechel 53a, 53173 Bonn, Germany
e-mail: *PET@oehr.info*

P. Paquet, MD, PhD
Department of Dermatopathology, CHU Sart-Tilman
4000 Liège, Belgium

Holger Palmedo, MD
Department of Nuclear Medicine
University Hospital Bonn
Sigmund-Freud-Strasse 25, 53127 Bonn, Germany
e-mail: *holger.palmedo@ukb.uni-bonn.de*

Gerald E. Piérard, MD, PhD
Department of Dermatopathology, CHU Sart-Tilman
4000 Liège, Belgium
e-mail: *gerald.pierard@ulg.ac.be*

Uwe Pietrzyk, PhD
Insitut für Medizin (ME)
Forschungszentrum Jülich GmbH
52425 Jülich, Germany
e-mail: *u.pietrzyk@fz-juelich.de*

Sven Reske, MD, PhD
Department of Nuclear Medicine
University Hospital Ulm
Robert-Koch-Straße 8, 89081 Ulm, Germany
e-mail: *sven.reske@medizin.uni-ulm.de*

Michael J. Reinhardt, MD
Department of Nuclear Medicine
University Hospital Bonn
Sigmund-Freud-Strasse 25, 53127 Bonn, Germany
e-mail: *michael.reinhardt@ukb.uni-bonn.de*

P. Rigo, MD, PhD
Service de Médecine Nucléaire
Centre Hospitalier Princesse Grace
BP 480 MC 980112 Monaco Cedex, Monaco
e-mail: *prigo@chpg.mc*

Hermann Rink, PhD
Haselweg 3
53340 Meckenheim
e-mail: *Hermann.Rink@t-online.de*

Jörn H. Risse, MD
Gemeinschaftspraxis
für Radiologie und Nuklearmedizin
von-Stauffenberg-Str. 9, 53606 Bad Honnef, Germany
e-mail: *Joern.Risse@freenet.de*

Holger Schirrmeister, MD
Department of Nuclear Medicine
University Hospital Kiel
Arnold-Heller-Straße 9, 24105 Kiel, Germany
e-mail: *hschirrmeister@wkk-hei.de*

Heinrich Schüller, MD
University of Bonn
Department of Radiology
Sigmund-Freud-Strasse 25
53105 Bonn, Germany
e-mail: *schueller@uni-bonn.de*

Marc Seltzer, MD
Division of Nuclear Medicine
UCLA School of Medicine
1245 16th Street, Suite 301
Santa Monica, CA 90404, USA
e-mail: *MSeltzer@mednet.ucla.edu*

Akira Shohtsu
HIMEDIC Imaging Center at Lake Yamanaka
Hirano 562–12, Yamanakako-mura, Minamitsuru-gun
Yamanashi, 401–0502, Japan

Oleg Shvarts, MD
Department of Urology, UCLA School of Medicine
10833 Le Conte Avenue, Los Angeles, CA, USA

Hans-Joachim Straehler-Pohl, MD
Department of Head and Neck Surgery
University of Bonn
Sigmund-Freud-Straße 25, 53105 Bonn, Germany
e-mail: *hans.straehler-pohl@ukb_uni-bonn.de*

Sigrid S. Stroobants, MD, PhD
Catholic University Leuven, PET-Center
(Department of Nuclear Medicine)
University Hospital Gasthuisberg
Herestraat 49, 3000 Leuven, Belgium
e-mail: *sigrid.stroobants@zu.kuleuven.ac.be*

Ruth D. Tesar
President, Imagemed Group, LLC
3195 Folsom Boulevard
Sacramento, CA 95816, USA
e-mail: *ruth.tesar@imagemedgroup.com*

David W. Townsend, PhD
University of Tennessee Medical Center
1924 Alcoa Highway, Box 41A
Knoxville, TN 37920, USA
e-mail: *dtownsend@mc.utmck.edu*

Timothy Turkington, PhD
Division of Nuclear Medicine
Department of Radiology, PET Facility
Duke University Medical Center
Durham NC 27710, USA
e-mail: *turki001@mc.duke.edu*

Johan F. Vansteenkiste, MD, PhD
Catholic University Leuven, Respiratory Oncology Unit
(Department of Pulmonology)
University Hospital Gasthuisberg
Herestraat 49, 3000 Leuven, Belgium
e-mail: *johan.vansteenkiste@uz.kuleuven.ac.be*

Rainer Wagner, PhD
Department of Neurology at the University of Cologne
MPI for Neurological Research, University of Cologne
Gleuelerstr. 50, 50931 Cologne, Germany
e-mail: *rainer@pet.mpin-koeln.mpg.de*

Gert Jacobus van der Westenhuizen, MD
Holston Valley Medical Center
Department of Radiology
130 W. Ravine Rd.
Kingsport, TN 37660, USA
e-mail: *gert@chartertn.net*

Terence Wong, MD
Division of Nuclear Medicine,
Department of Radiology, Room 1410
Duke Hospital North, Erwin Road
Duke University Medical Center
Durham NC 27710, USA
e-mail: *wong0015@mc.duke.edu*

Seiei Yasuda, MD
Department of Surgery
Tokai University School of Medicine
Kanagawa, 259-1193, Japan
e-mail: *yasuda@is.icc.u-tokai.ac.jp*

Sibylle I. Ziegler, PhD
Department of Nuclear Medicine
Technical University Munich, Klinikum rechts der Isar
Ismaninger Str. 22, 81675 Munich, Germany
e-mail: *S.Ziegler@lrz.tu-muenchen.de*

Michael Zimny, MD
Institut for Nuclear Medicine
Municipal Hospital Hanau
Leimenstr. 20, 63450 Hanau, Germany
e-mail: *Zimny@cybernuk.de*

PART I

Basics

CHAPTER 1

Physical Principles, Dedicated/Coincidence PET

S. Ziegler

Positron emission tomography (PET) is a nuclear medical modality that provides quantitative tomographic images and allows non-invasive determination of the time course of a radioactive substance in vivo. Positron emitters are used for labelling biochemical substances. After injection of the radioactive tracer, radiation from the body is registered in external detectors and tomographic images of the tracer distribution in the body are reconstructed using mathematical algorithms. Developments in PET instrumentation aim at improving resolution and sensitivity, in order to obtain precise measurements with as little radioactivity as possible. Another focus of technological advances is the development of cost-effective tomographs for fluoro-2-deoxy-D-glucose (FDG) imaging.

1.1 Physics Background

During β^+-decay, a positron and a neutrino are emitted from the nucleus. Depending on the nuclide, a certain amount of kinetic energy is shared by the positron and neutrino. The positron loses its kinetic energy in the surrounding tissue by ionization and excitation processes. Once the positron is slowed down, a positronium atom consisting of a positron and an electron is created. The positronium has a very short half-life of around 10^{-10} s and the masses of positron and its antiparticle electron are finally transferred into energy. For energy and momentum to be conserved, this annihilation results in two gamma rays, which are emitted back-to-back and which have an energy of 511 keV each. Decay events are detected by coincidence registration of the gamma quanta. Thus, it is not the location of positron emission but the location of positron annihilation that is detected in PET. This physical effect results in an uncertainty in localization, which can amount to as much as several millimetres. Since the energy is split between positron and neutrino, only very few positrons have the maximum energy, thus the spatial distribution of positron annihilation is strongly peaked around the positron emission (see Table 1). Table 1 summarizes the most commonly used positron emitters with their properties. Because of the short physical half-lives (minutes), it is necessary to produce them as close to the positron tomograph as possible.

Annihilation events are registered by coincidence detectors consisting of two opposing detector units. Only those events are counted that occur within the sensitive volume between the detectors and which emit gamma quanta along a line connecting the two detectors, so that they can be detected within a very short time interval (coincidence window) in both detectors. The connecting line between the two detectors represents a coincidence line. Thus, no lead collimators are needed, in contrast to single photon emission computed tomography (SPECT), as co-linearity of the gamma quanta is exploited and used as „electronic collimation". Intrinsic spatial resolution of a coincidence detector pair is defined by the size of the detectors and does not change much along a coincidence line. It corresponds to one half of the detector front face. Furthermore, sensitivity is independent of source position between the detectors as long as the source covers the detector face (Budinger 1998). Because of the limitations in the currently available detector materials, the coincidence timing window is 6–15 ns in modern tomographs. Therefore, there is a chance that two uncorrelated gamma rays are detected within the timing window. These random coincidences reduce the image contrast and developments in hard- and software aim at reducing this background. On their way through the body, one or both gamma rays can undergo Compton scattering. The flight direction of these gamma rays is changed and they lose some of their energy, therefore the count rate along a coincidence line is reduced depending on the scattering material. This at-

Table 1. Most commonly used positron emitters, radioactive half-life $T_{1/2}$, maximum positron energy E_{max}, and path length R_p in water within which 50 % (95 %) of the positrons are stopped (from Levin and Hoffman 1999)

	$T_{1/2}$ (min)	E_{max} (MeV)	R_p (mm)
^{15}O	2.05	1.72	0.7 (3.3)
^{13}N	9.9	1.19	0.5 (2.1)
^{11}C	20.4	0.97	0.3 (1.6)
^{18}F	109.7	0.64	0.2 (0.9)

tenuation effect can reduce the count rate dramatically for gamma rays originating in the centre of the body (e.g. factor 100). For quantitative measurements this effect needs to be corrected. Transmission measurements with external rod or point sources are used to determine the distribution of attenuation factors (Zaidi and Hasegawa 2003). These attenuation factors are then applied in the reconstruction process resulting in attenuation-corrected images. The quality of attenuation correction is strongly influenced by the count statistics of transmission measurements and segmentation of transmission data is a common remedy. Since emission and transmission scans are performed sequentially, artefacts can be generated by misregistration due to patient movement. Therefore, technological advances are aimed at reducing the scanning time.

Gamma rays that were scattered in the body may be detected and falsely assigned to another coincidence line. This background of scattered events can amount to more than 30% of the count rate and its elimination is one of the main issues in 3D tomographs.

The number of events measured in a coincidence line corresponds to the sum of all events along the direction of the coincidence pair through the object. In order to determine the activity distribution in the object, this integral information needs to be measured in many lines with different angles through the object. Therefore, detectors are arranged in a ring and coincidence events are logged for a number of opposing detector channels. As in SPECT acquisitions, radial as well as angular sampling must be provided for artefact-free reconstructions. The spatial distribution of the activity concentration within the field-of-view can be reconstructed from the measured projections using mathematical algorithms. Statistical, iterative methods yield superior image quality compared to filtered backprojection algorithms and are the standard processing for reconstructing whole-body PET images today (Leahy and Byrne 2000).

1.2 Detectors for PET

Similar to conventional nuclear medicine, scintillation crystals are used for the detection of annihilation quanta, which are read out by photomultiplier tubes. Currently, avalanche photodiodes as a semiconductor replacement for photomultiplier tubes are only used in prototype tomographs for animal studies (Lecomte et al. 1996; Ziegler et al. 2001).

For efficient detection of high energy gamma rays in PET, scintillation materials need to fulfil special requirements. High density and atomic number are necessary for high photo absorption at 511 keV. High scintillation light yield usually is involved with good energy resolution. Energy resolution is important for discriminating radiation, which has less than 511 keV after a scatter interaction. Energy thresholds of 350–450 keV are commonly used. Depending on the energy resolution, sensitivity, i.e. detection of unscattered rays, is more or less compromised if a high energy threshold is chosen in order to reduce the scatter fraction.

Table 2. Scintillation crystals used for PET

	NaI:Tl	BGO	LSO:Ce	GSO:Ce
Light yield (% NaI)	100	15	75	30
Wavelength (nm)	410	480	420	440
Scintillation light decay time (ns)	230	300	40	60
Attenuation length for 511 keV (mm)	30	11	12	15

NaI:Tl thallium-doped sodium iodide, BGO bismuth-germanate, LSO:Ce cerium-doped lutetium-oxyorthosilicate, GSO:Ce cerium-doped gadolinium-oxyorthosilicate

A short decay time of the scintillation light provides good timing and count-rate characteristics. It allows the use of short coincidence timing windows, reducing random background.

The first positron tomographs consisted of individual thallium-doped sodium-iodide (NaI:Tl) crystals coupled to photomultiplier tubes. This material, well known in nuclear medicine, has excellent characteristics for the detection of gamma rays with 140 keV energy, it is luminous and inexpensive. The biggest drawback with respect to positron imaging is its low detection probability for gamma rays with 511 keV (Table 2).

Bismuth germanate (BGO) has been the most commonly used crystal in PET, as it has a high atomic number and therefore high detection efficiency. The light yield of BGO, on the other hand, is low and the decay time is long, limiting the coincidence timing window width and the count-rate performance. Recently, new scintillators were characterized for the efficient and fast detection of 511 keV gamma rays. For PET, cerium-activated gadolinium oxyorthosilicate (GSO) and lutetium oxyorthosilicate (LSO) (Melcher et al. 1990; Melcher and Schweitzer 1992) are currently the most favourable scintillators (Table 2). Both have a short attenuation length for gamma rays with 511 keV. With LSO, the detection efficiency above 400 keV is 38% higher than in GSO because of a higher photo absorption probability. Although generally higher light output results in better energy resolution, this is not the case for LSO and energy resolution is worse than what is expected from photon statistics. The measured energy resolution is similar for LSO and GSO, although LSO emits much more light (Moszynski et al. 1998). Both LSO and GSO also meet the requirement of a short scintillation decay time.

1.3 Tomograph Design

After the introduction of tomographic reconstruction in CT, coincidence techniques were used for emission tomography for the first time in the seventies (Phelps et al. 1975). Since then, technological advances have aimed at improving resolution and sensitivity. In addition, dual-head coincidence cameras, capable of acquiring data in SPECT as well as in PET mode, were developed. Performance parameters such as resolution and sensitivity, but also scatter and random fraction influence the image quality that can be achieved. Standard procedures were defined in order to compare scanner performance and have been revised recently, trying to represent the clinical situation in whole-body imaging (NEMA 1994, 2001). When comparing the performance of different tomographs (offered at different costs) in a specific imaging situation, it is essential to be aware of their individual characteristics and adjust acquisition and processing parameters accordingly (Kadrmas and Christian 2002).

1.3.1 Dedicated PET

Ring tomographs consist of some ten thousand detection elements arranged in several (e.g. 31) rings. A small diameter ring covers a larger solid angle and is therefore more sensitive, it is also less expensive because less crystal material is needed. On the other hand, the fraction of scattered radiation that is detected is higher for smaller rings. Therefore, the choice of ring diameter is always a compromise. Typically, ring tomographs have detector diameters of 80–90 cm. The reconstructed image covers only about 50 % of the ring diameter, therefore the effect of spatially variant coincidence efficiency is limited. The axial extent of ring tomographs ranges from 15 to 18 cm. Annular lead shielding with an inner diameter equalling the patient port at the sides of the detector rings reduces the single event rate originating from activity outside the field-of-view. Since the number of random coincidences increases with the square of the singles count rate, this shielding effectively reduces random background.

Septa made of lead or tungsten between the detector slices were traditionally used in the 2D acquisition mode, allowing coincidences only within one slice or within direct neighbours. Scatter fraction in 2D mode is less than 20 %. For higher sensitivity, tomographs with retractable septa, offering 2D and 3D mode, were developed (Cherry et al. 1991). In 3D acquisitions, the axial acceptance angle is increased, allowing coincidences between all detector slices. Dedicated reconstruction algorithms are needed for the 3D data. It has been shown that statistical reconstruction algorithms applied after rebinning of the 3D into 2D data (Defrise et al. 1997) yield the best results for whole-body images (Lartizien et al. 2003). Sensitivity in 3D mode is increased by about a factor of 5 (Table 3), but more scattered and random events are detected, a fact that needs to be addressed in quantitative studies. The septa-less 3D mode is particularly susceptible to detection of gamma rays originating outside the field-of-view, thus side shielding becomes more important.

The characteristics of LSO and GSO are advantageous for 3D imaging: dead time per event is short because of their fast light decay time, thus the count-rate performance is adequate for the higher sensitivity. In addition, their good energy resolution is a prerequisite to eliminate some of the scattered radiation.

Three detector concepts, which differ in their crystal readout scheme, are implemented in the current commercial PET scanners. The most common scheme is the block detector (Casey and Nutt 1986), which uses scintillator blocks cut into small (e.g. 6 mm × 6 mm) subcrystals with light sharing between them for crystal identification. Thus, it is possible to pack small scintillation crystals in a dense matrix but only use a few photomultiplier tubes (e.g. 64 crystals read out by four pho-

Table 3. Characteristics of full-ring tomographs. Siemens/CTI ECAT EXACT HR+ (Brix et al. 1997), GE Advance (DeGrado et al. 1994; Lewellen et al. 1996), ADAC CPET (Adam et al. 2001), Siemens/CTI ECAT ART (Bailey et al. 1997), and a coincidence camera (ADAC MCD) (Sossi et al. 2001). If not otherwise stated, data were measured according to the NEMA NU-2 1994 protocol (NEMA 1994)

	EXACT HR+		Advance		ART	CPET	MCD[d]
	2D[a]	3D[b]	2D[a]	3D[c]			
Crystal material	BGO		BGO		BGO	NaI	NaI
Axial field-of-view (cm)	15.5	15.5	15.2	15.2	16.2	25.6	38
Resolution in the centre: transaxial FWHM (mm)	4.3	4.4	4.5	4.5	5.7	4.6	5.2
axial FWHM (mm)	4.2	4.1	4.0	6.0	6.0	5.7	5.0
Sensitivity (cps/Bq/ml)[e]	5.7	27.7	5.7	27.6	7.5	12.7	1.9
Scatter fraction (%)	17	33	9	36	37	25	37 (48)[e]

[a] With septa (2D), lower energy threshold 350 keV
[b] Without septa (3D), lower energy threshold 350 keV
[c] Without septa (3D), lower energy threshold 300 keV
[d] Acquisition in two energy windows (511 keV, 310 keV) 30 % width
[e] Measured according to NEMA NU-2 2001

tomultipliers). The crystal in which a gamma ray deposited energy is identified by centroid calculation of the photomultiplier signals. The size of the sub-crystals defines the resulting spatial resolution. Commercial scanners with BGO block detectors of various dimensions are available (Table 3) and offer 2D as well as 3D acquisition (Wienhard et al. 1992; DeGrado et al. 1994; Lewellen et al. 1996; Brix et al. 1997). LSO block detectors were introduced in the new tomograph ACCEL (CTI/Siemens), also offering 2D and 3D mode. Because of its superior count-rate performance, this scanner allows whole-body measurements including transmission scan in less than 20 min.

A recently introduced scheme is the continuous pixelated detector (Allegro, Philips Medical Systems) (Surti et al. 2000). In this case, small GSO crystals ($4 \times 6 \times 20\,mm^3$) are coupled to a continuous light guide, which is read out by a matrix of closely packed photomultiplier tubes. The advantage of this design is a more homogeneous light collection for all crystals, ensuring good system energy resolution, which is particularly important for this 3D-only scanner with large axial field-of-view (18 cm). Compared to block detectors, dead time is higher because the light of each event is read out by a larger number of photomultiplier tubes. Again, this scanner also allows the acquisition of whole-body images in a very short time.

The third detector principle uses continuous light guides in combination with large NaI detectors, which are read out like gamma cameras (Muehllehner and Karp 1986). This design has the advantage that NaI is less expensive than the other materials. In order to detect coincidence events efficiently, the crystals in this scanner are thicker (25 mm) than in a conventional gamma camera. Systems with six large area NaI detectors are operated in 3D mode for increased system sensitivity (Karp et al. 1990). This 3D-only scanner was recently improved by implementing curved crystals and fast electronics for higher sensitivity and better count-rate performance (C-PET, Philips Medical Systems) (Adam et al. 2001).

Another example for reduced system cost is a sector tomograph with less detector units than a full-ring tomograph. One of the commercial positron tomographs (ECAT ART, CTI/Siemens) consists of only one third of block detectors, which cover 165° and are continuously rotated around the patient (Townsend et al. 1993; Bailey et al. 1997). This tomograph is operated in 3D only, resulting in a system sensitivity similar to a full-ring tomograph in 2D mode.

1.3.2 Coincidence Cameras

Dual-head coincidence cameras (hybrid positron emission tomographs) provide two different imaging modes: SPECT (with collimators) and coincidence imaging (without collimators) (Patton 2000). They were introduced as a less expensive tomograph for FDG imaging. The NaI crystals in these cameras are thicker (5/8–1 inch) compared to conventional SPECT instrumentation in order to improve the detection probability at 511 keV. The thickness of the crystal can only be increased as long as the performance in single-photon detection is not compromised. This is accomplished by digital corrections or, in the case of 1-inch crystals, by special design of the light collection using slots in the crystal. The large area cameras rotate around the patient and acquire data in 3D mode, covering an axial field-of-view of about 40 cm. The characteristics of one coincidence camera are included in Table 3. While spatial resolution of coincidence cameras is very good (5 mm), low coincidence efficiency and elevated background levels result in low contrast in the reconstructed image, as compared to ring tomographs. Without additional shielding, a number of events originating from outside the coincidence field-of-view are detected in the large area detectors, increasing the singles detector rates and thus the chance for random events. This reduces the image contrast and several means to minimize this effect have been implemented (side shields, septa, graded absorbers). The ratio of coincidence versus singles events in a coincidence camera is 1–2%, depending on the crystal thickness. In order to register reasonable coincidence rates, single rates of more than 1 million counts per second need to be processed in a detector head. Fast electronics and pulse shaping is implemented in the modern systems to overcome the problem of a low sensitivity but nevertheless high count-rate camera. Furthermore, digital camera head technology allows use of different set-ups for coincidence or single photon mode, an option that was not available at the time of the first experimental coincidence cameras (Anger 1963).

Several schemes have been introduced for transmission measurement and attenuation correction in dual-head coincidence cameras (for an overview see Turkington 2000). These techniques provide better delineation of anatomical structures and, in combination with background correction algorithms, enhance lesion detectability (Zimny et al. 1999) as well as diagnostic accuracy in cardiac viability measurements (Nowak et al. 2000). Since coincidence cameras acquire with a large opening angle, 3D reconstruction taking into account the specific detector is essential (Levkovitz et al. 2001).

As coincidence cameras offer positron imaging at reduced hardware cost, it cannot be expected that their performance will be identical to that of dedicated PET, but their use needs to be defined within the clinical situation. Comparative studies have shown that coincidence cameras yield similar results to dedicated PET in the imaging situation of head and neck cancer. In general, although detectability of small lesions with low FDG uptake is compromised, metabolic characterization of lesions larger than 15 mm is feasible with dual-head coincidence cameras (for an overview see Ak et al. 2001).

References

Adam LE, Karp JS, Daube-Witherspoon ME, Smith RJ (2001) Performance of a whole-body PET scanner using curve-plate NaI(Tl) detectors. J Nucl Med 42:1821–1830

Ak I, Blokland JA, Pauwels EK, Stokkel MP (2001) The clinical value of 18F-FDG detection with a dual-head coincidence camera: a review. Eur J Nucl Med 28:763–778

Anger HO (1963) Gamma-ray and positron scintillation camera. Nucleonics 21:10–56

Bailey DL, Young H, Bloomfield PM, Meikle SR, Glass D, Myers MJ, Spinks TJ, Watson CC, Luk P, Peters AM, Jones T (1997) ECAT ART – a continuously rotating PET camera: performance characteristics, initial clinical studies, and installation considerations in a nuclear medicine department. Eur J Nucl Med 24: 6–15

Brix G, Zaers J, Adam LE, Bellemann ME, Ostertag H, Trojan H, Haberkorn U, Doll J, Oberdorfer F, Lorenz WJ (1997) Performance evaluation of a whole-body PET scanner using the NEMA protocol. J Nucl Med 38:1614–1623

Budinger TF (1998) PET Instrumentation: what are the limits? Semin Nucl Med 28:247–267

Casey ME, Nutt R (1986) Multicrystal two dimensional BGO detector system for positron emission tomography. IEEE Trans Nucl Sci 33:460–463

Cherry SR, Dahlbom M, Hoffman EJ (1991) 3D PET using a conventional multislice tomograph without septa. J Comput Assist Tomogr 15:655–668

Defrise M, Kinahan PE, Townsend DW, Michel C, Sibomana M, Newport DF (1997) Exact and approximate rebinning algorithms for 3-D PET data. IEEE Trans Med Imag 16:145–158

DeGrado TR, Turkington TG, Williams JJ, Stearns CW, Hoffman JM, Coleman RE (1994) Performance characteristics of a whole-body PET scanner. J Nucl Med 35:1398–1406

Kadrmas DJ, Christian PE (2002) Comparative evaluation of lesion detectability for 6 PET imaging platforms using a highly reproducible whole-body phantom with (22)Na lesions and localization ROC analysis. J Nucl Med 43:1545–1554

Karp JS, Muehllehner G, Mankoff DA, Ordonez CE, Ollinger JM, Daube-Witherspoon ME, Haigh AT, Beerbohm DJ (1990) Continuous-slice PENN-PET: a positron tomograph with volume imaging capability. J Nucl Med 31:617–627

Lartizien C, Kinahan PE, Swensson R, Comtat C, Lin M, Villemagne V, Trebossen R (2003) Evaluating image reconstruction methods for tumor detection in 3-dimensional whole-body PET oncology imaging. J Nucl Med 44:276–290

Leahy R, Byrne C (2000) Recent developments in iterative image reconstruction for PET and SPECT. IEEE Trans Med Imaging 19:257–260

Lecomte R, Cadorette J, Rodrigue S, Lapointe D, Rouleau D, Bentourkia M, Yao R, Msaki P (1996) Initial results from the Sherbrooke avalanche photodiode positron tomograph. IEEE Trans Nucl Sci 43:1952–1957

Levin CS, Hoffman EJ (1999) Calculation of positron range and its effect on the fundamental limit of positron emission tomography system spatial resolution. Phys Med Biol 44:781–799

Levkovitz R, Falikman D, Zibulevsky M, Ben-Tal A, Nemirovski A (2001) The design and implementation of COSEM, an iterative algorithm for fully 3D listmode data. IEEE Trans Med Imaging 20:633–642

Lewellen TK, Kohlmyer SG, Miyaoka RS, Kaplan MS, Stearns CW, Schubert SF (1996) Investigation of the performance of the General Electric ADVANCE positron emission tomograph in 3D mode. IEEE Trans Nucl Sci 43:2199–2206

Melcher CL, Schweitzer JS (1992) A promising new scintillator: cerium-doped lutetium oxyorthosilicate. Nucl Instr Meth 314: 212–214

Melcher CL, Schweitzer JS, Utsu T, Akiyama S (1990) Scintillation properties of GSO. IEEE Trans Nucl Sci 37:161–164

Moszynski M, Kapusta M, Wolski D, Szawlowski M, Klamra W (1998) Energy resolution of scintillation detectors readout with large area avalanche photodiodes and photomultipliers. IEEE Trans Nucl Sci 45:472–477

Muehllehner G, Karp JS (1986) A positron camera using position-sensitive detectors: PENN-PET. J Nucl Med 27:90–98

NEMA (1994) NEMA standards publication NU 2-1994: performance measurements of positron emission tomographs. National Electrical Manufacturers Association, Washington DC

NEMA (2001) NEMA standards publication NU 2-2001: performance measurements of positron emission tomographs. National Electrical Manufacturers Association, Rosslyn, VA

Nowak B, Zimny M, Schwarz ER, Kaiser HJ, Schaefer W, Reinartz P, vom Dahl J, Buell U (2000) Diagnosis of myocardial viability by dual-head coincidence gamma camera. Eur J Nucl Med 27:1501–1508

Patton JA (2000) Instrumentation for coincidence imaging with multihead scintillation cameras. Semin Nucl Med 30:239–254

Phelps M, Hoffman E, Mullani N, Ter-Pogossian M (1975) Application of annihilation coincidence detection to transaxial reconstruction tomography. J Nucl Med 16:210–224

Sossi V, Pointon B, Boudoux C, Cohen P, Hudkins K, Jivan S, Nitzek K, deRosario J, Stevens C, Ruth TJ (2001) NEMA NU-2-2000+ Performance measurements on an ADAC MCD Camera. IEEE Trans Nucl Sci 48:1518–1523

Surti S, Karp JS, Freifelder R, Liu F (2000) Optimizing the performance of a PET detector using discrete GSO crystals on a continuous lightguide. IEEE Trans Nucl Sci 47:1030–1036

Townsend DW, Wensveen M, Byars LG, Geissbuhler A, Tochon-Danguy HJ, Christin A, Defrise M, Bailey DL, Grootoonk S, Donath A, Nutt R (1993) A rotating PET scanner using BGO block detectors: design, performance and applications. J Nucl Med 34:1367–1376

Turkington TG (2000) Attenuation correction in hybrid positron emission tomography. Semin Nucl Med 30:255–267

Wienhard K, Eriksson L, Grootoonk S, Casey M, Pietrzyk U, Heiss W-D (1992) Performance evaluation of the positron scanner ECAT EXACT. J Comput Assist Tomogr 16:804–813

Zaidi H, Hasegawa B (2003) Determination of the attenuation map in emission tomography. J Nucl Med 44:291–315

Ziegler SI, Pichler BJ, Boening G, Rafecas M, Pimpl W, Lorenz E, Schmitz N, Schwaiger M (2001) A prototype high resolution animal positron tomograph with avalanche photodiode arrays and LSO crystals. Eur J Nucl Med 28:136–143

Zimny M, Kaiser HJ, Cremerius U, Reinartz P, Schreckenberger M, Sabri O, Buell U (1999) Dual-head gamma camera 2-[fluorine-18]-fluoro-2-deoxy-D-glucose positron emission tomography in oncological patients: effects of non-uniform attenuation correction on lesion detection. Eur J Nucl Med 26:818–823

CHAPTER 2

Dual-Modality PET/CT Acquisition Systems for Clinical Oncology

T. Beyer · D.W. Townsend

2.1 Adding Anatomical to Functional Information

In clinical oncology, diagnosis and staging of disease are traditionally based on conventional planar X-ray or computed tomography (CT) imaging. Both techniques provide information on the morphology of the patient with good anatomical detail – X-ray imaging in planar transmission mode and CT in tomographic transmission mode. In detecting disease, anatomical imaging techniques rely on significant alterations of the morphology of the patient. For example, specific criteria exist on the minimum size of a lesion seen on CT to be a candidate for harboring malignant disease (Ferguson et al. 1986; Jamis-Dow et al. 1996; Padhani 1998; Greene et al. 2002).

However, disease originates as a functional change, which typically precedes any related anatomical alterations (Fig. 1a). To detect, stage, and follow functional changes has been the domain of nuclear medicine since its inception. For example, with positron emission tomography (PET), cross-sectional images of the temporal and spatial distribution of positron-emitting radiopharmaceuticals can be obtained, thereby assessing biochemical and metabolic activity of organs and tissues in vivo (Valk et al. 2003). PET is therefore termed a functional imaging technique.

Positron emission tomography offers the ability to detect cancerous disease by tracing increased accumulation of 2-[^{18}F]fluoro-2-deoxy-D-glucose ([^{18}F]FDG), an ^{18}F-labeled glucose analogue (Biersack et al. 1997; Wahl 1997; Gambhir et al. 2001), an approach based on the hypothesis that cancer can be characterized by increased glucose uptake (Warburg 1931, 1956; Smith 1998). Inflammatory disease, however, can also result in increased glucose uptake, and therefore FDG may not be the most effective tracer to differentiate malignant from benign disease (Shreve 1998). In addition, variations of normal physiologic tracer uptake may complicate the interpretation of an FDG PET scan (Shreve et al. 1999).

An important aspect in diagnostic imaging in oncology is to detect the primary disease and to stage the patient with respect to metastatic spread of the malignancy. Whole-body FDG PET protocols have been developed to examine the entire patient from head to toe, or at least to examine the region from the cranium to the lower pelvis for primary and secondary disease (Hoh et al. 1993). In whole-body PET, the patient is administered a single dose of FDG (typically 300–500 MBq) and scanned in contiguous, overlapping steps through the axial field-of-view of the PET tomograph. After completion of the entire examination, the individual images (also termed bed positions) are assembled and available for viewing (Fig. 1b). The ability to identify malignant disease before anatomical changes become noticeable, and to examine the patient for disseminated disease without additional exposure from further radiotracer injections has contributed to the success of FDG PET imaging in oncology (Gambhir et al. 2001).

Nevertheless, the high sensitivity of FDG PET is frequently associated with a lower specificity as a result of the poor anatomical localization of lesions seen on the FDG PET images. The ability to differentiate malignant from physiologic uptake patterns, and to localize lesions is directly affected by the experience of the clinical reader. While FDG is metabolized in normal organs and tissues (e.g. liver, muscle) and excreted through the urinary system (e.g. high uptake in the bladder), little other detailed anatomical information can be extracted (Fig. 1b). Furthermore the lack of anatomical detail in PET images becomes critical when using highly specific tracers (Fig. 1c). The application of specific tracers may help to overcome the challenges of differentiating physiologic from non-physiologic uptake patterns in PET, by exclusively binding to malignant tumor cells without the typical physiologic background variants.

Therefore, with the growing acceptance of FDG PET, increased efforts have been made to overcome the lack of sufficient anatomical detail information by retrospectively registering and fusing the functional information with anatomical images (Hill et al. 2001). To illustrate the potential benefit of combined anatomical and functional information, these combinations are sometimes referred to as "anato-metabolic imaging" (Wahl et al. 1993). Over the past decade a number of software-based algorithms has been presented that allow the registration and combined display of CT and PET images. These retrospective image registration techniques

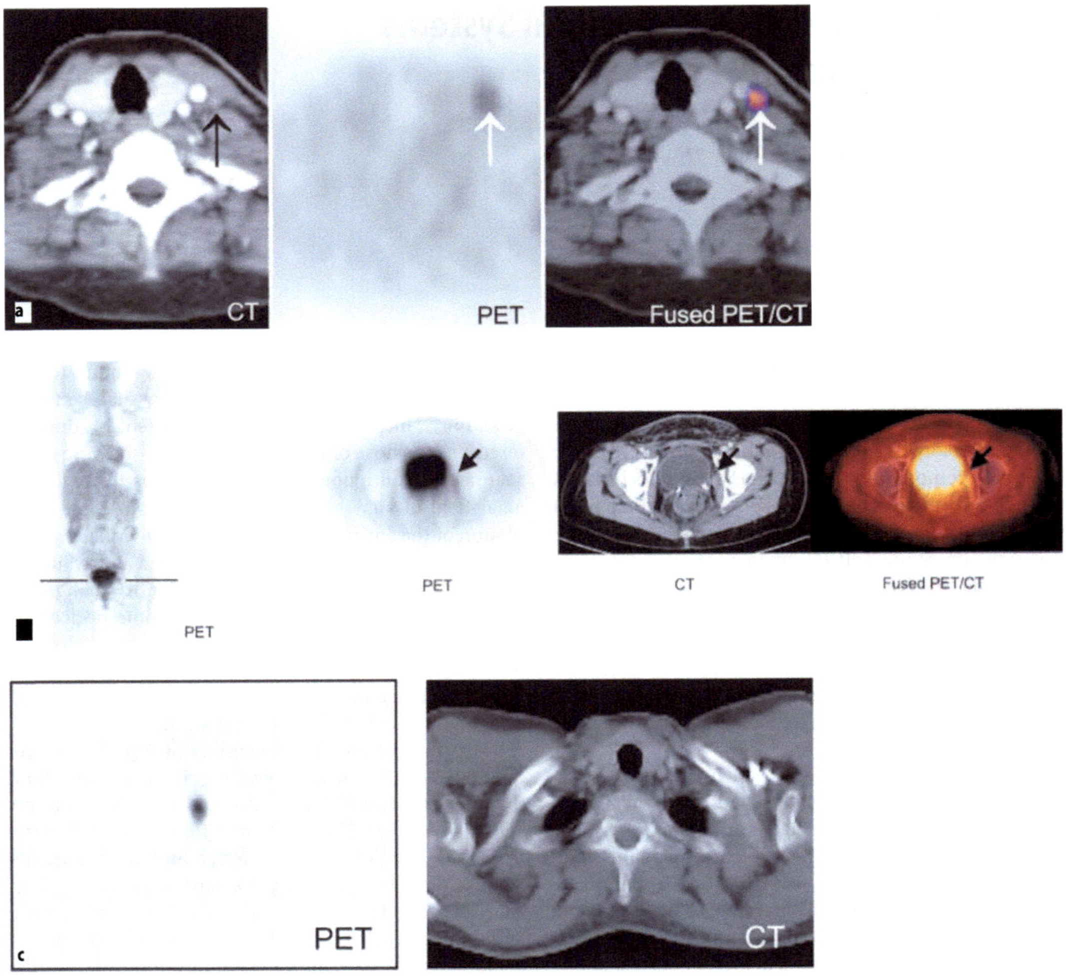

Fig. 1. Clinical PET imaging. **a** Patient with a head and neck metastasis. The CT was negative for disease with normal-sized lymph nodes. The corrected PET image shows a focal FDG accumulation (*arrow*) suspicious of malignancy in the left neck. The combined PET/CT image localizes the focal FDG uptake (*arrow*) to a lymph node in the left neck that was later confirmed to be a metastasis. (Data courtesy of Drs Thomas Egelhof and Gerald Antoch, University Hospital Essen, Germany.) **b** Whole-body FDG PET study of a female with recurrent cervical cancer. The coronal whole-body PET image shows a focal FDG uptake in the pelvis, which is difficult to interpret as either normal ureter uptake or a pelvic lymph node. Fused PET/CT images localized the focus to a pelvic sidewall node. (Courtesy of Dr Lutz Freudenberg, University Hospital Essen, Germany.) **c** Transverse PET image of the apex of the lungs of a cancer patient acquired 4 h after injection of 220 MBq [^{68}Ga]DOTATOC. (Courtesy of Dr Michael Hofmann, University of Hannover, Germany.) No anatomical detail is seen on the PET emission image of this highly specific tracer. The corresponding transverse CT is shown to the right

work well for the brain (Woods et al. 1998) but impose fairly high demands on the user when complementary image sets of extra-cranial structures are to be aligned (Pietrzyk et al. 1990; Wahl et al. 1993). Combining complementary whole-body image data sets retrospectively is challenging because of the difference in patient positioning and variable definitions of the axial examination ranges of the two imaging modalities. Normal variants of the position and metabolic activity of bowel and intestines at the time of the two scans, as well as dissimilar breathing patterns contribute to additional systematic differences in the two data sets. Though some of the positioning errors may be overcome by non-linear image warping techniques and 3D elastic transformations (Tai et al. 1997), these registration algorithms are typically limited to a single anatomical region such as the thorax (Wahl et al. 1993; Yu et al. 1994; Tai et al. 1997; Cai et al. 1999; Slomka et al. 2001; Slomka et al. 2003) and are often labor-intensive, thus making them less attractive for routine clinical use in high-throughput situations.

2.2 Anato-Metabolic Imaging: The Proof-of-Principle for Dual-Modality Imaging

2.2.1 Hardware Fusion: A Prototype PET/CT

An alternative approach to post hoc anato-metabolic image alignment is the fusion of the hardware components to allow the acquisition of anatomical and functional information in a single scan session without repositioning the patient between examinations. When combining functional imaging with CT, the CT transmission information could also be used for quantitative corrections of the emission data (LaCroix et al. 1994; Kinahan et al. 1998).

Two approaches exist for combined tomographic imaging: the use of a single detector system for both the transmission and the emission scan, and the combination of two separate tomographs in-line. In 1991, Hasegawa and colleagues presented a dual-modality imager based on a high-purity Ge-array detector (Hasegawa et al. 1990) that was capable of simultaneously acquiring CT and single photon emission computed tomography (SPECT) data. First studies of the myocardium of porcines were successful, but the limited transverse field-of-view of the system and the lengthy scan times limited the applicability of this correlated imaging device. A few years later the same group presented their vision of an in-line SPECT/CT system for use in humans, and discussed an approach to the quantification of SPECT-tracer concentrations in the myocardium and brain based on the available CT transmission information (Tang et al. 1999a).

In the mid-1990s similar instrumentational efforts by Townsend and co-workers in the field of complementary CT and PET imaging led to the design, construction and clinical operation of the first combined, dual-modality PET/CT tomograph (Townsend et al. 1998a, 1999a). It comprised two complementary and commercially available tomographs in-line. The PET components of the prototype PET/CT resembled those of a rotating, partial-ring PET tomograph, the ECAT ART, and were mounted on a common aluminum disk to the rear of the CT system, a Somatom AR.SP (Fig. 2). The entire assembly was housed inside a compact gantry, which was only slightly deeper than the CT gantry alone. Because of the increased depth of the combined system, the tilt option was disabled. Notably, all major hardware components were left unchanged, and therefore the performance of the prototype PET/CT was the same as that of the PET and CT separately (Beyer et al. 2000). A common patient support system was used for scanning, and mounted to the front of the combined gantry. With the prototype PET/CT tomograph, patients of up to 200 kg could be examined with a co-axial imag-

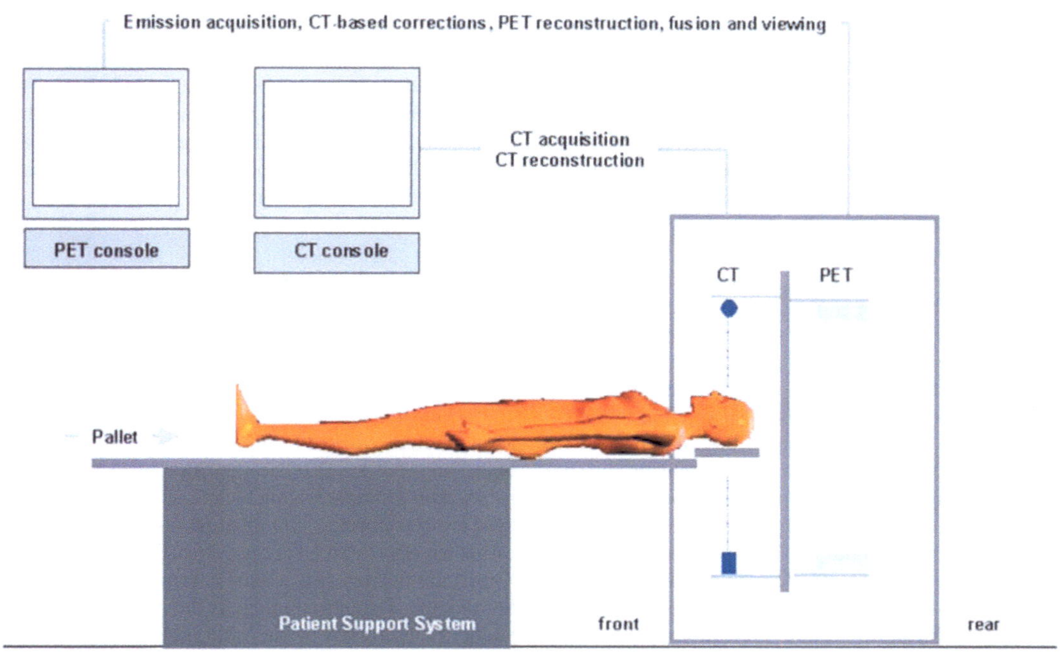

Fig. 2. Design of the prototype PET/CT tomograph (1998–2000). The PET components were mounted to the rear of the CT within a combined gantry. The prototype was operated from two independent consoles. Final data processing as well as image reconstruction and viewing were performed on the PET console

ing range of up to 100 cm, which is sufficient to cover a whole-body imaging range that typically extends from the head and neck to the thighs, depending on the size of the patient (Fig. 1b). The CT and the PET components of the prototype PET/CT were operated independently at the time. After the CT images were reconstructed, they were transferred to the PET console where further data processing and image reconstruction of the corrected emission data were performed. A typical whole-body PET/CT examination on the prototype would be completed in less than one hour, with the corrected PET and CT image being available for viewing shortly afterwards.

The prototype PET/CT tomograph was completed in 1998 and installed in May of the same year at the University of Pittsburgh Medical Center. More than 300 oncology patient studies were performed during the three years of operation of the prototype PET/CT. Physicians quickly appreciated the immediate access to intrinsically aligned whole-body PET and CT image sets for diagnosis and follow-up in cancer patients. First clinical results were very encouraging by demonstrating the gain in diagnostic accuracy and confidence with combined PET/CT imaging (Charron et al. 1999, 2000; Kluetz et al. 2001) that was anticipated during the prototype development.

2.2.2 FDG PET/CT Imaging Protocols

While the prototype PET/CT provided full functionality of both the CT and the PET components, it was almost exclusively used as a combined imaging device. With its introduction into the clinical environment, a standard PET/CT acquisition protocol was generated, which involved the acquisition of a topogram to define the examination range, a set of contiguous spiral CT scans, and a whole-body PET emission scan covering the same axial imaging range as the CT (Fig. 3). The individual scan ranges of the CT and PET examination were of course matched to ensure CT-based quantitative corrections (see Sect. 2.2.3) for the entire co-axial examination range.

All patients were injected with typically 350 MBq of FDG at least one hour prior to the start of the combined examination. At the beginning of the PET/CT scan the patient was positioned in head-first supine on the common table. In contrast to standard PET, where the definition of the examination range is based entirely on external laser markers and on the experience of the technologist, the PET examination range can be defined more accurately by using the topogram. The topogram is acquired during continuous table motion with the X-ray tube/detector-assembly locked in either frontal or lateral position (or any other position in between), thus generating an anatomical overview image, similar to a conventional X-ray, at a given projection (Fig. 3). After the definition of the axial examination range, the patient was automatically positioned in the CT field-of-view for the CT examination. Accounting for the limited tube heat capacity of the prototype design, up to four contiguous, spiral CT scans had to be defined, with intermittent tube cooling periods, to cover the extended axial examination range. The scan parameters for each spiral scan were similar to those of a stand-alone spiral CT scan of clinical quality.

After the completion of the last CT spiral, the patient was advanced to the field-of-view of the PET, to the rear of the combined gantry, where emission scanning commenced in the caudo-cranial direction, starting at the thighs. Depending on the axial co-scan range and the emission time allotted for an individual bed position (i.e. single emission scan), the combined scanning would be completed in about one hour. This time was too long for most patients to tolerate being positioned with their arms raised above their head for the duration of the combined scan, and therefore most patients were positioned on the bed comfortably with their arms close to their body. Unlike in standard CT practice, patients were allowed to breathe shallowly.

By the time the emission data acquisition was complete, the CT transmission images were reconstructed and transferred to the PET console, where they became available for attenuation and scatter correction of the emission data. Emission image reconstruction began after the completion of the last bed position of the PET scan. All emission images were routinely corrected for attenuation using the available CT transmission information and reconstructed iteratively (Defrise and Kinahan 1998). Special viewing tools were made available to view the reconstructed CT and corrected PET images, side-by-side, or in fused mode, with the PET images superimposed on the CT images.

2.2.3 CT-based Attenuation Correction

It was originally shown by La Croix and Tang that CT transmission data can be used for attenuation correction of complementary emission data, which are acquired at photon energies different from those of the X-ray photons emitted from the CT tube (LaCroix et al. 1994; Tang et al. 1999b). The algorithm by La Croix et al. is based on a simple scaling technique. First, the CT images are transformed into attenuation images at some estimated effective CT energy, which, depending on the X-ray tube characteristics, can be from 60 keV to 80 keV. Second, the attenuation image at the relevant emission energy is multiplied by the ratio of attenuation coefficients of water at that effective CT energy and the emission energy, respectively. This simple scaling approach works well for soft tissues, but serious overestimation

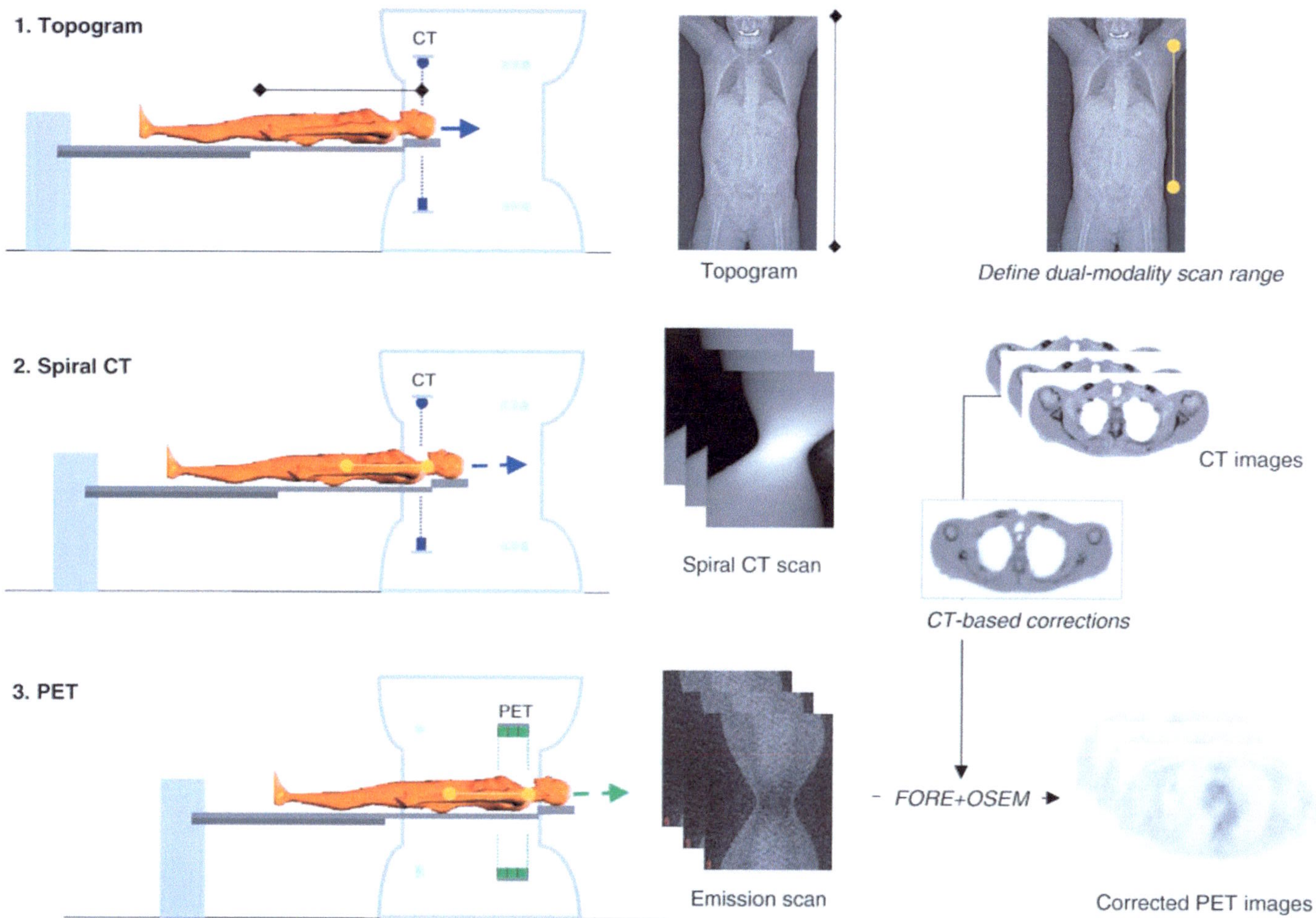

Fig. 3. Examination PET/CT protocol. Following the administration of the PET radiopharmaceutical (including some uptake time), the patient is positioned on the scanner bed, and a topogram scan (overview) is acquired to determine the range of the PET/CT examination (1). Subsequent CT data are typically acquired in spiral mode (2). After the completion of the CT examination, the patient is moved to the field-of-view of the PET, when emission scanning commences (3). CT images can be used for CT-based quantitative corrections of the PET emission data. At the end of the combined examination, co-registered CT and corrected PET images are available to the user, and can be viewed in fused mode, or separately

of the attenuation properties of cortical bone and ribs was observed, especially with increasing difference of the transmission and emission photon energies (LaCroix et al. 1994). Nevertheless, the overestimation of attenuation in bone translated into only a minor average overestimation of the tracer uptake in the corrected SPECT images due to the low fraction of voxels containing bone compared to other tissues.

The original scaling approach can therefore be extended to CT-based attenuation correction of PET emission data (Kinahan et al. 1998). Instead of a linear scaling approach with a single scale factor, a bi-linear scaling must be considered to account for both the photon energy difference between CT and PET, and the different attenuation properties of low-Z (soft tissues) and high-Z (bone) materials in the range of the lower energy X-ray photons (Fig. 4).

Today, bi-linear scaling methods (Fleming 1989; Kinahan et al. 1998) are widely accepted for clinical PET/CT imaging, and are, with small adaptations, used routinely for CT-based attenuation correction of the PET emission data (Beyer et al. 2002; Burger et al. 2002). The time for the acquisition of the attenuation data for a whole-body study can be reduced to 1 min, or less, by using a fast CT scan instead of a lengthy PET transmission measurement. Furthermore, CT transmission data acquired in post-injection scenarios are not noticeably affected by the emission activity inside the patient due to the high X-ray photon flux (Beyer et al. 2000). Therefore, corrective data processing as in post-injection PET transmission imaging (Smith et al. 1997; Watson et al. 1999) is not required.

Nevertheless, serious artifacts in the CT images may still be observed when, for example, metal implants, or other high-density materials, such as ceramic fillings, pacemakers, or chemotherapy infusion ports are present inside the CT field-of-view (de Man et al. 1999). These CT artifacts have been shown to propagate through CT-based attenuation correction into the corrected PET emission images where artificially increased tracer uptake patterns may then be generated (Antoch et al. 2002b; Goerres et al. 2002a). It is therefore recommended that PET/CT images are read with care when lesions are detected on PET that are close to visible artifactual structures on CT. For these cases, the additional evaluation of the emission data prior to CT-based attenuation correction is advisable.

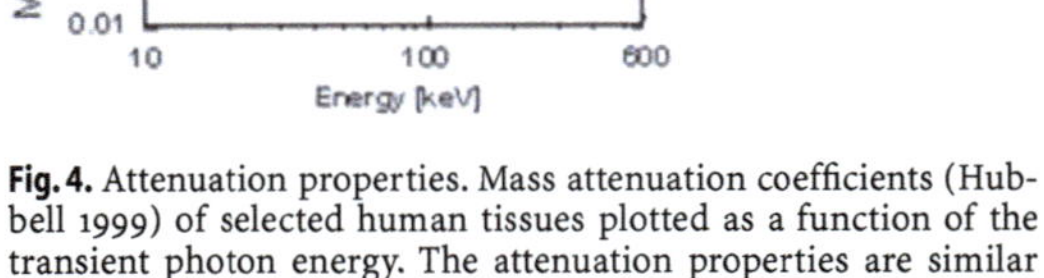

Fig. 4. Attenuation properties. Mass attenuation coefficients (Hubbell 1999) of selected human tissues plotted as a function of the transient photon energy. The attenuation properties are similar for low-Z tissues (blood, fat, muscle), which are significantly lower than those of high-Z tissues (bone), particularly at lower photon energies, as a result of the higher fraction of photoelectric absorption at these energies. The range of photon energies for CT, SPECT and PET are indicated as color bars above the graph

2.2.4 Limitations of the Prototype PET/CT

Future developments of dual-modality imaging systems and their acceptance by a broader clinical audience require the recognition and modification of a number of hardware limitations inherent to the prototype system (Table 1). For example, the PET components provided the clinical user with satisfactory image quality (Townsend et al. 1999b), but increased count-rate performance and higher absolute sensitivities (Townsend et al. 1998b) are needed to allow for faster imaging (less than 1 h) and potentially improved lesion detection. Similarly, performance increases of the CT system have to be considered. Extended durability of the X-ray tube and higher tube output levels are needed for extended spiral scanning of clinical quality that is accepted by the radiologists. In addition, faster gantry rotation times and multi-row detector technology help reduce the frequency of motion artifacts and allow for better contrast enhancement and multi-phase contrast enhancement studies of the liver, for example. The limitations of the transverse field-of-view to 45 cm frequently led to truncation artifacts in CT images and subsequent biases of the reconstructed emission data following CT-based attenuation correction (Beyer 2000). A larger measured, or reconstructed field-of-view of the CT is therefore desirable when scanning large patients, or patients with their arms parallel to the body. In view of an extension of the co-axial imaging range, the mechanical design of the patient positioning system has to be revised. A modified bed design should also eliminate any existing vertical deflection between the CT and PET systems in-line. Of course, when fusing the hardware components, similar integration is useful at the level of the acquisition and data analysis software. Therefore, new PET/CT designs mandate a unified user interface and computer power that is adaptable to the dual-acquisition requirements, data handling and processing.

Table 1.
Selected design parameters of the prototype PET/CT system, consequences for its performance, and PET/CT design goals

Prototype design	Consequences	Revised PET/CT design goals
PET components		
ECAT ART	Dedicated, low-end PET	Maximize PET performance
60 cm patient port	Limitations for use in RTP	Prepare for RTP use
CT components		
Somatom AR.SP	Early 1990s technology	Increase CT performance
30 rpm	Early 1990s technology	Sub-second rotation
45 cm field-of-view	Truncation artifacts	Increase CT field-of-view
PET/CT		
100 cm co-scan range	Limited whole-body scans	Extend imaging range
No bed support	Vertical deflection possible	Avoid relative bed deflection
Limited service access	Service challenges	Full service access
Dual acquisitions	Operation not integrated	Integrate acquisition system

RTP radiation therapy planning, rpm rotations per minute

2.3 PET/CT Design Considerations: The Second Generation of PET/CT Tomographs

Recognizing the success of the first prototype and responding to the potential of dual-modality PET/CT in clinical oncology, several manufacturers of medical imaging equipment have proposed their designs of PET/CT tomographs (Table 2). At the Society of Nuclear Medicine Meeting (SNM) in 2000 in St. Louis, CPS Innovations (Knoxville, TN, USA) introduced the first dedicated PET/CT tomograph that was cleared for marketing by the FDA. This tomograph was commercially released at the Radiological Society of North America (RSNA) Meeting later that year, and since then has been distributed as the biograph BGO through Siemens Medical Solutions, Inc. (Hoffman Estates, IL, USA) and as the ECAT REVEAL HD through CTI Molecular Imaging, Inc. (Knoxville, TN, USA). At the RSNA Meeting in 2000, GE Medical Systems also introduced a combined CT/PET system, now named the Discovery LS. Philips Nuclear Medicine presented their proposed design of a combined PET/CT tomograph, the Gemini, at the RSNA Meeting in 2001, and in a significantly revised version at the SNM 2002. In all three PET/CT tomographs the CT information is available for diagnostic purposes, anatomical landmarking and quantitative corrections of the complementary functional data. A fourth imaging device (Fig. 5a), the Discovery VH by GE Medical Systems (Bocher et al. 2000; Patton et al. 2000), also allows the acquisition of functional and anatomical data, but cannot be used for diagnostic CT evaluations because of its low-end X-ray components (Israel et al. 2000). It is therefore not considered a dual-modality PET/CT imaging device for the purpose of the following discussions.

In response to the major design goals in Table 1, several design changes have been implemented in this generation of commercially available PET/CT tomographs (Fig. 5b–d). For example, revised bed designs aim at avoiding any relative vertical offset of the patient and the pallet between the two complementary imaging modalities (Fig. 6). Vertical offsets in PET/CT images may arise from transiting a patient through the fields-of-view of the axially displaced imaging components while leaving the support structures of the patient pallet fixed with respect to the gantry (Fig. 6a). The vertical deflection depends on the axial position of the pallet inside the combined system and on the patient weight. Since the field-of-view of the CT and the PET are axially displaced (Fig. 2), a relative vertical deflection is thus created between the two image sets.

In one of the revised designs, the pallet is mounted to a post-type support structure that resides on a floor-mounted rail system (Fig. 5b). The patient is repositioned between scans by moving the entire post with the pallet attached (Fig. 6b). Alternatively, a standard patient bed (e.g. from CT) can be mounted to a rail system in the floor and moved to bridge the distance between the CT and the PET field-of-view (Fig. 5c). Then the vertical deflection would be the same for the CT and the PET scan, and the relative vertical deflection would be essentially zero, or limited to residual vertical non-linearities of the floor-mounted rail system. In another design the bed support system is fixed with respect to the gantry. The pallet moves on rails inside the combined system, where it is supported further by a post (Fig. 5d). The maximum co-axial imaging range with any of these patient handling systems is 145–195 cm (Table 2).

To meet the standards of radiology practice in oncology all available dedicated PET/CT tomographs employ commercial CT scanners in tandem with state-of-the-art PET technology. The CT modules of the combined tomographs offer sequential and spiral scanning modes with increased X-ray tube heat capacities and multiple CT detector row technology, which allows the simultaneous acquisition of up to four slices depending on the manufacturer (Table 2). Multi-row CT offers large vol-

Table 2. Design and performance parameters of PET/CT systems. PET performance parameters were acquired to NEMA-2000 standard

Manufacturer		CPS Innovations	CPS Innovations	CPS Innovations	CPS Innovations
Concept		Dedicated PET/CT	Dedicated PET/CT	Dedicated PET/CT	Dedicated PET/CT
Introduced		1998	2000	2001	2002
		1st generation	2nd generation		3rd generation
	Height/width/depth (cm)	168/170/110	188/228/170	188/228/170	200/228/168
	Inner tunnel length (cm)		100	100	106
	Patient port diameter	Uniform, 60 cm	Uniform, 70 cm	Uniform, 70 cm	Uniform, 70 cm
	Standard co-scan range	100 cm	145 cm	145 cm	182 cm
	PHS	Standard CT bed	Floor-mounted rail, fixed fulcrum	Floor-mounted rail, fixed fulcrum	Floor-mounted rail, fixed fulcrum
	Max patient weight	200 kg	204 kg	204 kg	204 kg
	Radiation therapy table attachment	No	Yes	Yes	Yes
CT system					
	System components	Somatom AR.SP	Somatom Emotion (Duo)	Somatom Emotion (Duo)	Somatom Sensation 16
	Spiral CT	Yes	Yes	Yes	Yes
	Max number of active detector rings	1	1 (2)	1 (2)	16
	Detector material	Xe	Ultrafast ceramics	Ultrafast ceramics	Ultrafast ceramics
	Detector design	Individual, tungsten septa	Matrix	Matrix	Adaptive pixel array
	Measured transverse FOV	45 cm	50 cm	50 cm	50 cm
	Min and max slice width (mm)	1 and 10	1 and 10 (1 and 10)	1 and 10 (1 and 10)	0.6 and 10
	Max rotation speed	30 rpm	75 rpm	75 rpm	143 rpm
CT performance	*High-contrast resolution, 0 % MTF*	0.4 mm	0.32 mm (15.5 lp/cm)	0.32 mm (15.5 lp/cm)	0.17 mm (30 lp/cm)
	Low-contrast resolution, spiral, CATPHAN 20 cm	2.5 mm/5 HU/1.9 s	5 mm/3 HU/0.8 s/ 15.8 mGy/90 mAs	5 mm/3 HU/0.8 s/ 15.8 mGy/90 mAs	5 mm/3 HU/0.75 s/ 20 mGy/190 mAs
	Center dose ($CTDI_{100}$, body phantom) per 100 mAs		6.7 mGy (130 kVp)	6.7 mGy (130 kVp)	6.5 mGy/112 mAs (140 kVp)
PET system					
	System components	ECAT ART	ECAT EXACT HR+	ECAT ACCEL	ECAT ACCEL
	PET acquisition mode	3D	3D	3D	3D
	Detector design	Partial ring, rotating	Full ring	Full ring	Full ring
	Septa	No	No	No	No
	Detector material	BGO	BGO	LSO	LSO
	Transmission sources	Two ^{137}Cs points (550 MBq)	No	No	No
	Transverse FOV	58 cm	58.5 cm	58.5 cm	58.5 cm
	Axial FOV	16.2 cm	15.5 cm	16.2 cm	16.2 cm
	Transverse images per bed	47	63	47	47
	Image plane separation	3.4 mm	2.4 mm	3.4 mm	3.4 mm
PET performance	*Axial resolution at center*	6 mm	4.2 mm	5.8 mm	5.8 mm
(NEMA 2000)	*Transverse resolution at center*	6.2 mm	4.5 mm	6.3 mm	6.3 mm
	Sensitivity	8 cps/Bq	28 cps/Bq	27 cps/Bq	27cps/Bq
	Peak NEC	39.5 kcps at 18 kBq/ml (NE-94)	40 kcps at 11 kBq/ml	50 kcps at 14 kBq/ml	50 kcps at 14 kBq/ml

CPS Innovations is a joint venture of Siemens Medical Solutions, Inc and CTI Molecular Imaging, Inc

Table 2. Continued

GE Medical Systems	GE Medical Systems	GE Medical Systems	Philips Medical Systems		Manufacturer
SPET/coincidence PET/CT	Dedicated PET/CT	Dedicated PET/CT	Dedicated PET/CT		Concept
1999	2000	2002	2002		Introduced
2nd generation	2nd generation	3rd generation	2nd generation		
210/155/175	208/235/198	192/236/109	206/210/602	*Height/width/depth (cm)*	
n.a.	142	100	206 with gap (30)	*Inner tunnel length (cm)*	
60 cm	Tapered, 70–60 cm	Uniform, 70 cm	70 cm CT, 63 cm PET	*Patient port diameter*	
160 cm	160 cm	160 cm	195 cm	*Standard co-scan range*	
Floor-mounted, table can swing sideways for collimator exchange	Floor-mounted pedestal	Floor-mounted pedestal	Floor-mounted, dual pallet	*PHS*	
200 kg	200 kg	200 kg	202 kg	*Max patient weight*	
No	No	Yes	Yes	*Radiation therapy table attachment*	
					CT system
Unique, not available separately	LightSpeed Plus	LightSpeed Range	Mx8000D	*System components*	
No	Yes	Yes	Yes	*Spiral CT*	
1	4, 8 or 16 (since 2002)	4, 8, 16	2	*Max number of active detector rings*	
Solid state	Solid state – Lumex	Solid state – Lumex	Solid state	*Detector material*	
Individual, CdW	Pixel array	Pixel array	2D solid state detector array	*Detector design*	
45 cm	50 cm	51 cm	50 cm	*Measured transverse FOV*	
10 mm	0.625 and 10 mm	0.625 and 10 mm	0.5 and 10	*Min and max slice width (mm)*	
2.6 rpm	120 rpm	120 rpm	120 rpm	*Max rotation speed*	
4 lp/cm	8.5 lp/cm	8.5 lp/cm	22 lp/cm	*High-contrast resolution, 0% MTF*	*CT performance*
3 mm at 2.5 %	5 mm/3 HU/n.a./ 34 mGy/n.a.	6 mm/3 HU/n.a./ 34 mGy/n.a.	4 mm/3 HU/ n.a./ 27 mGy/ n.a.	*Low contrast resolution, CATPHAN 20 cm*	
3 mGy	6.8 mGy (120 kVp)	6.8 mGy (120 kVp)	14–28 mGy (120 kVp)	*Center dose ($CTDI_{100}$, body phantom) per 100 mAs*	
					PET
Millennium VG	ADVANCE Nxi	Unique, not available separately	Allegro	*System components*	
2D and 3D	2D and 3D	2D and 3D	3D	*PET acquisition mode*	
Panels	Full ring	Full ring	Full ring	*Detector design*	
Yes	Yes	Yes	No	*Septa*	
NaI	BGO	BGO	GSO	*Detector material*	
No	Optional (^{68}Ge rods)	No	^{137}Cs point (740 MBq)	*Transmission sources*	
54 cm	55 cm	70 cm	57.6 mm	*Transverse FOV*	
40 cm	15.2 cm	15.2 cm	18 cm	*Axial FOV*	
46	35	47	90	*Transverse images per bed*	
4.2 mm	4.2 mm	3.2 mm	2 mm	*Image plane separation*	
2.5 mm (2D), 4.5 mm (3D)	6.3 mm (2D), 6.4 mm (3D)	5.2 mm (2D), 5.8 mm (3D)	5 mm	*Axial resolution*	*PET performance*
4.3 mm (2D), 4.5 mm (3D)	4.8 mm (2D), 4.8 mm (3D)	6.2 mm (2D), 6.2 mm (3D)	4.9 mm	*Transverse resolution at center*	*(NEMA 2000)*
0.16 cps/Bq (2D), 1.6 cps/Bq (3D)	1.3 cps/Bq (2D), 6.5 cps/Bq (3D)	2.1 cps/Bq (2D), 9.5 cps/Bq (3D)	24.8 cps/Bq*) (NE-94)	*Sensitivity*	
2.1 kcps	165 kcps at 130 kBq/ml (2D), 42 kcps at 8.5 kBq/ml (3D)	85 kcps at 40 kBq/ml (2D), 56 kcps at 10 kBq/ml (3D)	30.5	*Peak NEC*	

*) Trues + Scatter

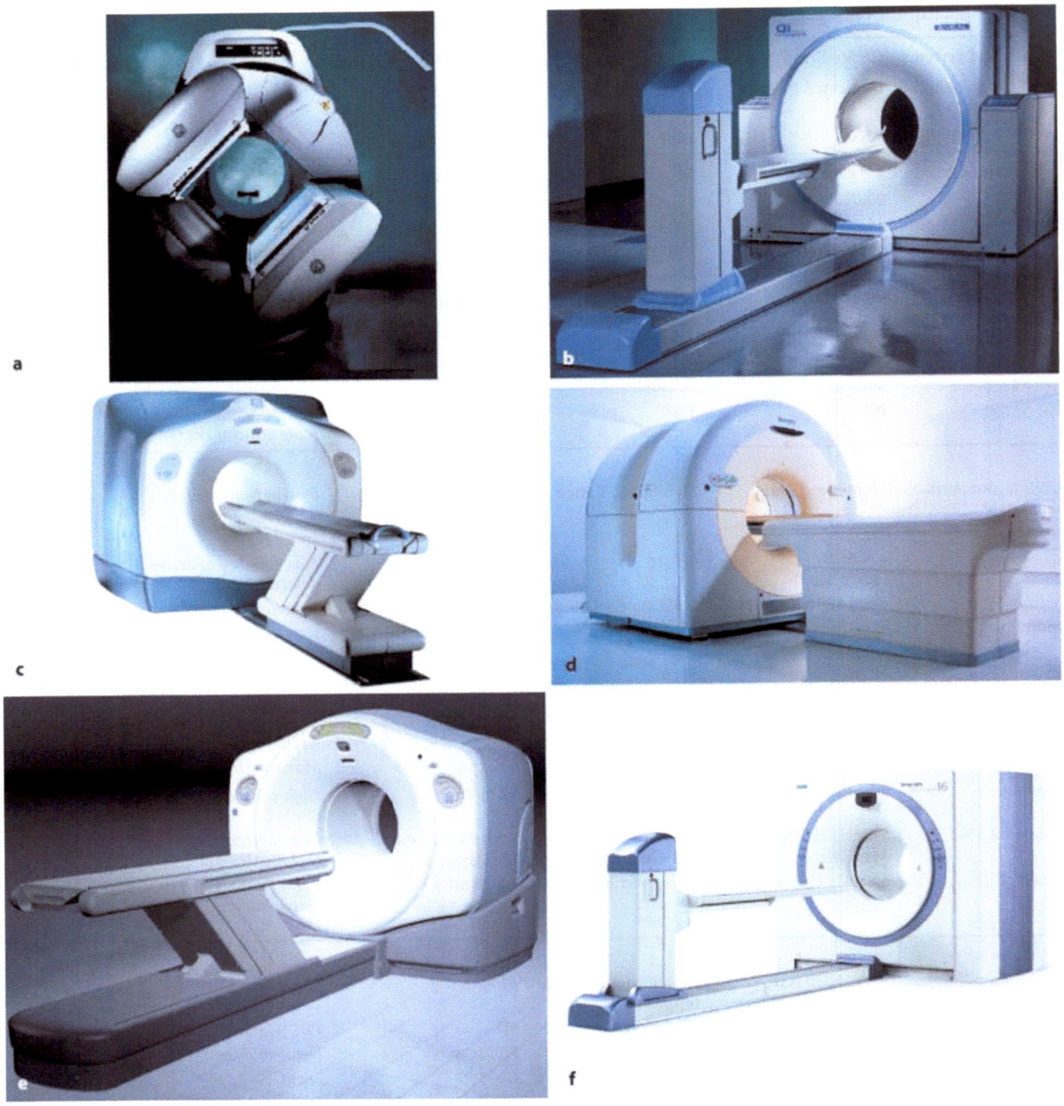

Fig. 5. Commercial dual-modality PET/CT tomographs. **a** Discovery VH by GEMS, **b** PET/CT-Duo tomograph manufactured by CPS Innovations (joint venture between Siemens Medical Solutions Inc. and CTI Molecular Imaging Inc.), **c** Discovery LS by GEMS, **d** Gemini by Philips Medical Systems, **e** Discovery ST by GEMS, and **f** ECAT ACCEL/Sensation 16 CT by CPS Innovations. The tomographs shown in (**b–d**) and (**e, f**) are second- and third-generation PET/CT systems, respectively

ume coverage in short scan times (McCollough and Zink 1999; Roos et al. 2002), a necessary prerequisite for oncology imaging when examining patients with only limited breath-hold capabilities. Alternatively, imaging ranges can be scanned with finer axial sampling within the same time that is needed with a single-row CT. Furthermore, when employing IV contrast agents, several organs can be imaged at peak contrast enhancement during a single spiral, or repeat CT examinations can be acquired for a single IV contrast injection over a single organ, such as the liver (Itoh et al. 2003). The use of spiral CT technology in combined PET/CT imaging therefore offers high-quality CT images for a variety of imaging conditions encountered in clinical oncology.

A major distinguishing feature of the combined PET/CT tomographs is the PET detector technology (Table 2). In the Discovery LS, for example, the PET tomograph is based on bismuth germanate (BGO), a scintil-

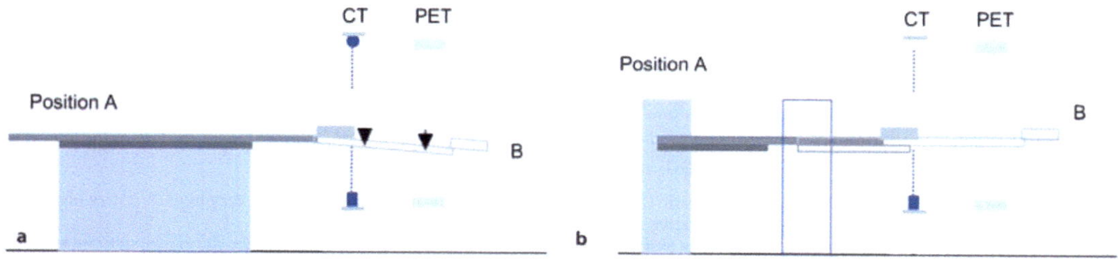

Fig. 6. Patient handling system and vertical bed deflection. A vertical offset (*arrows*) between the CT and PET data of the same examination is introduced when using a patient handling system with a center of gravity fixed with respect to the gantry (**a**). The relative vertical offset between the CT and PET data is eliminated when translating the entire patient handling system from position A to B, i.e. the patient is moved together with the support structure into the gantry (**b**)

lator that is the most widely employed detector material in PET. The ECAT HR+/Somatom Emotion (Duo) also uses BGO as the PET detector material of choice. However, alternative PET detector materials have been available for some time and are used for PET and PET/CT designs. For example, CPS Innovations offers a PET/CT model (ACCEL/Somatom Emotion (Duo), see Table 2), with the PET detector being based on lutetium oxyorthosilicate (LSO; Bruckbauer et al. 2001). LSO has several advantages over BGO: while LSO has a density similar to that of BGO, it offers an eight times faster decay time, and a five times higher light output (Melcher 2000). Accepting the potential for using faster crystals in PET imaging technology, Philips Medical Systems offer a combination of the gadolinium oxyorthosilicate (GSO)-based Allegro PET tomograph with a state-of-the-art CT scanner. GSO offers a five times shorter decay time and twice the light output of BGO, thus making it a good candidate next to LSO for a fast scintillator to replace BGO in fully 3D PET tomographs (Muehllehner et al. 2002). For a practical review of the advantages and disadvantages of faster scintillator materials for PET imaging, the reader is referred to Karp (2002) and Nutt (2002).

It is interesting to note that most commercial PET/CT designs favor the use of 3D-only emission acquisitions by eliminating the septa from the PET components. Assuming proper data processing, 3D PET offers a number of advantages over 2D PET, such as higher sensitivity and higher count rates at lower activity concentrations (Bendriem and Townsend 1998). Furthermore, the sensitivity advantage of 3D imaging and the fast scintillation properties of either GSO or LSO can be combined to result in high-quality PET images at reduced scan times and increased patient comfort.

Another difference of the second-generation PET/CT tomographs is the diameter of the combined gantry tunnel. In anticipation of the use of PET/CT imaging for the planning of radiation therapy, the patient port diameter of the combined gantry must be large enough to fit patients with therapy masks and other positioning devices on a standard flat treatment pallet. Therefore the patient port of the PET scanner should be increased to match the tunnel opening of the CT. In the design of the HR+/Somatom Emotion (Duo) and the ACCEL/Somatom Emotion (Duo), the tunnel diameter of the PET is increased from 56 cm to 70 cm by shortening the side shielding of the PET while keeping the detector ring diameter fixed. Using fast scintillators in conjunction with optimized detector electronics and shorter coincidence windows can compensate for the resulting increased fraction of random coincidences.

In summary, almost all PET/CT tomographs in use today are second-generation systems (Table 2) based on commercially available state-of-the-art CT in tandem with high-end PET components. This seeming imbalance of hardware components in favor of high-end PET modules originates from the primary motivation for combined PET/CT imaging devices: to complement clinically established PET imaging with intrinsically registered anatomical information (Townsend and Cherry 2001). The second-generation PET/CT designs clearly reflect the acceptance of PET imaging technology as the driving momentum in PET/CT devices. Compared to the prototype design, commercial PET/CT systems aim at higher performance of both the CT and the PET components without necessarily seeking a closer integration of the gantry components. A closer integration, however, has occurred at the level of the acquisition platforms, and unified consoles are available today to operate combined PET/CT either in dual-modality acquisition modes, or separately when desired.

2.4 Experiences with Existing PET/CT Technology

Over 200 combined PET/CT tomographs are operational worldwide today. An increasing number of publications demonstrate the benefits of PET/CT imaging and furthermore substantiate the hypothesis of its improved diagnostic accuracy and clinical value (Goerres et al. 2002c, 2002d; Hany et al. 2002; Cohade et al. 2003).

Table 3. Current scenarios of PET/CT imaging

Scenario	Methodology	Main focus	Demands on CT	Demands on PET
1	PET with CT for fast attenuation correction and anatomical labeling	Nuclear medicine	Low	High
2	Diagnostic CT with radiopharmaceutical (e.g., FDG) as alternative contrast agent	Radiology	High	High
3	Diagnostic CT with CT contrast agents and quantitative functional information	Cross-modality	Very high	Very high

Further discussion of the clinical experience can be found in Chap. 11.

There are three typical usage scenarios of these tomographs (Table 3): use the PET/CT as (1) a fast PET scanner with additional anatomical background information, (2) an anatomical imaging device with FDG, or any other radiopharmaceutical, acting essentially as a "new" CT contrast agent, or (3) a combined imaging device with high-quality CT and PET. Current PET/CT technology (Table 2) addresses most of the requirements of each scenario. However, the actual usage of the combined system will likely depend on the clinical and local preferences of the site of installation and the level of appreciation of the potential of combined imaging (Jager et al. 2003). Nonetheless a number of methodological issues are common to all clinical operations of PET/CT tomographs, and therefore shall be addressed briefly in the following sections.

2.4.1 CT Transmission Scanning and Attenuation Correction

Until recently the ability to correct PET emission data for attenuation routinely was opposed on the basis of noise propagation through measured attenuation correction (Wahl 1999). Noise propagation in whole-body PET imaging, however, can be minimized by spending one third and two thirds of the total scan time on the acquisition of the transmission and emission data, respectively (Holm et al. 1996; Beyer et al. 1997). For a seven-bed position whole-body PET examination (45 min), for example, transmission scanning then accounted for about 15 min, excluding the time to move the sources in and out of the field-of-view. Despite several efforts to reduce transmission scan time by introducing sophisticated segmentation techniques (Mix and Nitzsche 1999) and applying iterative reconstruction techniques to the attenuation data (Leahy and Qi 2000), transmission scan times cannot be reduced further in routine PET imaging. Therefore, whole-body PET imaging times are on the order of one hour, but could be reduced to, typically, 40 min when using faster detector materials, such as LSO or GSO. Nevertheless, given whole-body examination times of more than half an hour, most patients were positioned with their arms close to their body, thus introducing additional attenuation in the lateral direction for the thorax and abdomen.

With combined PET/CT tomographs, transmission scanning can be performed using the available CT and transmission scan times can be reduced to about 1 min (von Schulthess 2000). Further reductions of CT scan time can be achieved by using multi-row CT with large pitch factors (Kalender 2000) but little gain in overall scan times is thus expected; however, a reduction in axial image quality might be observed. Compared to standard PET, shorter transmission scanning results in shorter overall scan time and thus increased patient comfort. Today, with total scan times on the order of 20–30 min, patients can be asked to keep their arms above their head for the duration of the combined scan for better CT and PET image quality (Fig. 7a). Due to the high photon flux from the X-ray tube, CT transmission images are seemingly unaffected by contamination from the post-injection emission activity (Fig. 7b).

2.4.2 Respiration Protocols

Several PET/CT groups have described respiratory motion as a source of potential artifacts in corrected emission images after CT-based attenuation correction (Beyer 2000; Goerres et al. 2002b; Osman et al. 2002). These artifacts become dominant when standard breath-hold techniques are transferred directly from clinical CT to combined PET/CT examination protocols scanning without adaptations (Fig. 8a). In the absence of respiratory gating mechanisms for PET, alternatives have to be found to match the morphology of the patient, as captured by CT, with the PET tracer distribution that is imaged over several breathing cycles. Reasonable registration accuracy can be obtained with the spiral CT scan being acquired during shallow breathing (Goerres et al. 2002b, 2003a). Alternatively, when dealing with uncooperative patients a limited breath-hold protocol can be adopted, which requires the patient to hold their breath in expiration only for the time that the CT takes to cover the lower lung and liver (Beyer et al. 2003) (Fig. 8c). Very fast CT scanning together with a breath-hold command (in normal expiration, for example) may help reduce

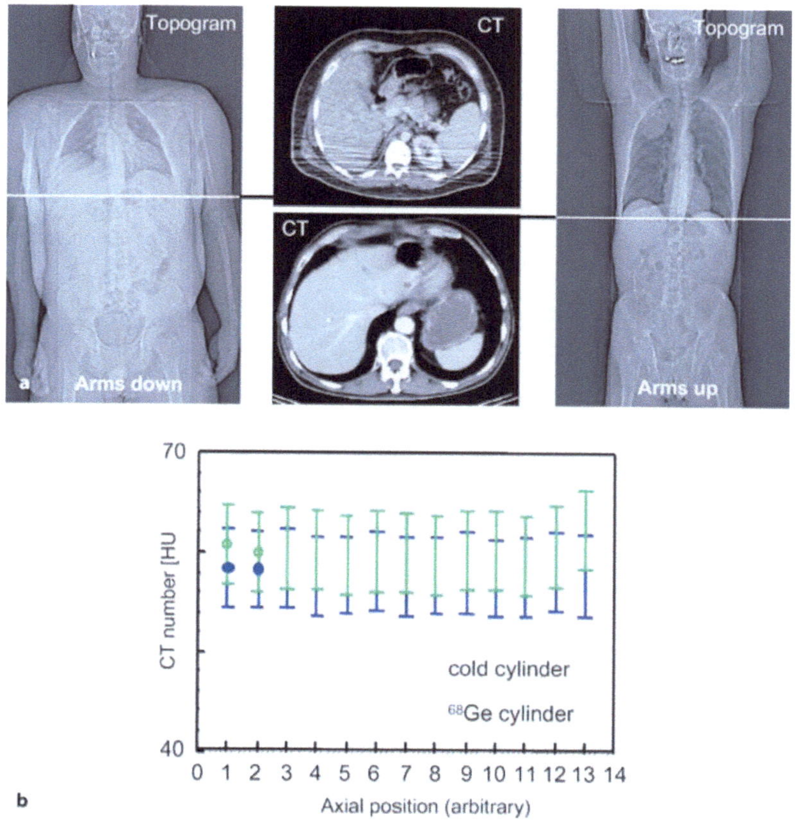

Fig. 7. Advantages of CT transmission scanning in combined PET/CT. Fast CT scanning capabilities reduce the overall scan time to less than 30 min. Therefore patients can be asked to keep their arms above their head to reduce otherwise well-known streak artifacts in the CT images (**a**). The high photon flux from the X-ray source (X-ray tube) renders the CT transmission images unaffected by contamination from annihilation photons in post-injection transmission scenarios. The average attenuation values of a cold and active (70 MBq) [^{68}Ge]resin-filled plastic cylinder scanned in standard CT transmission modes are shown in (**b**). No significant difference is seen

respiration mismatches over the entire whole-body examination range (Goerres et al. 2002b, 2003a).

Nevertheless, when respiration commands are not tolerated by the patient or when lesions are suspected in the area of the upper liver, it is recommended to reconstruct the emission data without attenuation correction and to review the two sets of fused PET/CT images very carefully (Osman et al. 2003).

2.4.3 Truncated Field-of-view

Spiral CT technology today offers a transverse field-of-view of 50 cm, and thus falls short 10 cm from the transverse PET imaging field (Table 2). This difference may lead to truncation artifacts in the CT images and to a systematic bias of the recovered tracer distribution when scanning very large patients, or positioning patients with their arms down (Fig. 9). If not corrected for truncation, CT images appear to mask the reconstructed emission data with the tracer distribution being only partially recovered outside the measured CT field-of-view (Fig. 9a).

To reduce the amount of truncation on CT and to minimize the frequency of these artifacts, whole-body or chest patients should be positioned according to CT practice with their arms raised above their head (Fig. 7a). By keeping the arms outside the field-of-view, the amount of scatter (Carney and Townsend 2002) and patient exposure are also much reduced. Given the short acquisition times of a PET/CT, most patients tolerate being scanned with their arms raised for the duration of the combined examination.

However, some patients may not tolerate such positioning well, even for very short total scan times. In these cases truncation may still occur and needs to be corrected. A number of algorithms have been suggested to extend artificially the truncated CT projections and to recover the truncated parts of the measured attenuation map (Fig. 9c). If applied to the CT images prior to CT-based attenuation correction, these correction algorithms will help to recover completely the tracer distributions measured with the complementary emission data (Schaller et al. 2002). Further work is needed, however, to make such algorithms routinely available for clinical diagnostics.

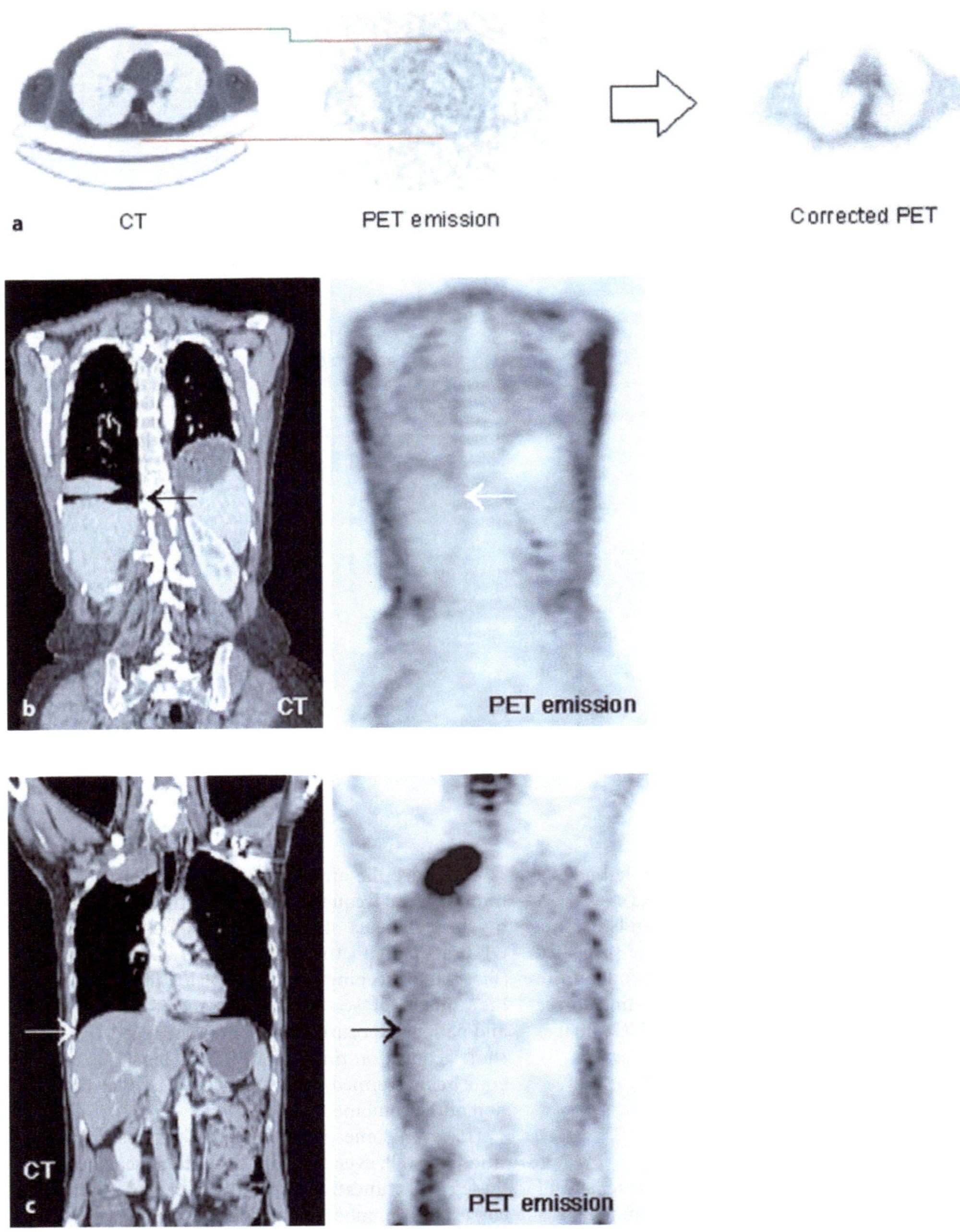

Fig. 8. Respiration mismatches. Mismatches in respiration between CT and PET can lead to serious artifacts (**a**): CT was acquired in full inspiration and PET was acquired during shallow breathing. Note the "disappearing chest wall". Serious artifacts may also be observed in the region of the diaphragm when uncoordinated breathing is accepted during the CT (**b**). These artifacts are not seen on the whole-body emission images generated over many respiratory cycles. Special breathing protocols have been proposed to minimize respiration-induced artifacts (**c**)

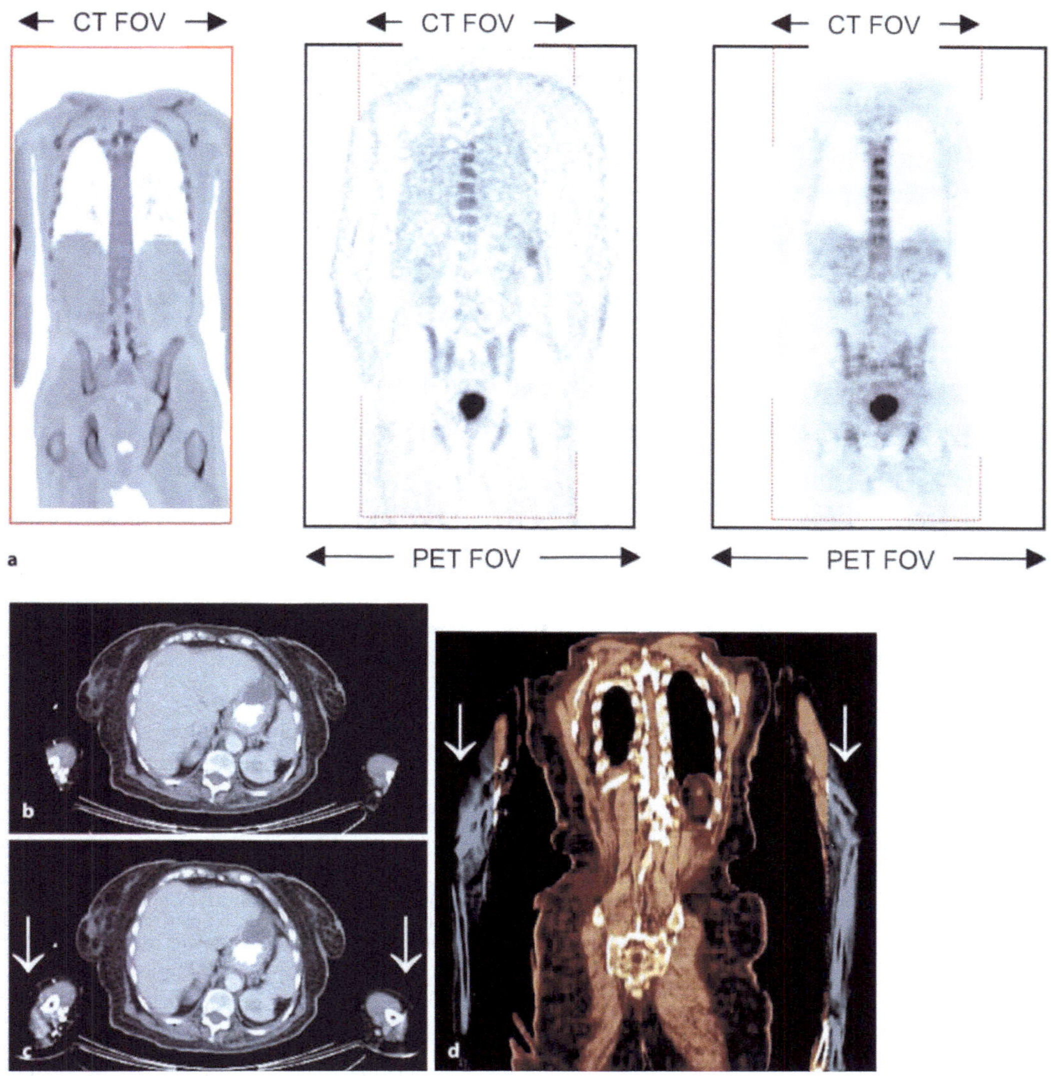

Fig. 9. Truncated field-of-view (FOV). The FOV of the CT is short 10 cm from the FOV of the PET. When positioning patients with arms down or partially outside the CT FOV (**a**), truncation artifacts may be observed on the CT and translate into the corrected PET with only a partially recovered tracer distribution. The truncated CT information (**b**) can be, at least partially, recovered (**c**) and attenuation information from the full PET FOV is available for CT-based attenuation correction (**d**). (Courtesy of Otto Sembritzki and Thomas Flohr, Siemens Medical Solutions, Forchheim, Germany)

2.4.4 The Use of CT Contrast Agents

A subject of debate in clinical PET/CT imaging is the use of CT contrast materials. These contrast agents represent high-density solutions, which are administered either intravenously or orally to enhance the vascular structures and digestive tract, respectively (Garrett et al. 1984; Mitchell et al. 1985). The debate on whether to use contrast agents in PET/CT imaging is based primarily on the fact that the bi-linear scaling approaches (Kinahan et al. 1998; Kamel et al. 2002a) do not account for the presence of CT contrast agents, and theoretically lead to an overestimation of the corrected emission activity (Fig. 10a). As indicated in Table 3, some user groups therefore argue that the use of contrast agents is not indicated in PET/CT and that CT images of lower diagnostic quality are acceptable (Hany et al. 2002; Kamel et al. 2002a).

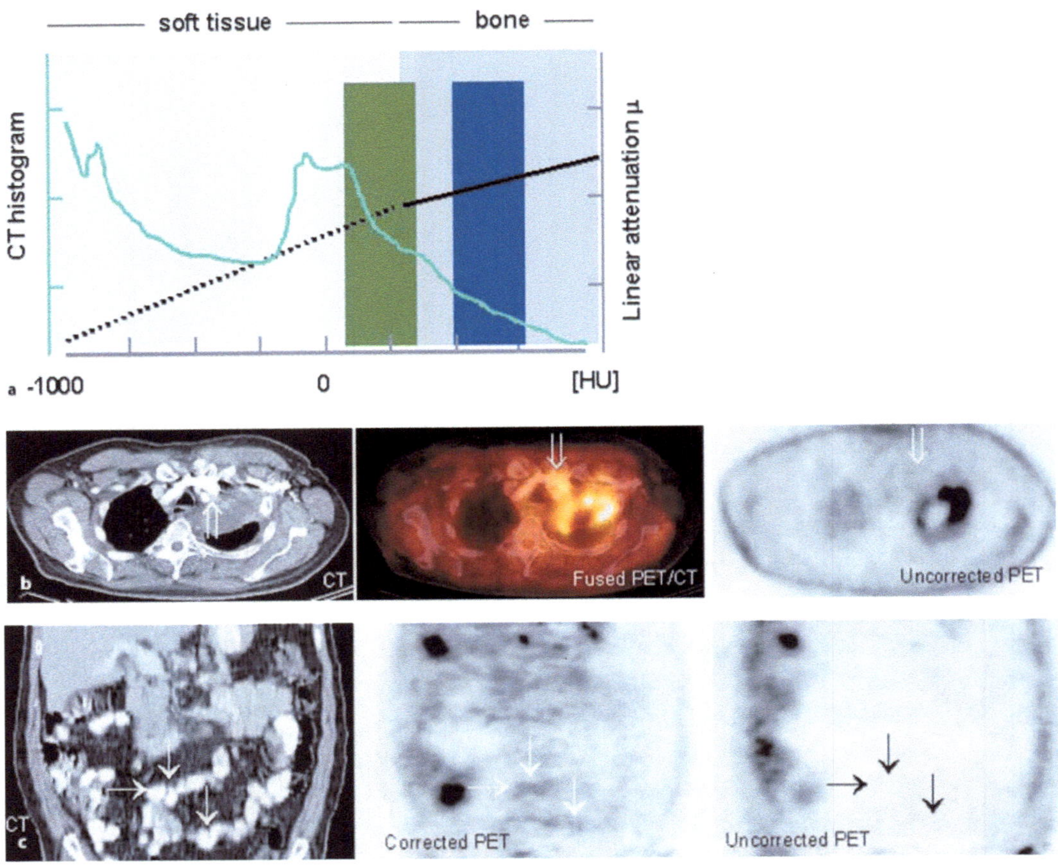

Fig. 10. CT-based attenuation correction in the presence of CT contrast agents. Standard CT-based attenuation correction is based on a bi-linear scaling model (**a**). The clinical ranges of contrast enhancement for IV (*green*) and oral (*blue*) CT contrast agents are indicated. Histogram-based separation of contrast-enhanced tissues from non-enhanced tissues is not feasible. Applying individual soft tissue or bone scale factors will overestimate the attenuation of contrast-enhanced tissues at 511 keV, thus potentially leading to artificially created tracer uptake patterns in the corrected emission images, as illustrated for a case with intravenous contrast (**b**) and with oral contrast (**c**)

As shown by others (Antoch et al. 2002a), the use of CT contrast agents together with standard-dose CT acquisition parameters is essential for high-quality diagnostic PET/CT imaging as well as in view of prospectively substituting a clinical CT examination with a PET/CT examination. In order to avoid overestimation of tracer uptake in contrast-enhanced tissues, the available CT-based attenuation correction algorithms should be modified. Furthermore, these modifications should account for patient-dependent contrast distribution and tissue enhancement.

To account for IV contrast agents (Fig. 10a), a third scale factor has been proposed (Beyer and Townsend 2001; Carney et al. 2002) but certain approximations are needed for the separation of non-enhanced and enhanced tissues that render such an approach problematic. Carney and colleagues have proposed a seed-growing segmentation technique to extract those anatomical regions that contain oral contrast and to replace their voxel value with a heuristic attenuation value at 511 keV (Carney and Townsend 2002; Carney et al. 2002). However, this approach is not reliable either, as the contrast distribution may vary significantly inside the patient. Other modifications to existing CT-based attenuation correction algorithms exist (Dizendorf et al. 2002), but generally these modifications require some significant user interaction, or are based on patient-independent assumptions that may leave some residual bias in the calculations.

In the absence of reliable correction algorithms, alternative contrast administration protocols have been proposed for PET/CT imaging. For example, high-density artifacts from bolus injection (Antoch et al. 2002b) may be avoided by applying the IV contrast volume with an adaptive pressure pump or, alternatively, by applying a second saline flush after the IV contrast agent has been injected. Oral contrast agents, on the other hand, are administered up to one hour prior to the examination. To avoid high-Z materials, which may lead to a potential overestimation of attenuation coefficients (Dizendorf et al. 2002), the use of negative oral contrast agents has been proposed for PET/CT imaging (Antoch et al. 2003).

In summary, there are several challenges for CT-based attenuation correction in combined PET/CT imaging. These include mismatches of morphology and function caused by respiratory or patient motion and the presence of truncation artifacts when scanning large patients. Furthermore, CT image artifacts originating from dental (Kamel et al. 2002b) and hip implants (Goerres et al. 2003b), or high-density CT contrast concentrations (Antoch et al. 2002b) may translate into artificially increased tracer uptakes in the corrected emission images. Therefore optimized acquisition protocols should be implemented routinely to minimize these artifacts, and adequate data processing schemes should be provided to correct for artifacts that cannot be avoided. The user should be aware of the potential pitfalls in PET/CT imaging and review the combined images prior to attenuation correction whenever artificial emission activities seem to originate from inconsistencies in the CT data.

2.5 Recent Developments and Trends for Tomorrow

Despite a number of methodological challenges, PET/CT imaging is increasingly accepted in clinical practice. While these challenges are well understood, general solutions to artifact-free combined imaging do not exist. Therefore a variety of optimized acquisition protocols are currently being considered to limit or partially avoid these artifacts. For example, limited breath-hold techniques have been shown to minimize effectively respiration-induced mismatches between CT and PET images. Alternative CT contrast injection schemes are being considered to avoid high-density contrast artifacts on CT that may translate into the corrected emission images. Nevertheless, high-quality PET/CT examinations cannot be performed routinely unless a number of CT correction algorithms become available in the PET/CT software to address streaking artifacts from high-density implants and non-standard patient positioning.

Current developments in improved acquisition and data-processing software go in hand with new hardware developments for updated combined tomograph designs, such as the Discovery ST from GE Medical Systems (Fig. 5e), and a combined LSO-PET/16-ring CT (Fig. 5f) from CPS Innovations. The ST, for example, is based on a revised full-ring BGO-PET system for routine whole-body imaging, together with a choice of 4-, 8-, or 16-ring CT technology.

By introducing 16-ring CT technology into combined PET/CT designs, the advantages of very fast and high-resolution volume coverage by CT are translated directly into the context of anato-metabolic imaging. Durable, high CT scan speeds (120 rpm and more) help to reduce respiration-induced artifacts and allow imaging of the anatomy of multiple organs at peak enhancement after IV contrast injection.

Although these fast scanning capabilities might result in an overall improved image and diagnostic quality of CT, the cost of combining a PET with the latest in multi-ring CT technology seems high unless dedicated applications are defined. Furthermore, the benefit of freezing motion during the acquisition of the CT, and imaging the anatomy of the patient at a particular point during involuntary periodic motion cycles (cardiac and respiration) is lost without adequate acquisition modes for the PET examination portion. Assuming the technical implementation of cardiac (and respiratory) gating of the emission scan in PET/CT tomographs, myocardial viability could be evaluated in a single examination by means of CT-angiography in combination with a PET viability study (Fig. 11). Imaging the heart, or substructures of it, however, requires sophisticated cardiac gating techniques that yet need to be developed for combined PET/CT imaging.

The efficacy of gating mechanisms in PET is frequently limited by insufficient analysis tools and, more importantly, by the significant increase in overall scan time to reach an acceptable level of statistical significance in the shorter time frames of interest. Using fast scintillator materials and appropriate detector electron-

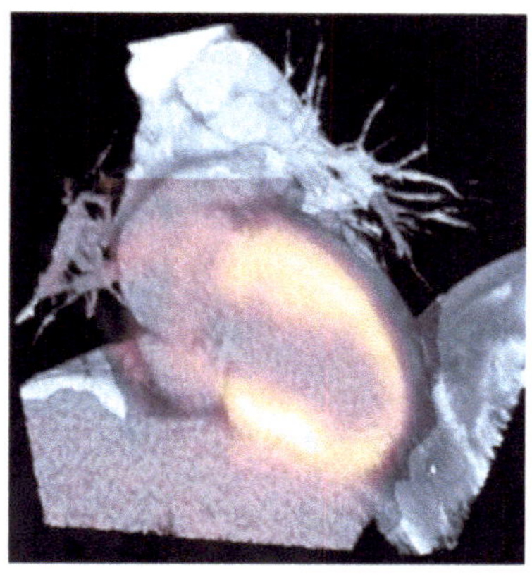

Fig. 11. Cardiac imaging with third-generation PET/CT. Male patient with hypometabolism in the apex of the myocardium. Fused 3D image of FDG PET and 16-ring CT scan. Data were acquired at the University Hospital Essen, Germany on an ECAT EXACT HR+ (non-gated mode) and a Somatom Sensation 16 (gated mode), respectively. (Image fusion courtesy of Stefan Käpplinger and Marc Rose, Siemens Medical Solutions, Erlangen, Germany)

ics allows the gating signal to be applied at higher count rates for improved noise characteristics of the gated emission frames.

Recently an innovative panel-based detector design for the next generation of PET tomographs has been proposed (Nahmias et al. 2002). Each panel measures 36 cm transverse by 52 cm in the axial direction, and is made up of 5 cm LSO detector blocks. Each LSO block consists of 12 by 12 individual crystals, each $4\times4\times25\,\text{mm}^3$ in size. The detector blocks and the photomultipliers mounted to the rear of the detectors are arranged in a quadrant-sharing mode, thus providing a cost-effective and high packing fraction. Panel-based PET tomographs are envisaged to employ three to five panels providing up to three times the peak noise equivalent count rate and about twice the volume sensitivity of a full-ring PET. First results with a prototype of the panel-based PET were shown to be effective in reducing whole-body (80 cm) scan times to 10 min or less (Nahmias et al. 2002).

The idea of covering large volumes in short scan times with either high sensitivities or high isotropic resolution is not new. Similar advances in CT technology have been pursued for several years now. In view of high-end applications in cardiology and oncology, in particular, a combination of a panel-based PET with a panel-based CT for ultra-fast scanning with very high sensitivity and isotropic spatial resolution certainly seems appealing. Until such a system becomes available we will witness a number of gradual design changes, such as the implementation of multi-row CT (16 and higher) in in-line PET/CT systems, and completely revised bed designs for extended volume coverage without any vertical deflection.

An application of great interest for current as well as future generations of PET/CT tomographs is image-guided radiotherapy (Wiele et al. 2003). With diagnostic information from both anatomical and functional imaging at hand, radiation therapy is likely to be more effective compared to using CT information only (Schmücking et al. 2001). It has been shown that respiratory gating can be used for the purpose of improved spatial resolution of lung lesions (Nehmeh et al. 2002a,b) and similar benefits can be expected for abdominal tumors. Being able to gate the CT and the PET acquisition in a combined PET/CT design will allow the target volumes to be defined more precisely, and additional safety margins are likely to be reduced if the actual radiotherapy is delivered in gated mode as well. Further studies are, of course, needed to provide the necessary acquisition schemes and data analysis tools before validating such a therapeutic approach.

In the near future significant enhancements of the PET/CT data handling and viewing software are expected to facilitate a broader clinical acceptance of this imaging modality by the diagnostic and referring physician and therapist. In the far future we expect to see a major leap in PET and CT performance based on new detector schemes, which is reflected in a major reduction in total scan time at optimized exposure levels. Assuming implementation of real-time 3D-reconstruction and on-line patient motion monitoring and correction, we can expect a complete diagnostic examination of oncology patients in five minutes or less. As the examination will then take less time than the actual image review, intelligent software tools are needed to direct the physicians to potentially malignant sites. Computer-aided diagnosis as an adjunct to 3D oncology imaging may revolutionize medicine again.

Acknowledgements. We are indebted to Dr Stefan Müller (Department of Nuclear Medicine, University Hospital Essen, Germany) for helpful discussions during the preparation of this manuscript. We gratefully acknowledge the support of Phil Vernon (General Electric Medical Systems), Drs York Hämisch and Matthias Egger (Philips Medical Systems), as well as Jonathan Frey and Dr Maxim Mamin (Siemens Medical Solutions) during the preparation of the summary in Table 2 and Fig. 5.

The PET/CT prototype project was supported by the National Cancer Institute (grants CA 65856).

References

Antoch G, Freudenberg L, Stattaus J, Jentzen W, Müller S, Debatin J, Bockisch A (2002a) Whole-body positron emission tomography-CT: optimized CT using oral and IV contrast materials. Am J Roentgenol 179:1555–1560

Antoch G, Ls LF, Egelhof T, Stattaus J, Jentzen W, Debatin J, Bockisch A (2002b) Focal tracer uptake: a potential artifact in contrast-enhanced dual-modality PET/CT scans. J Nucl Med 43:1339–1342

Antoch G, Kühl H, Kanja J, Lauenstein T, Schneemann H, Hauth E, Jentzen W, Beyer T, Goehde S, Debatin J (2003) Introduction and evaluation of a negative oral contrast agent to avoid contrast-induced artefacts in dual-modality PET/CT imaging. Radiology (in press)

Bendriem B, Townsend D (1998) The theory and practice of 3D PET. In: Cox PH (ed) Developments in nuclear medicine, vol 32. Kluwer Academic, Dordrecht

Beyer T (2000) Design, construction, and validation of a combined PET/CT tomograph for clinical oncology. Department of Physics, University of Surrey

Beyer T, Townsend D (2001) Dual-modality PET/CT imaging: CT-based attenuation correction in the presence of CT contrast agents. J Nucl Med 42:56P

Beyer T, Kinahan PE, Townsend DW (1997) Optimization of emission and transmission scan duration in 3D whole-body PET. IEEE Trans Nucl Sci 44:2400–2407

Beyer T, Townsend DW, Brun T, Kinahan PE, Charron M, Roddy R, Jerin J, Young J, Nutt R, Byars LG (2000) A combined PET/CT tomograph for clinical oncology. J Nucl Med 41:1369–1379

Beyer T, Townsend D, Blodgett T (2002) Dual-modality PET/CT tomography for clinical oncology. Quart J Nucl Med 46:24–34

Beyer T, Antoch G, Blodgett T, Freudenberg L, Akhurst T, Müller S (2003) Dual-modality PET/CT imaging: the effect of respiratory motion on combined image quality in clinical oncology. Eur J Nucl Med 30:588–596

Biersack HJ, Bender H, Ruhlmann J, Schomburg A, Grünwald F (1997) FDG PET in clinical oncology: review and evaluation of results of a private clinical PET center. In: Freeman LM (ed) Nuclear medicine annual 1997. Lippincott-Raven Publishers, Philadelphia, pp 1–29

Bocher M, Balan A, Krausz Y, Shrem Y, Lonn A, Wilk M, Chisin R (2000) Gamma camera-mounted anatomical X-ray tomography: technology, system characteristics and first images. Eur J Nucl Med 27:619–627

Bruckbauer T, Casey M, Valk PE, Rao J, Finley BR, Farboud B (2001) Optimizing 3D whole body acquisition for oncologic imaging on the ECAT ACCEL LSO PET system. EANM, Naples

Burger C, Goerres G, Schoenes S, Buck A, Lonn AHR, von Schulthess GK (2002) PET attenuation coefficients from CT images: experimental evaluation of the transformation of CT into PET 511-keV attenuation coefficients. Eur J Nucl Med 29:922–927

Cai J, Chu JCH, Recine D, Sharma M, Nguyen C, Rodebaugh R, Saxena VA, Ali A (1999) CT and PET lung image registration and fusion in radiotherapy treatment planning using the Chamfer-matching method. Int J Rad Oncol Biol Phys 43:883–891

Carney J, Townsend D (2002) CT-based attenuation correction for PET/CT scanners. In: Von Schultess G (ed) Clinical PET, PET/CT and SPECT/CT: combined amatomic-molecular imaging. Lippincott, Williams and Wilkins, Philadelphia

Carney J, Beyer T, Brasse D, Yap J, Townsend D (2002) Clinical PET/CT scanning using oral CT contrast agents. J Nucl Med 43:57P

Charron M, Beyer T, Kinahan PE, Meltzer CC, Dachille MA, Townsend DW (1999) Whole-body FDG PET and CT imaging of malignancies using a combined PET/CT scanner. J Nucl Med 40:256P

Charron M, Beyer T, Bohnen NN, Kinahan PE, Dachille M, Jerin J, Nutt R, Meltzer C, Villemagne V, Townsend DW (2000) Image analysis in patients with cancer studied with a combined PET and CT scanner. Clin Nucl Med 25:905–910

Cohade C, Osman M, Pannu HK, Wahl RL (2003) Uptake in supraclavicular area fat ("USA-Fat"): description on 18F-FDG PET/CT. J Nucl Med 44:170–176

Defrise M, Kinahan PE (1998) Data acquisition and image reconstruction for 3D PET. In: Bendriem B, Townsend DW (eds) The theory and practice of 3D PET. Kluwer Academic, Dordrecht, pp 11–54

DeMan B, Nuyts J, Dupont P, Marchal G, Suetens P (1999) Metal streak artifacts in X-ray computed tomography: a simulation study. IEEE Trans Nucl Sci 46:691–696

Dizendorf EV, Treyer V, von Schulthess GK, Hany TF (2002) Application of oral contrast media in coregistered positron emission tomography-CT. Am J Roentgenol 179:477–481

Ferguson MK, MacMahon H, Little AG, Golomb HM, Hoffman PC, Skinner DB (1986) Regional accuracy of computed tomography of the mediastinum in staging of lung cancer. J Thorac Cardiovasc Surg 91:498–504

Fleming JS (1989) A technique for using CT images in attenuation correction and quantification in SPECT. Nucl Med Commun 10:83–97

Gambhir SS, Czernin J, Schwimmer J, Silverman DHS, Coleman EE, Phelps ME (2001) A tabulated summary of the FDG PET literature. J Nucl Med 42 [Suppl]:1S–93S

Garrett P, Meshkov S, Perlmutter G (1984) Oral contrast agents in CT of the abdomen. Radiology 153:545–546

Goerres GW, Hany TF, Kamel E, von Schulthess GK, Buck A (2002a) Head and neck imaging with PET and PET/CT: artefacts from dental metallic implants. Eur J Nucl Med 29:367–370

Goerres GW, Kamel E, Heidelberg T-NH, Schwitter MR, Burger C, von Schulthess GK (2002b) PET-CT image co-registration in the thorax: influence of respiration. Eur J Nucl Med 29:351–360

Goerres GW, Kamel E, Seifert B, Burger C, Buck A, Hany TF, von Schulthess GK (2002c) Accuracy of image coregistration of pulmonary lesions in patients with non-small cell lung cancer using an integrated PET/CT system. J Nucl Med 43:1469–1475

Goerres GW, von Schulthess GK, Hany TF (2002d) Positron emission tomography and PET CT of the head and neck: FDG uptake in normal anatomy, in benign lesions, and in changes resulting from treatment. Am J Roentgenol 179:1337–1343

Goerres GW, Burger C, Schwitter MR, Heidelberg T-NH, Seifert B, von Schulthess GK (2003a) PET/CT of the abdomen: optimizing the patient breathing pattern. Eur Radiol 13:734–739

Goerres GW, Ziegler SI, Burger C, Berthold T, von Schulthess GK, Buck A (2003b) Artifacts at PET and PET/CT caused by metallic hip prosthetic material. Radiology 226:577–584

Greene FL et al (eds) (2002) AJCC – cancer staging manual, 6th edn. Springer, Berlin Heidelberg New York

Hany TF, Steinert HC, Goerres GW, Buck A, von Schulthess GK (2002) PET diagnostic accuracy: improvement with in-line PET-CT system: initial results. Radiology 225:575–581

Hasegawa B, Gingold E, Reilly S, Cann C (1990) Description of a simultaneous emission-transmission CT system. Proceedings of the Society of Photo-Optical Instrumentation Engineers (SPIE)

Hill DLG, Batchelor PG, Holden M, Hawkes DJ (2001) Medical image registration. Phys Med Biol 46:R1–R45

Hoh CK, Hawkins RA, Glaspy JA, Dahlbom M, Tse NY, Hoffman EJ, Schiepers C, Choi Y, Rege S, Nitzsche E, Maddahi J, Phelps ME (1993) Cancer detection with whole-body PET using 2-[18F]Fluoro-2-deoxy-D-glucose. J Comput Assist Tomogr 17: 582–589

Holm S, Toft P, Jensen M (1996) Estimation of the noise contributions from blank, transmission and emission scans in PET. IEEE Trans Nucl Sci 43:2285–2291

Hubbell J (1999) Review of photon interaction cross section data in the medical and biological context. Phys Med Biol 44:R1–R22

Israel O, Yefremov N, Mor M, Epelbaum R, Dann EJ, Gaitini D, Haim N, Guralnik L, Keidar Z (2000) Combined transmission and Ga-67 emission tomography (TET) in the evaluation of response to treatment and diagnosis of recurrence in patients with lymphoma. Eur J Nucl Med 27:1160

Itoh S, Ikeda M, Achiwa M, Ota T, Satake H, Ishigaki T (2003) Multiphase contrast-enhanced CT of the liver with a multislice CT scanner. Eur Radiol 13:1085–1094

Jager P, Slart R, Corstens F, Oyen W, Hockstra O, Teule J (2003) PET-CT: a matter of opinion. Eur J Nucl Med 30:470–471

Jamis-Dow CA, Choyke PL, Jennings SB, Lineham WM, Thakore KN, Walther MM (1996) Small (3 cm) renal masses: detection with CT versus US and pathologic correlation. Radiology 198: 785–788

Kalender WA (2000) Computed tomography. Publicis MCD, Munich

Kamel E, Hany TF, Burger C, Treyer V, Lonn AHR, von Schulthess GK, Buck A (2002a) CT vs 68Ge attenuation correction in a combined PET/CT system: evaluation of the effect of lowering the CT tube current. Eur J Nucl Med 29:346–350

Kamel EM, Burger C, Buck A, von Schluthess GK, Goerres GW (2002b) Impact of metallic dental implants on CT-based attenuation correction in a combined PET/CT scanner. Eur Radiol 13:724–728

Karp JS (2002) Is LSO the future of PET? Eur J Nucl Med 29:1525–1528

Kinahan PE, Townsend DW, Beyer T, Sashin D (1998) Attenuation correction for a combined 3D PET/CT scanner. Med Phys 25: 2046–2053

Kluetz PG, Meltzer CC, Villemagne MD, Kinahan PE, Chander S, Martinelly MA, Townsend DW (2001) Combined PET/CT imaging in oncology: Impact on patient management. Clin Positron Imaging 3:1–8

LaCroix KJ, Tsui BMW, Hasegawa BH, Brown JK (1994) Investigation of the use of X-ray CT images for attenuation correction in SPECT. IEEE Trans Nucl Sci 41:2793–2799

Leahy R, Qi J (2000) Statistical approaches in quantitative positron emission tomography. Statist Comput 10:147–165

McCollough CH, Zink FE (1999) Performance evaluation of a multi-slice CT system. Med Phys 26:2223–2230

Melcher CL (2000) Scintillation crystals for PET. J Nucl Med 41: 1051–1055

Mitchell D, Bjorgninsson E, terMeulen D, Lane P, Greberman M, Friedman A (1985) Gastrografin versus dilute barium for colonic CT examination: a blind, randomized study. J Comput Assist Tomogr 9:451–453

Mix M, Nitzsche EU (1999) PISAC: a post-injection method for segmented attenuation correction. J Nucl Med 40:297P

Muehllehner G, Karp K, Surti S (2002) Design considerations for PET scanners. Quart J Nucl Med 46:16–23

Nahmias C, Nutt R, Hichwa D, Czernin J, Melcher C, Schmand M, Andreaco M, Eriksson L, Casey M, Moyers C, Michel C, Bruckbauer T, Conti M, Bendriem B, Hamill J (2002) PET tomograph designed for five minute routine whole body studies. J Nucl Med 43 (6):S11

Nehmeh SA, Erdi YE, Ling CC, Rosenzweig KE, Schoder H, Larson SM, Macapinlac HA, Squire OD, Humm JL (2002a) Effect of respiratory gating on quantifying PET images of lung cancer. J Nucl Med 43:876–881

Nehmeh SA, Erdi YE, Ling CC, Rosenzweig KE, Squire O, Braban L, Ford EC, Sidhu K, Mageras G, Larson SM, Humm JL (2002b) Effect of respiratory gating on reducing lung motion artefacts in PET imaging of lung cancer. Med Phys 29:366–371

Nutt R (2002) Is LSO the future of PET? Eur J Nucl Med 29:1523–1524

Osman MM, Cohade C, Wahl RL (2002) Respiratory motion artifacts on PET emission images obtained using CT attenuation correction on PET-CT. J Nucl Med 43 :305P

Osman MM, Cohade C, Nakamoto Y, Marshall LT, Leal JP, Wahl RL (2003) Clinically significant inaccurate localization of lesions with PET/CT: frequency in 300 Patients. J Nucl Med 44: 240–243

Padhani AR (1998) Spiral CT: thoracic applications. Eur J Radiol 28:2–17

Patton JA, Delbeke D, Sandler MP (2000) Image fusion using an integrated, dual-head coincidence camera with X-ray tube-based attenuation maps. J Nucl Med 41:1364–1368

Pietrzyk U, Herholz K, Heiss W-D (1990) Three-dimensional alignment of functional and morphological tomograms. J Comput Assist Tomogr 14:51–59

Roos JF, Desbiolles LM, Willmann JK, Weishaupt D, Marincek B, Hilfiker PR (2002) Multidetector-row helical CT: analysis of time management and workflow. Eur Radiol 12:680–685

Schaller S, Semrbitzki O, Beyer T, Fuchs T, Kachelriess M, Flohr T (2002) An algorithm for virtual extension of the CT field of measurement for application in combined PET/CT scanners. Radiology 225 [Suppl]:497

Schmücking M, Baum RP, Przetak C, Lopatta EC, Niesen A, Plichta K, Leonhardi J, Wendt TG (2001) The role of F-18 FDG-PDET for 3-D radiation treatment planning of non-small cell lung cancer – first results of a prospective study. Nuklearmediziner 24:31–37

Shreve PD (1998) Focal fluorine-18 fluorodeoxyglucose accumulation in inflammatory pancreatic disease. Eur J Nucl Med 25: 259–264

Shreve PD, Anzai Y, Wahl RL (1999) Pitfalls in oncologic diagnosis with FDG PET imaging: physiologic and benign variants. Radiographics 19:61–77

Slomka P, Dey D, Przetak C, Baum R (2001) Nonlinear image registration of thoracic FDG PET and CT. J Nucl Med 42:11P

Slomka PJ, Dey D, Przetak C, Aladl UE und Baum RP (2003) Automated 3-Dimensional Registration of Stand-Alone 18F-FDG Whole-Body PET with CT. J Nucl Med 44 (7):p.1156–1167

Smith RJ, Joel SS K, Muehllehner G, Gualtieri E, Benard F (1997) Singles transmission scans performed post-injection for quantitative whole body PET imaging. IEEE Trans Nucl Sci 44:1329–1335

Smith TAD (1998) FDG uptake, tumour characteristics and response to therapy. A review. Nucl Med Commun 19:97–105

Tai YC, Lin KP, Hoh CK, Huang H, Hoffman EJ (1997) Utilization of 3-D elastic transformation in the registration of chest X-ray CT and whole body PET. IEEE Trans Nucl Sci 44:1606–1612

Tang HR, Brown JK, Silva AJD, Matthay KK, Price D, Huberty JP, Hawkins RA, Hasegawa BH (1999a) Implementation of a combined X-ray CT scintillation camera imaging system for localizing and measuring radionuclide uptake: experiments in phantoms and patients. IEEE Trans Nucl Sci 46:551–557

Tang HR, Schreck CE, Hasegawa BH, Hawkins RA (1999b) ECT attenuation maps from X-ray CT images. J Nucl Med 40:113P

Townsend DW, Cherry S (2001) Combining anatomy and function: the path to true image fusion. Eur Radiol 11:1968–1974

Townsend D, Beyer T, Kinahan P, Meltzer C, Brun T, Nutt R, Roddy R (1998a) The SMART scanner: a combined PET/CT tomograph for clinical oncology. Radiology 209:169–170

Townsend DW, Isoardi RA, Bendriem B (1998b) Volume imaging tomographs. In: Townsend DW, Bendriem B (eds) Theory and practice of 3D PET. Kluwer Academic, Dordrecht, pp 111–132

Townsend D, Beyer T, Kinahan P, Charron M, Meltzer C, Dachille M, Jerin J, Brun T, Roddy R, Nutt R, Byars L (1999a) Fusion imaging for whole-body oncology with a combined PET and CT scanner. J Nucl Med 40:148P

Townsend DW, Beyer T, Meltzer CC, Dashille MA, Derbyshire SWG, Jones AKP, Kelley DE, Luketich JT (1999b) The ECAT ART scanner for positron emission tomography 2. Research and clinical applications. Clin Posit Imaging 2:17–30

Valk PE, Bailey DL, Townsend DW, Maisey MN (2003) Positron emission tomography. Basic science and clinical practice. Springer, Berlin Heidelberg New York

Von Schulthess GK (2000) Cost considerations regarding an integrated CT-PET system. Eur Radiol 10 [Suppl 3]:S377–S380

Wahl RL (1997) Clinical oncology update: The emerging role of positron emission tomography, part I. PRO updates. Principles Pract Oncol 11:1–18

Wahl RL (1999) To AC or not to AC: that is the question. J Nucl Med 40:2025–2028

Wahl RL, Quint LE, Cieslak RD, Aisen AM, Koeppe RA, Meyer CR (1993) "Anatometabolic" tumor imaging: fusion of FDG PET with CT or MRI to localize foci of increased activity. J Nucl Med 34:1190–1197

Warburg O (1931) The metabolism of tumors. Smith, New York, pp 129–169

Warburg O (1956) On the origin of cancer cells. Science 123:306–314

Watson CC, Schäfer A, Luck WK, Kirsch C-M (1999) Clinical evaluation of single-photon attenuation correction for 3D whole-body PET. Trans Nucl Sci 46 (4):1024–1031

Wiele CVD, Lahorte C, Oyen W, Boerman O, Goethals I, Slegers G and Dierckx RA (2003) Nuclear Medicine imaging to predict response to radiotherapy: A rewiew. Int J Radiation Oncology Biol Phys. 55 (1):p.5–15

Woods RP, Grafton ST, Holmes CJ, Cherry SR, Mazziotta JC. (1998) Automated image registration I. General methods and intrasubject, intramodality validation. J Comput Assist Tomogr 22: 139–152

Yu JN, Fahey FH, Harkness BA, Gage HD, Eades CG, Keyes JW (1994) Evaluation of emission-transmission registration in thoracic PET. J Nucl Med 35:1777–1780

CHAPTER 3

Transport and Metabolism of Glucose and FDG

P. Oehr

The kinetics of the radiopharmaceutical 2-[^{18}F]fluoro-2-deoxy-D-glucose (2-[^{18}F]FDG), a glucose derivative, are determined by its distribution in the blood stream and tissues and by its metabolism.

In principle, only the distribution of the radionuclide ^{18}F is measured, although 2-[^{18}F]FDG is the pharmaceutical that is originally administered. Metabolic processes in the body can convert 2-[^{18}F]FDG into a different chemical form that has a different biological behavior. In order to develop a biokinetic model it is therefore necessary to know the possible chemical reactions that this radiopharmaceutical can undergo – including reactions under pathological conditions. The physiological determinants that are significant for tracer kinetics will be described in the following sections, and the possibilities for measuring those factors will be discussed.

3.1 Biological Functions of Carbohydrate Metabolism

3.1.1 Carbohydrate Requirements and Supply

The adult human organism has a minimum glucose requirement of 180 g per day. This amount of glucose is necessary in order to supply energy to those cells and organs that absolutely depend on glucose, namely the nervous system (144 g glucose per 24 h) and the red blood cells (36 g glucose per 24 h). The daily supply should even exceed 180 g of glucose-providing carbohydrates so that the other organs that have a minimum glucose requirement can also be supplied.

After all carbohydrate building blocks have been reabsorbed from the intestine, the glycogen supply (and later glucogenesis) is needed to provide glucose.

The monosaccharides glucose, fructose and galactose are the essential building blocks of our carbohydrate diet. With respect to glucose, the carbohydrate diet should not be formed by the direct supply of monosaccharides but by the supply and splitting of polysaccharides. In addition to the hexoses mentioned above, the pentoses (xylose, ribose, arabinose and xylitol) are of secondary importance quantitatively since they are present in food only in very small quantities. In diabetics the sugar substitutes fructose, sorbitol and xylitol can be of critical importance since they are utilized independently of insulin and are therefore used in the diet. The most important monosaccharide in the blood is glucose. The glucose pool in humans is approximately 0.11 mol and is distributed throughout a volume of about 28 liters. This corresponds to an average postprandial concentration of 5 mmol glucose per liter (90 mg/dl). Glucose is absorbed into the cells from the glucose pool by facilitated diffusion with the assistance of specific carrier types (GLUT 1-5).

3.1.2 Regulation Mechanisms

Glucose is broken down by the metabolic pathway called glycolysis (Fig. 1). This degradative pathway is present in all organs and cell systems. The breakdown of fructose, mannose, sorbitol and xylitol also involves glycolysis. Glycolysis can be followed by the pentose phosphate pathway, by glycogen synthesis, or by the formation of heteroglycans, as required.

The relative proportion of glycogen synthesis and pentose phosphate pathway differs from one cell type to another. Glycogen (see Fig. 1) is basically only formed in the liver and in muscle tissue. The throughput through the pentose phosphate pathway varies significantly (lactating mammary gland 60 %, liver 40 %, muscle tissue 5 %). The chief role of the pentose phosphate pathway is to provide NADPH for various metabolic pathways (reduced glutathione, synthesis of fatty acid, etc.) and also pentoses for the synthesis of nucleotides and nucleic acids. The glycogen concentration in the liver is 5–8 % on average, and in non-exercised muscle tissue it is generally less than 1 %. Only the glycogen in the liver is available for regulating blood sugar; the glycogen in the muscle is only able to satisfy the organ's own glucose requirements.

Gluconeogenesis occurs only in the liver and kidney. Synthesis of 1 mol glucose from 2 mol pyruvate requires 6 mol ATP and 2 mol NADH. The gluconeogenesis metabolic pathway represents a reversal of glycolysis, except for the fact that "gluconeogenetic enzymes" are involved instead of the enzymes hexokinase, phosphofructoki-

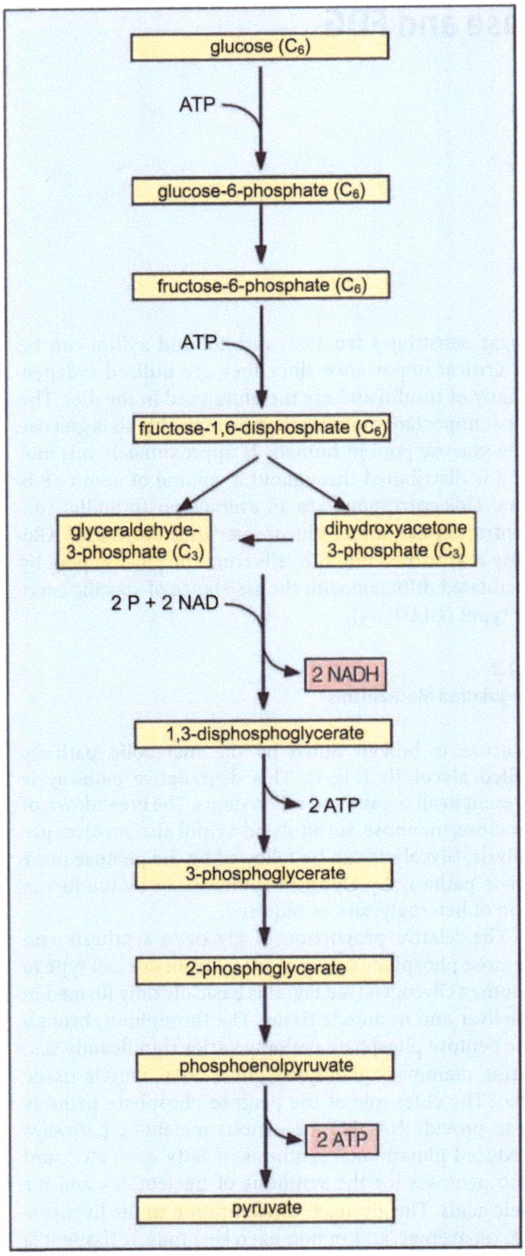

Fig. 1. Metabolism of glucose

nase and pyruvate kinase. Provision of a substrate for gluconeogenesis and control of the activity of the gluconeogenetic enzymes is affected by hormones.

3.1.3 Factors in Glucose Homeostasis

A precisely balanced system of hormones, enzymes and substrate streams is required in order to maintain homeostasis. Determination of the glucose concentration in peripheral blood relates only to the concentration in the extracellular glucose pool and does not provide any direct information about the rate of intracellular breakdown or of gluconeogenesis. The glucose flow rate or glucose conversion rate can be determined approximately under defined conditions by using the clamp technique. More accurate analyses can only be obtained by means of radioactively or non-radioactively labeled glucose molecules (tracer method).

An increase in glucose concentration in excess of 130 mg/dl in individuals with an empty stomach is referred to as hyperglycemia and is one of the primary symptoms of diabetes mellitus. A drop in glucose concentration below 50 mg/dl in combination with clinical symptoms is referred to as hypoglycemia. Serious cases of hypoglycemia have a negative effect on physical and mental performance and eventually lead to unconsciousness.

Euglycemia in individuals with an empty stomach is maintained when the consumption of 2 to 2.4 mg glucose/kg/min (132–170 mg/kg/h) is balanced out by an equally high rate of glucose production in the liver (glycogenolysis, gluconeogenesis). Fasting states that last for long periods of time result in an increase in gluconeogenesis in the liver and a decrease in glucose consumption in peripheral tissues. In chronic fasting states ketone bodies can compensate for some of the glucose consumption in the brain. The limitation of glucose utilization and reduced responsiveness to insulin that can be observed in longer-lasting fasting states, in Type II diabetes, and in the post-aggression state is referred to as insulin resistance. Insulin resistance can stem from reduced insulin sensitivity or a reduced metabolic response (unresponsiveness). An increase in glucogenesis and glycogenolysis with reduced consumption in the muscles and fatty tissue leads to an increase in the extracellular glucose pool and thus to hyperglycemia. Conversely, peripheral consumption in hyperinsulinism (insulinoma) can be increased so sharply that hypoglycemic metabolic conditions involving unconsciousness can occur if there is simultaneous inhibition of gluconeogenesis.

Insulin plays the key role in regulating glucose homeostasis. Because of its inhibiting effect on gluconeogenesis in the liver and the fact that it increases glucose uptake in skeletal and cardiac muscles and fatty tissue, dangerous reductions in the actual glucose concentration in the blood can result. Conversely, a lack of this hormone and consequently a predominance of catabolic hormones (adrenaline, cortisol, and glucagon) bring about an increase in hepatic glucose release and a decrease in peripheral glucose uptake in muscles and fat. In the post-aggression state and in Type II diabetes, an imbalance develops between hepatic glucose production and peripheral consumption, allowing hyperglycemic metabolic conditions to arise. The carbohydrate metabolism in the kidney is only of secondary importance for glucose homeostasis. The gluconeogenesis of the proximal tubule is again balanced out by insulin-independent glucose uptake in other sections of the nephron. Renal glucose production is only significant for lactic acidosis and for decompensation of gluconeogenesis in the liver.

Under hyperglycemic metabolic conditions the kidney has an important function as regards the elimination of glucose from the cardiovascular system. Normally 0.05% of the glomerular-filtered glucose volume is eliminated. If the reabsorption capacity of the tubules is exceeded (renal threshold), glycosuria is observed. Determination of glucose in the urine is an important diagnostic tool for monitoring hyperglycemia.

3.2 Metabolism of Glucose, 2-DG, 2-FDG and 3-FDG

3.2.1 Glucose

The metabolic process by which glucose is converted to pyruvate is referred to as glycolysis. In aerobic organisms glycolysis is a preliminary stage of the citric acid cycle and the respiratory chain, processes in which most of the free energy of glucose is released. The ten glycolysis reactions (see Fig. 1) take place in the cytosol. In the first stage glucose is converted to fructose-1,6-diphosphate by means of phosphorylation, isomerization, and then a second phosphorylation process. In these reactions two molecules of ATP are consumed for each glucose molecule, and then, in subsequent steps, net synthesis of ATP is initiated. In the second stage fructose-1,6-diphosphate is split by aldolase into dihydroxyacetone phosphate and glyceraldehyde-3-phosphate, which can easily be interconverted. Glyceraldehyde-3-phosphate is then oxidized and phosphorylated, yielding 1,3-diphosphoglycerate, an acylphosphate with a high phosphoryl group transfer potential. This is followed by the formation of 3-phosphoglycerate with simultaneous generation of ATP. Phosphoenol pyruvate, a second intermediate product with a high phosphoryl group transfer potential, is produced in the last stage of glycolysis through rearrangement of the 3-phosphoryl group and elimination of water. An additional ATP is formed during conversion of the phosphoenol pyruvate into pyruvate. This means that a total of 2 molecules of ATP are obtained through the formation of two pyruvate molecules from one glucose molecule. The electron acceptor in the oxidation of the glyceraldehyde-3-phosphate is NAD^+, which must be regenerated for continuation of glycolysis.

Glycolysis has 2 functions: it breaks down glucose for the purpose of ATP generation, and it provides building blocks for the synthesis of cell constituents. The rate of conversion of glucose to pyruvate is controlled so that these two chief cell requirements are taken into account. The glycolysis reactions are reversible under physiological conditions with the exception of the reactions that are catalyzed by hexokinase, phosphofructokinase and pyruvate kinase. Phosphofructokinase, the most important glycolysis control element, is inhibited by high ATP and citrate levels and activated by AMP and fructose-2,6-diphosphate. In the liver this diphosphate signals that there is an abundant amount of glucose. Phosphofructokinase is also active if either energy or building blocks are required. Hexokinase is inhibited by glucose-6-phosphate, which accumulates when phosphofructokinase is inactive. Pyruvate kinase, the other control point, is inhibited allosterically by ATP and alanine. Pyruvate kinase has its maximum activity therefore when the energy charge is low and intermediate glycolysis products accumulate. Pyruvate kinase is regulated by reversible phosphorylation, just like the tandem enzyme that controls the fructose-2,6-diphosphate level. A low glucose level in the blood promotes phosphorylation of liver pyruvate kinase, which reduces its activity and thus reduces glucose consumption in the liver.

3.2.2 Metabolism of 2-DG, 2-FDG and 3-FDG

As shown in Fig. 2, metabolism of the glucose derivatives described in this section, namely 2-deoxy-D-glucose (2-DG), 2-fluoro-deoxy-D-glucose (2-FDG) and 3-fluoro-deoxy-D-glucose (3-FDG), decreases in the order in which they are named. Phosphorylation of these molecules – with the exception of 3-FDG – takes place when the sugars are absorbed by the cell. One phosphate molecule with the alcohol group is added to the 6th carbon atom of a glucose or 2-FDG molecule. This requires the enzyme hexokinase, which is contained in the cells. In this case glucose, 2-DG and 2-FDG compete for the enzyme binding site. Glucose-6-phosphate and 2-DG-6-phosphate are metabolized further, but 2-FDG undergoes a reverse reaction to a limited extent by way of the enzyme glucose-6-phosphatase (see Fig. 3). Thus it can be transported out of the cell again. PET examinations take place 1–2 hours after injection of the tracer. Within this period it is still possible to disregard the reverse reaction. 3-FDG is not phosphorylated (see Fig. 2). Therefore it is not subject to the trapping mechanism and is eliminated more rapidly from the cells. Because of these different metabolic properties, the kinetics for accumulation in the cell are therefore very different for glucose, 2-DG, 2-FDG and 3-FDG (see below).

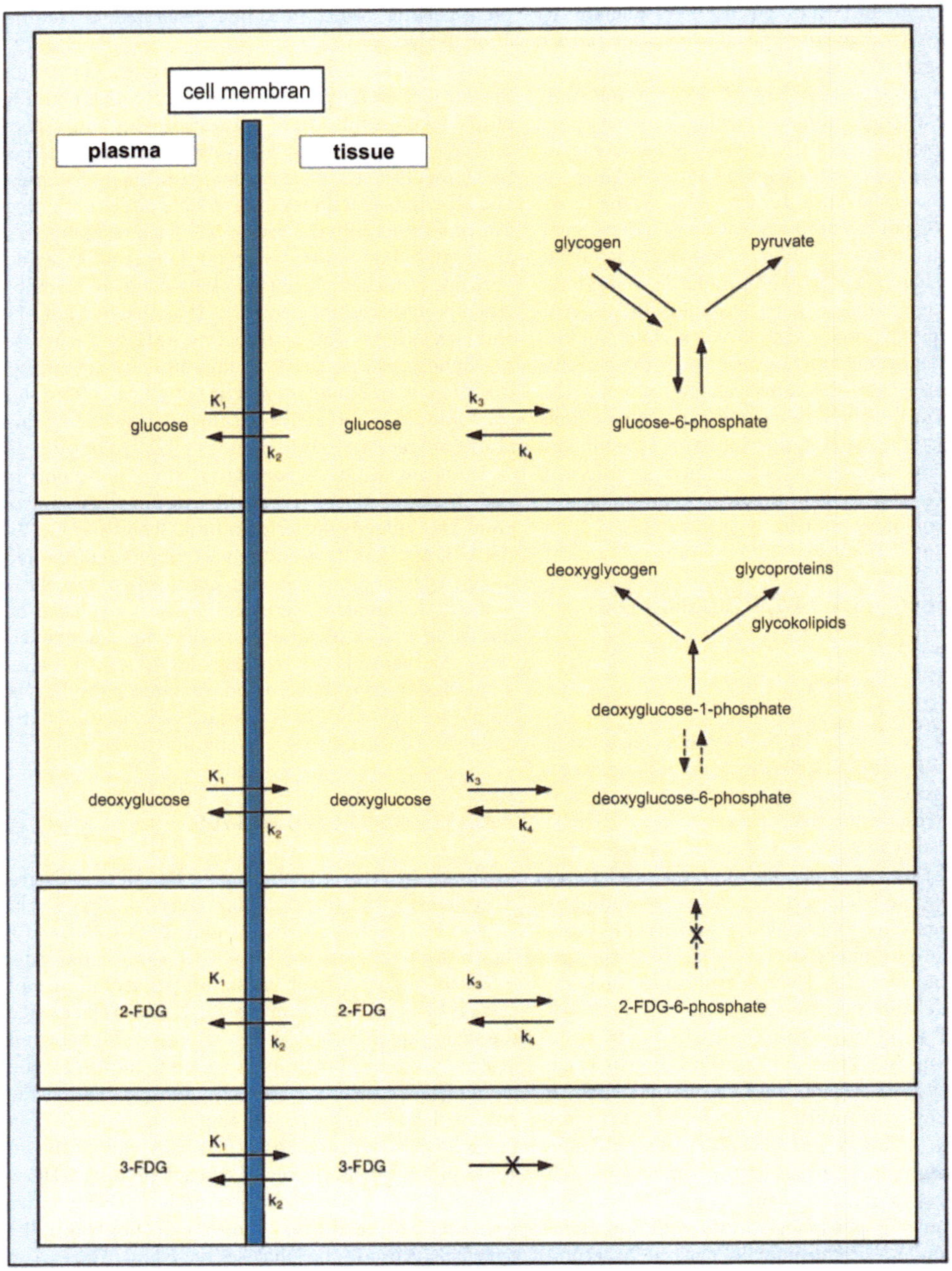

Fig. 2. Metabolism of glucose, 2-DG, 2-FDG and 3-FDG

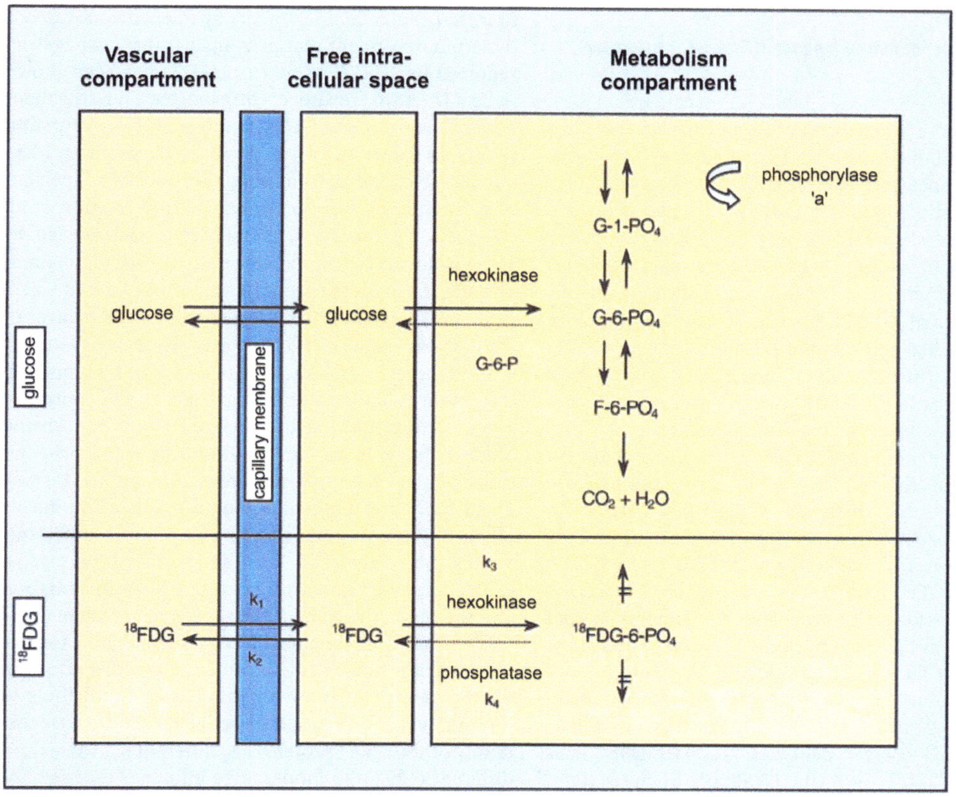

Fig. 3. Three-compartment model for calculating glucose metabolism using the [^{18}F]FDG method (after Sokoloff et al. 1977)

3.3 FDG Uptake

3.3.1 Glucose Transport Systems

A group of transport proteins makes it possible for glucose to enter or leave animal cells. Two principal mechanisms for glucose entry into (tumor) cells have been described: I. The Sodium-dependent Glucose Transporters (SGLT), and II. The Facilitative Sodium-independent Glucose Transporters (Class I-III).

The number of known glucose transporters has expanded considerably over the past 2 years. At least three, and up to six, Na+-dependent glucose transporters (SGLT1-SGLT6; gene name SLC5A) have been identified. Similarly, thirteen members of the family of facilitative sugar transporters (GLUT1-GLUT12 and HMIT; gene name SLC2A) are now recognized. These various transporters exhibit different substrate specificities, kinetic properties and tissue expression profiles. The number of distinct gene products, together with the presence of several different transporters in certain tissues and cells, indicates that glucose delivery into cells is a process of considerable complexity (Stuart Wood and Trayhurn 2003).

3.3.1.1 *The Sodium-dependent Glucose Transporters (SGLT)*

The SGLT transport glucose (and galactose), with different affinities, via a secondary active transport mechanism. The Na+-electrochemical gradient provided by the Na+ -K+ ATPase pump is utilized to transport glucose into cells against its concentration gradient.

SGLT1 has a limited tissue expression is expressed in the ciliated border of the small intestine tissue and in the proximal renal tubule, whereas SGLT2 is normally located distally in the renal tubule. Both sodium-glucose transporters are expressed even at low molar concentrations (Hediger and Rhoads 1994; Wright 2001; Wright and Turk 2003; Stuart Wood and Trayhurn 2003)

3.3.1.2 *The Facilitative Sodium-independent Glucose Transporters (Class I-III)*

The facilitative transporters (GLUT) utilize the diffusion gradient of Glucose (and other sugars) across plasma membranes and exhibit different substrate specificities, kinetic properties and tissue expression profiles. These transporters have a high degree of stereoselectivity, providing for the bidirectional transport of substrate, with passive diffusion down its concentration gradient. GLUTs function to regulate the movement of glucose between the extracellular and intracellular compartments maintaining a constant supply of glucose available for metabolism. Table 1 gives an overview and cites the corresponding literature.

On the basis of sequence similarities and characteristic elements, the extended GLUT family can be divided into three subfamilies, namely class I (the previously known glucose transporters GLUT1–4), class II (the previously known fructose transporter GLUT5, the GLUT7, GLUT9 and GLUT11), and class III (GLUT6, 8, 10, 12, and the myo-inositol transporter HMIT1). Functional characteristics have been reported for some of the novel GLUTs. Like GLUT1–4, they exhibit a tissue/cell-specific expression (GLUT6, leukocytes, brain; GLUT8, testis, blastocysts, brain, muscle, adipocytes; GLUT9, liver, kidney; GLUT10, liver, pancreas; GLUT11, heart, skeletal muscle). GLUT6 and GLUT8 appear to be regulated by sub-cellular redistribution, because they are targeted to intra-cellular compartments by dileucine motifs in a dynamin dependent manner. Sugar transport has been reported for GLUT6, 8, and 11; HMIT1 has been shown to be a H+/myo-inositol co-transporter. Thus, the members of the extended GLUT family exhibit a surprisingly diverse substrate specificity, and the definition of sequence elements determining this substrate specificity will require a full functional characterization of all members. Furthermore, the substrate transported by some isoforms has not yet been identified. Tissue- and cell-specific expression of the well-characterized GLUT isoforms underlies their specific role in the control of whole-body glucose homeostasis. Numerous studies with transgenic or knockout mice indeed support an important role for these transporters in the control of glucose utilization, glucose storage and glucose sensing. Much remains to be learned about the transport functions of the recently discovered isoforms (GLUT6–13 and HMIT) and their physiological role in the metabolism of glucose, myo-inositol and perhaps other substrates (Mueckler 1994; Joost and Thorens 2001; Joost et al. 2002; Uldry and Thorens 2003). More information and the respective publications are given in Table 1.

This family of transport proteins shows how isomeric forms of a single protein can have a lasting effect on the metabolic characteristics of cells and contribute to their variety and functional specialization. Because this family of transport proteins has different K_m values and different regulation modes, they influence the metabolic characteristics of cells in different organs.

Table 1. Expression and function of GLUT family members

Protein	Expression	Function	Reference
GLUT1	All tissues (abundant in brain, and erythrocytes)	Basal uptake	Hruz and Mueckler (2001); Mueckler (1994)
GLUT2	Liver, pancreatic islet cells, retina	Glucose sensing	Fukumoto et al. (1989); Watanabe et al. (1999)
GLUT3	Brain	Supplements GLUT1 in tissues in tissues with high energy demand	Kayano et al. (1990)
GLUT4	Muscle, fat, heart	Insulin responsive	Fukumoto et al. (1989)
GLUT5	testis, kidney, muscle, erythrocytes. small intestine, adipose tissue	Fructose transport	Rand et al. (1993); Concha et al. (1997); Hundal et al. (1998); Kayano et al. (1990)
GLUT6 (Formerly: GLUT9)	Spleen, leukocytes, brain		Doege et al. (2000b); Lisinski et al. (2001)
GLUT7	Liver		Joost and Thorens (2001)
GLUT8 (Formerly:GLUTX1)	Testis, brain		Doege et al. (2000a)
GLUT9 (Formerly: GLUTX)	Liver, kidney		Phay et al. (2000); Doege et al. (2000b)
GLUT10	Liver, pancreas		McVie-Wylie et al. (2001)
GLUT11 (Formerly: GLUT10)	Heart, muscle		Doege et al. (2001)
GLUT12 (Formerly: GLUT8)	Heart, prostate		Rogers et al. (2003)
Pseudogene (Formerly: GLUT6)			Kayano et al. (1990)

Glucose processing in mammals is complex due to the fact that many enzymes are involved. In many human tissues with physiological blood concentrations, transport through the cell membrane is the limiting factor (Baldwin et al. 1994) wherever the insulin concentration in tissues is low and wherever there are high-affinity transporters (low K_m value). When individuals have fasted for a long period of time and insulin is released either by injection or by the pancreas cells as the result of food intake, then the GLUT4 concentrations in the cell membranes of insulin-reactive heart and skeletal muscles increase to 5 to 40 times the normal concentrations. This is related to the transfluctuation of the transporter to the membrane by way of vesicles and results in correspondingly higher glucose transport (James 1994). Increased incorporation into heart and skeletal muscles is observed under these conditions when FDG is administered. It is for this reason that myocardial PET studies involving FDG are performed after a great deal of food has been consumed or after insulin has been administered.

3.3.2 Glucose Transporters in Cancer Diseases: Expression and Regulation

Higher rates of glucose metabolism have been observed in cancer cells for many years, and the significance of this fact for detection of increased metabolism by FDG has also been recognized (Warburg 1931; Som et al. 1980; Larson et al. 1981; Wahl et al. 1991). Many enzymatic changes have been described for cancer diseases in humans, including increased glucose transport rates, higher rates of glucose phosphorylation and generally very low rates of glucose-6-phosphate dephosphorylation (Weber et al. 1961; Monakhov et al. 1978; Hatanaka et al. 1970; Flier et al. 1987; Fukunaga et al. 1993; Graham et al. 1989). There are also a number of published papers that deal with the different changes in cell metabolism (Flier et al. 1987; Fukunaga et al. 1993; Graham et al. 1989).

Although tumors induce formation of new blood vessels to deliver nutrients and oxygen to the growing tumor, angiogenesis does not keep pace with the growth of the neoplastic cells. This results in large hypoxic areas throughout the tumor (Warburg 1931, 1956).

To form a three-dimensional multicellular mass, tumor cells must change their metabolism in order to survive and grow under these ischemic conditions (Dang and Semenza 1999). Tumor cells in these areas are not killed by ionizing radiation, which depends on oxygen, or by chemotherapeutic drugs, which do not reach these regions. A characteristic feature of these ischemic conditions is the production of large amounts of lactic acid from glycolysis in the presence of reduced oxygen concentrations (Warburg 1956). This is accompanied by an increased rate of glucose transport (Pedersen 1978; Birnbaum et al. 1987). It has also been shown that lactate causes translocation of GLUT1 and GLUT4 to the plasma membrane in isolated perfused hearts (Medina et al. 2002). It is possible that the lactate acid build-up in tumors is involved in translocation of the transporters to the plasma membrane which in turn causes an increase in glucose utilization by these cells. This demand for energy is satisfied by an increased sugar intake which is accomplished by an increase in glucose transporter expression and an increase in the translocation of the transporter to the plasma membrane (Medina and Owen 2002).

However, we should note that when FDG is used as an indicator for glucose metabolism, it cannot be handled by the cells in the same way as glucose because the affinity of the membrane transporters and the hexokinase and phosphatase enzymes for FDG and glucose may vary (Graham et al. 1989; Bell et al. 1993). Moreover, FDG is a poor substrate for phosphoglucoisomerase and other glycolytic enzymes.

3.3.2.1 *The Sodium-dependent Glucose Transporters (SGLT)*

Not much has been published regarding the relationship between SGLT transport systems and cancer. Since many years there is also the opinion that this does not play a big role in tumor-specific glucose transport (Hediger and Rhoads 1994). Ishikawa SGLT investigated SGLT gene expression in primary lung cancers and their metastatic lesions. They reported the differential gene expression of the GLUT family in primary and metastatic lesions of lung cancer. To investigate the role of Na(+)/glucose cotransporter (SGLT) genes in cancers, they examined the levels of expression of SGLT1 and SGLT2 genes in primary lung cancers and their metastatic lesions. Ninety-six autopsy samples (35 primary lung cancers, 35 corresponding normal lung tissues, 10 metastatic liver lesions, and 16 metastatic lymph nodes) from 35 patients were analyzed for SGLT1 and SGLT2 expression by reverse transcription (RT)-polymerase chain reaction (PCR). There were no significant differences in the level of expression of either gene between the primary lung cancers and normal lung tissues. The level of SGLT1 expression in the metastatic lesions and primary lung cancers did not differ significantly. The level of SGLT2 expression was, however, significantly higher in the metastatic lesions of both the liver and lymph node than in the primary lung cancers. The authors concluded that suggest that SGLT2 plays a role in glucose uptake in the metastatic lesions of lung cancer (Ishikawa et al. 2001).

3.3.2.2
The Facilitative Sodium-independent Glucose Transporters

The localization, expression and regulation of the GLUT family are tissue and often cell-specific. New GLUT isoforms are continually being discovered and characterized in various cell types. Their involvement in disease states is also continually under review. In cancer cells, which have broken free from the normally tight global regulation, aberrant expression of the GLUT family members provides the energy source required for further uncontrolled proliferation and metastasis. As every cell contains the genes for each GLUT family member we observe in cancer cells the expression of certain GLUT isoforms which, under normal conditions, would never have been expressed in these tissues (Medina and Owen 2002).

The majority of cancers and isolated cancer cell lines over-express the GLUT family members which are present in the respective tissue of origin under non-cancerous conditions. Moreover, due to the requirement of energy to feed uncontrolled proliferation, cancer cells often express GLUTs which under normal conditions would not be present in these tissues. This over-expression is predominantly associated with the likelihood of metastasis and hence poor patient prognosis (Medina and Owen 2002).

For many years cancer research paid great attention to the over-expression of glucose transporters of the facilitated diffusion type (Hatanaka et al. 1970; Lodish 1986/1987; Elsas and Longo 1992; Fukunaga et al. 1993; Bell et al. 1993; McGowan et al. 1995; Medina and Owen 2002). Some researchers have seen over-expression as a very general change in oncogenically transformed cells in vitro and in vivo in human cancer diseases. A multiple increase in transporters has been detected after transformations of cells containing oncogenes (Lodish 1986/1987; McGowan et al. 1995; Elsas and Longo 1992; Devaskar and Mueckler 1992; James 1994; Mueckler 1994; Ismail-Beigi 1993; Baldwin et al. 1994). Such observations concerning excessive expression of glucose transporters have been made using messenger-RNA analysis, direct immunohistochemical staining for glucose transporters, and direct measurement of glucose transport in transformed cells as compared with non-transformed parent cells (Lodish 1986/1987; McGowan et al. 1995; Elsas and Longo 1992; Devaskar and Mueckler 1992; James 1994; Mueckler 1994; Ismail-Beigi 1993; Baldwin et al. 1994; Brown and Wahl 1993; Nishioka et al. 1992; Yamamoto et al. 1990; Su et al. 1990; Mellanen et al. 1994; Mertens and Terriere 1993; Hediger and Rhoads 1994; Reske et al. 1997). In transformed cells the glucose influx is much higher than in normal cells. The membrane of transformed cells also contains a glucose transporter that has a higher affinity for glucose (i.e. a low K_m value); this transporter normally only occurs in brain cells and red blood cells. The rapid and high-affinity glucose uptake by the glucose transporter correlates with the high glucolytic activity of tumor cells.

A typical over-expression of the glucose transporter GLUT1 was detected in tissues of primary human mammary carcinomas as compared with normal mammary tissue (Brown and Wahl 1993). An overexpression of GLUT1 was also detected by Reske et al. (1997) in pancreas carcinoma. Over-expressions of the high-affinity transporters in cancer, namely GLUT1 and GLUT3, are typical in very different types of cancers, and the literature dealing with this phenomenon is rapidly increasing (Brown and Wahl 1993; Nishioka et al. 1992; Yamamoto et al. 1990; Su et al. 1990; Mellanen et al. 1994; Reske et al. 1997). It is also logical to develop radiopharmaceutical substances that can detect overexpressed glucose transporters (Mertens and Terriere 1993).

According to the review of Medina and Owen (2002), over-expression of GLUT1 in Human Cancer (refers to the level GLUT1 in relation to relevant non-cancerous tissue), and an association between GLUT1–5 with metastasis and or poor prognosis of the cancer has been reported by more than 50 authors. GLUT 1 over-expression was shown for bladder, breast, cervical, colorectal, embryonic, esophageal, lung and pancreatic (islet) cancer. GLUT 2 was reported to be over-expressed in gastric cancer, reduced in pancreatic cancer. GLUT 3 could be over-expressed in cancer of the brain (also no change reported), breast, head and neck, lung, and ovary as well as in gastric cancer and meningiomas. GLUT 4 was overexpressed in breast, lung and gastric cancer, GLUT 5 in cancer of the lung. More detailed information about over-expression is given in the review of Medina and Owen (2002).

3.3.3
Kinetics of Glucose Transport

The simplest substrates for transport measurements are those that are converted to phosphorylated compounds immediately after entry into the cell. The cell membrane is impermeable for intermediate phosphorylated products, and the substrate thus remains trapped inside the cell (trapping mechanism, see Fig. 3). D-glucose, 2-DG and 2-FDG fall into this category, since they are phosphorylated by hexokinase and ATP (Hatanaka et al. 1970; Renner et al. 1972; Gallagher et al. 1978; Minn et al. 1991). Of course they are transformed or broken down by further metabolic steps and can then leave the cell in different ways. Thus the path of glucose breakdown does not end with the third compartment.

2-FDG exhibits relatively limited reabsorption in the kidney in vivo compared with glucose and is therefore discharged into the urine virtually unchanged. Phosphorylated 2-FDG is therefore concentrated in vivo with the simultaneous clearance of non-phosphorylated 2-FDG. This provides a good contrast for the PET imaging technique (Gallagher et al. 1978). Because of the trapping mechanism the cell can concentrate the absorbed substrate in phosphorylated form in a substantially greater concentration than occurs in the surrounding milieu. This makes it possible to measure the accumulation over a certain time period within a constant transport rate and thus to determine the initial transport rates. The initial incorporation of the substrate by the cells follows normal Michaelis-Menten kinetics (see below). In the case of transport measurements over a longer period of time it is possible to determine that the incorporation rate decreases sharply and is even reversed. There are several reasons for this: 2-DG transport into the cell is faster than phosphorylation, for example, and a portion of the non-phosphorylated substrate is transported out again, i.e., flows out of the cell. A second reason may be that the metabolism of 2-DG does not provide new ATP for the phosphorylation reaction (as shown in Fig. 1). This is to be expected for the transport of 2-FDG alone, since later the substrate no longer appears to be metabolized (Gallagher et al. 1978; Minn et al. 1991). Measurements of the substrate transport from the cell can be determined using substances that are not metabolized by the cells. Substrate transport from the cell, like transport into the cell, is a process that is subject to saturation. 3-O-methyl-D-glucose, which is transported by the same carrier as glucose but is neither phosphorylated nor metabolized, has approximately the same K_m and V_{max} values for transport both into the cell and out of the cell (Renner et al. 1972). The same is probably true for 3-FDG (see Fig. 2). The K_m values for the various transport systems detected in humans with facilitated diffusion there are considerable different ranging from 2 to 60 mM. In addition to this variation, the number of carriers per cell may also vary, and one cell may be provided with one or more carriers. This makes it difficult to attribute kinetics specifically to one or more transport systems. Given this situation, the only way to determine the kinetics of the process absolutely is to carry out specific inhibition experiments with carrier-specific antibodies or other chemical inhibitors such as cytochalasin and phloretin (facilitated diffusion) or phlorizine and ouabain (Na^+/glucose symport) (Tetaud et al. 1997; Bissonnette et al. 1996). Furthermore it has been shown that after an irradiation dose of 10–50 gy the cells in cell cultures exhibit a manifold increase in 2-FDG uptake within some days (See also chapter 8, PET in Cell Culture).

3.3.4 Quantification of PET Measurements

3.3.4.1 *Compartment Models for [18F]FDG*

Radioactively labeled molecules such as [^{18}F]FDG can be traced in the living organism from the outside. In order to determine the relevant quantity (such as rate of metabolism) from the measured activity distributions and their course over time, it is necessary to use models to simplify complicated processes so that they can be described by simple mathematical equations. Linear compartment models have been used most widely. A compartment model consists of a number of spaces or regions; the labeled compound is distributed among these compartments in accordance with the constants that describe the kinetics ("rate constants"). It is assumed that the labeled compound is uniformly distributed within a compartment. It is further assumed that the amount of tracer that is transported per time unit from one compartment to an adjacent compartment is proportional to the total amount present in the compartment and can be described by a transport constant or "rate constant" having the dimension 1/time. The model is represented schematically by a number of sequentially numbered rectangles that are linked by arrows, beside which are written the transport constants k (see Figs. 2 and 3).

Most tissues can be divided into 4 compartments as regards FDG distribution:

1. FDG in the blood plasma
2. FDG in the interstitial tissue
3. FDG in the cell
4. FDG-6-P in the cell

The biochemical nature of radiopharmaceuticals can change in each of these compartments, whether by metabolism or unspecific bonding – to proteins, for example – or by specific bonding to enzymes. All diffusion and transport processes must also be analyzed bidirectionally. Major simplifications are necessary in order to model experimental data. Sokoloff et al., for example, developed a three-compartment model for calculating glucose metabolism using the [^{18}F]FDG method (Fig. 3).

When appropriately labeled substrate analogues are used it is not just the flow of blood or plasma that determines the amount of radioactivity that reaches the tissue but also (and more significantly) the cellular transport and/or intracellular metabolic reactions (e.g. transport and phosphorylation in the case of 2-FDG). The factors that determine the rates of transport and metabolism will be described below.

3.3.4.2
Passive Diffusion

Passive diffusion, such as through the capillary wall, is basically a symmetrical bidirectional process. It affects small molecules in particular – such as H_2O, O_2, CO_2, NH_3, ethanol, and similar non-dissociated molecules. Since radioactive indicators are generally injected by intravasation, the initial retention of a labeled endogenous substance in the section of tissue under examination is determined by the influx (in the direction of the substance concentration gradient through the membrane). The influx (unidirectional diffusion rate) is described by the following equation (after Henze et al. 1994):

$$N_i = Fc_p\left(1 - e^{PS/F}\right) \quad (1),$$

where N_i is the substrate, P is capillary permeability, S is the capillary surface per tissue mass, F is the blood flow per tissue mass, and c_p is the intra-arterial concentration of the substrate in the plasma. The influx of activity is obtained from the relation (generally time-independent) between the intravascular activity concentration (the labeled endogenous substance) and c_p.

The exponential term in Equation 1 should be disregarded with very high permeability. In such a case the influx rate becomes a linear function of perfusion. Perfusion thus becomes the limiting factor governing substrate uptake by the tissue. Diffusion between extra- and intracellular space can also be analyzed in analogy to Equation 1.

3.3.4.3
Carrier-Supported Transport

Michaelis-Menten Constant

Carrier-supported transport (facilitated diffusion) is also a process that is passive (i.e., independent of metabolic energy) and bidirectional and is determined by the direction of the concentration gradient through the membrane. Of course the transport rate is a function of the properties of the carrier in the membrane. This type of transport system can be saturated and inhibited just like active transport (with consumption of metabolic energy in the direction of an electrochemical gradient). The molecular process that takes place in a transport system is similar to that of an enzyme-catalyzed chemical reaction and can therefore be described in accordance with the theory of Michaelis and Menten:

$$N_i = \left(v_{max} \times c_p\right) / \left(K_m + c_p\right) \quad (2),$$

where N_i is again the substrate uptake rate, v_{max} is the maximum transport rate, and K_m is the Michaelis-Menten constant; c_p is the concentration of the free substrate in the plasma. Equation 2 expresses the fact that the transport system must be saturated by high substrate concentrations. The chemical kinetics must be described in similar fashion, i.e., the dependence of the reaction rate v (metabolic rate) on substrate concentration in the case of constant enzyme concentration

$$N = \left(v_{max} \times c_s\right)\left(K_m + c_s\right) \quad (3).$$

Here v_{max} is the maximum reaction rate reached at saturation and c_s is the substrate concentration (Fig. 4); K_m is the substrate concentration at which $v = 1/2\ v_{max}$ (Michaelis-Menten constant).

Lineweaver-Burk Diagram

In order to determine the Michaelis-Menten constant experimentally, the reciprocals of v and c_s are plotted (Lineweaver-Burk diagram, Fig. 5). This diagram permits simple graphic determination of the quantities that characterize the kinetics, K_m and v_{max}.

The reciprocal of the Michaelis-Menten constant indicates to what extent the dynamic reaction equilibrium is on the side of the reaction product. v_{max} is a measure of the amount of the enzyme required for the reaction or – analogous to carrier-supported transport – for the number of carriers per volume unit (Henze et al. 1994).

Eadie-Hofstee Plot

Another form of linear representation of Michaelis-Menten kinetics is the Eadie-Hofstee plot, Fig. 6. It indicates the presence of various system components better than the Lineweaver-Burk plot by deviating from linearity. It is obtained from the following equation:

$$v = K_m \times v / c_s + v_{max} \quad (4)$$

The diagram shows that the characterization of transport systems and enzymatic processes requires measurements at a minimum of two substrate concentrations (Henze et al. 1994).

Tumor-Standardized Uptake Value

Visual qualitative representation of PET studies is normally sufficient for evaluation. However, in many cases a quantitative evaluation is advantageous. This is the case with carcinoma of the breast, for example. In order to be able to compare the PET images of different patients, the PET data calibrated to activity concentration are normalized for image analysis with respect to injected activity and patient weight. The resulting transversal parametric slices represent a standardized measure of the regional tracer concentration at the point of uptake. This is referred to as the "standardized uptake value" (SUV) (Strauss and Conti 1991).

$$\mathrm{SUV} = \frac{\text{activity concentration in tissue [Bq/g]}}{\text{administered activity} \quad \text{Bq / body weight (g)}}$$

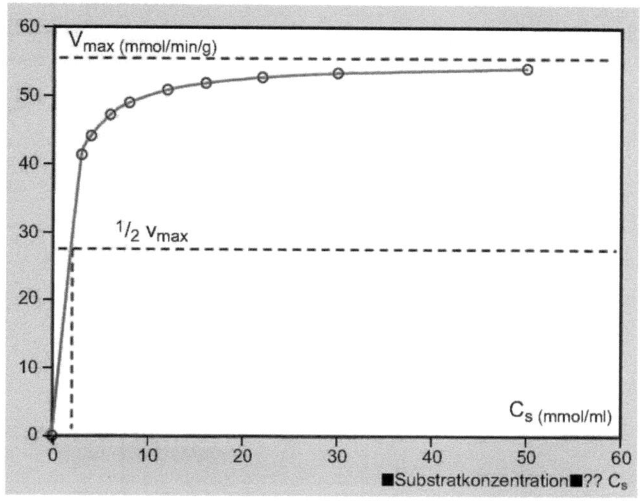

Fig. 4.
Reaction rate v as a function of substrate concentration c_s in an enzyme-catalyzed chemical reaction. v_{max} = maximum rate (with saturation), K_m = Michaelis-Menten constant

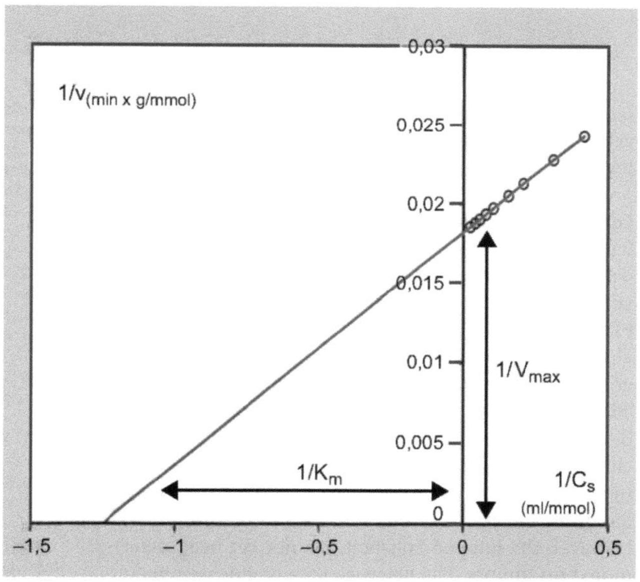

Fig. 5.
Lineweaver-Burk diagram. The coordinates show the reciprocals of the variables in Fig. 3-4. 1/v is plotted as a function of $1/c_s$

These data are used for both visual and quantitative evaluation. SUV-normalized diagrams of FDG distribution are recorded on X-ray film for the purpose of visual evaluation of PET scans. SUV values from zero to five for examination of the mammary glands or from zero to four for images of the axillae are represented by a linear gray-value display (Römer et al. 1997).

Positron emission tomography permits absolute activity measurement in vivo and therefore quantification of tracer concentration in addition to qualitative evaluation of the distribution of glucose in the body. The regional FDG image (SUV value) is determined using the "region of interest" (ROI) technique. The average SUV value within a ROI is used for evaluation. Quantitative image analysis is also affected by tumor size. Because of partial volume effects, tumors less than 2 cm in diameter yield a SUV value that is too low. However, partial volume correction is possible using the "recovery coefficient," a correction factor determined by phantom measurements (Römer et al. 1997; Sokoloff et al. 1977; Patlak and Blasberg 1985). Although the idea is simple, the SUV method is difficult to use because it involves many corrections (Lowe et al. 1994; Zasadny and Wahl 1993; Fischmann and Alpert 1993; Minn et al. 1995; Gatenby 1995). It is also difficult to standardize since many variable factors such as glucose concentration, body weight, time after injection, ROI size, and the resolution capability of the PET unit play a role (Lindholm et al. 1994; Minn et al.

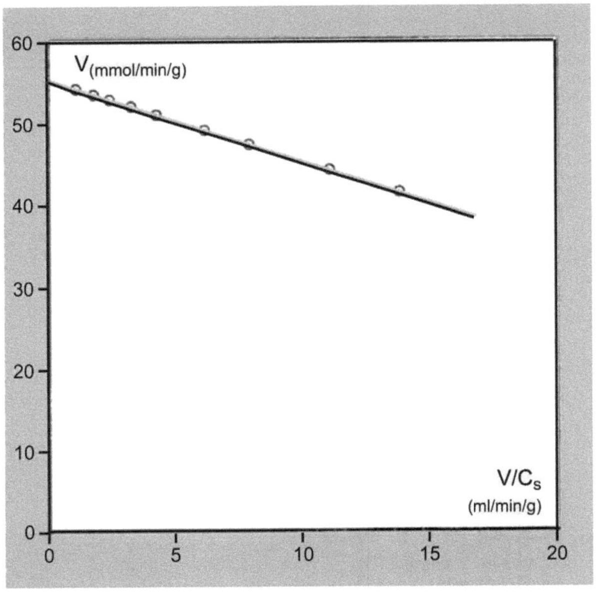

Fig. 6.
Eadie-Hofstee plot

1994; Keyes 1995). It is hardly possible to compare SUV values from different institutes using different PET systems and different working protocols.

Complex Compartment Models and the Lumped Constant

Relatively complex compartment models designed to determine glucose consumption are available for measurements of the transport of glucose and different FDG derivatives (Patlak and Blasberg 1985; Sokoloff et al. 1977; Phelps et al. 1979; Huang and Phelps 1986; Becker et al. 1998). Here we should also mention the term "lumped constant." This constant functions as a calibration factor between 2-FDG and glucose and hardly changes at the local level. The lumped constant is used in the Patlak-Gjedde method for quantitative determination of 2-[^{18}F]FDG influx (Patlak and Blasberg 1985). However, the lumped constant has not yet been determined for tumors. The heterogeneity of glucose uptake in tumors, among other things, makes it difficult to determine this value. In conclusion it can be noted that the scientific development of complex compartment models is still an open area of research.

References

Baldwin SA, Kan O, Whetton AD et al (1994) Regulation of the glucose transporter Glut-1 in mammalian cells. Biochem Soc Trans 22:814–817

Becker G, Piert M, Bares R, Machulla HJ (1998) Konzentrationsabhängigkeit des Transports von 3-[18F] FDG in der Schweineleber. Nuklearmedizin 37:68

Bell GI, Burant CF, Takeda J, Gould GW (1993) Structure and function of mammalian facilitative sugar transporters. J Biol Chem 268:19161–19164

Birnbaum MJ, Haspel HC, Rosen OM (1987) Transformation of rat fibroblasts by FSV rapidly increases glucose transporter gene. Science 235:1495–1498

Bissonnette P, Gagné H, Coady MJ, Benabdallah K, Lapointe JY, Berteloot A (1996) Kinetic separation and characterization of three sugar transport modes in Caco-2 cells. Am J Physiol 270: G833–G843

Brown RS, Wahl RL (1993) Overexpression of glut-1 glucose transporter in human breast cancer. Cancer 72:2979–2985

Brown RS, Fisher SJ, Wahl RL (1993) Autoradiographic evaluation of the intra-tumoral distribution of 2-deoxy-D-glucose and monoclonal antibodies in xenografts of human ovarian adenocarcinoma. J Nucl Med 34:75–82

Concha II, Velasquez FV, Martinez JM, Angulo C, Droppelmann A, Reyes AM, Slebe JC, Vera JC, Golde DW (1997) Human erythrocytes express GLUT5 and transport fructose. Blood 89:4190–4195

Dang CV, Semenza GL (1999) Oncogenic alterations of metabolism. Trends Biochem Sci 24:68–72

Devaskar SU, Mueckler MM (1992) The mammalian glucose transporters. Pediatr Res 31:1–13

Doege H, Schurmann A, Bahrenberg G, Brauers A, Joost HG (2000a) GLUT8, a novel member of the sugar transport facilitator family with glucose transport activity. J Biol Chem 275: 16275–16280

Doege H, Bocianski A, Joost HG, Schurmann A (2000b) Activity and genomic organization of human glucose transporter 9 (GLUT9), a novel member of the family of sugar-transport facilitators predominantly expressed in brain and leucocytes. Biochem J 350:771–776

Doege H, Bocianski A, Scheepers A, Axer H, Eckel J, Joost HG, Schurmann A (2001) Characterization of the human glucose transporter GLUT11, a novel sugat transport facilitator specifically expressed in heart muscle. Biochem J 359:443–449

Elsas LJ, Longo N (1992) Glucose transporters. Annu Rev Med 43: 377–393

Fischmann AJ, Alpert NM (1993) FDG-PET in oncology: there's more to it than looking at pictures. J Nucl Med 34:6–11

Flier JS, Mueckler MM, Usher P, Lodish HF (1987) Elevated levels of glucose transport and transporter messenger RNA are induced by ras or src oncogenes. Science 235:1492–1495

Fukumoto H, Kayano T, Buse JB, Edwards Y, Pilch PF, Bell GI, Seino S (1989) Cloning and characterization of the major insulin-responsive glucose transporter expressed in human skel-

etal muscle and other insulin-responsive tissues. J Biol Chem 264:7776–7779
Fukunaga T, Enomoto K, Okazumi S, Isono K (1993) Analysis of glucose metabolism in patients with esophageal cancer by FDG-PET: estimation of hexokinase activity in the tumor and prediction of prognosis: clinical PET in oncology. Proceedings of 2nd international symposium on PET in oncology. World Scientific, Singapore, pp 87–90
Gallagher BM, Fowler JS, Gutterson NI, MacGregor RR, Wan CN, Wolf AP (1978) Metabolic trapping as a principle of radiopharmaceutical design: some factors responsible for the biodistribution of [18F] 2-deoxy-2-fluoro-D-glucose. J Nucl Med 19:1154–1161
Gatenby RA (1995) Potential role of FDG-Pet imaging in understanding tumor-host interaction. J Nucl Med 36:839–899
Graham MM, Spence AM, Muzi M, Abbott GL (1989) Deoxyglucose kinetics in a rat brain tumor. J Cereb Blood Flow Metab 9:315–322
Hatanaka M, Augl C, Gilden RV (1970) Evidence for a functional change in the plama membrane of murine sarcoma virus-infected mouse embryo cells. Transport and transport-associated phosphorylation of 14C-2-deoxy-D-glucose. J Biol Chem 245:714–717
Hediger MA, Rhoads DB (1994) Molecular physiology of sodium-glucose cotransporters. Physiol Rev 74:993–1026
Henze E, Knapp H, Meyer GJ, Müller S (1994) 5: Prinzipien der Diagnostik. In: Büll U, Schicha H, Biersack HJ, Knapp WH, Reiners C, Schober O (eds) Nuklearmedizin. Thieme, Stuttgart, pp 114–138
Huang SC, Phelps ME (1986) Principles of tracer kinetic modeling in positron emission tomography and autoradiography. In: Phelps ME, Maziotta JC, Schelbert HR (eds) Positron emision tomography and autoradiography: principles and applications for the brain and heart. Raven, New York
Hundal HS, Darakhshan F, Kristiansen S, Blakemore SJ, Richter EA (1998) GLUT5 expression and fructose transport in human skeletal muscle (review). Adv Exp Med Biol 441:35–45
Hruz PW, Mueckler MM (2001) Structural analysis of the GLUT1 facilitative glucose transporter (review). Mol Membr Biol 18: 183–193
Ishikawa N, Oguri T, Isobe T, Fujitaka K, Kohno N (2001) SGLT gene expression in primary lung cancers and their metastatic lesions. Jpn J Cancer Res 92:874–879
Ismail-Beigi F (1993) Metabolic regulation of glucose transport. J Membr Biol 135:1–10
James DE (1994) Targeting of the insulin-regulatable glucose transporter (GLUT-4). Biochem Soc Trans 22:668–670
Joost HG, Thorens B (2001) The extended GLUT-family of sugar/polyol transport facilitators: nomenclature, sequence characteristics, and potential function of its novel members (review). Mol Membr Biol 18:247–256
Joost HG, Bell GI, Best JD, Birnbaum MJ, Charron MJ, Chen YT, Doege H, James DE, Lodish HF, Moley KH, Moley JF, Mueckler M, Rogers S, Schurmann A, Seino S, Thorens B. (2002) Nomenclature of the GLUT/SLC2A family of sugar/polyol transport facilitators. Am J Physiol Endocrinol Metab 2:E974–E976
Kayano T, Burant CF, Fukumoto H, Gould GW, Fan YS, Eddy RL, Byers MG, Shows TB, Seino S, Bell GI (1990) Human facilitative glucose transporters. Isolation, functional characterization, and gene localization of cDNAs encoding an isoform (GLUT5) expressed in small intestine, kidney, muscle, and adipose tissue and an unusual glucose transporter pseudogene-like sequence (GLUT6). J Biol Chem 265:13276–13282
Keyes JW Jr (1995) SUV: standard uptake or silly useless value? J Nucl Med 36:1836–1839
Larson SM, Weiden PL, Grunbaum Z et al (1981) Positron imaging feasibility studies. II. Characteristic of deoxyglucose uptake in rodent and canine neoplasms: concise communication. J Nucl Med 22:875–879
Lindholm P, Leskinen-Kallio S, Kirvela O et al (1994) Head and neck cancer: effect of food ingestion on uptake of C-11 methionine. Radiology 193:863–867
Lisinski I, Schurmann A, Joost HG, Cushman SW, Al-Hasani H. (2001) Targeting of GLUT6 (formerly GLUT9) and GLUT8 in rat adipose cells. Biochem J 358:517–522
Lodish HF (1986/1987) Anion-exchange and glucose transport proteins: structure, function and distribution. Harvey Lect 82:19–46
Lowe VJ, Hoffmann JM, DeLong DM et al (1994) Semiquantitativ and visual analysis of FDG-PET images in pulmonary abnormalities. J Nucl Med 35:1771–1776
Lowe VJ, Hoffmann JM, DeLong DM et al (1994) Semiquantitativ and visual analysis of FDG-PET images in pulmonary abnormalities. J Nucl Med 35:1771–1776
McGowan KM, Long SD, Pekala PH (1995) Glucose transporter gene expression: regulation of transcription and mRNA stability. Pharmacol Ther 66:465–505
McVie-Wylie AJ, Lamson DR, Chen YT (2001) Molecular cloning of a novel member of the GLUT family of transporters, SLC2a10 (GLUT10), localized on chromosome 20q13.1: a candidate gene for NIDDM susceptibility. Genomics 72:113–117
Medina RA, Owen GI (2002) Glucose transporters: expression, regulation and cancer (review). Biol Res 35:9–26
Medina RA, Southworth R, Fuller W, Garlick PB (2002) Lactate-induced translocation of GLUT1 and GLUT4 is not mediated by phosphatidylinositol-3-kinase pathway in the rat heart. Basic Res Cardiol 97:168–176
Mellanen P, Minn H, Grénman R, Härkönen P (1994) Expression of glucose transporters in head-and-neck tumors. Int J Cancer 56:622–629
Mertens J, Terriere D (1993) 3-radioiodo-phloretin – a new potential radioligand for in vivo measurement of glut proteins: a SPECT alternative for [18F]FDG. J Nucl Biol Med 37:158–159
Minn H, Kangas L, Knuutila V, Paul R, Sipilä H (1991) Determination of 2-fluoro-2-deoxy-D-glucose uptake and ATP level for evaluating drug effects in neoplastic cells. Res Exp Med 191:27–35
Minn H, Nuutila P, Lindholm P et al (1994) In vivo effect of insulin on tumor and skeletal muscle glucose metabolism in patients with lymphoma. Cancer 73:1490–1498
Minn H, Zasadny KR, Quint LE et al (1995) Lung cancer: reproducibility of quantitative measurements for evaluating 2-[F-18]-fluoro-2-deoxy-D-glucose uptake at PET. Radiology 196: 167–173
Monakhov NK, Neistadt EL, Shavlovskii MM et al (1978) Physicochemical properties and isoenzyme composition of hexokinase from normal and malignant human tissues. J Natl Cancer Inst 61:27–34
Mueckler M (1994) Facilitative glucose transporters. Int J Biochem 219:713–725
Nishioka T, Oda Y, Seino Y et al (1992) Distribution of the glucose transporters in human brain tumors. Cancer Res 52:3972–3979
Patlak CS, Blasberg RG (1985) Graphical evaluation of blood-to-brain transfer constants from multiple-time uptake data. Generalisations. J Cereb Blood Flow Metab 5:584–590
Pedersen PL (1978) Tumor mitochondria and the bioenergetics of cancer cells. Prog Exp Tumor Res 22:190–274
Phay JE, Hussain HB, Moley JF (2000) Cloning and expression analysis of a novel member of the facilitative glucose transporter family, SLC2A9 (GLUT9). Genomics 66:217–220
Phelps ME, Huang SC, Hoffmann EJ (1979) Tomographic measurement of local cerebral glucose metabolic rate in humans with (F-18) 2-fluoro-2-deoxy-D-glucose: validation of method. Ann Neurol 6:371–388
Rand EB, Depaoli AM, Davidson NO, Bell GI, Burant CF (1993) Sequence, tissue distribution, and functional characterization of the rat fructose transporter GLUT5. Am J Physiol 264:G1169–G1176
Reske SN, Grillenberger KG, Glatting G, Port M, Hildebrandt M, Gansauge F, Beger HG (1997) Overexpression of glucose transporter 1 and increased FDG uptake in pancreatic carcinoma. J Nucl Med 38:1344–1348
Rogers S, Docherty SE, Slavin JL, Henderson MA, Best JD (2003) Differential expression of GLUT12 in breast cancer and normal breast tissue. Cancer Lett 193:225–233
Römer W, Avril N, Schwaiger M (1997) Einsatzmöglichkeiten der Positronen-Emissions-Tomographie beim Mammakarzinom. Acta Med Austr 24:60–62
Sokoloff L, Reivich M, Kennedy C, Des Rosiers MH, Patlak CS, Pettigrew KD, Sakurada O, Shinohara M (1977) The [14C]-de-

oxyglucose method for the measurement of local cerebral glucose utilization: theory, procedure, and normal values in the conscious and anesthetized albino rat. J Neurochem 28: 897–916

Som P, Atkins HL, Bandoypadhyay D et al (1980) A fluorinated glucose analog, 2-fluoro-2-deoxy-D-glucose (18F): nontoxic tracer for rapid tumor detection. J Nucl Med 21:670–675

Strauss LG, Conti PS (1991) The applications of PET in clinical oncology. J Nucl Med 32:623–648

Stuart Wood I, Trayhurn P (2003) Glucose transporters (GLUT and SGLT): expanded families of sugar transport proteins (review). Br J Nutr 89:3–9

Su TS, Tsai TF, Chi CW, Han SH, Chou CK (1990) Elevation of facilitated glucose-transporter messenger RNA in human hepatocellular carcinoma. Hepatology 11:118–122

Tetaud E, Barrett MP, Bringaud F, Baltz T (1997) Kinetoplastid glucose transporters. Biochem J 325:569–580

Uldry M, Thorens B (2003) The SLC2 family of facilitated hexose and polyol transporters. Pflugers Arch (epub ahead of print)

Wahl RL, Hutchins GD, Buchsbaum DJ, Liebert M, Grossman HB, Fisher S (1991) 18F-2-deoxy-2-fluoro-D-glucose uptake into human tumor xenografts: feasibility studies for cancer imaging with PET. Cancer 67:1544–1550

Warburg O (1931) The metabolism of tumors. Smith, New York, pp 129–169

Watanabe T, Nagamatsu S, Matsushima S, Kondo K, Motobu H, Hirosawa K, Mabuchi K, Kirino T, Uchimura H (1999) Developmental expression of GLUT2 in the rat retina. Cell Tissue Res 298:217–223

Warburg OH (1956) On the origin of cancer cells. Science 123:309–314

Weber G, Banerjee G, Morris HP (1961) Comparative biochemistry of hepatomas. I. Carbohydrate enzymes in morris hepatoma 5123. Cancer Res 21:933–937

Wright EM (2001) Renal Na(+)-glucose cotransporters. Am J Physiol Renal Physiol 280:F10–F18

Wright EM, Turk E (2003) The sodium/glucose cotransport family SLC5. Pflugers Arch (epub ahead of print)

Yamamoto T, Seino Y, Fukumoto H, Koh G, Yano H, Inagaki N, Yamada Y, Inoue K, Manabe T, Imura H (1990) Overexpression of facilitative glucose transporter genes in human cancer. Biochem Biophy Res Commun 170:223–230

Zasadny KR, Wahl RL (1993) Standardized uptake values of normal tissues at PET with 2-(fluorine-18)-fluoro-2-deoxy-D-glucose: variations with body weight and a method for correction. Radiology 189:847–850

CHAPTER 4

Radiopharmaceutical Production and Safety of [^{18}F]FDG

P. Oehr

4.1 Radiopharmaceutical Chemistry of [^{18}F]FDG

4.1.1 Production of Positron Emitters

An advantage of positron emission tomography (PET) involves the existing positron emitters (Table 1). Most biomolecules can be labeled using carbon (^{11}C), nitrogen (^{13}N), oxygen (^{15}O) and fluorine (^{18}F), so that their biochemical properties are practically unaltered. In addition, the metabolism of these tracers is frequently known. This means that for 2-[^{18}F]fluoro-2-deoxy-D-glucose ([^{18}F]FDG), the glucose metabolism can be calculated from the basic activity distribution (modeling, Patlak plot). As a calculation of this type requires the input function, which is obtained using blood samples, it is often customary in clinical studies to limit calculations to quantification based on the standard uptake value. For this purpose, the activity measured in a pixel is normalized for the injected activity and the weight of the patient.

As shown in Table 1, all positron emitters have a relatively short half-life. Only ^{18}F, which has a half-life of 110 min, can be transported over certain distances. Otherwise on-site production in a cyclotron is required. The shorter-lived positron emitters such as ^{11}C, ^{13}N or ^{15}O must be produced on site or very close to their intended use.

Twenty years ago the short-lived radionuclides were available only in the large physics research centers with access to particle accelerators or nuclear reactors. The increasing clinical applications of cyclotron-produced radioisotopes and radiopharmaceuticals have led to the rapid rise in the number of compact cyclotrons throughout the world. To date, up to 121 medical cyclotrons have been established worldwide.

Companies producing cyclotrons commercially are: General Electric Medical Systems, CTI Cyclotron Systems, EBCO, IBA, NNK/Oxford Instruments, and Japan Steel Works. The majority of these machines are now negative-ion systems, which allow the option of dual irradiation of two targets. All have a modular design, which allows the system to be customized to a particular facility's needs (McCarthy and Welch 1998). Different cyclotrons suitable for sustaining a major program for PET research and clinical application are shown in Table 2. Figure 1 gives an example of a cyclotron that can be installed in larger diagnostic institutions. This cyclotron is a high-energy, negative-ion cyclotron, which permits not just high-yield [^{18}F]FDG production, but also offers optional ^{11}C, ^{13}N, ^{15}O and ^{18}F F2 targets, as well as precursor/tracer chemistry for ^{13}N-,^{15}O- and ^{11}C-labeled compounds. According to GE Medical Systems, it completes start-up in less than 10 minutes, and particle/production-mode changes in less than 3 minutes. The vacuum pump system enables beam operation within 20 minutes after short ventings to air of the cyclotron's interior. The cyclotron can be equipped with dual irradiation capability, which allows simultaneous production in two targets. Using simultaneous beam extraction allows concurrent production of multiple isotopes.

Table 1. Characteristics of the most common positron emitters

Positron emitter	Half-life (min)	Product	Maximum energy of positron (MeV)	Maximum linear range (mm)	Mean linear range (mm)
11C	20.4	11B	0.96	5.0	0.3
13N	9.9	13C	1.19	5.4	1.4
15O	2.1	15N	1.72	8.2	1.5
18F	110	18O	0.64	2.4	0.2
68Ga	68	68Zn	1.89	9.1	1.9
82Rb	1.3	82Kr	3.35	15.6	2.6

Table 2.
Overview: cyclotrons for production of positron emitters

Company	Name	Self-shielded	Beam current (μA)	Energy deuterons (MeV)	Energy protons (MeV)
GE	PET trace	–	75	8.4	16.5
IBA	Cyclone 10/5	–	60	5	10
	Cyclone 18/5	+	80	5	18
JSW	BC2010 N	+	70	10	20
NKK/Oxford	NKK/Oxford	+	50–100		12
CTI	RDS-112	+	50		11
EBCO	TR19	+ (opt.)	>150	9 (opt.)	13–19

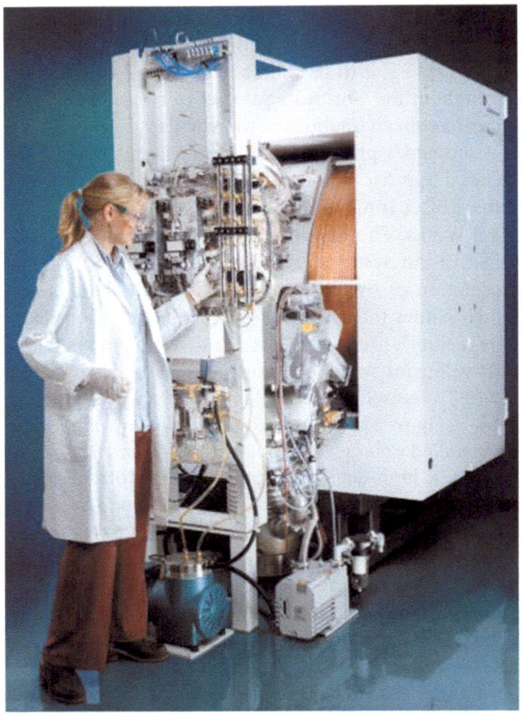

Fig. 1. PET trace cyclotron (GE Medical Systems)

4.1.2 Synthesis of [^{18}F]FDG

4.1.2.1 *Historical Development*

2-[^{18}F]fluoro- 2-deoxy-D-glucose was developed in 1976 in a collaboration between scientists at the National Institutes of Health, the University of Pennsylvania, and Brookhaven National Laboratory. It was developed for the specific purpose of mapping brain glucose metabolism in living humans, thereby serving as a tool in the basic human neurosciences. Using [^{18}F]FDG, it was possible for the first time to measure regional glucose metabolism in the living human brain. Around the same time, the use of [^{18}F]FDG for studies of myocardial metabolism and as a tracer for tumor metabolism was reported. After the first synthesis of [^{18}F]FDG via an electrophilic fluorination with ^{18}F gas (produced via the ^{20}Ne(d,alpha)^{18}F reaction), small-volume enriched water targets were developed that made it possible to produce large quantities of [^{18}F]fluoride ion via the high-yield ^{18}(p,n)^{18}F reaction. This was followed by a major milestone, the development of a nucleophilic fluorination method that produced [^{18}F]FDG in very high yield. These advances and the remarkable properties of [^{18}F]FDG have largely overcome the limitations of the 110-minute half-life of ^{18}F, so that [^{18}F]FDG is now available from many central production sites. This avoids the need for an on-site cyclotron and chemistry laboratory and has opened up the use of [^{18}F]FDG to institutions that have a PET scanner (or other imaging device) but no cyclotron or chemistry infrastructure. Currently, [^{18}F]FDG is used by many hospitals as an off-the-shelf radiopharmaceutical for clinical diagnosis in heart disease, seizure disorders, and oncology, the area of most rapid growth. However, it remains an important tool in human neuroscience and in drug research and development (Gallagher et al. 1977; Ido et al. 1978; Hamacher et al. 1986; Fowler and Ido 2002).

[^{18}F]FDG can be obtained commercially in Europe from several different centers. The production procedures differ somewhat from center to center, and only limited information is available about these procedures (Wienhard et al. 1989; Ido et al. 1978; Hamacher et al. 1986). It is therefore impossible to describe all the production techniques in this book. General guidelines are given in the literature. The currently authorized methods for Europe and the United States are described in detail in the european Pharmacopeia (EP) and the U.S. Pharmacopeia (USP). The quality assurance requirements listed in the USP and the draft Chemistry, Manufacturing, and Controls (CMC) issued by the U.S. Food and Drug Administration (FDA), and the EP are compared by Hung (Meyer et al. 1993; Meyer et al. 1995, Eur. Ph. 4th Edition 2002; Hung 2002).

4.1.2.2
Modern Radiochemistry Modules

Radiolabeling of compounds involves considerable amounts of radioactivity and must be performed by remote control in lead-shielded hot cells. About 3 Ci of ^{18}F are needed to synthesize about 1 Ci of [^{18}F]FDG, sufficient for more than 20 patient investigations at various distances from the cyclotron.

^{18}F-Radiolabeling is performed in fully automated synthesis modules. An example is given in Fig. 2, demonstrating an automated synthetic apparatus "FDG MicroLab", a PET trace module from GE. [^{18}F]FDG is synthesized by a solid-phase ^{18}F-fluorination. Its quality and reproducibility were evaluated by Kuge et al. in order to assess feasibility of the apparatus for routine clinical production of [^{18}F]FDG. For five consecutive [^{18}F]FDG syntheses, target irradiation was carried out at 15 microA for 60 min. [^{18}F]FDG was obtained in 50 min after EOB with an end-of-synthesis yield of 9.34 +/− 1.06 GBq. Radiochemical yield and purity were 47 +/− 3% (decay corrected) and 98.0 +/− 0.5%, respectively (Kuge et al. 1999).

4.1.3
Quality Control

Since [^{18}F]FDG can be synthesized using different methods, different amounts of impurities are present in the products supplied by the various producers. For this reason the individual producers are also required to document the purity of their products.

The product is a sterile, colorless to light-yellow, non-combustible radioactive liquid, which contains [^{18}F]FDG in aqueous solution. The [^{18}F]FDG solutions that are distributed must fall within specific limits. A distinction is made between radiochemical, isomeric, radionuclidic, chemical and biological purity.

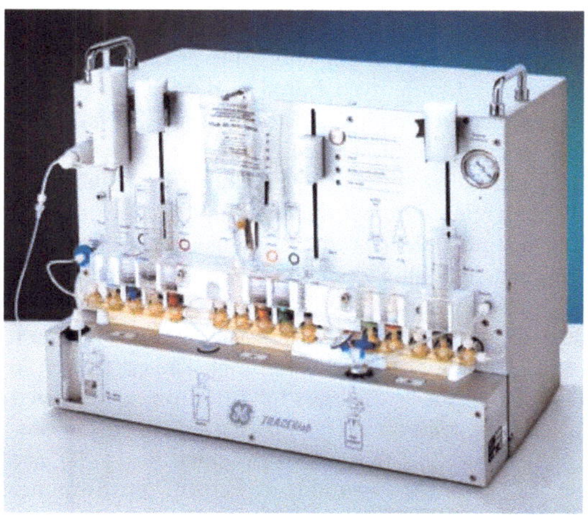

Fig. 2. "FDG MicroLab" (GE Medical Systems)

The aim of quality control is to supply a product that is physiologically absolutely safe. The European Pharmacopoeia 1997/99 lists the various syntheses, the characterizations and the respective methods of quality control for [^{18}F]FDG. Also listed are the permissible concentrations of the constituents in milligrams per dose. Quality control of the [^{18}F]FDG refers to three sectors:

1. Analysis of the chemical composition (HPLC, thin-layer chromatography)
2. Determination of radiochemical data (HPLC and activity detector, thin-layer chromatography, TLC scanner, half-life determination, gamma ray spectrum)
3. Bacteriologic examination (endotoxin tests (rabbit temperature control after i.v. injection of the FDG solution, limulus-amebocytes-lysate test) and sterility tests (blood culture system).

It is remarkable that the results of sterility testing often come a week after the patient was injected with the respective FDG solution.

4.2
[^{18}F]FDG Pharmacokinetics, Toxicity and Interactions

Several things occur when [^{18}F]FDG is injected intravenously in humans (a 30 s bolus injection, for example). Non-metabolized [^{18}F]FDG is eliminated by glomerular filtration without complete reabsorption into the urine. When the kidneys are functioning normally, approximately 16% of the administered glucose is eliminated with the urine after 60 minutes, and 50% is eliminated after 135 minutes (Gallagher et al. 1977, 1978; Woosley et al. 1970). Cellular uptake of [^{18}F]FDG is made possible by tissue-specific transport systems that are partially dependent on insulin. [^{18}F]FDG reacts inside the cell with the enzyme hexokinase and is phosphorylated to form [^{18}F]FDG-6-phosphate (Gallagher et al. 1977, 1978). Because the administered concentration of [^{18}F]FDG is very low (in the nmol range, see Table 3), it can be assumed that the normal metabolism of glucose is not affected, since the plasma glucose concentration is 1–4 mmol/l. Subsequent dephosphorylation by intracellular phosphatases is rather slow, and therefore the [^{18}F]FDG-6-phosphate will be retained in the tissues for several hours.

In the animal experiments of Reivich et al. in 1979, multiple doses of FDG were administered intravenously to mice (three injections of 14.3 mg/kg each) and to dogs (three injections of 0.72 mg/kg each). No effects were detected either microscopically or macroscopically in the blood, urine or cerebrospinal fluid, or in tissues such as the brain, heart, spleen, liver, kidneys, lungs, ovaries or intestines. There were no signs of toxicity

Table 3. Specific amounts of [^{18}F]FDG per administered patient dose. Column 1 describes the case involving maximum specific activity at the lowest chemical concentration, and column 2 shows the possible case of minimum specific activity and average chemical concentration. Column 3 shows the maximum dose of chemical concentration. Column 4 describes the case in which activity has decayed to the extent that 10 ml must be injected to reach a single dose of 370 MBq, which can result in the maximum possible chemical concentration of 652 μg per patient

	Maximum specific activity	Minimum specific activity	Activity limit	Maximum volume (10 ml)
Activity (MBq/batch in 14.5 ml)	50,750	5,075		360
Specific activity MBq (μmol)	10,000	1,000	1,000	100
Injected/patient (MBq)	180	360	450	360
μmol/patient	0.018	0.36	0.45	3.6
μg/patient (1 μmol FDG = 181.14 μg)	3.26	65.21	81.51	652.00
μg/kg patient (patient = 70 kg)	0.046	0.93	1.16	9.30

within a time span of 3 weeks. In humans (see Table 3) the administered dose of FDG is normally about 0.05–1 μg/kg and in extreme cases 9.3 μg/kg. The normal FDG dose is therefore 1,000 times lower than the concentration that appeared to be harmless in animals. Similar results were reported by Som et al. in 1980. These researchers injected mice with a FDG concentration that was 1,000 times the normal concentration. They were unable to detect either acute or chronic toxicity during a period of 3 weeks after injection. Even the maximum possible dose for humans (10 ml) is almost 100 times lower than this limit. It can be deduced that there is a large safety margin. Substance-related toxic side effects can be ruled out for these small doses and for this reason have not been described in the literature.

The [^{18}F]FDG dose that is administered for diagnostic purposes is therefore not expected to cause any pharmacological effects or substance-related side effects. No overdoses have been reported in the international literature to date.

Interactions with Other Substances. Any substance or therapeutic measure that reduces cell vitality will affect glucose metabolism indirectly. General examples are chemotherapy and external irradiation. It has been observed that a decrease in glucose utilization or [^{18}F]FDG uptake during or after chemotherapy or irradiation is associated with tumor regression – whereas glucose utilization is unchanged or increases with tumor progression. This observation forms the basis for [^{18}F]FDG therapy prognosis and can be used for therapy monitoring. However, chemotherapeutic agents can also result in a reduction in cellular [^{18}F]FDG uptake (probably as a function of tumor vitality). Radiation therapy can cause an increase in glucose uptake depending on the dose (see Chap. 8 for more details). Cortisone inhibits glucose utilization in lymphomas and can thus yield false-negative findings. It is therefore recommended that no cortisone be administered for a period of about 4 weeks before a [^{18}F]FDG PET examination.

4.3 [^{18}F]FDG Activity Dosages and Radiation Exposure

[^{18}F]FDG is administered at the various PET centers in activity dosages ranging from 185 to 740 MBq, although the majority of centers use dosages of 185–370 MBq. The relationship between administered dose and cumulative concentration in the target organ and surrounding tissue (background), on the one hand, and the resulting image quality (e.g. detectability of small lesions), on the other hand, depends on the particular diagnostic system and must be determined from case to case.

Concentration Phase. Emission scans are normally begun 30–60 minutes after injection, as long as the tissue scan of [^{18}F]FDG has reached an activity plateau and there is still sufficient activity for adequate count statistics.

Administered Activity. The activity administered to patients by i.v. injection normally ranges from to 185 to 370 MBq for all indications. Children receive smaller doses of 96 MBq or less. The time interval between two injections should be long enough to ensure that the radioactivity has decayed (physical decay) and the substance has been eliminated (biological clearance). No side effects are known that might be caused directly by one or more [^{18}F]FDG injections. Emission scans should begin no sooner than 40 minutes after injection. It is also possible to wait even longer before initiating scanning. The filling volume is generally 10 ml with a fluctuation in total activity from 5.075 to 50.750 MBq, depending on synthesis technique, and a maximum specific activity of 1–100 GBq/μmol. The data given in Table 3 are used as the basis for determining the specific volume per administered dose.

^{18}F decays to ^{18}O by positron emission (97 %) and electron capture (3 %) and has a half-life of 110 minutes. Positrons with an energy of 0.9 MeV are emitted primarily. The radiation detected in a PET camera is not direct positron radiation, however. Only after a positron has combined with a negatively charged electron and the two particles are annihilated, bringing about a conversion of the combined mass to energy (two times 511 keV), is there emission of two gamma quanta or photons of 511 keV each at an angle of virtually 180°.

The dosimetry for [^{18}F]FDG has been estimated by various authors. The effective equivalent dose (whole body) is 21–27 μSv/MBq (Meyer et al. 1995). For an activity dose of 370 MBq, the total dose can be calculated as 7.8–10 mSv. Other publications give estimates ranging between 4 and 10 mSv. The range of natural radiation exposure in Germany is 1–6 mSv, and the mean value is 2.4 mSv.

The estimated radiation exposures in an adult (weighing 70 kg) after injection of 185 MBq or 370 MBq [^{18}F]FDG are listed in Table 4. These estimates were calculated based on patient data and on [^{18}F]FDG data supplied by the MIRD Commission. According to these data, the bladder wall, with an equivalent dose of 120–170 μSv/MBq (80–100 mrem/mCi), must be considered as a critical organ (Dowd et al. 1991; Mejia et al. 1991; Meyer et al. 1995).

There is no risk of non-stochastic radiation damage (such as the first clinically detectable effects of irradiation) even after multiple injections or a single accidental administration of the entire contents of a multiple-dose vial, considering that the threshold dose is 250 mSv after acute whole-body irradiation.

Table 4. Estimated radiation dose with intravenous administration of [^{18}F]FDG in a patient weighing 70 kg

Organ	mGy/185 MBq	rad/5 mCi
Bladder wall	31.45	3.15
Bladder[a]	11.00	1.10
Bladder[b]	22.00	2.20
Heart	12.03	1.20
Brain	4.81	0.48
Kidneys	3.88	0.39
Uterus	3.70	0.37
Ovaries	2.78	0.28
Testes	2.78	0.28
Adrenal bodies	2.59	0.26
Small intestine	2.40	0.24
Gastric wall	2.22	0.22
Liver	2.22	0.22
Pancreas	2.22	0.22
Spleen	2.22	0.22
Breast	2.04	0.20
Lungs	2.04	0.20
Red bone marrow	2.04	0.20
Other tissues	2.04	0.20
Bone surface	1.85	0.18
Thyroid	1.79	0.18

[a] Bladder voided 1 h after administration
[b] 2 h after administration

The risk of dying from a radiation-induced late malignancy (leukemia and carcinoma) is currently estimated to be approximately 5–6 in 10,000 for a radiation exposure of 10 mSv (1 rem). The mean latency period must also be considered, which for carcinomas is 20–25 years, for example. The life expectancy for patients with a malignancy is significantly limited, and diagnostic information is essential in choosing a treatment that might improve the quality of life and/or extend life expectancy. From this perspective radiation risk is negligible.

The genetic risk after exposure to 10 mSv is estimated to be 1–2 in 100,000 for dominant mutations and 5–10 in 100,000 for recessive mutations.

4.4 Conclusions

[^{18}F]FDG, when administered systemically in the recommended diagnostic doses, is a safe substance with no apparent side effects. The estimated effective equivalent dose of approximately 10 mSv for an administered dose of 185–370 MBq is within the range of average radiation exposure when compared with other nuclear medical and radiological methods. Acute radiation damage is not expected, and the possibility of chronic radiation damage can be considered minimal.

References

Baudot P, Jaque M, Robin M (1977) Effect of a diazo-polyoxa-macroobicyclic complexing agent on the urinary elimination of lead in lead-poisoned rats. Toxicol Appl Pharmacol 41:113–115

Baumann M, Schäfer E, Grein H (1984) Short term studies with the cryptating agent hexaoxa-diaza-bicyclo-hexacosane in rats. Arch Toxicol 55 [Suppl 7]:427–429

Berry JJ, Hoffman JM, Steenbergen C, Baker JA, Floyd C, van Trigt P, Hanson MW, Coleman RE (1993) Human pathologic correlation with PET in ischemic and nonischemic cardiomyopathy. J Nucl Med 34:39–47

Dowd MT, Chin-Tu C, Wendel MJ, Faulhaber PJ, Cooper MD (1991) Radiation dose to the bladder wall from 2-(18F) fluoro-2-desoxy-D-glucose in adult humans. J Nucl Med 32:707–712

Fowler JS, Ido T (2002) Initial and subsequent approach for the synthesis of 18FDG. Semin Nucl Med 32:6–12. Review.

Gallagher BM, Ansari A, Atkins H, Casella V, Christman DR, Fowler JS, Ido T, MacGregor RR, Som P, Wan CN, Wolf AP, Kuhl DE, Reivich M (1977) Radiopharmaceuticals XXVII. 18F-labeled 2-desoxy-2-fluoro-D-glucose as a radiopharmaceutical for measuring regional myocardial glucose metabolism in vivo: tissue distribution and imaging studies in animals. J Nucl Med 18:990–996

Gallagher BM, Fowler JS, Gutterson NI, MacGregor RR, Wan CN, Wolf AP (1978) Metabolic trapping as a principle of radiopharmaceutical design: some factors responsible for the biodistribution of 2-deoxy-2-[18F]fluro-D-glucose. J Nucl Med 19: 1154–1161

Hamacher K, Coenen HH, Stöcklin G (1986) Efficient stereospecific synthesis of no-carrier-added 2-[18F] flouro-2-deoxy-D-glucose using aminopolyether supported nucleophilic substitution. J Nucl Med 27:235–238

Huiting JM, Visser FC, van Leeuwen GR, van Lingen A, Bax JJ, Heine RJ, Teule GJJ, Visser CA (1955) Influence of high and low plasma insulin levels on the uptake of fluorine-18 fluorodeoxyglucose in myocardium and femoral muscle, assessed by planar. Eur J Nucl Med 22:1141–1148

Hung JC (2002) Comparison of various requirements of the quality assurance procedures for (18)F-FDG injection. J Nucl Med. 2002 43:1495–1506

Ido T, Wan CN, Casella V, Fowler JS, Wolf AP (1978) Labeled 2-deoxy-D-glucose analogs. 18F-labeled 2-deoxy-2fluoro-D-glucose, 2-deoxy-2fluoro-D-mannose and 14C-2-deoxy-2-fluoro-D-glucose. J Label Comp Radiopharm 14:175–183

Kuge Y, Tsukamoto E, Katoh C, Seki K, Ohkura K, Ohmiya Y, Nishijima K, Tanaka A, Sasaki M, Tamaki N (1999) Synthesis of 18F-FDG with FDG MicroLab system: basic studies for clinical application. Kaku Igaku 36:873–878

Jones SC, Alavi A, Christman D, Montanez I, Wolf AP, Reivich M (1982) The radiation dosimetry of 2-F-18 fluoro-2-deoxy-D-glucose in man. J Nucl Med 23:613–617

Knuuti MJ, Nuutila P, Ruotsalainen U, Saraste M, Härkönen R, Ahonen A, Teräs M, Haarparanta M, Wegelius U, Haapanen A, Hartiala J, Voipio-Pulkki LM (1992) Euglycemic hyperinsulemic clamp and oral glucose load in stimulating myocardial glucose utilisation during positron emission tomography. J Nucl Med 33:1255–1262

McCarthy TJ, Welch MJ (1998) The state of positron emitting radionuclide production in 1997. Semin Nucl Med 28:235–246

Mejia AA, Nakamura T, Mastoshi I, Hatazawa J, Masaki M, Shoichi W (1991) Estimation of absorbed doses in humans due to intravenous administration of fluorine-18F-fluorodeoxyglucose in PET studies. J Nucl Med 32:699–706

Meyer GJ, Coenen HH, Waters SL (1993) Quality assurance and quality control of short lived radiopharmaceuticals for PET. In Stöcklin G, Pike V, eds. Radiopharmaceuticals for positron emission tomography: methodological aspects. Dordrecht Boston London: Kluwer Academic: 91–150

Meyer GJ, Waters SL, Coenen HH, Luxen A, Maziere B, Langström B (1995) PET radiopharmaceuticals in Europe: current use and data relevant for the formulation of summaries of product characteristics (SPCs). Eur J Nucl Med 22:1420–1432

Reivich M, Kuhl D, Wolf A, Greenberg J, Phelps M, Ido T, Casella V, Fowler J, Hoffman E, Alavi A, Som P, Sokoloff L (1979) The [18F] fluorodeoxyglucose method for the measurement of local cerebral glucose utilization in man. Circ Res 44:127–137

Schwaiger M, Büll U, Hör G, Hundeshagen H, Müller-Gärtner HW, Knapp WH, Notohamiprodjo G, Reiners C, Reske SN, Schicha H, vom Dahl J, Nienaber C, Sechtem U, Wolpers HG, Zimmermann R (1996) Indikationen für die klinische Anwendung der Positronen-Emissions-Tomographie in der Kardiologie. Positionsbericht der Arbeitsgruppe PET-Kardiologie der Deutschen Gesellschaft für Nuklearmedizin und des Arbeitskreises Nuklearkardiologie der Deutschen Gesellschaft für Kardiologie Z. Kardiol 85:453–468

Som P, Atkins HL, Bandoypadhyay D, Fowler JS, MacGregor RR, Matsui K, Oster ZH, Sacker DF, Shiue CY, Turner H, Wan CN, Wolf AP, Zabinki SV (1980) A fluorinated glucose analog, 2-fluoro-2-deoxy-D-glucose (F-18): nontoxic tracer for rapid tumor detection. J Nucl Med 21:670–675

Thomas DG, Duthie HL (1968) Use of 2 deoxy-D-glucose to test for the completeness of surgical vagotomy. Gut 9:125–128

Wienhard K, Wagner R, Heiss WD (1989) Grundlagen und Anwendung der Positronen-Emissions-Tomographie. Springer Verlag, Berlin

Woosley RL, Kim YS, Huang KC (1970) Renal tubular transport of 2-deoxy-D-glucose in dogs and rats. Pharmacol Exp Ther 173: 13–20

CHAPTER 5

Image Fusion

U. Pietrzyk

5.1 Introduction

Oncology is one of the important fields that significantly benefits from combining information from different sources. The combination of positron emission tomography (PET) images with those from computed tomography (CT) and magnetic resonance imaging (MRI) is the main example of image fusion, but there are also other combinations, such as the fusion of single photon emission computed tomography (SPECT) with CT or MR images. From these two examples it becomes obvious that image fusion most frequently combines functional images with images from CT and MRI, which provide primarily structural information. Exploiting the possibilities of image fusion increases the reliability of localizing a tumour precisely and differentiating it from other signals, which are probably not specified exactly by a single modality.

Despite the undoubted advantages, which have been expressed in numerous publications, the number of actual applications in a clinical setting is still rather limited and concentrates mostly on radiotherapy and surgery planning.

This chapter will attempt to contribute to a better understanding of the application of image fusion and its benefits, but will also outline major obstacles, which apparently prevent many clinicians from investing the extra effort to exploit image fusion techniques.

5.2 Basic Remarks

As a means of tracing radioactively labelled isotopes within living organisms and bodies, PET dominates the field of molecular imaging because of its unchallenged sensitivity to even the smallest amounts of tracer. Being a tomographic device, PET is able to detect small radiotracer concentrations in three-dimensional space, applying systems capable of imaging whole human brains or other parts of the body. Hence, PET provides both the advantage of a highly sensitive imaging device to detect signals from outside a living subject, while measuring this signal in a way that allows reconstruction of the spatial distribution of such tracers without superposition of signals from other surrounding tissue. The primary interest in applying PET is to measure a tracer distribution and to determine quantitatively the time course of the tracer concentration present at a specified location, rather than to delineate the exact boundaries and location of a morphological or anatomical structure of the subject or organ under study. The limited resolution of the imaging principle underlying PET does not allow a highly sensitive measurement of a tracer concentration, while at the same time determining precisely its position in space. Nevertheless, PET images may exhibit sufficient information, which can be useful for a primary spatial orientation within the imaged volume. This largely depends on the tracer being used during the PET study. Some typical uptake patterns may help to guide computerized algorithms or the human visual system during the comparison of multiple images obtained from the same subject but with different tracers or by different imaging devices.

In general, however, a direct comparison of PET with MR or CT images, placing one image from PET beside another from MRI or CT is not possible, as an exact spatial relation between the different images is not maintained. It is the process of image fusion that enables a direct comparison to be made, which in recent years has become a common procedure in the field of research and also to some extent in clinical work-up.

In the scientific literature, the process of visual presentation of multiple different medical images on a computer screen is called „image fusion“ or sometimes “image integration”. The technical procedures to obtain appropriate images, which are useful for image fusion, are usually discussed under the topic of „image registration“. Image registration algorithms and methods yield images, which then can be fused into a combined representation, usually in a single display on a computer screen. To avoid confusion, we will use the term image fusion as the final goal of the attempt to combine information from different images and to amplify the usefulness of exploring complementary information in the form of functional and morphological images. This term includes the technical prelude of obtaining images suitable for image fusion.

5.3 Properties of PET, SPECT, CT and MR Images Relevant for Image Fusion

Before discussing some technical details of image fusion, we will summarize the major properties of the various imaging techniques. Table 1 shows the properties that are most important for image fusion, including image resolution, matrix size, axial coverage and primary orientation. The most serious problem, and a clear limitation for the application of image fusion and the image quality in general, is the possible and frequent unintentional movement of the subject during image acquisition, or more precisely, during a certain time frame. This is true for both brain and extra-cranial imaging and can only be avoided in brain scanning by applying a rigid head fixation, which, however, is only tolerable for timely correlated surgical interventions. In extra-cranial imaging, i.e. during scans of the thorax or the abdomen, the respiratory motion usually leads to artefacts, but the fact that the relative position of the organs also changes when moving from one examination to another without remaining on the same patient support, has led to the development of combined imaging devices such as those for PET/CT applications. Even then, fast imaging by CT is currently compromised by lengthy PET acquisitions of 30 min or more and, therefore, it is necessary to pursue protocols that respect the limitations of every modality but which are also optimized to yield good quality images helpful to draw meaningful diagnoses.

5.4 Technical Issues in Image Fusion

Many details concerning the technical issues in image fusion have been presented in recent reviews (Hill et al. 2001; Hutton et al. 2002) and books (Hajnal et al. 2001), which also include a discussion of the basic principles and historical development of the techniques; for a comprehensive overview of this field, the interested reader is referred to this literature. Here, we will focus on those aspects most pertinent in applying image fusion to PET in relation to CT and MRI, summarizing the principles involved and emphasizing the benefit of using image fusion for better understanding and interpretation of medical images.

The task to be solved before applying image fusion is to find a transformation, which spatially aligns a set

Table 1. Properties of imaging modalities

	PET	SPECT	CT	MRI
Medical relevance	Function	Function	Morphology	Morphology
Information carrier	Radio-isotope/positron emitters	Radio-isotopes/photon emitters	X-rays	Radio waves
Physical phenomena	e^+e^--Annihilation	Photon detection	X-ray detection	Nuclear magnetic resonance
Measured parameter/contrast	Time course of activity distribution	Time course of activity distribution	Electron density; attenuation coefficient μ	Distribution of protons; relaxation times
Temporal resolution	Min/s	Min	<1 s per slice	Up to 20 images per s
Limitations	Unknown density; photon attenuation; motion artefacts	Unknown density; photon attenuation; motion artefacts	μ dependency on density, element number Z, photon energy; motion artefacts	Magnetic field inhomogeneities; flow artefacts; motion artefacts
Matrix size	128×128	64×64	256×256	256×256
(pixels)	(256×256)	(128×128)	(512×512)	(512×512)
Pixel size (mm^2)	2×2	3×3	1×1	1×1
Slice distance (mm)	2–6	3	2–8	1–8
Slice thickness (mm)	3–7	3	2–8	1–8
Primary orientation	Transaxial	Transaxial	Transaxial	User defined
Axial coverage, single scan (cm)/ special protocols	15–20/whole body (multiple bed pos.)	15–40	15/40 (helical scan)	20/50 (coil dependent)
Resolution (mm FWHM)				
Axial (z)	5–8	6–12	1	1
Transaxial (x-y)	3–8	6–12	0.5–1	0.5–1
No. of slices (typically useful slices)	30–60	30–60	30–50	20–200
Dynamic range (bit)	16	8/16	10–12	12–16
Contrast Low/high uptake	1 : 4	1 : 2		

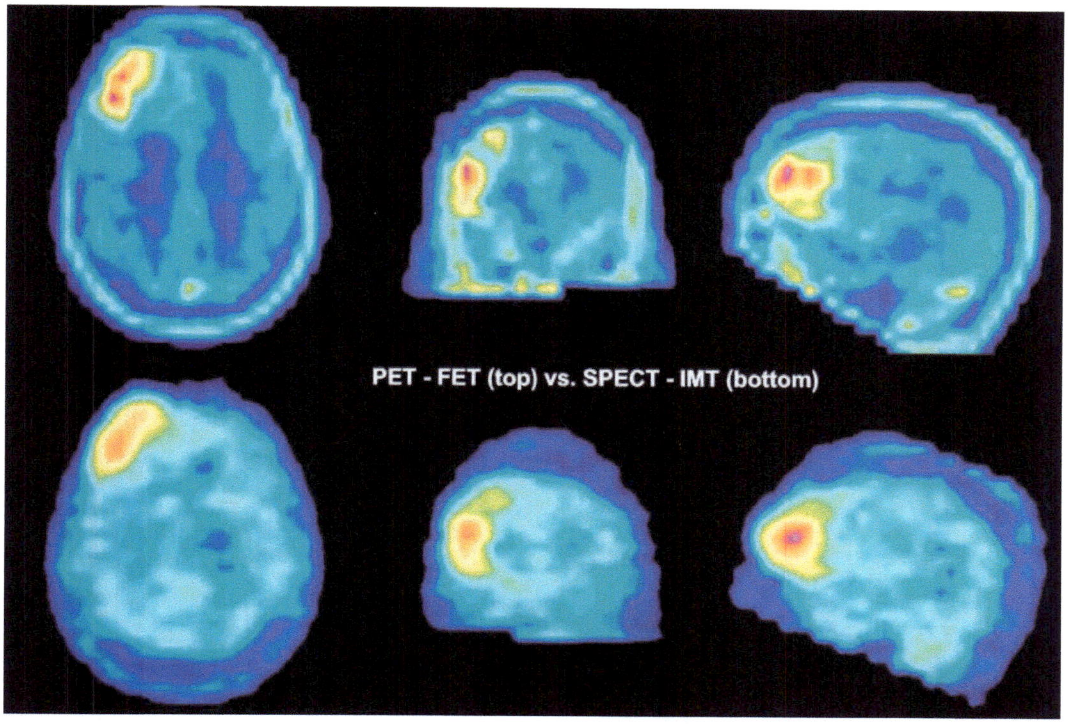

Fig. 1. Image fusion of PET (*top row*) and SPECT (*bottom row*) images. PET data were acquired with O-(2-[^{18}F]fluoroethyl)-l-tyrosine and SPECT images with 3-[^{123}I]iodo-alpha-methyl- l-tyrosine. Although spatial resolution would favour PET imaging, the outline of the tumour tissue is very similar in both modalities. (Courtesy of K.-J. Langen and D. Pauleit, Institute of Medicine, Research Centre Jülich, Germany)

of images with respect to a reference set. A set of images corresponds to a stack of tomograms covered by the field-of-view (FOV). When these images originate from the same subject, a rigid body transformation can be assumed, leaving the number of parameters to be determined with three for rotation and three for translation. Different tracers may yield quite different uptake patterns, thus influencing the strategy to register them. Images of the same type but from different devices, like those from PET and SPECT, are a relevant combination for image fusion (Fig. 1). The classic type of multimodality image fusion, however, encompasses the combination of PET with MRI or X-ray CT, with some diversity in the selection of tracer in PET and pulse sequence in MRI, influencing the contrast and uptake pattern in PET and tissue and contrast differentiation in MRI, respectively. This type of image registration requires a different strategy from those used in PET vs PET registration. As pointed out before, image fusion requires exact registration of the included images. As PET and MRI or CT images provide different, mainly complementary information, this is exactly why fusing them is interesting. However, there is no direct correlation between the images, so a straight line should not be expected when plotting the intensity of all pixel pairs for one image set on the *x*-axis and that of the other image set on the *y*-axis (Fig. 2C). In other words, the signals of white matter tissue in MRI (Fig. 2B) have a different intensity distribution from those of white matter tissue in a PET image (Fig. 2A), disregarding the state of registration. Robust similarity measures have been suggested, mainly with the background of information theory. They can evaluate such two-dimensional distributions (Fig. 2C) and have been applied to determine the transformation to achieve exact spatial registration. One of the most successful measures suggested independently by several authors as described in Hajnal et al. (2001) is „mutual information". It explores both the joint (Fig. 2C) and the two marginal distributions (Fig. 2D, E). For a detailed description the reader is referred to an excellent review by D.J. Hawkes (Hajnal et al. 2001, Chap. 2), which also includes a discussion of a number of other similarity measures proposed in the literature and applied to solve the PET–MRI or PET–CT registration issue.

Evaluating the 2D voxel-intensity histogram is not the only method currently applied for image registration. Prospective techniques follow strict protocols in patient handling, such as marker or head-frame mount-

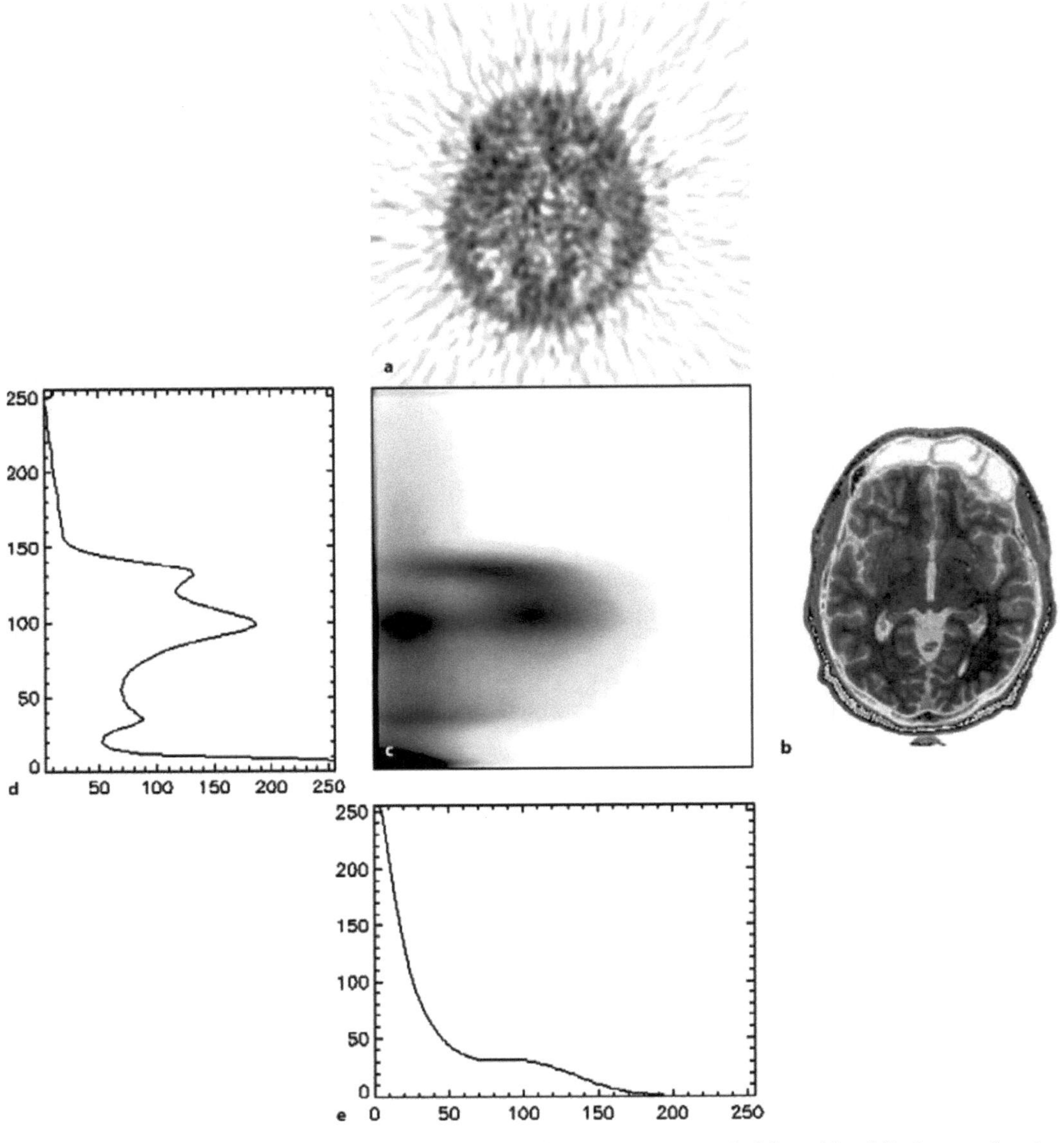

Fig. 2. The centre part (**c**) shows a two-dimensional histogram of intensities of both images, PET (A) and MRI (**b**). The joint distribution in (**c**) and both marginal distributions, (**d**) and (**e**), are used to calculate similarity measures such as „mutual information". Robust measures are required for multimodality image registration such as PET versus MRI, as a simple correlation, which would follow the diagonal shown in (**c**), is not applicable

ing and so far have provided the most precise registration results, required during pre-surgical diagnostics and surgery. Retrospective techniques allow for more freedom in planning the various steps for image fusion. Also, they are easily applicable in situations in which patients are undergoing multiple studies, especially in cases where one imaging modality yields non-conclusive results and requires supplementation by another. Both approaches require detailed logistics in solving the issue of data transfer and data format. This extra effort might explain the reluctance in applying image fusion in a clinically oriented environment, considering the many publications about image registration and image fusion compared to the number of applications for clinical studies.

New systems emerging in the field of medical imaging devices may compensate for this extra logistical effort by combining structural and functional imaging in a single system, such as the combination of PET and CT, which is now provided by a number of manufacturers. This issue is discussed further in Chap. 11.

5.5 Image Fusion in Brain Imaging

The application of image fusion to brain images is relatively easy and has gained considerable interest. In most cases, image registration of brain images from the same subject approximates well to the determination of a rigid body transformation to map the PET image onto the underlying anatomy, based on the solutions mentioned in the previous paragraph. The most frequent applications of image fusion in brain research are (a) pre-surgical diagnostics in tumour studies, (b) uptake pattern of new ligands in receptor studies, (c) early lesion detection in blood flow and metabolic studies, and (d) functional anatomical brain mapping in neuroscience studies. Technically the registration step is mostly solved either prospectively by applying head-frames (a) or by visually controlled real-time interactive procedures (a–c), while automated protocols tend to find application in nearly all fields, when robust algorithms are available. Automated protocols also have an advantage, when a large number of image sets needs to be processed. In a recent study, Thiel and colleagues (Thiel et al. 2001) showed that image fusion between PET images from a language activation study and corresponding MR images is feasible even under clinical conditions. Following a strict protocol applied to more than 60 patients, they were able to extract interesting findings concerning a hypothesized disinhibition phenomenon in patients with frontal or posterior temporal lesions. Figure 3 shows the case of a left-handed female patient with a tumour and an activation (after word repetition) definitely in tumour tissue. Image fusion was obtained after automated registration of a sequence of PET images and interactive registration of PET and MR images. Results from fused images may indeed influence the planning of therapy, including surgery, radiation and chemotherapy. Figure 4 shows a case where image fusion could guide the optimal location for tissue biopsy. MR images showed an extended area of solid tumour mass. PET images, obtained with O-(2-[F-18]fluoroethyl)-L-tyrosine (FET), in contrast, showed focal uptake only in a much smaller volume.

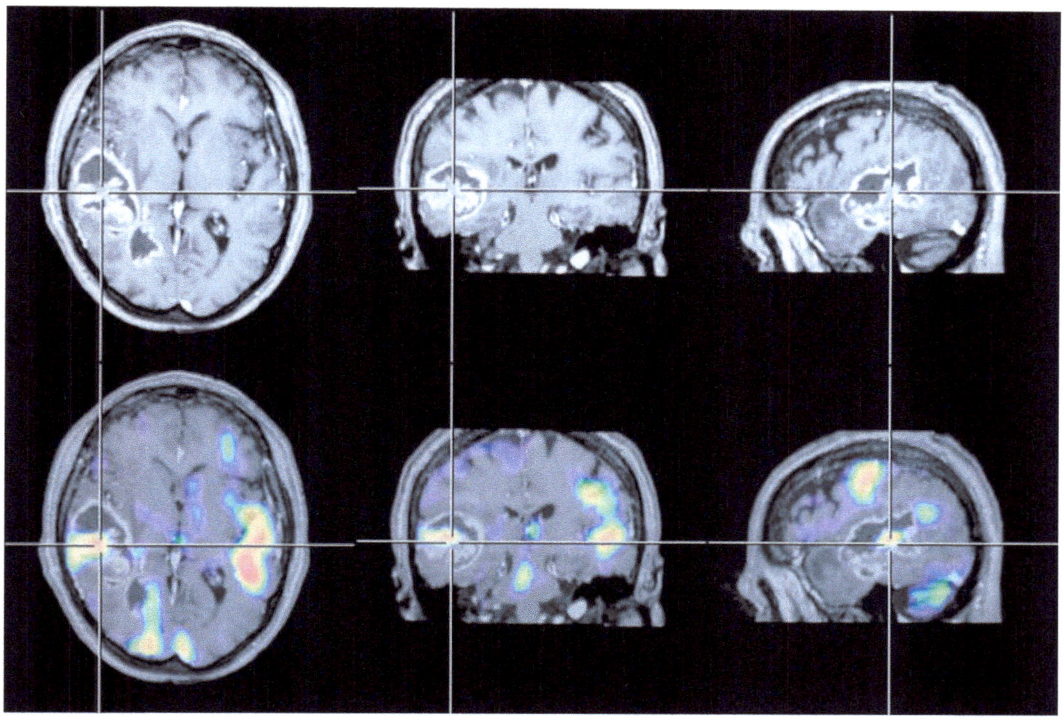

Fig. 3. A „classic" type of multimodality image fusion (MRI, *top row*; PET, *bottom row*), which is often applied in oncological studies within the course of pre-surgical diagnostics. It shows the case of a left-handed female patient with a tumour and an activation (after word repetition), which definitely lies within tumour tissue. (Courtesy of A. Thiel and K. Herholz, Neurological Clinic, University of Cologne and Max-Planck Institute of Neurological Research, Cologne, Germany)

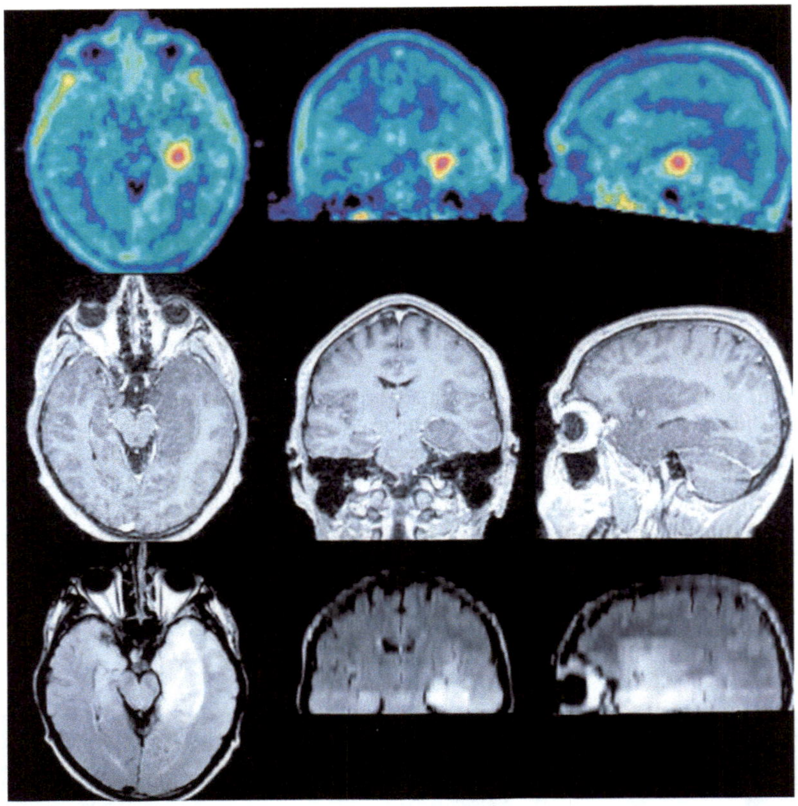

Fig. 4.
PET and MRI fusion: MR (MPRAGE, *middle row*; FLAIR, *bottom row*) images show an extended area of pathology. In contrast, PET images, obtained with O-(2-[^{18}F]fluoroethyl)-l-tyrosine, show a focal tracer uptake in a much smaller volume providing guidance for biopsy. (Courtesy of K.-J. Langen and D. Pauleit, Institute of Medicine, Research Centre Jülich, Germany)

5.6 Image Fusion Strategies for Extra-cranial Images

The situation with extra-cranial images is far more complicated and has not yet entered clinical routine work-up, at least when images originate from separate imaging systems. The reasons for this are manifold. First, the imaging protocols applied at the separate imaging devices are quite different. The FOV in MR imaging is limited to yield good resolution and sampling of the region of interest. In contrast, PET can image larger parts of the body, albeit with multiple bed positions and, hence, is prone to movement artefacts. Second, respiratory movement of the diaphragm, the cardiac cycle and relatively longer data acquisition times combined with variable patient positioning are the main obstacles that hamper a straightforward application of image fusion.

Yet, by carefully adjusting the protocols it was possible to obtain good image fusion results (Wahl et al. 1993; Theissen et al. 2000). Since PET imaging is not meant primarily to provide anatomical information, it was necessary to look for other means to help combining PET images showing patterns of focal uptake with structural images from CT and MRI. Another type of PET image, which resembles low-resolution images from CT, was found to be useful. Such images result from transmission scans, a separate acquisition to obtain an attenuation map required to compensate for photon absorption within the patient's body. These transmission scans are obtained by operating the PET scanner with external sources rotating around the FOV and, hence, are acquired with the patient lying on the same support in an identical manner as for the normal PET emission scans. Such images reconstructed from transmission scans show a clear outline of the body and may serve as a means to link PET images (from standard emission scanning) to CT and MR images. This notion was first described in 1966 by David Kuhl and colleagues (Kuhl et al. 1966). An application using this intermediate set is shown in Fig. 5. By carefully selecting the appropriate acquisition protocols, i.e. similar positioning of the patient's arms and including images from the transmission scan, it was possible to adjust the translations and rotations of the MR images with respect to the PET transmission images and, hence, to the emission images. The problem of identical positions of arms and legs, which might influence the shape of the thorax, can also be solved by introducing an identical support

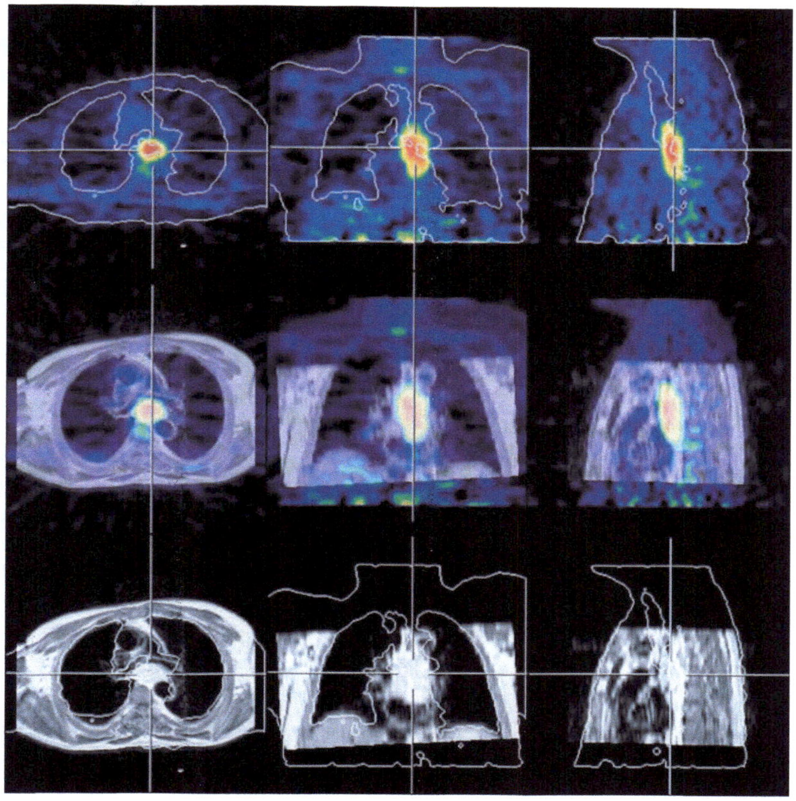

Fig. 5.
Study of the thorax (oesophageal carcinoma) with PET emission images (*top row*), fused images obtained from PET and MRI (*middle row*) and MR images (*bottom row*). Contours shown in the top and bottom parts originate from the PET transmission images and provide essential clues for registration. (Courtesy of P. Theissen, Department of Nuclear Medicine, University of Cologne, Germany)

or coil (for MRI), as was used during the study shown in Fig. 6. For this study of a patient with suspected breast carcinoma, the appropriate coil was used during the MR study and also during the PET examination. Nearly identical positioning was achieved as can be deduced from the contour overlay, with red contours extracted from PET transmission images and white contours extracted from the MR images.

5.7 Combined Devices for Functional-Anatomical Imaging (PET/CT)

A few years ago, a new type of imaging device revolutionized the field of image fusion. It is the combination of PET and X-ray CT in a single system, which allows the study of patients using both types of techniques in close temporal relation. A typical application of a PET/CT system is shown in Fig. 7, with both PET and CT scans covering the same range of the patient's body. The clear outline of anatomical structures and pathologies is helpful in relating to the focal tracer uptake in the PET images. Townsend and Cherry (2001) have provided a recent overview, which also covers the development of such systems. These devices, which may play a very important role in future multimodal tomographic imaging, are discussed further in Chap. 11. Therefore, we have to discuss image fusion from combined devices with the earlier standard of applying software-based solutions. In another example, shown in Fig. 8, it becomes obvious that a single modality alone cannot provide all the necessary clues to obtain a proper diagnosis. In the PET image obtained from a coincidence PET camera, combined with CT imaging capabilities (Bocher et al. 2000), focal tracer uptake is easily detected, although it is not possible to localize precisely where this focus is anatomically. In contrast, anatomical imaging sometimes does not show a significant contrast between healthy and pathologic tissue. Software-based solutions would be difficult to apply in such cases, as there might not be enough structural information on PET emission images to guide the algorithm or the observer to the best solution to register both sets of images.

The combined devices are primarily applied in oncological studies, which frequently aim to examine the whole or larger parts of the body in the search for local tracer uptake as a sign of tumours or metastasis. Most problems apparent with separate imaging systems

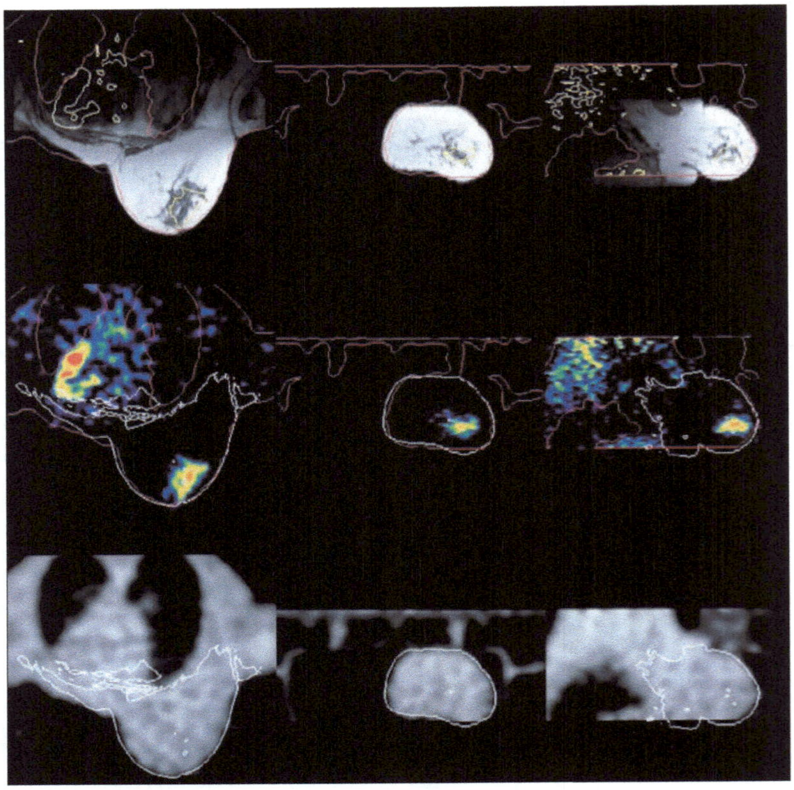

Fig. 6. Image fusion of PET (*top row*) and MR (*bottom row*) images of a patient with breast carcinoma. Image registration was obtained by applying the same positioning system (MRI coil) in both modalities. In addition, PET transmission images were introduced to warrant exact relative positioning, as they provide a clear body outline to be compared to MR images. Red contours are extracted from PET transmission images and white contours originate from MRI. (Courtesy of W. Eschner, K. Scheidhauer and P. Theissen, Department of Nuclear Medicine, University of Cologne, Germany)

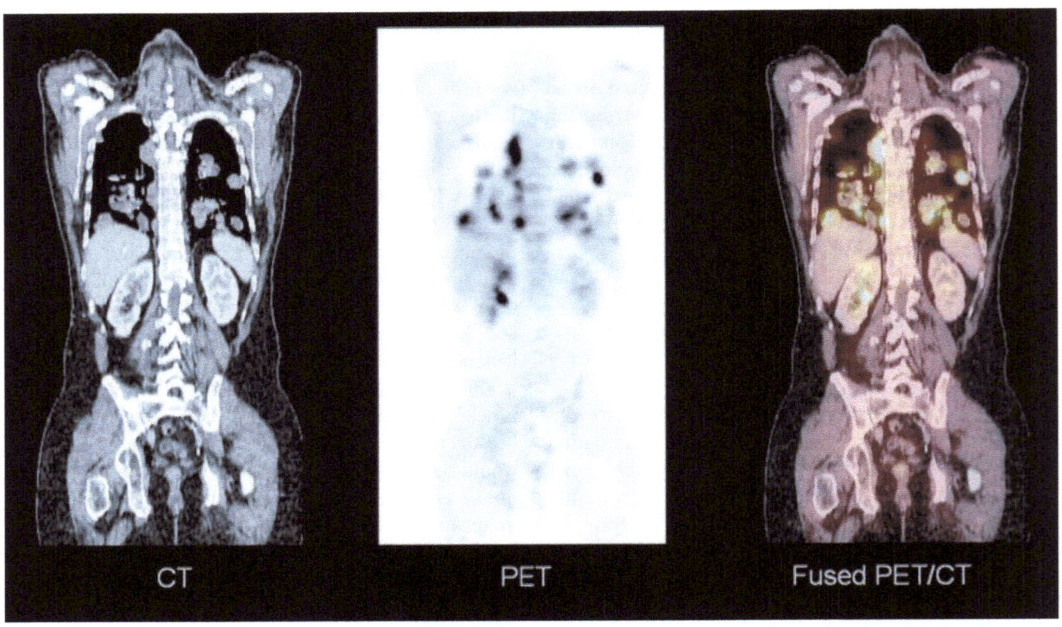

Fig. 7. Typical application of image fusion using a combined PET/CT system. Multiple metastases can be localized precisely as a result of optimal positioning of the patient, who underwent the study in a single session. (Courtesy of L. Freudenberg and G. Antoch, University of Essen, Germany)

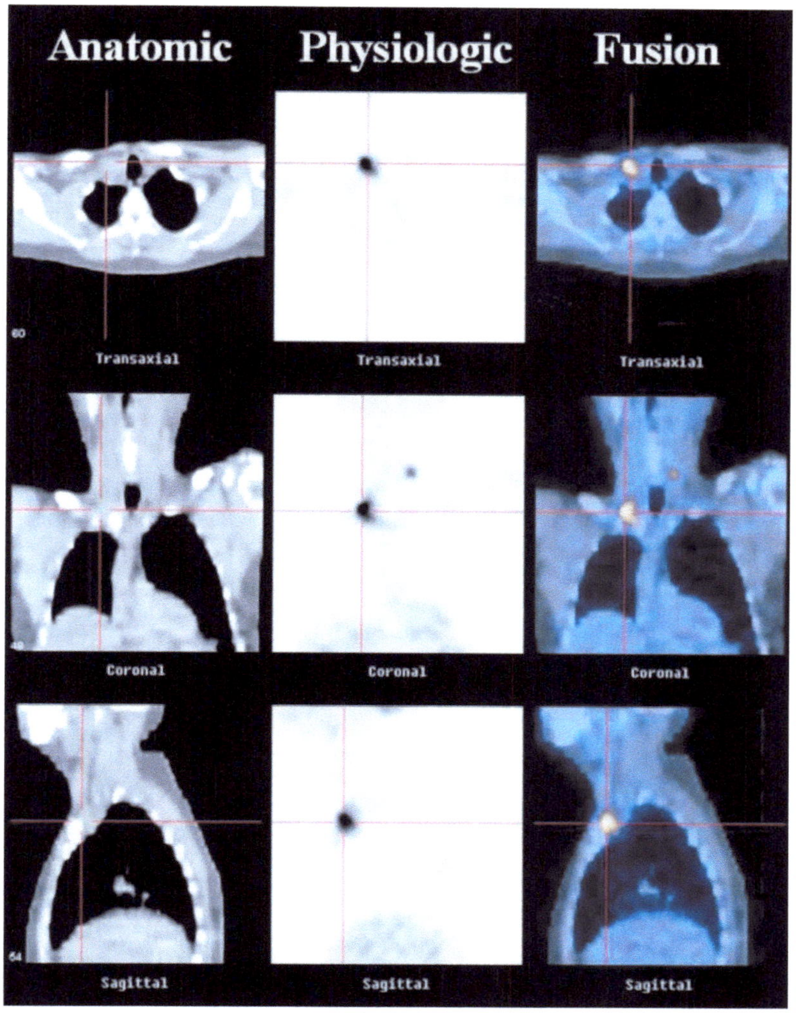

Fig. 8.
When only focal uptake is visible on PET images, it is difficult to correlate such findings to the underlying anatomy. In this example, there is no clear body outline to guide an exact registration. Combined PET/CT systems are a major benefit in such cases. (Courtesy of R. Chisin, Medical Biophysics and Nuclear Medicine, Hadassah University Hospital, Jerusalem, Israel)

could be solved, such as using an identical patient support and the fact that the patient does not need to move from one system to another. Still, there are points to be borne in mind, which require a critical discussion of protocols and results. During imaging with PET the patient has to rest quietly for 60 min or longer, with only the respiratory motion being tolerable. An examination with X-ray CT only lasts minutes at most and needs to be adjusted so as not to cause too many differences in the position of the arms and the diaphragm, which would result in mismatch, invalidating the image fusion. Despite such limitations, these combined devices establish a major progress in image fusion. A second-generation version of the current systems should allow shorter acquisition times for PET imaging by constructing larger detector heads, enabling us to cover a larger fraction of the body at a single bed position.

Software-based solutions for image registration will also remain important with combined PET/CT devices, especially for follow-up studies, where independent sets of images are to be fused. Further developments will also include the option of elastic, non-linear transformations to take into account the position dependence of the patient‘s body shape.

References

Bocher M, Balan A, Krausz Y, Shrem Y, Lonn A, Wilk M, Chisin R. (2000) Gamma camera mounted anatomical X-ray tomography. Eur J Nucl Med 27:619–627

Hajnal JV, Hill DLG, Hawkes DJ (eds) (2001) Medical image registration. CRC Press, Boca Raton

Hill DLG, Batchelor PG, Holden M, Hawkes DJ (2001) Medical image registration. Phys Med Biol 46:1–45

Hutton BF, Braun M, Thurfjell L, Lau DYH (2002) Image registration: an essential tool for nuclear medicine. Eur J Nucl Med 29: 559–577

Kuhl DE, Hale J, Eaton WL (1966) Transmission scanning: a useful adjunct to conventional emission scanning for accurately keying isotope deposition to radiographic anatomy. Radiology 87:278–284

Theissen P, Pietrzyk U, Dietlein M, Schicha H (2000) Image fusion of PET and MRI examinations of chest, abdomen, and pelvis. Eur J Nucl Med 27:S201

Thiel A, Herholz K, Koyuncu A, Ghaemi M, Kracht L, Habedank B, Heiss W-D (2001) Plasticity of language networks in patients with brain tumors: a positron emission tomography activation study. Ann Neurol 50:620–629

Townsend DW, Cherry SR (2001) Combining anatomy and function: the path to true image fusion. Eur Radiol 11:1968–1974

Wahl RL, Quint LE, Cieslak RD, Aisen AM, Koeppe RA, Meyer CR (1993) Anatometabolic tumor imaging: fusion of FDG PET with CT and MRI to localize foci of increased activity. J Nucl Med 34:1190–1197

CHAPTER 6

PET Scanner Quality Control

T.-G. Turkington

6.1 Quality Control Issues

The quality control (QC) related to PET instruments includes specific procedures that are performed on the systems, monitoring of the routine data acquisition process, and inspection of the data produced by the system. As with all QC, a limited amount of time can be spent on a system that is being used effectively. The effort, to be most helpful, should be geared toward uncovering any operational problems in the system, with emphases on those malfunctions that are most likely to occur, and those malfunctions that are most likely to result in problems in the interpretation of the resulting images.

Quality control procedures have been established for specific systems (Spinks et al. 1989; Daghighian et al. 1989; van Balen et al. 1999). A strong emphasis should be placed on understanding the specifics of the particular system being used. PET systems have differences that can impact how best to perform QC procedures. Each manufacturer will provide suggestions and tools for doing QC on its systems, hopefully in a way that will be as effective as possible, while requiring as little labor as possible. Since the details of each system differ, and since the tools provided for performing QC differ, we will not attempt in this chapter to provide details on how to perform QC on each type of PET system. Instead, we will explain some features and procedures that are common to many of the existing systems, and describe some evaluation that be done on the images resulting from any system to assure proper function.

6.2 Basic Ring Function and the Sinogram

A ring-based PET system, as shown in Fig. 1, counts the number of times each pair of detectors is hit simultaneously during the scan. A pair of detectors measures

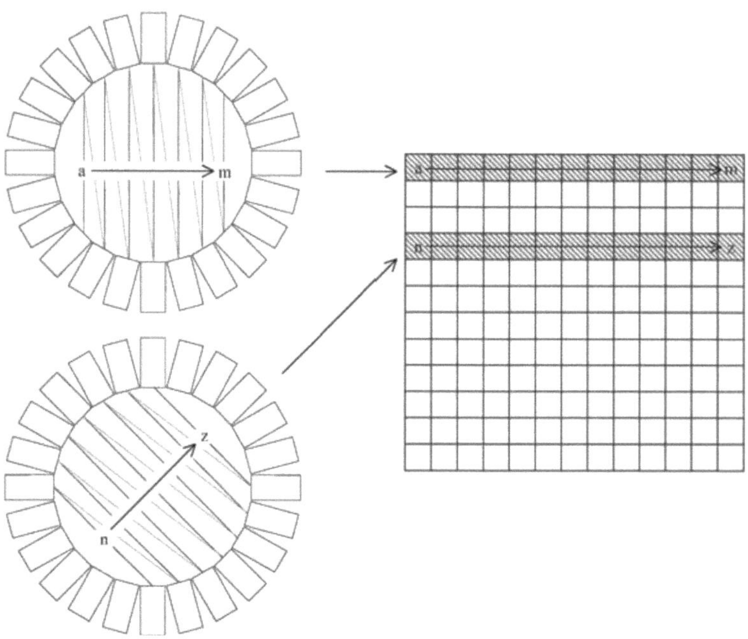

Fig. 1. Relationship between detector pairs (*lines of response*) and sinogram elements. The first sinogram row is filled with numbers representing the counts obtained in the lines representing a vertical projection (*above left*), consisting of appropriate detector pairs. Subsequent rows represent increasing projection angles. In this illustration, adjacent angles are interleaved into a single sinogram row

the amount of radioactivity on the line of response between the detectors. If a ring consists of n detectors, there are $n(n-1)/2$ pairs of detectors (e.g., for 600 detectors there are ~180k pairs). Some of these pairs (for example, neighboring detectors) would measure radiation coming from outside the field of view, which is a cylinder significantly smaller than the ring of detectors itself, so the number of lines of response measured by the system is typically about half of $n(n-1)/2$.

The most common representation of the raw data is the sinogram, a matrix of pixels representing the number of counts measured on each line of response. Each horizontal row of pixels represents a projection angle, that is, all of the parallel lines of response at a specific projection angle. The relationship between lines of response in the detector ring and the pixels in the sinogram is shown in Fig. 1. Increasing the number of detectors in the ring will increase both the number of angles (and therefore, number of rows in the sinogram) and the number of lines of response at each angle (columns in the sinogram).

In Fig. 1, two slightly different angles are interleaved into each sinogram row. Within the central part of the field of view, the slightly rotated angle (represented by dashed lines) samples lines of response between those sampled by the solid light lines, so it reasonable to represent them in interleaved form. An alternate way of forming the histogram would be to make the first row from the solid lines, the second row from the dashed lines, and so on. This representation would have twice as many rows with half as many columns. The first representation yields an approximately square sinogram, with the actual aspect ratio depending on how much of the area within the detector ring is the field of view.

If a detector malfunctions, errors will result in all lines of response associated with that detector. In Fig. 2, the fan of lines associate with a single detector and the corresponding pixels in the sinogram are marked. Each detector in the ring is represented by a diagonal line or by a pair of diagonal lines (as in this case) in the sinogram. A dead detector would give no counts along these lines. A detector with a small gain shift would detect some of the expected counts, but not all. A detector with electronic noise problems might yield more counts than neighboring detectors.

The most common PET system design uses detector blocks (Casey and Nutt 1986) with arrays (e.g., 6×6 or 8×8) of small scintillator crystals read out by four photomultiplier (PMT) channels (either four PMTs, two dual-cathode PMTs, or a single quad-cathode PMT). The sum of the pulses from all four channels indicates the incident photon energy. The system determines which crystal within the block was hit from the relative pulse heights measured in the four channels. A calibration is performed on each block to define a position map, which is the assignment from calculated Anger-like x,y to crystal number. Since PMTs are the most common element within a PET system to malfunction, it is usually expected that a sinogram corresponding to a whole block will demonstrate problems, rather than for a single crystal element.

Figure 3 shows the variety of ways a gain drift in a PMT channel can affect detector performance. In the top row, the relative pulses in the PMTs are shown for photon interactions in four of the six crystal elements. Based on these pulse heights and using the position map, the system can correctly determine which crystal was hit in each case. In the lower row, pulse heights are shown for the situation in which the PMT on the right has reduced gain, and all pulses from it are therefore reduced in amplitude. For the left-most crystal, there is little effect. For the right-most crystal, enough of the total signal (sum of all PMTs) is lost that the event is not considered to be above the energy threshold. For the middle two situations, there may still be enough total pulse height to pass the energy requirement (lower-energy thresholds can be as low as 300 keV, which is much lower than the 511 keV incidence energy). However, the relative pulse heights may cause the event to be assigned to a crystal closer to the left than the actual hit

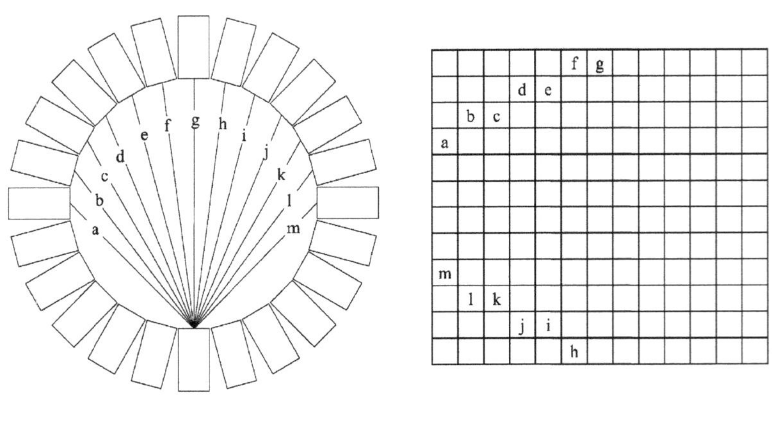

Fig. 2.
Lines of response and sinogram elements associated with a specific detector block

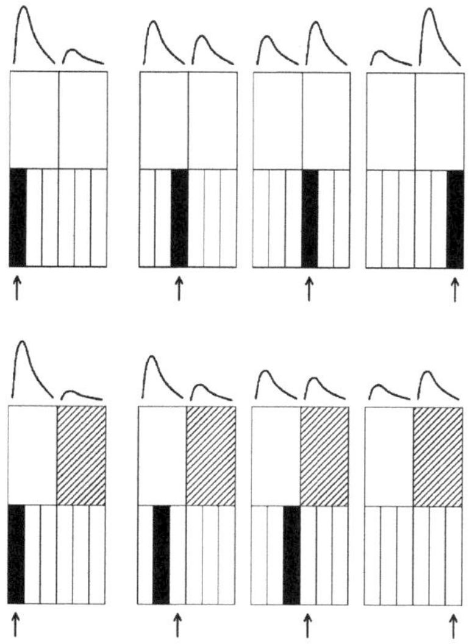

Fig. 3. How PMT gain affects positioning. In the upper row, PMT pulse heights are shown for photons entering four different crystal elements within the block (*indicated by the arrows*). The relative pulse heights are used then to determine which crystal was hit (*indicated by the blackened crystal*). The sum of the pulses provides an energy estimate. In the lower row, the effect of reduced gain in the right PMT is shown. At right, the event is not recorded because the total energy measured is too low. At left, there is little effect. In the middle two cases, the event is recorded, but the crystal is misidentified

location. Therefore, a malfunctioning PMT can lead to lost events as well as mislocated events and the shift of some events away from the malfunctioning PMT may actually lead to higher counts than expected in some of the crystals.

6.2.1 Blank Scan

The blank scan is a transmission scan performed without any attenuating medium (i.e., the patient body) in the field of view of the scanner. It serves two purposes in routine PET operation. One purpose is to provide a reference for the subsequent transmission scans performed on patients. The ratio of the transmission count rate to blank count rate on a line of response is the attenuation factor, which is then used to attenuation-correct the emission counts measured on the same line.

$$A = T/B$$
$$E_c = E_r/A$$

Here, T is the number of transmission counts on a line of response, B is the number of blank counts, A is the attenuation factor (having a value between 0 and 1). E_r is the number of emission counts measured on that line (raw) and E_c is the attenuation-corrected data for that line. (In many cases, instead of this direct correction, the attenuation factors are first used to produce an attenuation image, which is then segmented to reduce noise, and new, lower-noise attenuation factors are calculated from the segmented image.)

The blank scan is also used routinely as a flood scan to determine that all detectors in the system are functioning correctly. A blank scan sinogram from one slice is shown in Fig. 4. The entire sinogram is shown, as well as an enlarged region. The sinogram has some inherent non-uniformities. First, there are more counts on the sides than in the center, for all angles. This is due to the higher sensitivity to radiation from the transmission source for lines of response at the edge. In addition,

Fig. 4. An example blank sinogram, with expanded corner

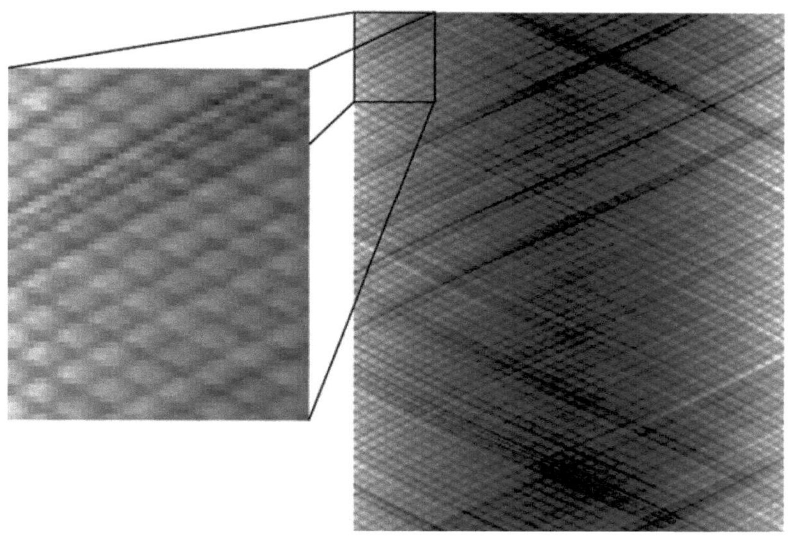

there is a regular pattern of diagonal lines in both directions. These lines are inherent to the block detectors of this scanner. Within a block, edge crystals tend to yield fewer counts than central crystals. All lines of response corresponding to an edge crystal, then, will show fewer counts, resulting in a diagonal sinogram pattern such the one in Fig. 2. Since the scanner from which this sinogram was produced has 6 crystals per block, the lower-intensity lines due to edge crystals repeat every 12 pixels across the sinogram (rather than 6, because of the interleaving of angles.) Lines of response corresponding to two edge crystals (at the intersection of two weak diagonal lines in the sinogram) are particularly weak.

In addition to these expected patterns, this sinogram demonstrates additional non-uniformity. Some of the diagonal lines correspond to an entire detector block giving too few counts. Other lines, such as those seen in the expanded section, correspond to part of a block, indicating that a PMT may have gain problems but not enough reduce the counts everywhere in the block.

Figure 5 shows the evolution of a detector problem over several days. By day five, an obvious band of decreased counts is seen. On the earlier days, the same detector is yielding a much more subtle pattern, with some crystals showing too many counts and some too few, as might happen from misassignment of events from a small gain problem. On the evening of the eighth day, the gains were adjusted, which fixed the problem.

6.3 Impact of Malfunctioning Detectors

The impact of malfunctioning detectors is difficult to predict (Buchert et al. 1999). A block yielding too few counts will not have the severe impact that even a modest PMT problem can have in SPECT, were a small non-uniformity gets amplified into a ring artifact. In Fig. 6, an extreme case is shown, in which the electronic unit processing signals from six adjacent detector blocks was malfunctioning. This yields a broad diagonal band in the blank sinogram with zero counts. Most sites would elect to not use a PET scanner with such an extreme malfunction. The impact on reconstructed images varies, depending on the reconstruction algorithm and

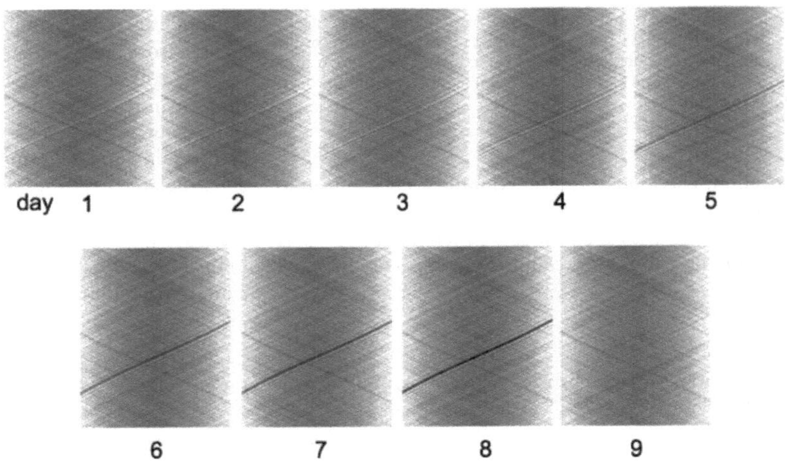

Fig. 5. Evolution of a detector block with drifting PMT. A gain calibration was performed in the evening of day 8, fixing the problem

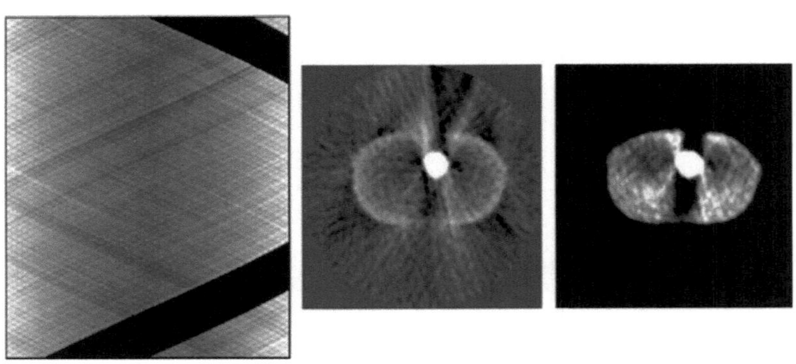

Fig. 6. Images obtained from a system with a severe problem. The blank sinogram indicates that no counts are being collected from several neighboring block detectors. Reconstructed images of an oval phantom with a hot sphere show resulting artifacts. The image in the middle was reconstructed with filtered back-projection and no attenuation correction. The image at right was reconstructed with OS-EM and segmented attenuation correction

the way corrections are performed. Example images are shown for two different reconstructions in Fig. 6. The phantom has an oval cross section, and includes a hot sphere. In either case, a malfunction this severe causes noticeable artifacts, and image quality would have to be considered unacceptable, although many of the regions within the images may still be interpretable. While some correction and reconstruction algorithms may cope better with severe detector problems such as this, no algorithm can completely recover the missed data, and any resulting images should be viewed very cautiously.

6.4 A Simple Daily Protocol

A very basic protocol to demonstrate proper PET system performance for systems with radionuclide-based transmission scanning consists of performing a blank scan and recording the coincidence count rate and scanner room temperature during this acquisition. Any large problems that affect the system globally will cause the count rate to deviate substantially (>5%) from the previous day. Since the count rate can be monitored accurately on a very short time scale, it is possible to discover severe problems within the first minute of the blank scan. Smaller changes in the count rate may be due a small number of detectors drifting or malfunctioning or a small shift in gains throughout the system, such as may be caused by a temperature fluctuation in the scanner room. Problems with individual detectors will show up as non-uniformities in the blank sinograms, so inspecting them is the next step toward diagnosing problems and assuring proper system function.

Unlike on a gamma camera used for SPECT, where small non-uniformities can amplify into noticeable ring artifacts in the reconstructed SPECT images, small non-uniformities in a PET system are generally not only benign, but practically inevitable, and should not prohibit use of the system. It is important, however, to notice changes in the blank quality, since PMT drifts can be gradual, and early detection can allow better planning for maintenance. A useful method for monitoring small changes in the blank scan is to subtract blank images obtained on different days, as shown in Fig. 7. In this case, the subtraction (in most regions dominated by noise) shows that there is a small decrease in the counts obtained from one block detector over the five days between these scans.

Keeping a daily log of blank count rates and on-line sinograms from blanks for several weeks can very helpful if the system is powered down for some period. Whether the power-down was intentional or not, there will be some wait time until the system can be used again. A simple protocol is to wait until the blank count rate is within the range of values obtained over the previous days. Once the rate is up to normal, perform short (5 min.) blank scans until the sinograms are as uniform (disregarding statistical noise) as previous days. Once this level of uniformity is achieved, perform the routine blank at the normal duration.

6.5 Quantitative Accuracy

The raw data of a PET scan consist of the number of counts measured on each line of response during the scan. Images are reconstructed from the raw data, and these images can be scaled so that pixel values represent the radioactivity concentration. For this to happen, several corrections must be in place. By far the most important correction is the attenuation correction. In scans of the abdomen of a large patient, both photons from an emission in the body will make it through all the tissue in fewer than 5% of the events. Very large attenuation correction factors (>20x) are required for each line of response. Smaller, but necessary corrections include correction for detector and system dead-time (a multiplicative factor), correction for random events (a subtraction), and correction for scatter (a subtraction). These three corrections are relatively small (<20%) in clinical imaging in 2D mode, but can become quite large (over 50% of the measured counts can be scattered or random events) in 3D mode.

Just as attenuation causes the largest quantitative inaccuracies of all physical factors, it also causes the most

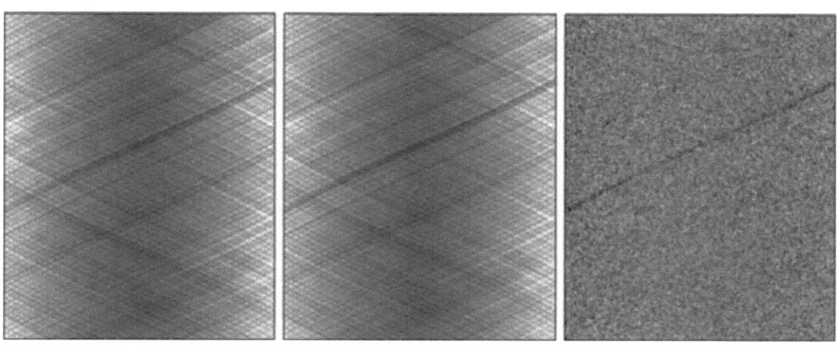

Fig. 7. Blank scan subtraction. A blank scan sinogram from one day (*left*) is subtracted from the blank sinogram obtained five days later (*middle*) and the result is presented on the right. The main difference is statistical noise, but this sensitive test shows that the number of counts measured in one block has decreased slightly

problematic qualitative artifacts. Therefore, large errors in the quantitative accuracy of the images a PET system is producing can indicate problems in the corrections that can also yield qualitative inaccuracy. It is therefore useful to do some QC on the system's quantitation even if high levels of accuracy (< 5 % errors) are not required. Uptake of fluorodeoxyglucose (FDG) in the normal brain is consistent enough that it provides an easy assessment of quantitative accuracy. For example, a 400 MBq dose should yield about 40 kBq/cc in gray matter, within a factor of two or so. Larger discrepancies may indicate problems in the corrections, most likely to be attenuation correction. Even the count rate during a brain scan should be within a relatively small range (compared to the larger range of count rates from the body, depending greatly on patient size).

6.6 Determining Whether or Not to Scan

In some cases, problems with a PET scanner will inherently keep it from being used, such as problems with data acquisition, motion, or computers. In these cases, there is no decision to be made, and the system must be repaired as quickly as possible.

The issue of whether or not to use a PET system whose function is compromised in a less severe way is not as straightforward. Several factors must be considered in making the decision, including the likelihood that the system, in its compromised state, will lead to erroneous interpretation, the relative benefit vs. harm to the patients involved, and the urgency of the studies to be performed. In many cases, a problem can be noted before it is too severe. Appropriate measures can be taken to schedule service for the system. In other cases, a problem appears suddenly overnight, or even during the scanning day. Detector blocks with PMT drifts yielding too-few counts are generally not considered a reason to not scan, but may warrant more frequent blank acquisitions, both the monitor the system, and to provide more appropriate reference for transmission scans if the system is changing during the day. Bigger problems, such as completely malfunctioning detectors or groups of detectors, would generally dictated delaying use of the scanner, though even then special cases will warrant cautious use, such as a patient already having been injected with radiotracer before the problem appears.

References

Buchert R, Bohuslavizki KH, Mester J, Clausen M (1999) Quality assurance in PET: evaluation of the clinical relevance of detector defects. J Nucl Med 40:1657–1665

Casey ME, Nutt R (1986) A multicrystal 2-dimensional BGO detector system for positron emission tomography. IEEE Trans Nucl Sci 33:460–463

Daghighian F, Hoffman EJ, Huang SC (1989) Quality-control in PET systems employing 2-D modular detectors. IEEE Trans Nucl Sci 36:1034–1037

Spinks T, Jones T, Heather J, Gilardi M (1989) Quality control procedures in positron tomography. Eur J Nucl Med 15:736–740

Van Balen S, Hoving BG, Boellaard R, Lammertsma AA (1999) Quality control and calibration of the ECAT HR plus PET scanner. Eur J Nucl Med 26:OS248

PART II

Experimental Oncology

CHAPTER 7

Introduction to Experimental PET in Oncology

P. Oehr

7.1 PET and Molecular Imaging

Positron emission tomography (PET) and single photon emission computed tomography (SPECT) are molecular imaging techniques that use radiolabeled molecules to image molecular interactions of biological processes in vivo. PET imaging technologies have been developed to provide a pathway to the patient from the experimental paradigms of biological and pharmaceutical sciences in genetically engineered and tissue-transplanted mouse models of disease. PET provides a novel way for molecular therapies and molecular diagnostics to come together in the discovery of molecules that can be used in low mass amounts to image the function of a target and, by elevating the mass, pharmacologically to modify the function of the target. In both cases, the molecules are the same as or analogs of each other. PET can be used to titrate drugs to their sites of action within organ systems in vivo and to assay biological outcomes of the processes being modified in the mouse and the patient. The goal is to provide an innovative way of discovery and to accelerate the approval of radiopharmaceuticals and pharmaceuticals. Extending this relationship into clinical practice can improve drug use by providing molecular diagnostics in concert with molecular therapeutics. Diseases are biological processes, and molecular imaging with PET is sensitive and informative to these processes. This sensitivity is exemplified by the detection of disease using PET without evidence of anatomic changes on computed tomography (CT) and magnetic resonance imaging (MRI). These biological changes are seen early in the course of disease, even in asymptomatic stages, as illustrated by the metabolic abnormalities detected with PET and fluoro-2-deoxy-D-glucose (FDG) in Huntington's and familial Alzheimer's diseases 7 and 5 years, respectively, before symptoms appear. Differentiation of viable from non-viable tissue is basially a question of metabolism, as shown by the use of PET to differentiate patients with coronary artery disease who will benefit from revascularization from those who will not. Although beginning within a specific organ, cancer is a systemic disease, the most devastating consequences of which result from metastases. Whole-body PET imaging with FDG enables inspection of glucose metabolism in all organ systems in a single examination to improve the detection and staging of cancer, selection of therapy, and assessment of therapeutic response. In lung and colorectal cancers, melanoma, and lymphoma, PET FDG improves the accuracy of detection and staging from 8% to 43% over conventional work-ups and results in treatment changes in 20–40% of the patients, depending on the clinical question. Approximately 65% are upstaged because unsuspected metastases are detected, and 35% are downstaged because a structural diagnosis of lesions is changed from malignant to benign. Similar results are now being shown for other cancers. The main difference between CT, sonography, MRI, and PET or SPECT is not technologic but, rather, a difference between detecting and characterizing a disease by its anatomic features as opposed to its biology. The importance and success of developing new molecular imaging probes is increasing as PET becomes integral to the study of the integrative mammalian biology of disease and as molecular therapies targeting the biological processes of disease are developed (Phelps 2000).

7.2 Assay Models for Experimental PET

7.2.1 Cell Culture PET

Tumor cells in monolayer culture, which have been treated under different experimental conditions, are incubated in Petri dishes with [^{18}F]FDG or other tracers during tumor imaging for a defined period of time and under different experimental conditions. The reactions can be stopped (e.g. glucose accumulation) by rinsing the cells with tracer-free medium. Quantitative determination of tracer-accumulation/tissue/time culture is performed after locating the Petri dishes on trays in the gantry of a conventional PET scanner (Fig. 1). Photon emission per Petri dish per culture or even per cell can be determined in a single bed position for the entire set of Petri dishes of a complete experiment. More than 100 Petri dishes (3 cm diameter) can be evaluated in a single session. Tracer uptake per cell is calculated by evaluat-

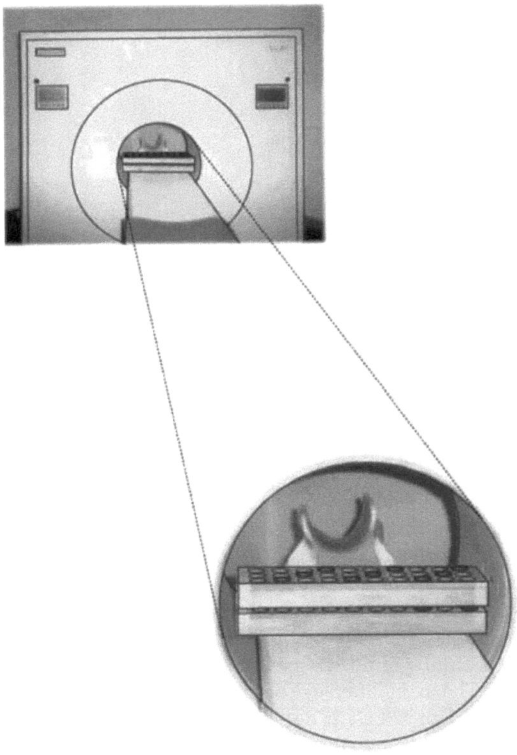

Fig. 1. System for measurement of ^{18}F accumulation in tumor cells grown on Petri dishes, which are located on trays and positioned in the gantry of a PET scanner

ing the regions of interest (ROI) made for each monolayer culture (Fig. 2). Counting the cell number per Petri dish, including a tracer standard, and keeping a defined molarity, allows the number of ^{18}F-FDG-tracer molecules accumulated per cell to be calculated, for example (compare Chap. 8).

7.2.2 Small-Animal Models

While first applications of animal PET were studies of larger animals such as monkeys or dogs, modern molecular biology has shifted the focus towards imaging of laboratory mice and rats. Rats and non-human primates are favorable for research in the field of neuroscience. The capability of the technology in modern molecular biology to "knock out" or disable genes in mice and to "knock in" or insert new genes and to create herewith many types of transgenic mice has made the mouse a preferred model for a large variety of studies. It has also led to new challenges in small-animal PET detector technology and data handling, in the development of radioactive tracers as well as in animal handling.

Yet mice may not be the best model for many human diseases. Breast cancer, for example, is best studied in rats. Tumors in the rat show spectra of hormonal responses that are similar to the human response. The rat is a widely used model in biomedical research and is often the preferred rodent model in many areas of physiological and pathobiological research. Rats are also bigger than mice – making them easier to work with – and their physiology and behavior are well understood.

Mice knockouts are created when genetically modified stem cells are implanted into pregnant females and allowed to develop. Rat stem cells are more difficult to culture, and fail to develop in the womb. Although many genetic tools are available for the rat, methods to produce gene-disrupted knockout rats are greatly needed. A recent important development, however, is the first production of knockout rats using N-ethyl-N-nitrosourea (ENU) mutagenesis and a yeast-based screening assay. By these means the stem-cell approach was bypassed by injecting male rats with a chemical that causes DNA to change at random. The rats were allowed to reproduce, and the mutations were passed on to their offspring. By screening the offspring's DNA, the researchers were able to pinpoint changes in key genes. Zan et al. developed protocols for creating ENU-induced germline mutations in several rat strains. F(1) pre-weanling pups from mutagenized Sprague-Dawley (SD) male rats were then screened for functional mutations in Brca1 and Brca2 using a yeast gap-repair, ADE2-reporter truncation assay. As a result, knockout rats for each of these two breast cancer suppressor genes could be produced (Zan et al. 2003). Women with similar faulty genes (brca1 and brca2) have an increased risk of developing breast cancer.

This new experimental approach might make rats an important tool for future investigation of cancer with small-animal PET scanners.

7.2.3 Small-Animal PET Scanners

Small-animal PET can provide a complete description of the kinetics of the radiotracer in a single animal. This leads to a reduction in the number of animals used, which might be of special importance when using unique, lesioned or genetically altered animals. The potential of small-animal PET to reduce the number of animals could be demonstrated for occupancy studies where a saturation curve produced using post-mortem dissection would require a minimum of three to four animals at each of eight dose points to produce a relatively poorly defined curve. It could be shown that the saturation curves of two ligands for the dopamine transporter were sufficiently well described with a small-animal PET using only 12 animals each. The data could be biomathematically modeled and in vivo dissociation constants could be estimated (Hume et al. 1997; Myers 2001).

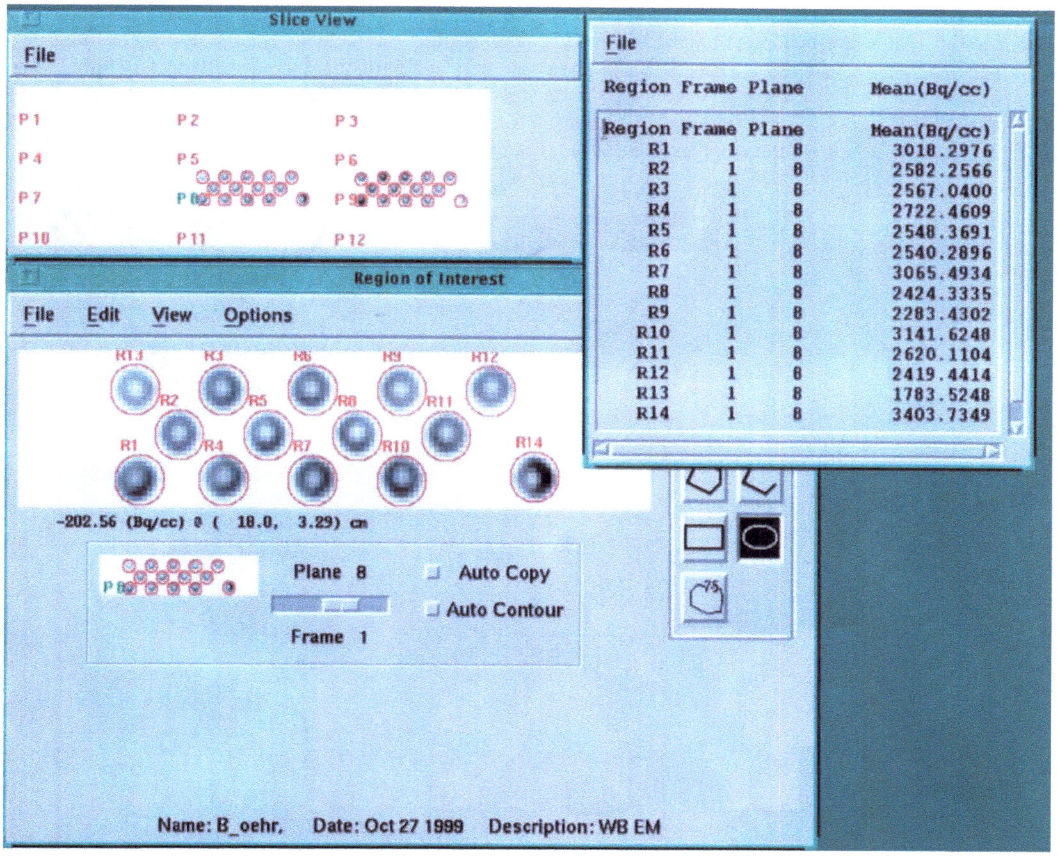

Fig. 2. Quantitative determination of glucose uptake per Petri dish on a tray by evaluating the regions of interest defined for each cell culture. Here, 14 Petri dishes are located on a tray. Six to eight trays can be evaluated in one bed position. The system can be used to calculate the number of glucose molecules accumulated per cell under various experimental conditions

The design of the first-generation animal PET systems has been dominated by the need to improve significantly the detector spatial resolution. Early work was carried out at Sherbrooke University in Canada, where the first animal PET system using solid-state photodetectors was developed (Lecomte et al. 1990). The application of PET technology to small animals such as mice and rats requires dedicated scanners, which have been developed in recent years.

There are four commercially available small-animal PET scanners: the microPET, the quad-HIDAC system, the A-PET and the YAP-(S)PET scanner.

7.2.3.1
The MicroPET

This scanner is marketed by Concorde Microsystems (Knoxville, USA).

7.2.3.2
The Quad-HIDAC System

This scanner has been developed by Oxford Positron Systems (Weston-on-the-Green, UK).

Both the microPET and the quad-HIDAC systems are described in Chap. 9, Fig. 1A and B.

7.2.3.3
The A-PET

A new system, the A-PET, is now available at Philips Medical Systems. The A-PET consists of a discrete $2 \times 2 \times 10\,mm^3$ GSO Anger-logic detector for use in a high resolution, high sensitivity, and high count-rate animal PET scanner. This detector uses relatively large 19 mm diameter photomultiplier tubes (PMT), but nevertheless achieves good crystal separation and energy resolution. The scanner has a port diameter of

21 cm, transverse field-of-view of 12.8 cm, axial length of 12.8 cm, and operates in 3D volume imaging mode. The absolute coincidence sensitivity is expected to be 2.3% for a point source. Due to the use of large PMTs in an Anger design, the encoding ratio (number of crystals/PMT) is high, which reduces the complexity and leads to a cost-effective scanner. Simulation results show that this scanner can achieve NEC rates significantly higher than many of the current generation animal scanners for small cylindrical phantoms due to its high sensitivity and reduced dead time. The scanner is shown in Fig. 3.

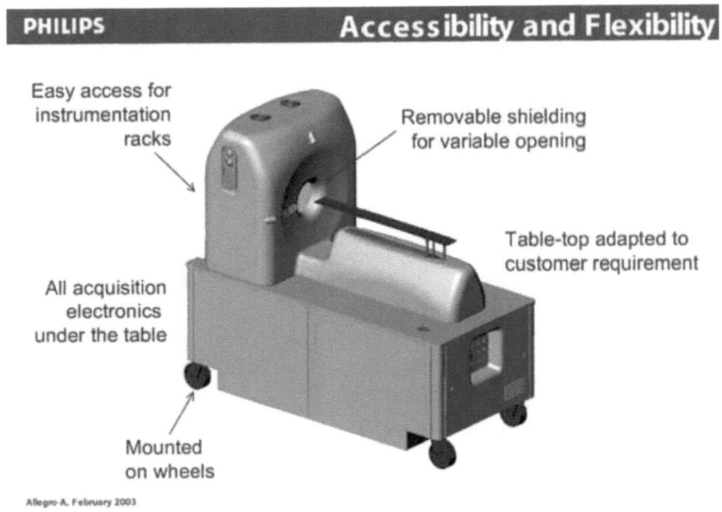

Fig. 3.
The A-PET, Philips Medical Systems animal PET scanner

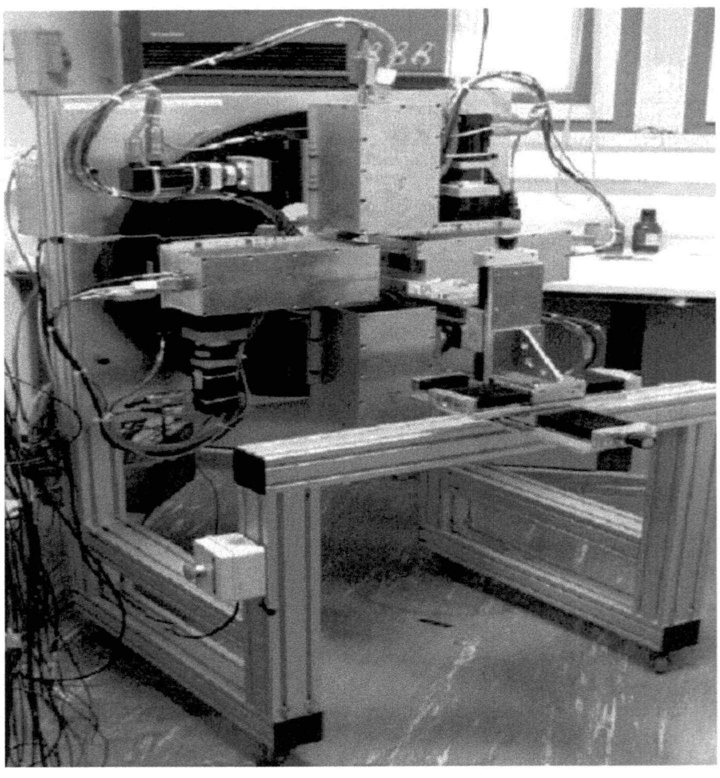

Fig. 4.
The YAP-(S)PET scanner

7.2.3.4
The YAP-(S)PET scanner

The "small-animal scanner" is based on the YAP:Ce detector technology, originally developed by the team of researchers lead by Del Guerra at the University of Ferrara (Italy). The first production unit of the YAP-(S)PET scanner has been installed at the University of Naples "Federico II". Another unit has been installed at the "Ambisen" interdepartmental research center in Pisa, where it will be used to promote cooperation with research teams from other centers in the fields of medicine and oncology, biology and drug research.

The YAP-(S)PET scanner uses the YAP:/Ce pixelized crystal matrix approach, conveniently coupled with position-sensitive photomultiplier technology. This technology has now become commercially available in an affordable off-the-shelf product. The outstanding characteristic of the YAP-(S)PET scanner is the ability to execute both PET and SPECT with the same equipment. This is due to the fact that the YAP:Ce crystal matrix is effective in detecting 511 keV radiation for PET, and also generates enough light for detecting low-energy gammas for SPECT. This provides an accurate and versatile instrument for all functional imaging investigations on mice and rats, for laboratory studies.

The YAP-(S)PET scanner is shown in principle in Fig. 4. However, different scanner configurations are available:

1) YAP-PET-2: This configuration includes two detector heads, coincidence electronics and software for PET scans and analyses;
2) YAP-SPET-2: Equivalent to the above, but includes two removable lead collimators, electronics and software suited for both PET and SPECT analysis;
3) YAP-PET-4: This configuration includes four detector heads, coincidence electronics and software for PET scans and analyses;
4) YAP-SPET-4: Equivalent to the above, but includes four removable lead collimators, electronics and software suited for both PET and SPECT analysis.

7.2.4
Multimodal Mouse Phantom for Fusion Imaging

Isotope Products Laboratories new multimodal mouse phantom is a true multimodal lesion phantom in a sealed source. Designed for quantitative CT/PET and CT/SPECT fusionimaging, it requires no mixing, filling or assembly (Fig. 5). Fillable phantom lesions are surrounded by "cold" capsules, reducing accuracy and limiting the size of the spot. Isotope Products Laboratories technique embeds the hot spot directly in the background activity, allowing true quantitative QC of hot spots as small as 1×1 mm. Also embedded in the background matrix is a bone-equivalent "skeleton" featuring "bones" as small as 0.5 mm diameter. It is so far the only sealed-source phantom with CT visibility and multimodal imaging QC capability. The specifications are shown in Table 1.

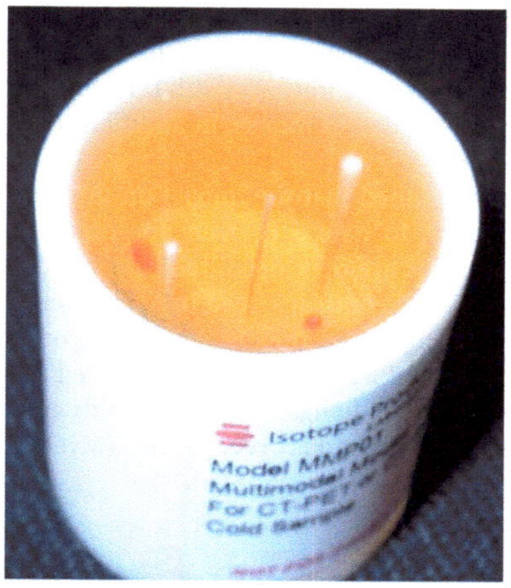

Fig. 5. The mouse PET phantom

Table 1. Specifications of the IPL multimodal mouse phantom for fusion imaging

PET/SPECT lesions	1×1 mm, 2×2 mm, 3×3 mm, imbedded directly in the background activity
CT targets	0.5 mm, 1.3 mm, 2.0 mm, bone-equivalent „skeleton“
Background activity	74 kBq/ml (2 μCi/ml)
Hot-spot activity	740 kBq/ml (20 μCi/ml)
Total activity	2.8 MBq nominal (75 μCi)
Nuclides available	Co-57 for CT/SPECT and Ge-68 for CT/PET
Active dimensions	3.5 cm diameter × 3.5 cm high

7.3
Conclusions

According to the improvements described above, the prospect of in vivo imaging of small animals becomes attractive. Purpose-built PET scanners capable of imaging individual tissues are now in routine experimental use. The study of small animals in this way does have intrinsic problems and constraints associated with it. For example, the animal must be completely immobilized, stable ligand within the radiolabeled preparation may be limiting and anatomical definition may be poor. In spite of this, consistent, semi-quantitative data can be produced and in vivo radio-imaging can provide a genuine and unique complement to more conventional techniques. Animal numbers can be significantly reduced and the quality of data improved due to reduced inter-animal variation, and longitudinal studies, to monitor disease progression, are feasible. As the resolution of imaging systems improves still further, such studies could be extended to mouse, in addition to rat, models of disease.

It has to be mentioned that the impact on the pharmaceutical industry, to date, has been anecdotal. As new chemical entities are developed, radiotracers that aid in characterizing these drugs need to be developed rapidly to have an impact on the development process. The combined use of PET and gene-manipulated animal models to validate radioligands quickly holds great promise for accelerating the discovery process (Myers et al. 1999; Eckelman 2003; Zan et al. 2003).

References

Eckelman WC (2003) The use of PET and knockout mice in the drug discovery process. Drug Discov Today 8:404–410

Hume SP, Brown DJ, Ashworth S, Hirani E, Luthra SK, Lammertsma AA (1997) In vivo saturation kinetics of two dopamine transporter probes measured using a small animal scanner. J Neurosci Methods 76:45–51

Lecomte R, Cadorette J, Jouan A, Heon M, Rouleau D, Gauthier G (1990) High resolution positron emission tomography with a prototype camera based on solid state scintillation detectors. IEEE Trans Nucl Sci 37:805–811

Myers R (2001) The biological application of small animal PET imaging. Nucl Med Biol 28:585–593

Myers R, Hume S, Bloomfield P, Jones T (1999) Radio-imaging in small animals. J Psychopharmacol 13:352–357

Phelps ME (2000) PET: the merging of biology and imaging into molecular imaging (review). J Nucl Med 41:661–681

Zan Y, Haag JD, Chen KS, Shepel LA, Wigington D, Wang YR, Hu R, Lopez-Guajardo CC, Brose HL, Porter KI, Leonard RA, Hitt AA, Schommer SL, Elegbede AF, Gould MN (2003) Production of knockout rats using ENU mutagenesis and a yeast-based screening assay. Nat Biotechnol 21:645–651

CHAPTER 8

PET in Cell Cultures: Oncology, Genetics, and Therapy

P. Oehr · N. Gilbert · H. Lemmoch · M. Ludwig
R. Wagner · H. Schüller · H. Rink

The aim of the studies was to investigate the effects of irradiation and/or chemotherapy in tumor cells and in radiosensitive wild-type mutants as a tool to understand the biological base and mechanisms of modulation of 2-[^{18}F]fluoro-2-deoxy-D-glucose accumulation.

8.1 Introduction

2-[^{18}F]Fluoro-2-deoxy-D-glucose ([^{18}F]FDG) has been shown to be a useful radiopharmaceutical for the quantitative determination of regional glucose metabolism, and it localizes in the brain, heart and in tumors. Higher rates of glucose metabolism have been observed in cancer cells for many years, and the significance of this fact for detection of increased cellular metabolism by [^{18}F]FDG in cancer cells has also been recognized. A group of transport proteins enables glucose and glucose derivatives to enter or leave animal cells (see Chap. 3). [^{18}F]FDG is now the most frequently used radiopharmaceutical in positron emission tomography (PET). Administered doses, scan parameters and evaluation protocols have generally been determined empirically and optimized as a result of pragmatic considerations.

The relationship between administered dose and cumulative concentration in the target organ and in the surrounding tissue (background), on one hand, and the resulting image quality (e.g. detectability of small lesions), on the other hand, depends on the mechanism of [^{18}F]FDG accumulation in cells and the clearance rate of the body by the urogenital system.

When appropriately labeled substrate analogues are used, it is not just the flow of blood or plasma that determines the amount of radioactivity that reaches the tissue but also (and more significantly) the cellular transport and/or intracellular metabolic reactions (e.g. transport and phosphorylation in the case of FDG).

A similarity exists in the metabolic pathways of glucose and of glucose and FDG when the sugars are accumulated by the cell. One phosphate molecule with the alcohol group is added to the sixth carbon atom of a glucose or FDG molecule. This requires the activity of the enzyme hexokinase, which is localized in the cells. In this case glucose and FDG compete for the enzyme binding site. The phosphorylated molecules, glucose-6-phosphate and 2-FDG-6-phosphate, cannot leave the cell. This biochemical pathway of 2-FDG has been called the trapping mechanism (Horton et al. 1973; Gallagher 1978). Due to the trapping mechanism and the increased accumulation in tumors, FDG-6-phosphate can be called a tumor marker.

In patients with cancer, the [^{18}F]FDG method is used for diagnostics and follow-up studies.

In both cases it is important to know whether increased accumulation of ^{18}F activity is caused only by cell proliferation or whether other mechanisms could induce increased uptake as well.

We investigated the dose-dependent change of [^{18}F]FDG uptake in the presence of an irradiation-induced inhibition of cell growth after irradiation under different experimental conditions in different cell culture systems.

8.2 Material and Methods

HeLa cell lines, and wild-type AA8 (not radiation sensitive) or mutant EM9 (radiation sensitive) Chinese hamster cells originated from ATCC, Manassas, Virginia (USA), and [^{18}F]FDG in physiological NaCl solution came from the Forschungszentrum Karlsruhe, or from MPI fuer neurologische Forschung Koeln, Germany).

Cells were irradiated by an X-ray tube (Müller RT 200) with a 200 kV, 0.5 mm Cu filter and a focus distance of 25 cm. These parameters result in a dose rate of 3.75 Gy/min.

Irradiation experiments over a period of several days were started at the onset of the growth phase with 0–30 Gy, with and without chemotherapy, and stopped after 72 hours. For in vitro tumor cell [^{18}F]FDG uptake assays, the cell lines were cultured in plastic Petri dishes containing Dulbecco's Modified Eagle's Medium at 36°C with 10% fetal calf serum. Assays were made by incubations of the monolayer cultures in triplicate with [^{18}F]FDG in phosphate-buffered saline (PBS) buffer, pH 7.2. The reactions were started or stopped by washing the cells three times with PBS buffer.

[^{18}F]FDG uptake was simultaneously determined in a PET gantry, evaluation was made by regions of interest. Cell-bound ^{18}F activity was counted by measurement of the photon emission in the gantry of a Siemens EXACT ECAT 927/47 camera.

8.3 Results

When HeLa cells are incubated with [^{18}F]FDG for 30 minutes, a constant accumulation of ^{18}F activity is observed (Fig. 1). This kind of assay shows that HeLa cells can transport and accumulate [^{18}F]FDG.

Irradiation of HeLa cells shows an inverse relation of cell numbers to increasing X-ray doses (Fig. 2). Proliferation is reduced at 5 Gy, and the cell number decreases at 10–50 Gy.

Accumulation of ^{18}F activity/cell by irradiated cells after 30 minutes incubation with [^{18}F]FDG increased in the cultures within 48 hours. This increase was correlated to the increase of irradiation dose. This can be demonstrated by plotting the relation of ^{18}F accumulation by irradiated cells in relation to the accumulation by the non-irradiated cells (Fig. 3).

Basic data in untreated AA8 and EM9 cells were similar. Irradiation of the cells led to a dose-dependent strong inhibition of cell proliferation, increased ^{18}F accumulation/cell and hexokinase activity/cell, which were higher in radiation-sensitive cells compared to the wild-type (Figs. 4, 5). Chemotherapy could inhibit the irradiation effects.

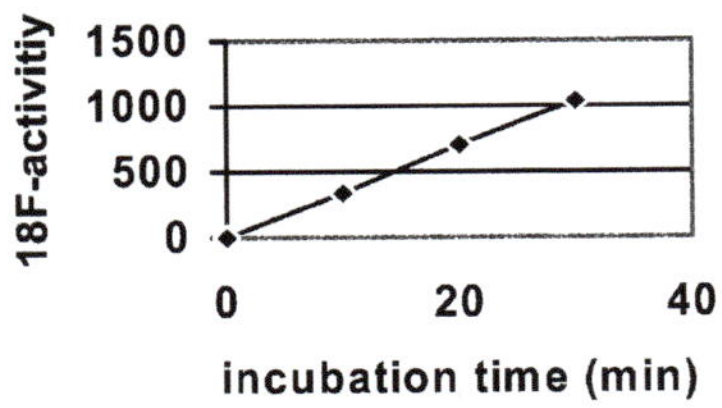

Fig. 1. Accumulation of [^{18}F]FDG in HeLa tissue culture (becquerels/cubic centimeter)

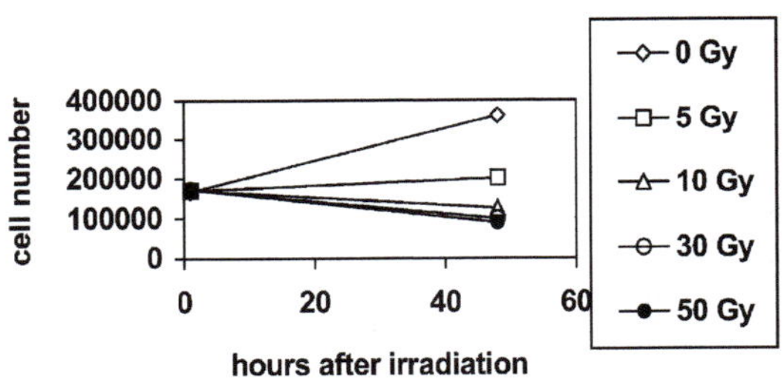

Fig. 2. Effect of irradiation on HeLa cell proliferation

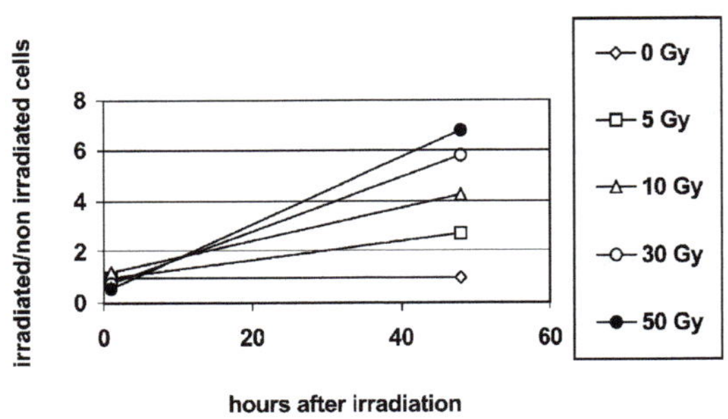

Fig. 3. Effect of irradiation on [^{18}F]FDG accumulation/cell: relationship of irradiated/not irradiated cells (HeLa)

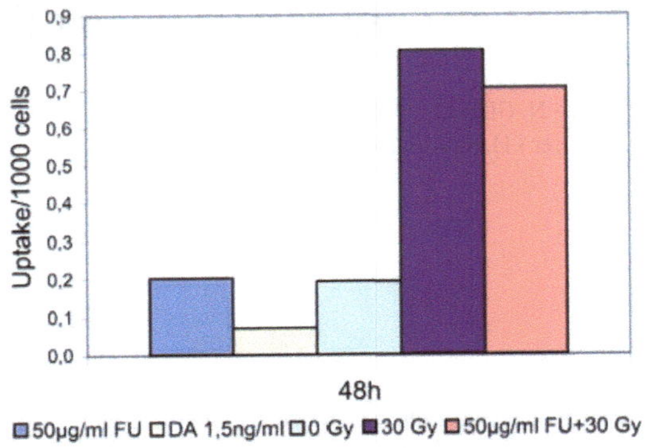

Fig. 4. [^{18}F]FDG uptake (nCi/cc) in EM9 cells (radiation-sensitive mutant cells)

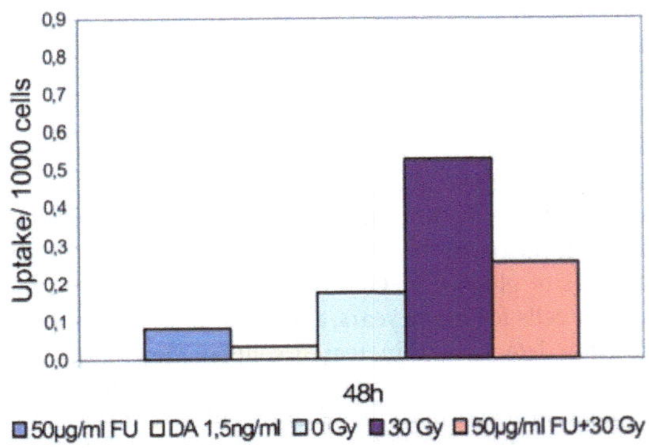

Fig. 5. [^{18}F]FDG uptake (nCi/cc) in AA8 cells (insensitive cells)

8.4 Discussion

The clinical significance of [^{18}F]FDG is based on the fact that tumor cells take up more glucose in comparison with normal cells. An increased uptake of [^{18}F]FDG in tumor cells and the detection of this uptake using PET permit a quantitative analysis. The mechanisms of FDG uptake have not yet been fully explained. Discussion centers on whether they are controlled by the proliferative activity of cells or by other parameters. We investigated the change in [^{18}F]FDG uptake after irradiation with doses of different strengths.

The experimental studies on [^{18}F]FDG uptake in HeLa cells were carried out with FDG concentrations of less than 1 μmol/l and focused on a time period of 30 minutes. Under these conditions, no inhibition of cell growth can be expected. The linearity of the [^{18}F]FDG uptake within a time period of 30 minutes demonstrates that the measurement reflects the period of maximum uptake, and the measured uptake activity reflects the [^{18}F]FDG transport into the cells. In tumor cells, therefore, an increase in the radiation dose brings about an increase in [^{18}F]FDG transport in particular. The dose-dependent change in [^{18}F]FDG uptake is an indication of the proliferation-independent mechanism of [^{18}F]FDG uptake, especially when [^{18}F]FDG uptake increases concomitantly with inhibition of cell division caused by radiation. Since an inflammatory reaction can be excluded as the source of the increased [^{18}F]FDG uptake, it seems obvious to consider repair processes with their increased energy requirements as an explanation for the changed behavior of the cells. The dose-dependent increase suggests an increasing need for repair.

Similar results were obtained with the [^{18}F]FDG PET examination of a patient with two lymph node tumors of a papillary thyroid cancer; the patient received a total dose of 30/60 Gy, respectively. On the basis of this therapy, there was a short-term increase in ^{18}F uptake. Additional examinations featuring an antigranulocytic scan showed an additional increase in [^{18}F]FDG uptake, caused by inflammation, in the area of the metastases (Hautzel et al. 1997).

On the other hand, experimental studies on spheroids from a human adenocarcinoma cell line showed a balance of increased [^{18}F]FDG uptake in surviving cells and an absence of uptake in dead cells after a single irradiation of 6 Gy, with the result that there was no significant change in [^{18}F]FDG uptake per volume unit of the spheroids (Senekowitsch-Schmidtke et al. 1998). In studies involving rats with tumor transplants, it has been observed that after a single irradiation of 10 Gy, radiation-sensitive tumor cells demonstrated a significant two- to threefold increase in the accumulation of ^{18}F within a period of 2–6 hours after irradiation, whereas radiation-insensitive tumors showed an insignificant and low increase of ^{18}F activity (Furuta et al. 1997). If [^{18}F]FDG PET studies are carried out at shorter intervals after the beginning of radiation therapy, clear increases in ^{18}F uptake can be detected. In four patients with intracranial tumors who received 15–27.5 Gy, there was an increase in glucose uptake of 25–42 % 1 day after irradiation; this receded 7 days later and then remained within the range of 10 % above to 12 % below the pretherapeutic basic uptake level (Rozental et al. 1991).

In other studies with 44 and 21 patients, respectively, it was reported that in many patients a decrease in ^{18}F uptake was detectable 3 months after radiation therapy, but that in some cases it was not possible to differentiate between proliferation, repair processes, inflammation and remaining vital tumor tissue (Haberkorn et al. 1991; Engenhart et al. 1992).

8.5 Conclusion

It is possible to detect the dose-dependent increase in [^{18}F]FDG accumulation in HeLa tumor cells using a simple system of cell culture, X-ray tube and PET. It is also possible to investigate these effects in mutants having different radiation sensitivity with and without simultaneous addition of drugs used in therapy of tumors.

This observed increased uptake is triggered by a mechanism independent of cell proliferation, and can presumably be traced to the increased energy requirements of cells during repair processes. These can be differently influenced by drugs interfering with nucleotide or protein synthesis.

Basic data in untreated AA8 and EM9 cells demonstrated that irradiation of the cells led to a dose and genetic disposition-dependent inhibition of cell proliferation. Increased [^{18}F]FDG accumulation/cell and hexokinase activity/cell were higher in radiation-sensitive cells compared to the wild-type. Chemotherapy could inhibit the irradiation effects. As a conclusion, increased irradiation-induced [^{18}F]FDG uptake in the investigated cells may be related to a proliferation-independent increase of hexokinase activity. This uptake increases to levels above those of non-irradiated proliferating tumor cells, is related to the genetic disposition of radiosensitivity and seems to be based on a network of dose- and time-dependent intracellular stress mechanisms, which can be inhibited by chemical drugs. The results give rise to the assumption that there are limits to make reliable FDG PET diagnostics based on the hypothesis of cell proliferation-dependent FDG uptake during radio- and/or chemotherapy.

The user of PET should also be conscious of the fact that the signal he receives from a treated tissue is dependent on the cell number and uptake of radiotracer per cell. PET alone can only refer to the signal of radioactive decay; it provides, however, no information about the cell mass or number of cells. PET-CT may be an approach that partially solves this problem.

From the experimental and clinical studies discussed here, it emerges that three factors can lead to an increase in [^{18}F]FDG uptake after irradiation of tumors in patients: proliferation, inflammation and repair processes. Accordingly, during the [^{18}F]FDG PET examination it must be clarified whether an increased ^{18}F uptake after radiation therapy occurs as a result of the dose, or whether the tumor tissue has proliferated independent of therapy and more [^{18}F]FDG is being taken up for this reason. It is therefore important to determine the point in time at which an increase in [^{18}F]FDG uptake that is independent of tumor growth no longer appears in patients. Further systematic studies of irradiated cell cultures can provide information on this point.

References

1. Engenhart R, Kimming BN, Strauss LG, Hover KH, Romahn J, Haberkorn U, van Kaick G, Wannenmacher M et al (1992) Therapy monitoring of presacral recurrences after high-dose irradiation: value of PET, CT, CEA and pain score. Strahlenther Onkol 168:203–212
2. Furuta M, Hasegawa M, Hayakawa K, Yamakawa M, Ishikawa H, Nonaka T, Mitsuhashi N, Niibe H et al (1997) Rapid rise in FDG uptake in an irradiated human tumour xenograft. Eur J Nucl Med 24:435
3. Gallagher BM, Fowler JS, Gutterson NI, MacGregor RR, Wan CN, Wolf AP (1978) Metabolic trapping as a principle of radiopharmaceutical design: some factors responsible for the biodistribution of [18F] 2-deoxy-2-fluoro-D-glucose. J Nucl Med 19:1154–1161
4. Haberkorn U, Strauss LG, Dimitrakopoulou A, Engenhart R, Oberdorfer F, Ostertag H, Romahn J, van Kaick G et al (1991) PET studies of fluorodeoxyglucose metabolism in patients with recurrent colorectal tumors receiving radiotherapy. J Nucl Med 32:1485–1490
5. Hautzel H, Muller-Gartner HW et al (1997) Early changes in fluorine-18-FDG uptake during radiotherapy. J Nucl Med 38:1384–1386
6. Horton RW, Meldrum BS, Bechelard HS (1973) Enzymatic and cerebral metabolic effects of 2-deoxy-D-glucose. J Neurochem 21:506–520
7. Rozental JM, Levine RL, Metha MP, Kinsella TJ, Levin AB, Algan O, Mendoza M, Hanson JM, Schrader DA, Nickles RJ et al (1991) Early changes in tumor metabolism after treatment: the effects of stereotactic radiotherapy. Int J Radiat Oncol Biol Phys 20: 1053–1060
8. Senekowitsch-Schmidtke R, Matzen K, Truckenbrodt R, Mattes J, Heiss P, Schwaiger M et al (1998) Tumor cell spheroids as a model for evaluation of metabolic changes after irradiation. J Nucl Med 39:1762–1768

CHAPTER 9

Small-Animal PET in Oncology

M. Honer · M. Brühlmeier
I. Novak-Hofer · S. Ametamey

9.1 Dedicated Small-Animal PET Cameras

9.1.1 Commercial Small-Animal PET Systems

The application of positron emission tomography (PET) technology to small animals such as mice and rats requires dedicated scanners, which have been developed in recent years. Two types are commercially available so far: the microPET (Fig. 1a) marketed by Concorde Microsystems (Knoxville, USA), and the quad-HIDAC system (Fig. 1b) developed by Oxford Positron Systems (Weston-on-the-Green, UK). Similar to clinical PET tomographs, the microPET camera is based on scintillation crystals arranged in a detector ring (Chatziioannou et al. 1999). The microPET system uses lutetium oxyorthosilicate as scintillation crystals coupled by optical fibers to multichannel photomultiplier tubes. The scanner has a volumetric resolution of approximately 6 mm^3 in the center of the field-of-view, which extends 10 cm axially. The camera's raw detection efficiency is 2.4%.

The quad-HIDAC system consists of high-density avalanche chamber (HIDAC) detector modules and multiwire proportional chambers (Jeavons et al. 1999). Four detector banks rotate 180° forward and backward to cover all angles and to guarantee uniform acquisition. The field-of-view is 28 cm axially and 17 cm in diameter, allowing whole-body imaging of even large rats with a single bed position. The geometry of the detectors and the size of the field-of-view result in a solid angle of 70%, which contributes to the sensitivity of the camera. The quad-HIDAC system features a raw detection efficiency of 1.5% and a spatial resolution of less than 1 mm^3 as demonstrated in instrumental validation experiments (Missimer et al. 2001).

9.1.2 Resolution Versus Sensitivity

The main advantage of dedicated small-animal PET cameras compared to clinical PET systems is their superior intrinsic resolution. High spatial resolution in small-animal imaging is of great importance since the size of the regions of interest in a tumor mouse (e.g. the tumor itself) may be only of the order of a few millimeters. High-resolution imaging is particularly indispensable to visualize tumor heterogeneity. Figure 2 exemplifies resolution and image quality of a representative 2-[^{18}F]fluoro-2-deoxy-D-glucose ([^{18}F]FDG) PET scan acquired in a human using a state-of-the-art PET system for human application (*left*; GE Advanced, PET Zurich;

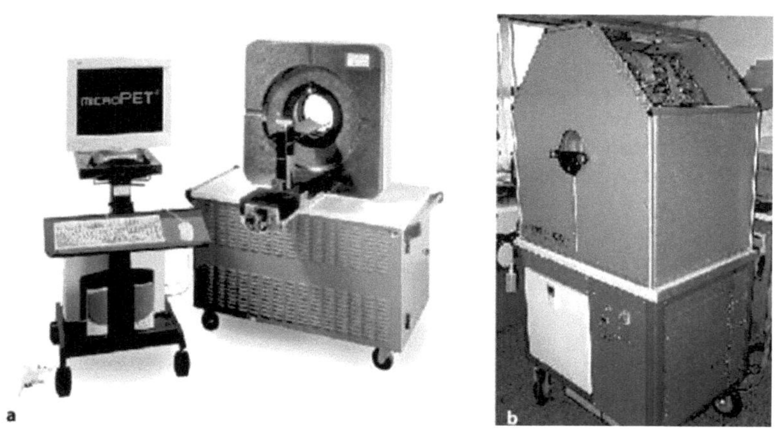

Fig. 1. The microPET camera (**a**) and the quad-HIDAC tomograph (**b**)

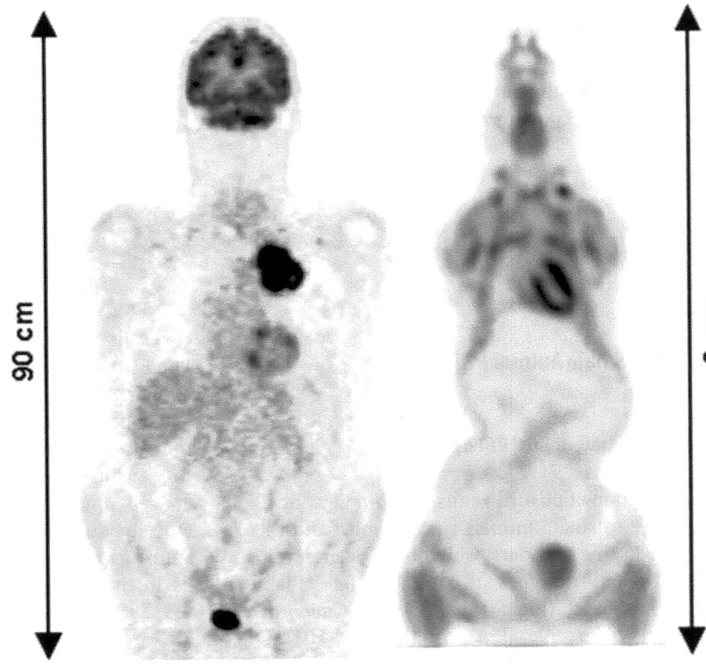

Fig. 2.
Coronal [^{18}F]FDG images using a clinical tomograph (human *left*) and the quad-HIDAC system (mouse *right*)

image courtesy of Dr G. Goerres) and in a mouse using the dedicated small-animal tomograph quad-HIDAC (*right*). The excellent resolution of the quad-HIDAC system is highlighted by the comparable detail of both PET scans in spite of a great difference in target size.

The limited sensitivity of small-animal PET systems compared to clinical cameras requires high doses of injected radioactivity to yield count statistics sufficient to reconstruct small volumes. However, high doses of radioactivity imply the injection of a significant mass of stable compound, which may lead to a saturation of transporters, enzymes or receptors, depending on the nature of the tracer. For oncological applications, however, metabolic tracers such as [^{18}F]FDG are often used, and in these cases the injected mass of the tracer is less critical. If the metabolic tracer has relatively slow kinetics at equilibrium, static scanning with longer acquisition times can be performed to compensate for low system sensitivity. Moreover, long-lived PET nuclides such as fluorine-18 (half-life = 110 min) are less demanding of system sensitivity than carbon-11-labeled PET tracers (half-life = 20 min) in small-animal PET investigations.

9.1.3 Practical Issues and Limitations

The necessity of using anesthesia in order to immobilize mice and rats during image acquisition represents a major difference between PET scanning of humans and small animals. In general, anesthesia should be administered at a superficial level to minimize effects on circulation and metabolism, and to permit long-term anesthesia and/or repetitive scanning of the animal. The most consistent and convenient anesthetic regimen involves isoflurane inhalation anesthesia and spontaneous breathing instead of intubation and artificial ventilation. Despite tight restraint of the animal, small motion artifacts caused by breathing cannot be avoided. For reliable monitoring of anesthesia, the breathing rate is the best parameter and can be simply measured by a thorax belt. Body temperature has to be regulated by a rectal probe and an automated feedback temperature control system, which is linked to an appropriate heating device.

The effect of anesthesia on perfusion, uptake and metabolism of any PET tracer has to be evaluated in detail. Cross-comparisons between anesthetized and non-anesthetized animals need to be performed using alternative techniques, e.g. classical post-mortem tissue sampling. However, in many cases, the negative effects of anesthesia can be avoided by allowing the animal to remain conscious during uptake and accumulation of the radioactive probe. After tracer uptake is complete and a steady state has been reached, the animal is anesthetized immediately before initiation of PET scanning. [^{18}F]FDG is a good example of a tracer that can be used in this manner.

In every small-animal PET experiment, the injection of the radiotracer is a compromise among numerous demands and limitations. In general, vascular access in mice and rats may be complicated by anesthesia and the restricted accessibility of the animal if it is positioned inside the quad-HIDAC tomograph, for example. The most important limitation, however, is the injection volume, which cannot exceed 200 µl for a mouse. In practice, the injected activity is determined by the injection volume. The injected activity must accommodate for scanner performance in two ways. The activity must be sufficient to yield enough count statistics to reconstruct small volumes, but should not exceed the maximum coincidence count rate of the system. For the 16-module variant of the quad-HIDAC camera, the optimum injected activity ranges between 4 and 23 MBq.

9.2 Applications of Small-Animal PET in Oncology

Experimental tumors in small animals are commonly used as biological models in oncological research. Dedicated small-animal PET systems such as the quad-HIDAC system have a sub-millimeter resolution, which is sufficient to visualize small tumors or even heterogeneity of tracer uptake within a tumor. The analysis of tumor xenografts is simplified by the ability to place the tumor away from major organs in the shoulder or the back of the animal. Whole-body PET also allows the identification and monitoring of the spread of metastatic disease. However, tumor xenografts differ from spontaneous human tumors in various aspects, e.g. the tumor size in mice commonly does not exceed 20 mm, the growth is relatively fast and a final tumor stage is reached only after a few weeks. Often, the xenografts show a solid pattern with a relatively low stromal portion, and the density of tumor vasculature in xenografts is lower than in spontaneous tumors. These differences in tumor micro-architecture may be of relevance for the kinetics of diagnostic or therapeutic agents and may also affect tumor uptake of a PET tracer.

Small-animal PET has the major advantage of non-invasiveness, permitting serial and longitudinal studies in the same animal, e.g. for long-term monitoring of chemo- or radiotherapy or the testing of new anti-cancer drugs. At the same time, the intra-individual variation of tumor size and physiology (which is particularly pronounced in animal tumor models) is avoided by repeated analysis of the same tumor in the same mouse. Thus, each animal can be used as its own control, which leads to better statistics of the data and a significant reduction of required animal numbers.

Numerous well-characterized PET tracers permit investigation of tumor biology and biochemistry under various experimental conditions. However, PET probes targeted on altered glucose metabolism ([^{18}F]FDG), oxygen metabolism ([^{18}F]fluoromisonidazole, [^{18}F]FMISO), protein synthesis ([^{11}C]methionine) or cell proliferation (3'-deoxy-3'-[^{18}F]fluorothymidine) of cancer cells are relatively non-specific for tumors in animal models. For example, some tumors are characterized by very low growth rates and may show even lower glucose or amino acid consumption than non-malignant tissue (e.g. inflammatory cells). The development of novel probes for tumor-specific targets such as cell surface antigens or receptors is expected to improve tumor visualization. PET also allows assessment of the pharmacokinetics of PET probes and enables a complete kinetic data set of tracer dynamics to be obtained from a single animal. Particularly, the optimal time point after tracer injection with highest tumor to non-tumor ratio is of interest to optimize tumor visualization. Moreover, the examination of whole-body biodistribution of the PET probe helps to identify critical organs with high radioactive burden, which may prove useful for the extrapolation of dosimetry data from small animals to clinical PET studies.

Some examples of applications and approaches of small-animal PET in oncology are described in the following sections.

9.2.1 Tumor Glucose Metabolism

While [^{18}F]FDG is widely used for tumor imaging in clinical oncology, it has also been applied to measure glucose metabolism in tumor xenografts of small animals, usually by post-mortem autoradiography or by gamma-counting (Chung et al. 1999; Furuta et al. 1997). However, regarding [^{18}F]FDG uptake, experimental xenografts derived from human tumor cell lines may behave differently from spontaneous tumors in humans, even if the tumor cell line is the same. In Fig. 3, [^{18}F]FDG was used to measure glucose metabolism in a nude mouse carrying a KB-31 epidermoid cell xenograft (tumor mouse courtesy of Dr T. O'Reilly, Novartis). This tumor cell line has been isolated from human squamous cervix carcinoma, which exhibits marked [^{18}F]FDG uptake in most cases (Belhocine et al. 2002). In contrast to human squamous cervix carcinoma, the KB-31 cell xenograft in a mouse shows virtually no accumulation of [^{18}F]FDG, suggesting low glucose metabolism.

In Fig. 4, another mouse KB-31 xenograft displays faint uptake of [^{18}F]FDG, significantly lower than in normal tissue, e.g. in muscles. There are notable differences of normal [^{18}F]FDG distribution in nude mice compared to humans. Highest uptake is found in brown fat, which is typically located in-between the shoulder blades and plays a role in thermoregulation by glucose burning. Variable [^{18}F]FDG uptake is found in muscles, being highest in the region of the shoulders and the pelvis. The latter may be a result of muscle activation of the animals, which were injected without anesthesia and were allowed to move in their housing during the [^{18}F]FDG uptake phase. Interestingly, the [^{18}F]FDG up-

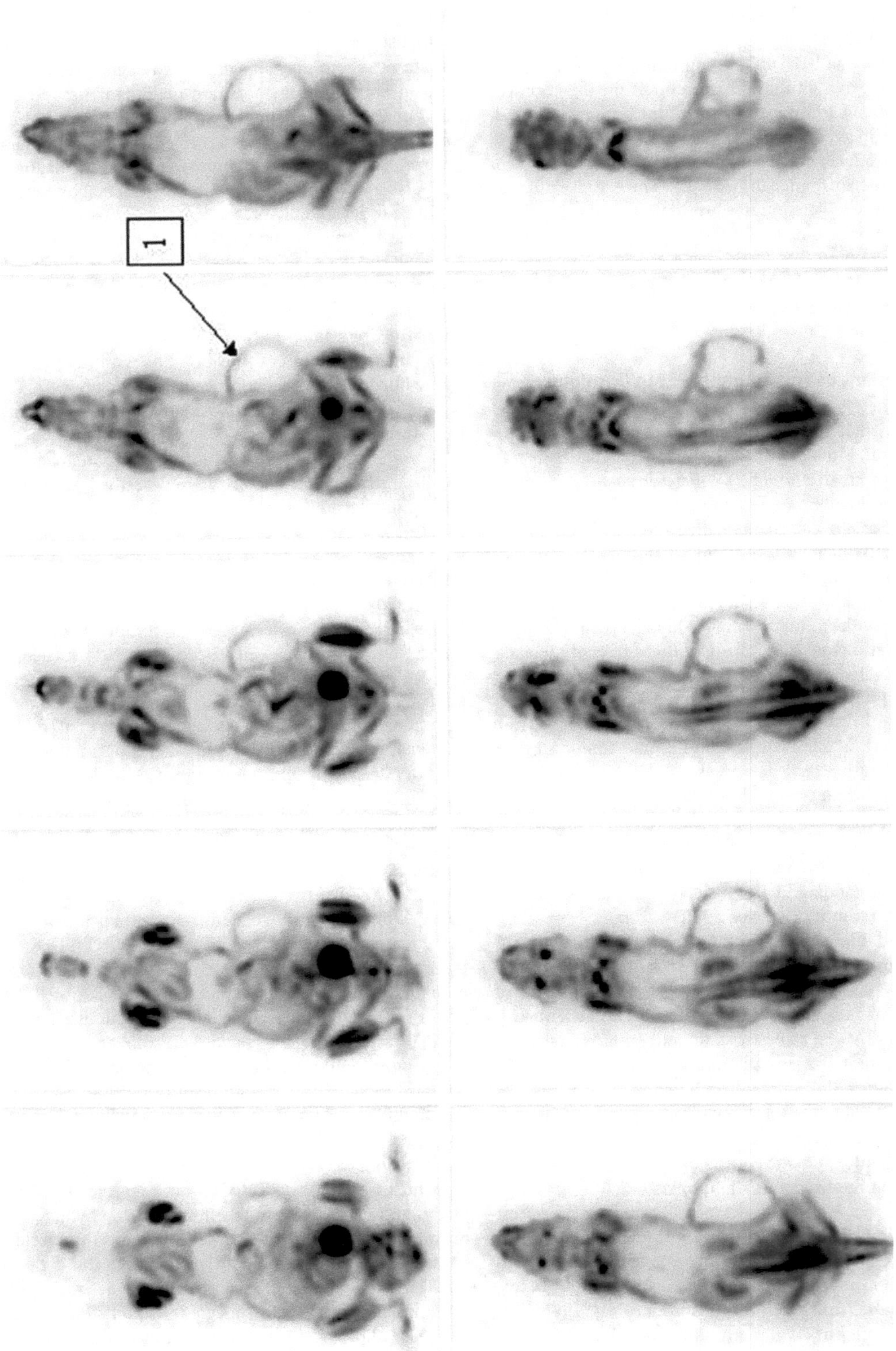

Fig. 3. Series of coronal [18F]FDG images (ventral to dorsal) showing a KB-31 epidermoid cell tumor xenograft (*1*) in a nude mouse without uptake of [^{18}F]FDG

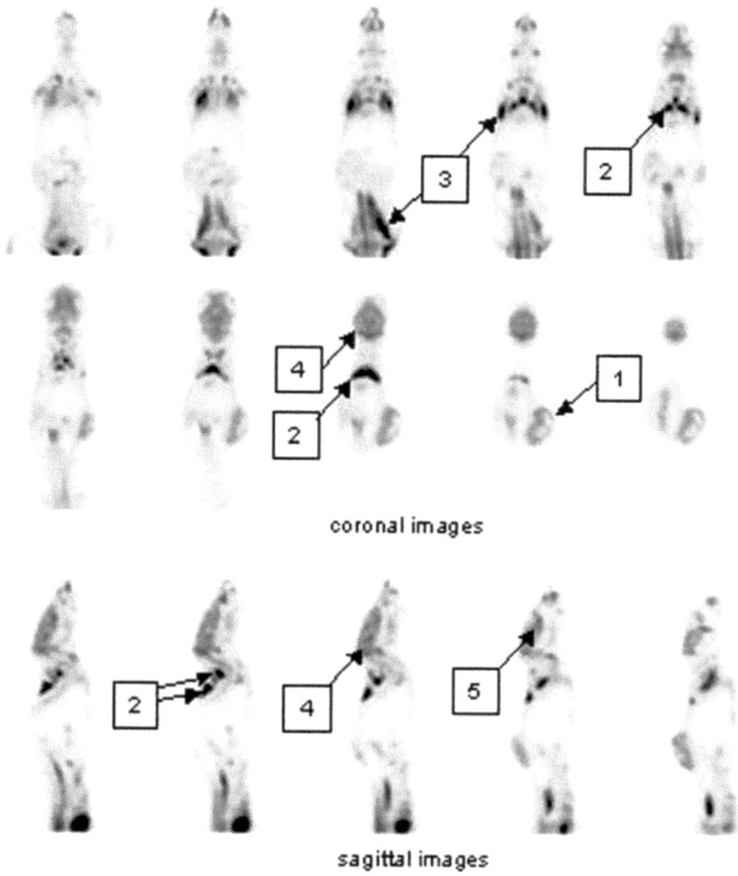

Fig. 4.
Series of coronal [^{18}F]FDG images (ventral to dorsal) of a nude mouse with a KB-31 epidermoid cell tumor xenograft showing low glucose metabolism in the tumor (*1*), but high uptake in brown fat tissue (*2*) and in muscle (*3*), while brain uptake (*4*) is rather low and considerably less intense than in the lacrimal glands (*5*)

take into the mouse brain is significantly lower than in humans, as observed in Fig. 4, showing low uptake in the cerebral cortex, the striatum and the cerebellum.

9.2.2 Tumor Oxygen Metabolism

The presence of hypoxic tissue in malignant tumors is associated with impaired prognosis as such tumors show a more aggressive biological behavior and poor response to radio- or chemotherapy. While the invasive measurement of tissue oxygenation by polarographic needle electrodes represents a gold standard to detect hypoxia, there has been a considerable effort in developing non-invasive methods for the same purpose. A variety of substances has been evaluated to detect tumor hypoxia in vivo by PET imaging (Chapman et al. 1998). Many of these agents are radiolabeled derivatives of the nitroimidazole group. [^{18}F]FMISO is a representative substance that has been used in humans by several research groups (Rasey et al. 1996; Rischin et al. 2001). In the presence of severe tissue hypoxia (pO_2<5 mmHg), [^{18}F]FMISO forms bioreductive metabolites, which accumulate in tissue and can be detected as increased radioactivity by PET. [^{18}F]FMISO PET images of a KB-31 epidermoid cell tumor xenograft of approximately 16 mm × 13 mm size are shown in Fig. 5, where the sub-millimeter resolution of the dedicated small-animal PET scanner allows visualization of tumor heterogeneity and enables hypoxic and normoxic tumor areas to be distinguished.

9.2.3 Double Tracer PET Studies

Double tracer studies may be needed if different parameters of tumor biology are to be assessed. Invasive methods such as organ gamma-counting or autoradiography have the disadvantage of being non-repeatable experiments. Consequently the tumor uptake of both tracers has to be measured simultaneously, usually requiring two tracers with different radionuclides for energy discrimination. Meanwhile, PET as a non-invasive method permits repetitive measurements in the same animal and assures greater experimental flexibility.

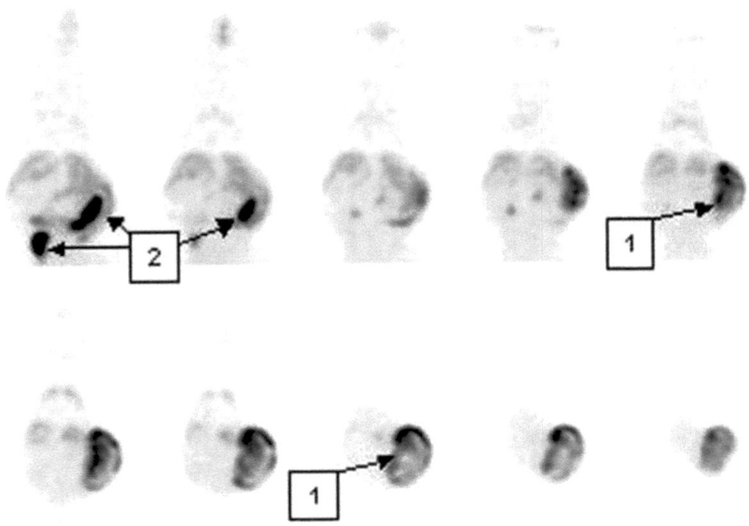

Fig. 5.
Series of coronal [^{18}F]FMISO images (ventral to dorsal) of a nude mouse with a KB-31 epidermoid cell tumor xenograft displaying heterogeneous tumor uptake (*1*), which indicates hypoxia. Radioactivity in the bowel (*2*) by hepato-biliary clearance is a disadvantage of [^{18}F]FMISO, which may interfere with tumor imaging in the abdomen

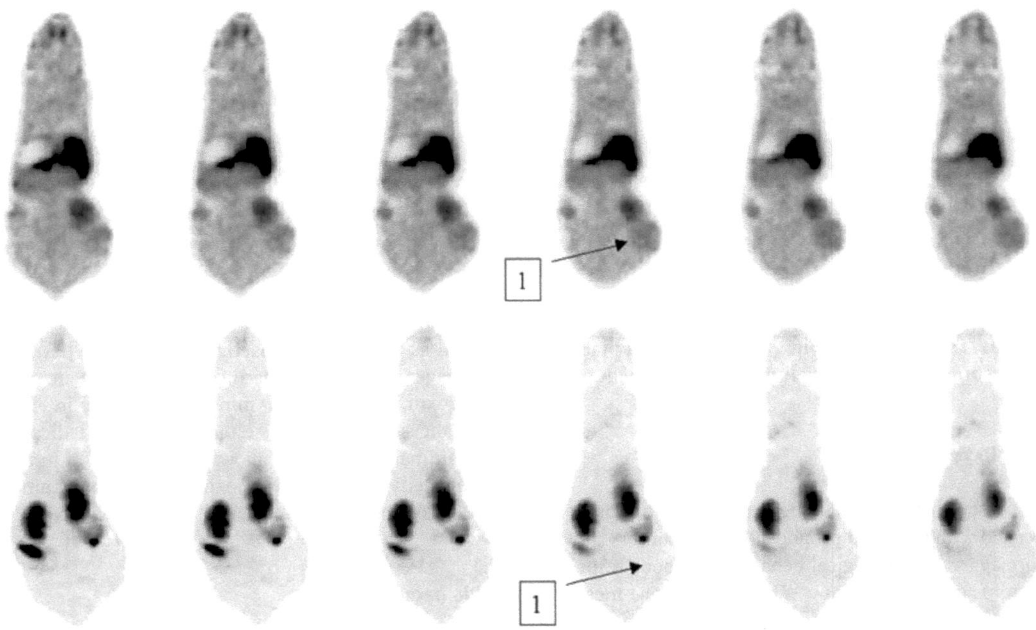

Fig. 6. Series of coronal [^{11}C]methionine (*upper row*) and [^{18}F]FMISO (*lower row*) images (ventral to dorsal) of a nude mouse with a SK-N-AS neuroblastoma tumor (*1*)

In the experiment shown in Fig. 6, PET images of the tracers [^{11}C]methionine and [^{18}F]FMISO were obtained for a combined measurement of tumor amino-acid metabolism and hypoxia in a SK-N-AS neuroblastoma xenograft in a nude mouse. The neuroblastoma tumor was not hypoxic and consequently exhibited no accumulation of [^{18}F]FMISO (in contrast to the KB-31 tumor in Fig. 5). However, the neuroblastoma was visualized by a moderate uptake of [^{11}C]methionine, indicating a slightly increased amino-acid metabolism compared to normal tissue.

9.2.4 Tumor-Associated Receptors and Antigens

Antibodies binding to tumor-associated cell surface antigens are of potential use for cancer therapy. The efficacy of antibody treatment is, however, limited by tumor heterogeneity, for a number of reasons. Elements contributing to heterogeneous tumor uptake are diffusion and penetration of antibodies (or other tumor-seeking molecules) into the tumor, and these factors can be studied to a certain degree in tumor xenografts. Alternatively, heterogeneous uptake of tumor cell specific antibodies may be also caused by cellular heterogeneity, changes in expression of antigen and/or by a variable spread and composition of connective tissue in various tumors, but these factors are *not* well accessible in the xenograft model.

Antibodies reach the tumor through blood vessels, and each tumor is vascularized to a different extent. For instance, some human tumor cell xenografts such as colon or renal carcinoma xenografts are densely packed and only moderately vascularized. In contrast, many neuroblastoma xenografts are disperse aggregates of cells and highly vascularized. Perfusion markers (e.g. [^{64}Cu]PTSM) can be used to detect areas of limited tracer access within tumors. The counteracting interstitial pressure within tumors slows down the exit of tumor-seeking molecules from the blood vessels and the diffusion within the tumor. Diffusion of large molecules such as antibodies is also limited by their size. Figure 7 illustrates limited access of antibody to the inside of a human renal carcinoma (Caki-2) xenograft. The high-affinity chCE7 antibody binds to L1-CAM, a cell surface protein, which is overexpressed in some renal carcinomas and in neuroblastomas (Meli et al. 1999). High-resolution PET imaging reveals that the distribution of the radiocopper-labeled antibody within this compact xenograft is heterogeneous, with the rim of the tumor showing highest accumulation of radioactivity. In this case, permeability into the tumor is limited by the size of the antibody conjugate and by perfusion.

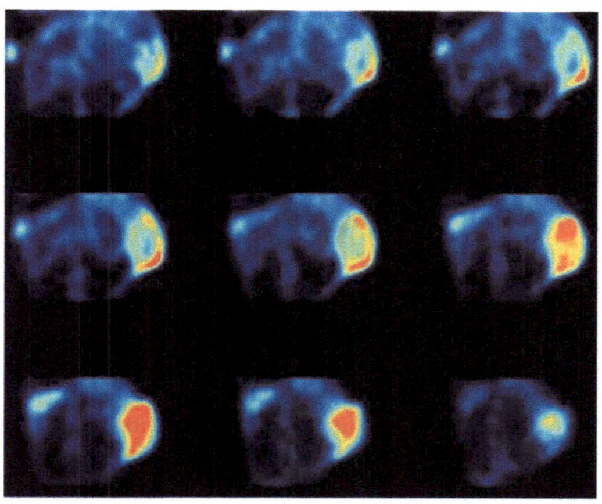

Fig. 7. Series of sections through a renal cell carcinoma tumor showing heterogeneous tracer uptake. The mouse was injected with ^{64}Cu-labeled chCE7 monoclonal antibody

Efficacy of anti-tumor substances is increased by their uniform distribution within tumors, allowing effectors (radionuclides or cytotoxic molecules) to reach tumor cells in the interior of tumors. Similarly to "real" tumors, larger xenografts develop necrotic areas within the tumor. These regions lack antigen-binding sites and the less well perfused inner regions contain more radio-resistant and chemoresistant hypoxic cells, which are difficult to be reached and targeted. As a consequence, tumors tend to regrow both in model systems and in the clinical setting. In the search for more effective targeting molecules, small-animal PET imaging can be used to evaluate tumor penetration of small antibody fragments or receptor-binding peptides in comparison to intact antibody molecules. PET imaging can also serve to follow antibody distribution during the course of therapies such as radioimmunotherapy or treatment with angiogenesis inhibitors.

9.2.5 Biodistribution of Established and New Radiotracers for PET or Therapy

During the process of developing new radiotracers for tumor diagnosis or therapy, molecules with high accumulation in the tumor and low levels of radioactivity in normal tissues are desired. PET imaging can give more detailed information than classical post-mortem biodistribution studies measuring radioactivity of dissected tissues. A main advantage is also seen in dynamic PET imaging, since a single animal may be sufficient to find the optimal time point for tumor visualization. At the same time, a rapid assessment of clearance of radioactivity from normal tissues is possible. Figure 6 (*lower row*) shows uptake of the hypoxia tracer [^{18}F]FMISO in a nude mouse with a SK-N-AS tumor xenograft with highest levels of radioactivity in bowel and kidneys, indicating that these organs receive the highest radiation dose. In the case of [^{11}C]methionine (*upper row*), liver and spleen are identified as putative critical organs (Fig. 6).

The monoclonal chCE7 antibody, which targets neuroblastomas and some renal carcinomas (Meli et al. 1999), shows therapeutic efficacy in the mouse xenograft model when applied in ^{131}I-labeled form (Hoefnagel et al. 2001). ^{67}Cu-labeled chCE7 is a potentially even more effective agent, due to the excellent physical properties of the ^{67}Cu nuclide. Radiocopper-labeled antibodies show high tumor to non-tumor ratios in biodistribution studies (Novak-Hofer et al. 2002) and degradation in liver and spleen by hepatocytes and cells of

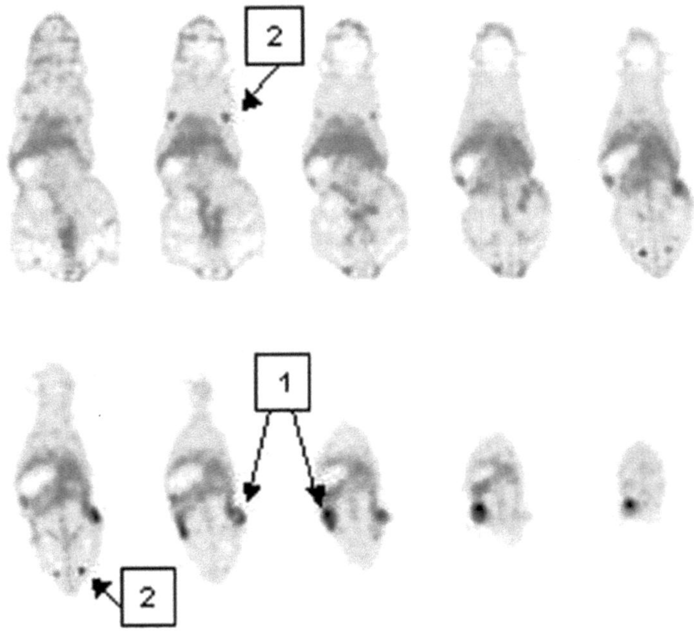

Fig. 8.
Series of coronal ^{64}Cu-labeled chCE7 images of a nude mouse with two renal cell carcinoma tumors. High radioactivity levels are identified in the tumors (*1*) and in lymph nodes (*2*)

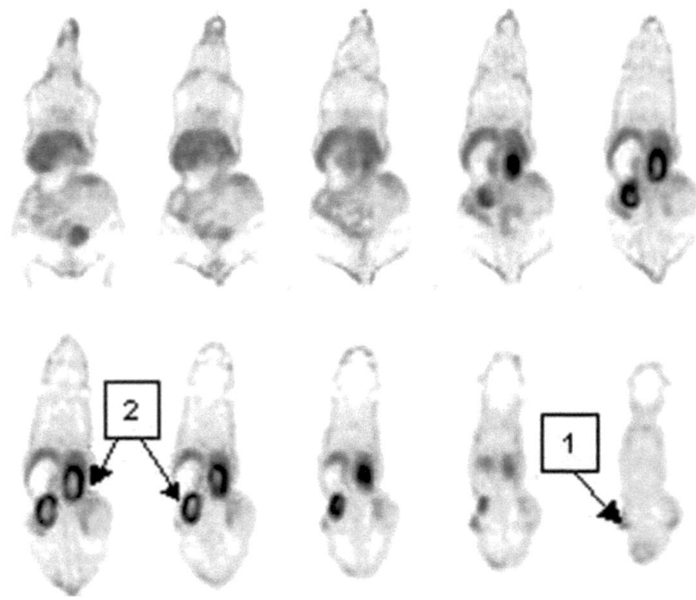

Fig. 9.
Series of coronal sections of ^{64}Cu-labeled antibody $F(ab')_2$-fragments in a mouse with a neuroblastoma tumor (*1*). Highest radioactivity is found in the renal cortex (*2*)

the reticuloendothelial system. Figure 8 displays a series of coronal sections through a nude mouse carrying two renal carcinoma xenografts imaged after injection of ^{64}Cu-labeled chCE7 antibody. Next to the tumor, liver and spleen show highest radioactivity levels due to accumulation of radioactive metabolites. Interestingly, the PET images also reveal high accumulation of radioactivity in various lymph nodes, which contain cells of the reticuloendothelial system. Mouse lymph nodes are tiny structures that are usually not dissected when performing biodistribution studies. The radiocopper accumulation detected in lymph nodes by PET imaging may thus be relevant for clinical radioimmunotherapy with ^{67}Cu-labeled antibodies.

During the development of antibody-based therapeutics, recombinant antibody fragments are evaluated in the search for agents that clear more rapidly from blood and tissues such as liver and spleen than intact antibody molecules. Figure 9 shows biodistributions of ^{64}Cu-labeled $F(ab')_2$-fragments of the chCE7 antibody. In contrast to the favorable biodistributions observed with the intact antibody (Fig. 8), radiocopper-labeled antibody fragments show high levels of radioactivity in the kidneys. This unwanted effect is caused by the uptake and retention of terminal degradation products consisting of amino acid-linked copper complexes in the proximal tubule cells of the kidney (Novak-Hofer et al. 1997). PET imaging shows that the renal cortex accumulates the highest levels of radioactivity. Current efforts are directed to reduce radioactivity in the kidneys by chemical modification of copper chelators or by blocking uptake sites in the kidneys with basic amino acids.

References

Belhocine T, Thille A, Fridman V, Albert A, Seidel L, Nickers P, Kridelka F, Rigo P (2002) Contribution of whole-body 18FDG PET imaging in the management of cervical cancer. Gynecol Oncol 87:90–97

Chapman JD, Engelhardt EL, Stobbe CC, Schneider RF, Hanks GE (1998) Measuring hypoxia and predicting tumor radioresistance with nuclear medicine assays. Radiother Oncol 46:229–237

Chatziioannou AF, Cherry SR, Shao Y, Silverman RW, Meadors K, Farquhar TH, Pedarsani M, Phelps ME (1999) Performance evaluation of microPET: a high-resolution lutetium oxyorthosilicate PET scanner for animal imaging. J Nucl Med 40:1164–1175

Chung JK, Lee YJ, Kim C, Choi SR, Kim M, Lee K, Jeong JM, Lee DS, Jang JJ, Lee MC (1999) Mechanisms related to [18F]fluorodeoxyglucose uptake of human colon cancers transplanted in nude mice. J Nucl Med 40:339–346

Furuta M, Hasegawa M, Hayakawa K, Yamakawa M, Ishikawa H, Nonaka T, Mitsuhashi N, Niibe H (1997) Rapid rise in FDG uptake in an irradiated human tumour xenograft. Eur J Nucl Med 24:435–438

Hoefnagel CA, Rutgers M, Buitenhuis CK, Smets LA, de Kraker J, Meli M, Carrel F, Amstutz H, Schubiger PA, Novak-Hofer I (2001) A comparison of targeting of neuroblastoma with mIBG and anti L1-CAM antibody mAb chCE7: therapeutic efficacy in a neuroblastoma xenograft model and imaging of neuroblastoma patients. Eur J Nucl Med 28:359–68

Jeavons AP, Chandler RA, Dettmar CAR (1999) A 3D HIDAC-PET camera with sub-millimetre resolution for imaging small animals. IEEE Trans Nucl Sci 46:468–473

Meli ML, Carrel F, Waibel R, Amstutz H, Crompton N, Jaussi R, Moch H, Schubiger PA, Novak-Hofer I (1999) Anti-neuroblastoma antibody chCE7 binds to an isoform of L1-CAM present in renal carcinoma cells. Int J Cancer 83:401–408

Missimer J, Honer M, Ametamey S, Schubiger PA (2001) Performance of 16-module quad-HIDAC PET camera. High resolution imaging in small animals. Rockville, MD, USA, 9–11 Sept 2001

Novak-Hofer I, Zimmermann K, Maecke HR, Amstutz HP, Carrel F, Schubiger PA (1997) Tumor uptake and metabolism of copper-67-labeled monoclonal antibody chCE7 in nude mice bearing neuroblastoma xenografts. J Nucl Med 38:536–544

Rasey JS, Koh WJ, Evans ML, Peterson LM, Lewellen TK, Graham MM, Krohn KA (1996) Quantifying regional hypoxia in human tumors with positron emission tomography of [18F]fluoromisonidazole: a pretherapy study of 37 patients. Int J Radiat Oncol Biol Phys 36:417–428

Rischin D, Peters L, Hicks R, Hughes P, Fisher R, Hart R, Sexton M, D'Costa I, von Roemeling R (2001) Phase I trial of concurrent tirapazamine, cisplatin, and radiotherapy in patients with advanced head and neck cancer. J Clin Oncol 19:535–542

CHAPTER 10

Small-Animal PET in Neuro-oncology and Gene Therapy

A.H. Jacobs · W.-D. Heiss

10.1 Introduction

Glioblastomas are the most common types of brain tumors, constituting ~20% of all intracranial neoplasms. Although sophisticated regimens of conventional therapies are being carried out, the disease invariably leads to death over months or years. Therefore, development of new treatment strategies for patients with glioblastomas is highly important. The first successful gene therapy paradigms for experimental brain tumors were conducted more than 10 years ago, and they were thought to revolutionize the treatment of patients with gliomas. Application of gene therapy has been quickly forced into clinical trials, the first patients being enrolled in 1994. However, overall results have been disappointing. Only a few patients seemed to benefit from gene therapy, showing long-term treatment response, and most of these patients had small glioblastomas. Whereas the gene therapy itself has been sophisticated, limited attention has been paid to technologies that (i) allow identification of viable target tissue in heterogeneous glioma tissue and (ii) enable assessment of successful vector administration and vector-mediated gene expression in vivo. These measures are a prerequisite for the development of successful gene therapy in the clinical application. As biological treatment strategies such as gene- and cell-based therapies hold promise to correct disease pathogenesis selectively, successful clinical implementation of these treatment strategies relies on the establishment of molecular imaging technology allowing the non-invasive assessment of endogenous and exogenous gene expression in vivo. Imaging endogenous gene expression will allow the characterization and identification of target tissue for gene therapy. Imaging exogenously introduced cells and genes will allow the determination of the "tissue dose" of transduced cell function and vector-mediated gene expression, which in turn can be correlated to the induced therapeutic effect. Only these combined strategies of non-invasive imaging of gene expression in vivo will enable the establishment of safe and efficient vector administration and gene therapy protocols for clinical application. One of the potential applications of small-animal PET lies in the further design of new treatment strategies for gliomas.

10.2 Gliomas – General and Molecular Aspects

Gliomas are divided histologically into astrocytomas, oligodendrogliomas and mixed gliomas. Grading is performed according to the World Health Organization (WHO), taking into account the presence of nuclear changes (WHO grade I), mitotic activity (WHO grade II), endothelial proliferation (WHO grade III), and necrosis (WHO grade IV) [55, 61]. Glioblastoma, corresponding to WHO grade IV, is the most fatal and most common primary brain neoplasm, with an incidence of 3–6 in 100,000. Approximately 50% of all gliomas and 20% of all primary intracranial tumors are glioblastomas. Together with all intracranial neoplasms, the glioblastoma is the second most common cause of death as a result of an intracranial disease, after stroke. Despite aggressive multimodal treatment strategies (surgery, radiation, chemotherapy), median survival of patients with gliomas is limited, depending on grade and age at diagnosis, varying from 1 year for glioblastoma, to 2–3 years for grade III and to 5–10 years for a grade II glioma.

Magnetic resonance imaging is widely used to assess the extent of blood–brain barrier disruption as an indirect measure for active tumor growth and response to therapy. However, the overall goal within the next years is to make positron emission tomography (PET) imaging modalities more readily available. PET allows the detection of metabolically active tumor and the assessment of response to therapy. Both measures are highly important variables in the development of new biological treatment regimens.

Moreover, to develop potential specific molecular therapeutic targets, glial tumorigenesis has to be fully understood. A complex series of molecular changes occurs, which results in dysregulation of the cell cycle, alterations of apoptosis and cell differentiation, in neovascularization as well as tumor cell migration and invasion throughout the brain parenchyma. Genetic alterations that play an important role in glioma development include a loss or mutation of the tumor suppressor gene TP53 and other genes involved in the regulation of the cell cycle, as well as activation or amplification of growth factors and/or their receptors, such as CDKN2A/p16, EGFR, PDGFR, PTEN and TGF-ß [6; 66]. During progression from low-grade astrocytoma (WHO grade II) to anaplastic astrocytoma (WHO grade III) and to glioblastoma multiforme (WHO grade IV), a step-wise accumulation of genetic alterations occurs. While TP53 mutation and overexpression of PDGF and PDGFR represent early changes during low-grade glioma development, progression to anaplastic astrocytoma is associated with RB alteration and loss of heterozygosity (LOH) of 19q, further malignant progression to glioblastoma including LOH 10q and mutations of the PTEN gene [54]. These secondary glioblastomas, which develop from better differentiated astrocytomas, can be distinguished from primary de novo glioblastomas on the basis of molecular genetic findings [59], with amplification and/or overexpression of the EGFR, p16 deletion, PTEN mutation, RB alteration and LOH 10p and 10q associated with primary glioblastoma. Most importantly, molecular alterations have been identified that indicate the therapeutic response of patients and, thus, are prognostically relevant: anaplastic oligodendrogliomas with LOH 1p and/or LOH 19q are characteristically sensitive to PCV chemotherapy, and patients' survival is significantly prolonged [13, 17, 81].

10.3 Gene Therapy for Gliomas – Current Status and Future Perspectives

Gene therapy is based on the transduction of therapeutic genes into diseased target tissue to induce a therapeutically valuable alteration of tissue phenotype. In general, the design of effective gene therapy strategies relies on concerted research (i) to define alterations in molecular tumor genetics and tumor biology, (ii) to develop safe and efficient vectors and application systems to achieve efficient, targeted and regulated alteration of specific gene expression, and (iii) to develop technology that will non-invasively identify target tissue in vivo (by imaging endogenous gene expression) and will follow the biological treatment effects (by imaging exogenous and endogenous gene expression).

In terms of gene therapy of gliomas, transduction of tumor cells with "therapeutic" genes may influence their biological properties (i) by rendering them sensitive to prodrugs, (ii) by altering the expression of cell-cycle-regulating proteins, (iii) by inhibiting angiogenesis, (iv) by stimulating the immune response, or (v) by introducing selectively replicating viral vector particles (so-called virus therapy). A promising strategy for successful gene therapy of glioblastomas is a *multimodal* approach combining the synergistic effects of various prodrug activating systems [2, 78] with immunomodulation [7, 92] mediated by selectively replicating adeno- or herpes viral vectors (reviewed by [47]).

Suicide gene therapy based on the retrovirus vector-mediated expression of herpes simplex virus type 1 thymidine kinase (HSV-1-*tk*) and subsequent ganciclovir (GCV) application was successful in various experimental brain tumor models. Clinical studies revealed that this approach as an adjuvant to the surgical resection of recurrent high-grade gliomas can be performed safely, although clinical responses were observed in only a few patients with small brain tumors [53, 75, 76, 83]. The lack of therapeutic efficiency of replication-deficient retrovirus vector systems in clinical settings may be the result of (i) the inability to distribute vector-producer cells throughout the tumor, (ii) vector-producer cell instability, (iii) the low transduction efficiency of retrovirions, and (iv) the heterogeneity of glioma tissue. To circumvent some of these problems and to serve improved distribution of vector particles within tumor tissue, replication-competent oncolytic herpes viral vectors [63, 77] as well as vector application by means of stereotactically guided convection-enhanced delivery [93] are being used, and are being evaluated in combination with improved prodrug–suicide gene systems as part of a multimodal gene therapy approach [1, 51, 78].

The discrepancy between successful experimental gene therapy protocols and the limited efficiency in their clinical application highlights the importance of developing assays (i) that allow a non-invasive determination of viable target tissue, which might benefit from a biological treatment paradigm as well as assays (ii) for the assessment of the transduced "tissue dose" of a therapeutic gene in patients in vivo. The clinical gene therapy trials for glioblastoma performed so far have all suffered from a lack of ability to investigate the magnitude and extent of transduced therapeutic gene expression in vivo, the only qualitative information being obtained from biopsied tissue samples [30, 70, 71]. Therefore, one of the most important issues for making gene therapy widely applicable to humans is the establishment of gene therapy protocols, which include molecular imaging technology including metabolic imaging of target tissue and non-invasive monitoring of the location, magnitude and duration of vector-mediated gene expression in vivo [48, 49, 51, 91]. This is in line with the Recombinant DNA Advisory Committee of the NIH, which, as a reaction to the first gene therapy death, called for better assays for measuring transgene expression in cells and tissues.

10.4 Small-Animal PET – Imaging of Endogenous Gene Expression for Characterization of Target Tissue

In most of the clinical gene therapy studies, magnetic resonance imaging (MRI) has been used to localize the tumor and to follow gene therapeutic effects, although MRI reveals only indirect measures of tumor activity. Besides a determination of the size and localization of the tumor, MRI assesses secondary phenomena such as edema and signs of increased intracranial pressure at high spatial resolution. Gadolinium (Gd)-enhanced MRI is used widely as a surrogate marker (i) to follow tumor progression, (ii) to guide surgery or focal radiation therapy, and (iii) to follow changes induced by gene therapy. The contrast-enhancing lesion in T1-weighted MRI (T1+Gd) corresponds histologically to a hypercellular region with neovascularization; a central hypointense area (T1) is mainly caused by tumor necrosis. In the computed tomography era, biopsies from signal changes in areas surrounding the contrast-enhancing tumor revealed the presence of migrating tumor cells, which should be the target for gene therapy. However, a major problem of MRI after therapy is the assessment of residual active tumor, and differentiation from treatment-induced (resection, radiation, gene therapy) enhancement is often impossible. This differentiation may only become possible by molecular PET imaging technology.

PET reveals highly specific quantitative information on the metabolic state of a glioma [38, 50, 74]. Depending on the radiotracer used, various molecular processes can be visualized by PET, most of them relating to an increased cell proliferation within gliomas (Fig. 1). Radiolabeled 2-[^{18}F]fluoro-2-deoxy-D-glucose ([^{18}F]FDG), methyl-[^{11}C]-L-methionine ([^{11}C]MET) and 3'-deoxy-3'-[^{18}F]fluoro-L-thymidine ([^{18}F]FLT) are being incorporated into proliferating gliomas depending on their tumor grade as a reflection of increased activity of membrane transporters for glucose ([^{18}F]FDG), amino acids ([^{11}C]MET) and nucleosides ([^{18}F]FLT), as well as increased expression of cellular hexokinase ([^{18}F]FDG) and thymidine kinase ([^{18}F]FLT) genes, which specifically phosphorylate [^{18}F]FDG and [^{18}F]FLT, respectively. [^{18}F]FDG PET can monitor the rate of glucose uptake and has been used to detect the metabolic differences between normal brain tissue, low-grade and high-grade gliomas, and radionecrosis [27, 32, 34, 36, 37]. Increased intratumoral glucose consumption correlates to tumor grade, cell density, biological aggressiveness and patient survival [5, 19, 28, 36, 52, 72]. [^{18}F]FDG PET is able to guide stereotactic tumor biopsy to identify the most malignant tumor part with high accuracy, and malignant progression of low-grade gliomas is indicated by a newly appearing hypermetabolism. However, because of relatively high background levels of cortical glucose consumption, more specific radiotracers for glioma diagnosis have been developed. The radiolabeled amino acid [^{11}C]MET has been shown to be a more specific tracer in tumor detection, tumor delineation, and differentiating benign from malignant lesions as a result of its low uptake in normal brain [14, 18, 35, 52, 68, 69, 82]. The increased methionine uptake is related to increased transport mediated by type L amino acid carriers [41, 60]. [^{11}C]MET uptake correlates to cell proliferation in vitro, to Ki-67 expression and to proliferating cell nuclear antigen expression and microvessel density, indicating its role as a marker for active tumor proliferation. The third parameter that can be assessed non-invasively by PET is the incorporation of nucleosides into DNA in proliferating cells. Radiolabeled thymidine ([^{3}H]TdR) is the gold standard for determination of cell proliferation in cell culture, and to date ^{11}C- and ^{18}F-labeled thymidine compounds have been radiosynthesized to allow a non-invasive assessment of tumor proliferation as well as early response to chemotherapy by PET. [^{18}F]FLT

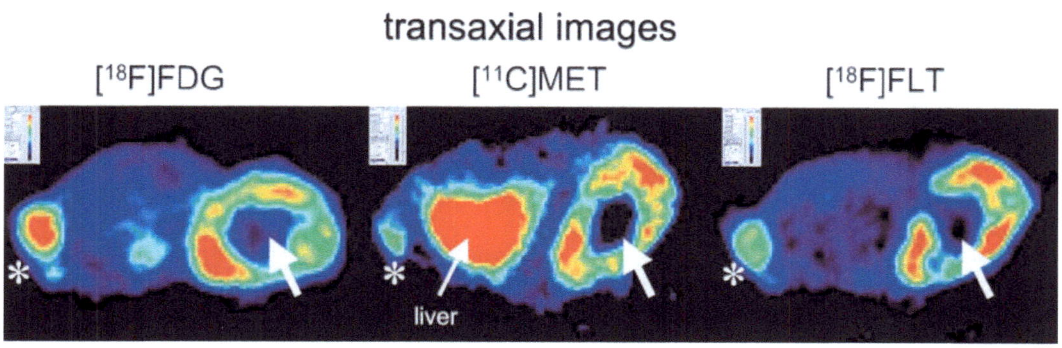

Fig. 1. Molecular imaging parameters of interest for the identification of target tissue for gene therapy in experimental glioma models. Signs of increased cell proliferation can be observed by means of multi-tracer microPET imaging using [^{18}F]FDG, [^{11}C]MET and [^{18}F]FLT as specific tracers for glucose consumption, amino acid transport and DNA synthesis, respectively. Figures represent transaxial images through the body of an experimental rat bearing subcutaneously growing rat F98 gliomas. The small tumor on the left (*) shows homogeneous radiotracer uptake, indicating biologically active tumor tissue. The larger tumor on the right shows the signs of central necrosis (*arrow*). Vector application into the central necrotic tumor tissue (*arrow*) will be of no benefit, and vector application into the surrounding active tumor rim will be difficult and not successful. Therefore, small-animal PET is directly involved in the planning of successful vector application and gene therapy strategies

is stable in vivo and has been used for the evaluation of tumor proliferation primarily in extracranial tissues [84]. Unpublished results in patients with gliomas indicate that [^{18}F]FLT is a promising tracer to study glioma proliferation, especially in areas with high [^{18}F]FDG background. Relative [^{18}F]FLT uptake within gliomas is greater than relative [^{11}C]MET uptake, indicating the possible role of [^{18}F]FLT as a more specific tumor marker than [^{18}F]FDG and [^{11}C]MET [57, 58, 62, 64, 84].

In gene therapy, imaging the expression of endogenous genes by [^{18}F]FDG, [^{11}C]MET, and [^{18}F]FLT as direct measures for the respective gene expression and as surrogate markers for proliferation and tumor cell density will (i) identify the biological active tumor portion as proper target tissue and (ii) measure the response to gene therapy [49]. As indicated in Fig. 1, in experimental glioma models, microPET reveals homogeneous radiotracer uptake in small gliomas, where gene therapy vectors can be applied directly into the tumor. However, in larger tumors the signs of central necrosis are present, indicating that vector application into the surrounding active tumor ring will be difficult. Therefore, small-animal PET is directly involved in the proper planning of vector application.

10.5 Small-Animal PET – Imaging of Expression of Exogenously Introduced Genes

As described above, PET allows the quantitative localization of expression of endogenous or exogenous genes coding for enzymes or receptors by measuring the accumulation or binding of the respective enzyme substrates or receptor-binding compounds [33, 73, 85]. The unique ability of HSV-1-*tk* selectively to incorporate radiolabeled nucleoside analogues into DNA [23, 79, 91, 94] allows the non-invasive imaging of tk-gene expression in distinct regions within a transduced tissue [22–24, 31, 39, 65, 86, 87, 89, 91]. Saito et al. (1982) were the first to propose that the HSV-1-*tk* gene might be used as a marker gene for the early detection of herpes encephalitis by using specific radiolabeled nucleoside analogues as marker substrates [79, 80]. However, with the development of gene therapy strategies based on HSV-1-*tk* as suicide gene, the HSV-1-*tk* gene became attractive as a PET marker gene to follow gene therapy non-invasively. Tjuvajev et al. (1995) demonstrated for the first time, that in retrovirally transduced, stably TK-expressing rat RG2 glioma clones, the accumulation rate of the specific HSV-1-*tk* marker substrate, 2'-fluoro-2'-deoxy-1ß-D-arabinofuranosyl-5-[^{131}I]iodouracil ([^{131}I]FIAU), correlated with the level of tk-mRNA expression [91].

The quantitative determination of TK expression by PET is based on the same principles as the measurement of local cerebral glucose utilization, as described by Sokoloff et al. [85]. As reviewed previously [11, 26], quantification is performed by measuring the accumulation rates of specific viral thymidine kinase substrates, such as [^{124}I]FIAU [10, 12, 44, 48, 49, 86] and the acyclic guanosine derivatives 8-[^{18}F]fluoro-ganciclovir ([^{18}F]FGCV [22, 23]), 8-[^{18}F]fluoro-penciclovir ([^{18}F]FPCV [24, 42]), 9-[(3-[^{18}F]fluoro-1-hydroxy-2-propoxy)methyl]guanine ([^{18}F]FHPG [12, 16, 39, 40]), 9-[4-[^{18}F]fluoro-3-(hydroxymethyl)butyl]guanine ([^{18}F]FHBG [3, 4, 95]) and recently also by 1-(2-fluoro-2-deoxy-ß- D-ribofuranosyl)5-[^{123}I]iodouracil ([^{123}I]FIRU [67]), as marker substrates by wild-type or mutated HSV-1-*tk* genes as marker genes [9, 25]. The chemical structures of the various specific HSV-1-*tk* marker substrates are summarized in Fig. 2. Most importantly, various levels of TK expression could be distinguished non-invasively in vivo by PET after retroviral [39, 43, 86, 89], adenoviral [23, 87] and herpes viral [8, 48] vector-mediated tk-gene transfer into liver or subcutaneous glioma mod-

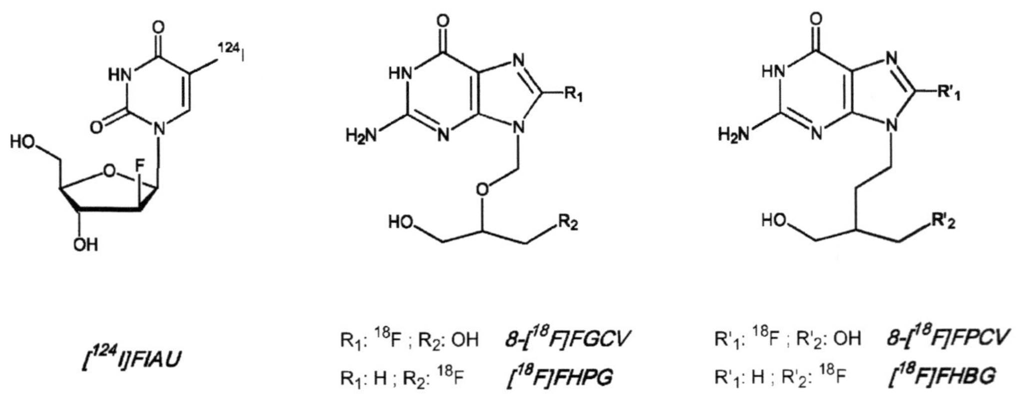

Fig. 2. Specific PET marker substrates for localization of exogenous HSV-1-*tk* gene expression. *[^{124}I]FIAU* 2'-fluoro-2'-deoxy-1ß-d-arabinofuranosyl-5-[^{124}I]iodouracil, *8-[^{18}F]FGCV* 8-[^{18}F]fluoro-ganciclovir, *8-[^{18}F]FPCV* 8-[^{18}F]fluoro-penciclovir, *[^{18}F]FHPG* 9-[(3-[^{18}F]fluoro-1-hydroxy-2-propoxy)methyl]guanine, *[^{18}F]FHBG* 9-[4-[^{18}F]fluoro-3-(hydroxymethyl)butyl]guanine

els in rodents (Figs. 3–5). Incorporating the tk gene as a PET marker gene into a gene therapy vector allows non-invasive detection of the location, level and duration of vector-mediated tk-gene expression. These parameters determine the transduced "tissue-dose" of vector-mediated therapeutic gene expression, which can be correlated to the induced therapeutic response. It is important to note that this has already been achieved in the clinical application. In a phase I/II clinical trial of liposomal vector-mediated gene therapy of recurrent glioblastoma, a modern vector administration method (stereotactic convection-enhanced delivery) was combined with modern PET technology to determine the biologically active target tissue together with vector-mediated therapeutic HSV-1-*tk*-gene expression [49]. A comparison of accumulation rates of [^{124}I]FIAU, [^{18}F]FHPG and [^{18}F]FHBG in HSV-1-*tk* transduced tumors in experimental models [12;88] indicates that [^{124}I]FIAU and [^{18}F]FHBG might be the marker substrates of choice for clinical application [4, 49, 88, 95].

Recently, a tkgfp dual reporter gene [45] was used to monitor transcriptional activation of p53-dependent

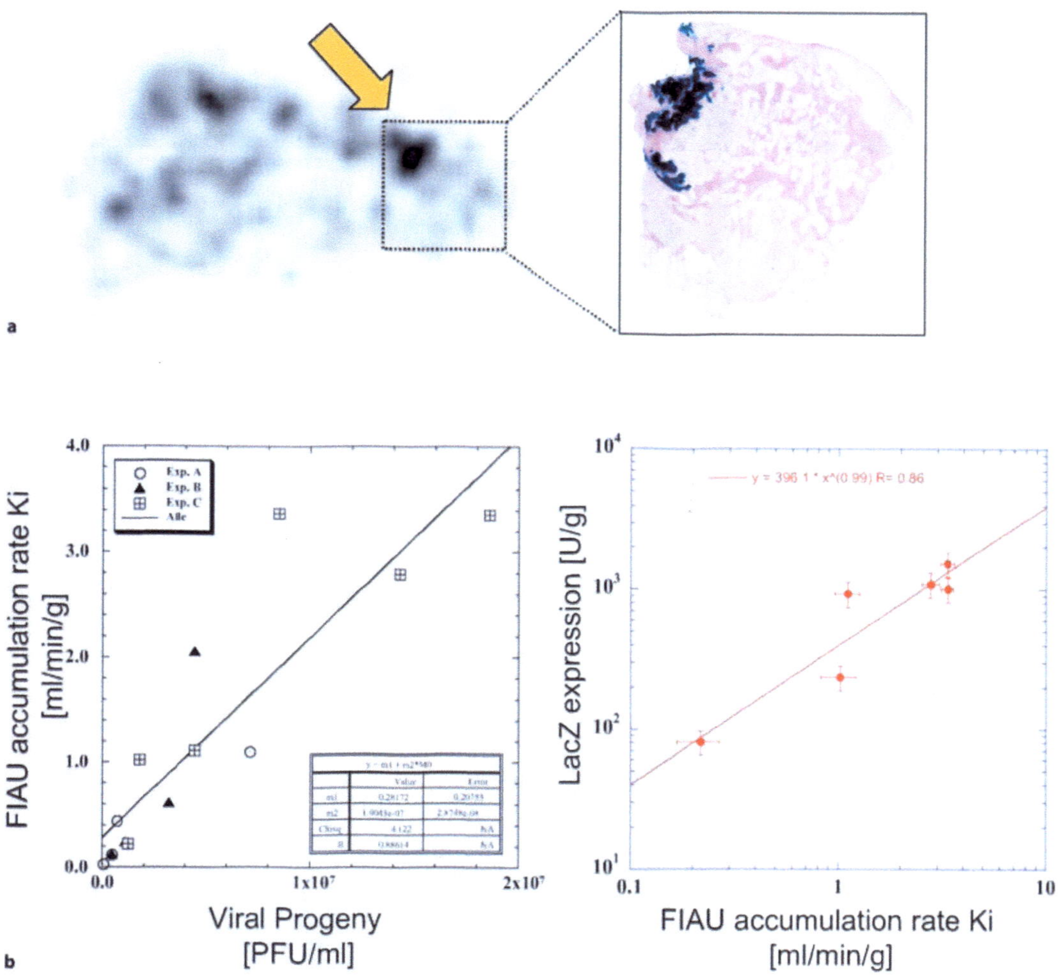

Fig. 3. Indirect localization (**a**) and quantification (**b**) of a second, proportionally co-expressed gene by [^{124}I]FIAU PET. HSV-1-tk gene expression was studied in a subcutaneous human U87dEGFR glioma model in nude rats after intratumoral injection of the replication-conditional HSV-1 vector hrR3. This vector expresses HSV-1-*tk* and lacZ genes under immediate early promoters. Co-registration of transaxial [^{124}I]FIAU PET images of HSV-1-*tk* expression (**a**, left) with histochemical analysis of LacZ expression (**a**, right) revealed co-localization of both genes. Quantitative assays in cell culture revealed that the rate of accumulation of FIAU not only reflects the level of HSV-1-*tk* expression, but also correlates to secondary measures of this vector, such as viral progeny and level of LacZ expression. These results indicate that indirect localization and quantification of any gene of interest that is proportionally co-expressed with a PET marker gene is possible. From Jacobs et al. (2001), with permission [48]

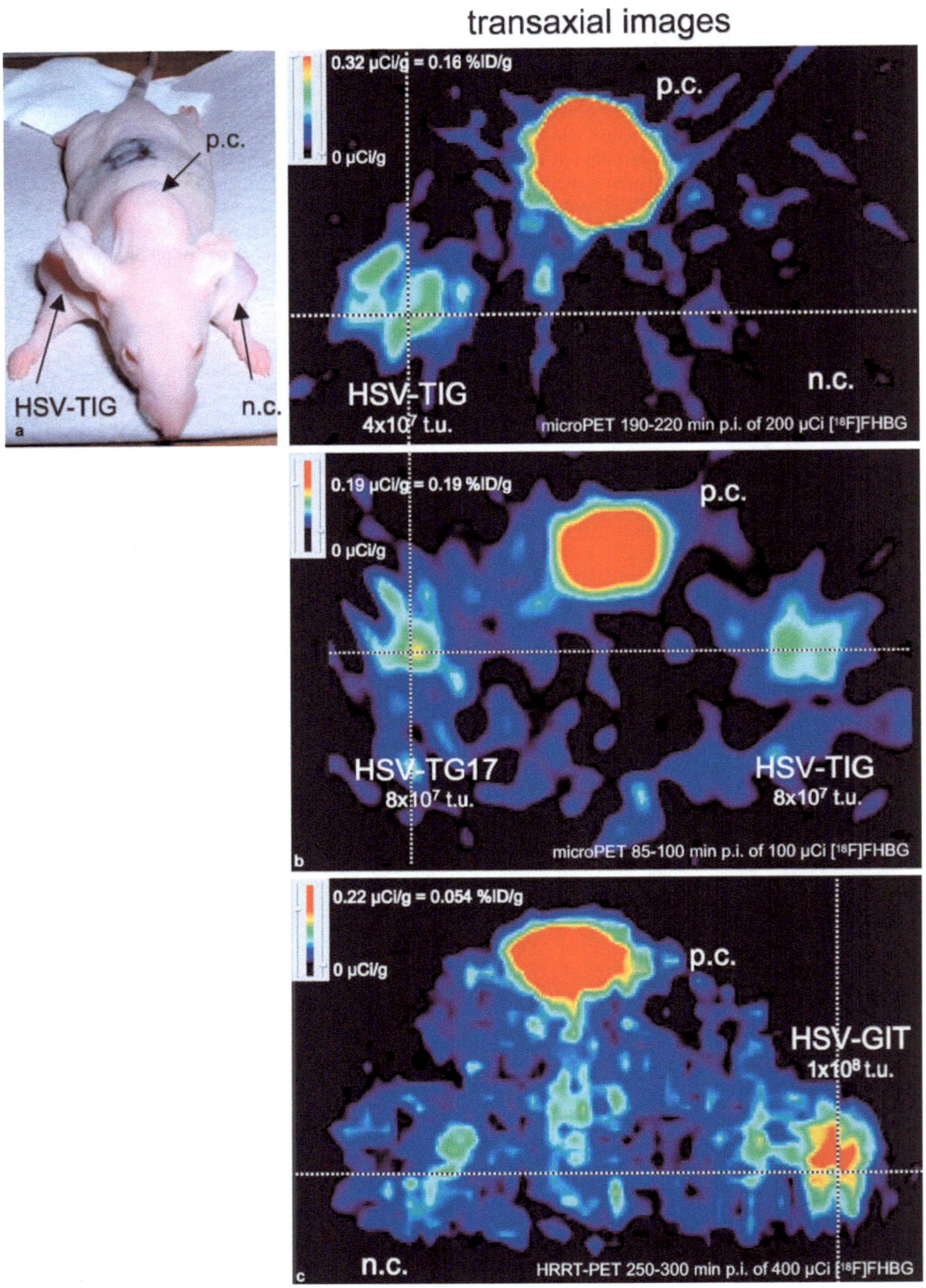
transaxial images
p.c.
HSV-TIG
n.c.
a
0.32 µCi/g = 0.16 %ID/g
0 µCi/g
p.c.
HSV-TIG
4x10⁷ t.u.
n.c.
microPET 190-220 min p.i. of 200 µCi [18F]FHBG
0.19 µCi/g = 0.19 %ID/g
0 µCi/g
p.c.
HSV-TG17
8x10⁷ t.u.
HSV-TIG
8x10⁷ t.u.
microPET 85-100 min p.i. of 100 µCi [18F]FHBG
b
0.22 µCi/g = 0.054 %ID/g
0 µCi/g
p.c.
HSV-GIT
1x10⁸ t.u.
n.c.
HRRT-PET 250-300 min p.i. of 400 µCi [18F]FHBG
c

◀ **Fig. 4.** HSV-1 amplicon vector-mediated tk-gene expression in vivo in nude mice (**a**, **b**) and nude rats (**c**) bearing subcutaneous Gli36dEGFR gliomas. Each animal had two subcutaneous Gli36dEGFR-wt gliomas at both upper flanks and one Gli36dEGFR-TG17-R6 tumor in the neck, which served as positive control (*p.c.*; photomicrograph in **a**). HSV-1 amplicon vectors HSV-TIG (**a**, **b**), HSV-TG17 (**b**) and HSV-GIT (**c**) were injected at doses ranging from 4×10^7 to 1×10^8 transducing units directly into Gli36dEGFR-wt gliomas along the cranio-caudal axis of the animal. In (**a**) and (**c**) one tumor served as negative control (*n.c.*) and the other tumor was transduced, in (**b**) both wild-type tumors were transduced by HSV-1 amplicon vectors 24 hours prior to PET imaging. [^{18}F]FHBG PET imaging was performed by microPET (**a**, **b**) and HRRT PET (C) at 30 min to 5 hours after i.v. administration of 100–400 μCi [^{18}F]FHBG. Transaxial PET images (**a–c**) demonstrate regions of TK-related radioactivity primarily around injection sites. Positive control tumors growing in the neck demonstrated 4.0–5.7-fold higher levels of TK expression, respectively. Radioactivity concentration in transduced tumors was assessed from PET images and background activity (mediastinum) was subtracted. Note that, even after HSV-GIT transduction (**c**), specific [^{18}F]FHBG-related radioactivity could be observed, indicating that HSV-1 amplicon-mediated tk expression can be imaged even with the tk gene located at the weak position downstream from the IRE site. *TG17* tkgfp fusion gene, *TIG* tkIRESgfp coexpression construct, *GIT* gfpIRESTk co-expression construct. From Jacobs et al. [51], with permission

genes for non-invasive characterization of a signal transduction pathway [20]. Human U87 glioma and SaOS-2 osteosarcoma cells were transduced retrovirally with a cis-p53/TKGFP reporter system, in which the tkgfp marker gene was placed under control of an artificial cis-acting p53-specific enhancer. In rat xenografts the DNA damage-induced up-regulation of p53 transcriptional activity correlated with the expression of p53-dependent downstream genes in U87 (wild-type p53), but not in SaOS-2 osteosarcoma (p53 -/-) cells and with the level of p53-dependent TKGFP expression as assessed by [^{124}I]FIAU-PET. These data indicate that PET is sufficiently sensitive to image the transcriptional regulation of genes in certain signal transduction pathways. This molecular imaging strategy will enable non-invasive assessment of the activity of signal transduction pathways, of the expression of different endogenous genes and of novel molecular therapeutic targets in vivo [20].

As not all genes of interest (GOI) carry an enzymatic function that could be used for an enzymatic radionuclide assay in vivo, the general attempt is proportionally to co-express any GOI with an imaging marker gene. Therefore, to enable indirect and quantitative assessment of the expression of any GOI, gene co-expression strategies are being used. Apart from coordinately promoter-based co-expression ([48]; Fig. 3), strategies serving a proportional co-expression of a PET- or MRI-marker gene and a GOI make use of gene fusion [45] (Figs. 4, 5), an internal ribosome entry site (IRES) derived from encephalomyocarditis virus [51, 90, 97](Fig. 4) or the proteolytic 2A-element derived from picornavirus [15]. In addition, co-administration of two distinct but otherwise identical adenovirus vectors has been shown to result in proportional co-expression of PET marker genes expressed by these vectors [96]. In single-cell-derived retrovirally transduced tumor clones, it was demonstrated that PET imaging of HSV-1-*tk* expression could be used to monitor the topology and activity of the lacZ gene as the second gene under the transcrip-

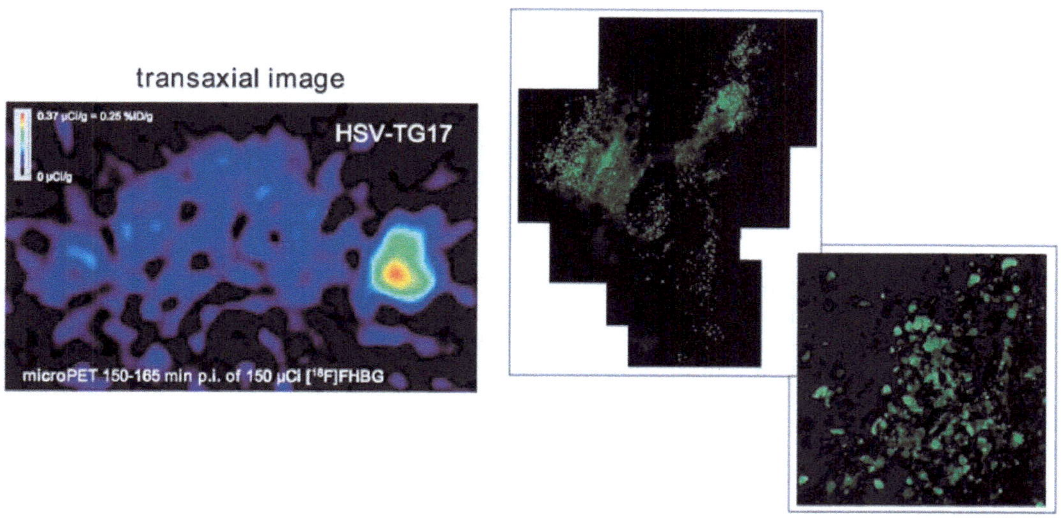

Fig. 5. Co-registration between HSV-TG17-mediated tg17-gene expression in vivo as assessed by [^{18}F]FHBG microPET and histology/fluorescence microscopy. After microPET imaging, the animal was killed and the HSV-TG17-transduced tumor processed for fluorescence microscopy. For fluorescence microscopy, a set of representative pictures (10×) acquired at the laser scanning microscope in the same transaxial plane was put together, the figure on the right demonstrating a part at higher magnification (63×). Both microPET and fluorescence microscopy demonstrate efficient tg17-gene transduction within the tumor. From Jacobs et al. [51], with permission

tional control of a single promoter within a bicistronic unit that includes an IRES [90]. In a similar approach the activity of proportionally co-expressed renilla luciferase and a dopamine type 2 receptor could be quantified and localized by PET [97].

The applicability of this "indirect" imaging method has been translated into a model of vector application in vivo employing recombinant HSV-1 vectors, which are commonly used for virus therapy of gliomas ([8, 46–48]; Fig. 3). In the first (hrR3) and second (MGH-1) generation HSV-1 vectors, the PET marker gene HSV-1-*tk* and the marker gene lacZ are under transcriptional control of early gene, and hence, timely coordinately active promoters [29, 56]. The level and location of PET-based imaging of hrR3- and MGH-1-mediated TK expression in vivo reflected indirectly the level and location of LacZ expression and also the viral progeny of these vectors ([48]; Fig. 3). However, the propensity of replication-conditional vectors eventually to disrupt cellular functions interferes with the enzymatic radiotracer assay, so that the PET-imageable TK expression mediated by these vectors identifies only the viable portion of infected tumor tissue.

To circumvent HSV-1 vector-induced toxicity interfering with the PET imaging of these vectors, helper virus-free HSV-1 amplicon vectors [21] were engineered and functionally characterized. These vectors bear transcriptionally linked genes of interest for proportional co-expression of three gene functions: (i) a marker gene for HSV-1 vector generation in culture (gfp); (ii) the HSV-1-*tk* as PET marker gene for assessment of HSV-1 vector-mediated gene expression in vivo; (iii) a therapeutic gene (*E. coli* cytosine deaminase; cd) for suicide gene therapy of gliomas [51]. Functional proportional co-expression of the PET marker gene HSV-1-*tk* and the linked gfp and therapeutic *E. coli* cd gene could be observed irrespective of the location of genes within the constructs (Figs. 4, 5). These HSV-1 amplicon vectors carrying the HSV-1-*tk* as PET marker gene and a linked therapeutic gene will enable the indirect non-invasive localization of the distribution of therapeutic gene expression by PET and, hence, will allow the correlation of the primary transduction efficiency of these vectors with their induced therapeutic response.

Further marker gene/marker substrate combinations suitable for small-animal PET imaging have been developed for various applications that are not relevant to the application in gliomas. They include: (i) the aromatic L-amino acid decarboxylase (AADC) gene, which was used to restore dopaminergic function and to image AADC gene expression by 6-[^{18}F]-fluoro- L-m-tyrosine and PET; (ii) a wild-type or mutated dopamine-2-receptor using the specific dopamine-2-receptor binding compounds [^{11}C]raclopride and 3-(2'-[^{18}F]fluoroethyl)-spiperone; (iii) an ^{18}F-labeled glycopeptide used non-invasively to assess endogenous alpha$_v$ß$_3$ integrin expression on melanoma cells for tumor detection and therapy monitoring; (iv) the sodium/iodide symporter gene used as marker and therapeutic gene to induce expression of the thyroid-derived iodide concentrator.

10.6 Summary and Conclusion

In summary, small-animal PET will allow the further development and, finally, a successful implementation of molecular therapies for patients with glioblastomas. Both viral and non-viral vectors applied by direct injection or convection-enhanced delivery appear to be safe in clinical application. Until now, only a few patients with glioblastomas have shown a significant gene therapeutic benefit, as deduced from the small number of long-term survivors. Non-invasive imaging by PET for the identification of viable target tissue and for monitoring the distribution of transgene expression over time will help to identify patients who might benefit from molecular therapies. Therefore, PET will have a critical impact on the development of standardized gene therapy protocols and on efficient and safe vector applications in humans.

Acknowledgements. This work is supported in part by the Ministerium für Schule, Wissenschaft und Forschung NRW (MSWF 516-40000299), the Center for Molecular Medicine Cologne (CMMC-TV46) and the Max-Planck Society, Germany.

References

1. Aghi M, Chou TC, Suling K, Breakefield XO, Chiocca EA (1999) Multimodal cancer treatment mediated by a replicating oncolytic virus that delivers the oxazaphosphorine/CYP2B1 and ganciclovir/HSV-TK gene therapies. Cancer Res 59:3861–3865
2. Aghi M, Kramm CM, Chou TC, Breakefield XO, Chiocca EA (1998) Synergistic anticancer effects of ganciclovir/thymidine kinase and 5- fluorocytosine/cytosine deaminase gene therapies. J Natl Cancer Inst 90:370–380
3. Alauddin MM, Conti PS (1998) Synthesis and preliminary evaluation of 9-(4-[18F]-fluoro-3- hydroxymethylbutyl)guanine ([18F]FHBG): a new potential imaging agent for viral infection and gene therapy using PET. Nucl Med Biol 25:175–180
4. Alauddin MM, Shahinian A, Gordon EM, Bading JR, Conti PS (2001) Preclinical evaluation of the penciclovir analog 9-(4-[18F]fluoro-3-hydroxymethylbutyl)guanine for in vivo measurement of suicide gene expression with PET. J Nucl Med 42: 1682–1690
5. Barker FG, Chang SM, Valk PE, Pounds TR, Prados MD (1997) 18-Fluorodeoxyglucose uptake and survival of patients with suspected recurrent malignant glioma. Cancer 79:115–126
6. Barker FG, Israel MA (1999) Molecular Genetics. In: Berger MS, Wilson CB (eds) The gliomas. Saunders, Philadelphia, pp 39–51
7. Benedetti S, Pirola B, Pollo B, Magrassi L, Bruzzone MG, Rigamonti D, Galli R, Selleri S, di Meco F, De Fraja C, Vescovi A, Cattaneo E, Finocchiaro G (2000) Gene therapy of experimental brain tumors using neural progenitor cells. Nat Med 6:447–450
8. Bennett JJ, Tjuvajev J, Johnson P, Doubrovin M, Akhurst T, Malholtra S, Hackman T, Balatoni J, Finn R, Larson SM, Federoff H, Blasberg R, Fong Y (2001) Positron emission tomography imaging for herpes virus infection: Implications for oncolytic viral treatments of cancer. Nat Med 7:859–863

9. Black ME, Newcomb TG, Wilson HM, Loeb LA (1996) Creation of drug-specific herpes simplex virus type 1 thymidine kinase mutants for gene therapy. Proc Natl Acad Sci USA 93:3525–3529
10. Blasberg RG, Tjuvajev JG (1999) Herpes simplex virus thymidine kinase as a marker/reporter gene for PET imaging of gene therapy. Q J Nucl Med 43:163–169
11. Blasberg RG, Tjuvajev JG (2002) Molecular-genetic imaging: a nuclear medicine-based perspective. Mol Imaging 1:280–300
12. Brust P, Haubner R, Friedrich A, Scheunemann M, Anton M, Koufaki ON, Hauses M, Noll S, Noll B, Haberkorn U, Schackert G, Schackert HK, Avril N, Johannsen B (2001) Comparison of [18F]FHPG and [124/125I]FIAU for imaging herpes simplex virus type 1 thymidine kinase gene expression. Eur J Nucl Med 28:721–729
13. Cairncross JG, Ueki K, Zlatescu MC, Lisle DK, Finkelstein DM, Hammond RR, Silver JS, Stark PC, Macdonald DR, Ino Y, Ramsay DA, Louis DN (1998) Specific genetic predictors of chemotherapeutic response and survival in patients with anaplastic oligodendrogliomas. J Natl Cancer Inst 90:1473–1479
14. Chung JK, Kim YK, Kim SK, Lee YJ, Paek S, Yeo JS, Jeong JM, Lee DS, Jung HW, Lee MC (2002) Usefulness of 11C-methionine PET in the evaluation of brain lesions that are hypo- or isometabolic on 18F-FDG PET. Eur J Nucl Med Mol Imaging 29:176–182
15. De Felipe P, Martin V, Cortes ML, Ryan M, Izquierdo M (1999) Use of the 2A sequence from foot-and-mouth disease virus in the generation of retroviral vectors for gene therapy. Gene Ther 6:198–208
16. De Vries EF, van Waarde A, Harmsen MC, Mulder NH, Vaalburg W, Hospers GA (2000) [11C]FMAU and [18F]FHPG as PET tracers for herpes simplex virus thymidine kinase enzyme activity and human cytomegalovirus infections. Nucl Med Biol 27:113–119
17. DeAngelis LM, Burger PC, Green SB, Cairncross JG (1998) Malignant glioma: who benefits from adjuvant chemotherapy? Ann Neurol 44:691–695
18. Derlon JM, Bourdet C, Bustany P, Chatel M, Theron J, Darcel F, Syrota A (1989) [11C]L-methionine uptake in gliomas. Neurosurgery 25:720–728
19. Di Chiro G, DeLaPaz RL, Brooks RA, Sokoloff L, Kornblith PL, Smith BH, Patronas NJ, Kufta CV, Kessler RM, Johnston GS, Manning RG, Wolf AP (1982) Glucose utilization of cerebral gliomas measured by [18F] fluorodeoxyglucose and positron emission tomography. Neurology 32:1323–1329
20. Doubrovin M, Ponomarev V, Beresten T, Balatoni J, Bornmann W, Finn R, Humm J, Larson S, Sadelain M, Blasberg R, Gelovani TJ (2001) Imaging transcriptional regulation of p53-dependent genes with positron emission tomography in vivo. Proc Natl Acad Sci USA 98:9300–9305
21. Fraefel C, Song S, Lim F, Lang P, Yu L, Wang Y, Wild P, Geller AI (1996) Helper virus-free transfer of herpes simplex virus type 1 plasmid vectors into neural cells. J Virol 70:7190–7197
22. Gambhir SS, Barrio JR, Phelps ME, Iyer M, Namavari M, Satyamurthy N, Wu L, Green LA, Bauer E, MacLaren DC, Nguyen K, Berk AJ, Cherry SR, Herschman HR (1999) Imaging adenoviral-directed reporter gene expression in living animals with positron emission tomography. Proc Natl Acad Sci USA 96:2333–2338
23. Gambhir SS, Barrio JR, Wu L, Iyer M, Namavari M, Satyamurthy N, Bauer E, Parrish C, MacLaren DC, Borghei AR, Green LA, Sharfstein S, Berk AJ, Cherry SR, Phelps ME, Herschman HR (1998) Imaging of adenoviral-directed herpes simplex virus type 1 thymidine kinase reporter gene expression in mice with radiolabeled ganciclovir. J Nucl Med 39:2003–2011
24. Gambhir SS, Bauer E, Black ME, Liang Q, Kokoris MS, Barrio JR, Iyer M, Namavari M, Phelps ME, Herschman HR (2000) A mutant herpes simplex virus type 1 thymidine kinase reporter gene shows improved sensitivity for imaging reporter gene expression with positron emission tomography. Proc Natl Acad Sci USA 97:2785–2790
25. Gambhir SS, Bauer E, Black ME, Liang Q, Kokoris MS, Barrio JR, Iyer M, Namavari M, Phelps ME, Herschman HR (2000) A mutant herpes simplex virus type 1 thymidine kinase reporter gene shows improved sensitivity for imaging reporter gene expression with positron emission tomography. Proc Natl Acad Sci USA 97:2785–2790
26. Gambhir SS, Herschman HR, Cherry SR, Barrio JR, Satyamurthy N, Toyokuni T, Phelps ME, Larson SM, Balatoni J, Finn R, Sadelain M, Tjuvajev J, Blasberg R (2000) Imaging transgene expression with radionuclide imaging technologies. Neoplasia 2:118–138
27. Glantz MJ, Hoffman JM, Coleman RE, Friedman AH, Hanson MW, Burger PC, Herndon JE, Meisler WJ, Schold SC Jr (1991) Identification of early recurrence of primary central nervous system tumors by [18F]fluorodeoxyglucose positron emission tomography. Ann Neurol 29:347–355
28. Goldman S, Levivier M, Pirotte B, Brucher JM, Wikler D, Damhaut P, Stanus E, Brotchi J, Hildebrand J (1996) Regional glucose metabolism and histopathology of gliomas. A study based on positron emission tomography-guided stereotactic biopsy. Cancer 78:1098–1106
29. Goldstein DJ, Weller SK (1988) Herpes simplex virus type 1-induced ribonucleotide reductase activity is dispensable for virus growth and DNA synthesis: isolation and characterization of an ICP6 lacZ insertion mutant. J Virol 62:196–205
30. Harsh GR, Deisboeck TS, Louis DN, Hilton J, Colvin M, Silver JS, Qureshi NH, Kracher J, Finkelstein D, Chiocca EA, Hochberg FH (2000) Thymidine kinase activation of ganciclovir in recurrent malignant gliomas: a gene-marking and neuropathological study. J Neurosurg 92:804–811
31. Haubner R, Avril N, Hantzopoulos PA, Gansbacher B, Schwaiger M (2000) In vivo imaging of herpes simplex virus type 1 thymidine kinase gene expression: early kinetics of radiolabelled FIAU. Eur J Nucl Med 27:283–291
32. Heiss WD, Heindel W, Herholz K, Rudolf J, Bunke J, Jeske J, Friedmann G (1990) Positron emission tomography of fluorine-18-deoxyglucose and image-guided phosphorus-31 magnetic resonance spectroscopy in brain tumors. J Nucl Med 31: 302–310
33. Heiss WD, Pawlik G, Herholz K, Wagner R, Goldner H, Wienhard K (1984) Regional kinetic constants and cerebral metabolic rate for glucose in normal human volunteers determined by dynamic positron emission tomography of [18F]-2-fluoro-2-deoxy-D-glucose. J Cereb Blood Flow Metab 4:212–223
34. Herholz K, Heindel W, Luyten PR, denHollander JA, Pietrzyk U, Voges J, Kugel H, Friedmann G, Heiss WD (1992) In vivo imaging of glucose consumption and lactate concentration in human gliomas. Ann Neurol 31:319–327
35. Herholz K, Holzer T, Bauer B, Schroder R, Voges J, Ernestus RI, Mendoza G, Weber-Luxenburger G, Lottgen J, Thiel A, Wienhard K, Heiss WD (1998) 11C-methionine PET for differential diagnosis of low-grade gliomas. Neurology 50:1316–1322
36. Herholz K, Pietrzyk U, Voges J, Schroder R, Halber M, Treuer H, Sturm V, Heiss WD (1993) Correlation of glucose consumption and tumor cell density in astrocytomas. A stereotactic PET study. J Neurosurg 79:853–858
37. Herholz K, Rudolf J, Heiss WD (1992) FDG transport and phosphorylation in human gliomas measured with dynamic PET. J Neurooncol 12:159–165
38. Herholz K, Wienhard K, Heiss WD (1990) Validity of PET studies in brain tumors. Cerebrovasc Brain Metab Rev 2:240–265
39. Hospers GA, Calogero A, van Waarde A, Doze P, Vaalburg W, Mulder NH, de Vries EF (2000) Monitoring of herpes simplex virus thymidine kinase enzyme activity using positron emission tomography. Cancer Res 60:1488–1491
40. Hustinx R, Shiue CY, Alavi A, McDonald D, Shiue GG, Zhuang H, Lanuti M, Lambright E, Karp JS, Eck SL (2001) Imaging in vivo herpes simplex virus thymidine kinase gene transfer to tumour-bearing rodents using positron emission tomography. Eur J Nucl Med 28:5–12
41. Ishiwata K, Enomoto K, Sasaki T, Elsinga PH, Senda M, Okazumi S, Isono K, Paans AM, Vaalburg W (1996) A feasibility study on L-[1-carbon-11]tyrosine and L-[methyl-carbon-11]methionine to assess liver protein synthesis by PET. J Nucl Med 37:279–285
42. Iyer M, Barrio JR, Namavari M, Bauer E, Satyamurthy N, Nguyen K, Toyokuni T, Phelps ME, Herschman HR, Gambhir SS

(2001) 8-[18F]Fluoropenciclovir: an improved reporter probe for imaging HSV1-*tk* reporter gene expression in vivo using PET. J Nucl Med 42:96–105
43. Iyer M, Wu L, Carey M, Wang Y, Smallwood A, Gambhir SS (2001) Two-step transcriptional amplification as a method for imaging reporter gene expression using weak promoters. Proc Natl Acad Sci USA 98:14595–14600
44. Jacobs A, Braunlich I, Graf R, Lercher M, Sakaki T, Voges J, Hesselmann V, Brandau W, Wienhard K, Heiss WD (2001) Quantitative kinetics of [124I]FIAU in cat and man. J Nucl Med 42:467–475
45. Jacobs A, Dubrovin M, Hewett J, Sena-Esteves M, Tan C, Slack M, Sadelain M, Breakefield XO, Tjuvajev JG (1999) Functional co-expression of HSV-1 thymidine kinase and green fluorescent protein: implications for non-invasive imaging of transgene expression. Neoplasia 1:154–161
46. Jacobs A, Fraefel C, Breakefield XO (1999) HSV-1 based vectors for gene therapy of neurological diseases and brain tumors, part I. HSV-1 structure, replication and pathogenesis. Neoplasia 1:387–401
47. Jacobs A, Fraefel C, Breakefield XO (1999) HSV-1 based vectors for gene therapy of neurological diseases and brain tumors, part II. Vector systems and applications. Neoplasia 1:402–416
48. Jacobs A, Tjuvajev JG, Dubrovin M, Akhurst T, Balatoni J, Beattie B, Joshi R, Finn R, Larson SM, Herrlinger U, Pechan PA, Chiocca EA, Breakefield XO, Blasberg RG (2001) Positron emission tomography-based imaging of transgene expression mediated by replication-conditional, oncolytic herpes simplex virus type 1 mutant vectors in vivo. Cancer Res 61:2983–2995
49. Jacobs A, Voges J, Reszka R, Lercher M, Gossmann A, Kracht L, Kaestle C, Wagner R, Wienhard K, Heiss WD (2001) Positron-emission tomography of vector-mediated gene expression in gene therapy for gliomas. Lancet 358:727–729
50. Jacobs AH, Dittmar C, Winkeler A, Garlip G, Heiss WD (2002) Molecular imaging of gliomas. Mol Imaging 1:309–335
51. Jacobs AH, Winkeler A, Hartung M, Slack M, Dittmar C, Kummer C, Knoess S, Galldiks N, Vollmar S, Wienhard K, Heiss WD (2003) Improved HSV-1 amplicon vectors for proportional co-expression of PET marker and therapeutic genes. Hum Gene Ther 14:277–297
52. Kaschten B, Stevenaert A, Sadzot B, Deprez M, Degueldre C, Del Fiore G, Luxen A, Reznik M (1998) Preoperative evaluation of 54 gliomas by PET with fluorine-18-fluorodeoxyglucose and/or carbon-11-methionine. J Nucl Med 39:778–785
53. Klatzmann D, Valery CA, Bensimon G, Marro B, Boyer O, Mokhtari K, Diquet B, Salzmann JL, Philippon J (1998) A phase I/II study of herpes simplex virus type 1 thymidine kinase "suicide" gene therapy for recurrent glioblastoma. Study Group on Gene Therapy for Glioblastoma. Hum Gene Ther 20:2595–2604
54. Kleihues P, Burger PC, Collins VP, Newcomb EW, Ohgaki H, Cavenee WK (2000) Glioblastoma. In: Kleihues P, Cavenee WK (eds) Pathology and genetics of tumours of the nervous system. World Health Organisation Classification of Tumours. IARC Press, Lyon, pp 29–39
55. Kleihues P, Soylemezoglu F, Schauble B, Scheithauer BW, Burger PC (1995) Histopathology, classification, and grading of gliomas. Glia 15:211–221
56. Kramm CM, Chase M, Herrlinger U, Jacobs A, Pechan PA, Rainov NG, Sena-Esteves M, Aghi M, Barnett FH, Chiocca EA, Breakefield XO (1997) Therapeutic efficiency and safety of a second-generation replication- conditional HSV1 vector for brain tumor gene therapy. Hum Gene Ther 8:2057–2068
57. Krohn KA, Mankoff DA, Eary JF (2001) Imaging cellular proliferation as a measure of response to therapy. J Clin Pharmacol [Suppl] 96S-103S
58. Kubota K, Ishiwata K, Kubota R, Yamada S, Tada M, Sato T, Ido T (1991) Tracer feasibility for monitoring tumor radiotherapy: a quadruple tracer study with fluorine-18-fluorodeoxyglucose or fluorine-18-fluorodeoxyuridine, L-[methyl-14C]methionine, [6-3H]thymidine, and gallium-67. J Nucl Med 32:2118–2123
59. Lang FF, Miller DC, Koslow M, Newcomb EW (1994) Pathways leading to glioblastoma multiforme: a molecular analysis of genetic alterations in 65 astrocytic tumors. J Neurosurg 81:427–436
60. Langen KJ, Muhlensiepen H, Holschbach M, Hautzel H, Jansen P, Coenen HH (2000) Transport mechanisms of 3-[123I]iodo-alpha-methyl-L-tyrosine in a human glioma cell line: comparison with [3H]methyl]-L-methionine. J Nucl Med 41:1250–1255
61. Louis DN, Holland EC, Cairncross JG (2001) Glioma classification: a molecular reappraisal. Am J Pathol 159:779–786
62. Mankoff DA, Dehdashti F, Shields AF (2000) Characterizing tumors using metabolic imaging: PET imaging of cellular proliferation and steroid receptors. Neoplasia 2:71–88
63. Markert JM, Medlock MD, Rabkin SD, Gillespie GY, Todo T, Hunter WD, Palmer CA, Feigenbaum F, Tornatore C, Tufaro F, Martuza RL (2000) Conditionally replicating herpes simplex virus mutant, G207 for the treatment of malignant glioma: results of a phase I trial. Gene Ther 7:867–874
64. Mier W, Haberkorn U, Eisenhut M (2002) [18F]FLT; portrait of a proliferation marker. Eur J Nucl Med Mol Imaging 29:165–169
65. Morin KW, Knaus EE, Wiebe LI (1997) Non-invasive scintigraphic monitoring of gene expression in a HSV-1 thymidine kinase gene therapy model. Nucl Med Commun 18:599–605
66. Morrison RS (1999) Growth factor mediated signaling pathways. In: Berger MS, Wilson CB (eds) The gliomas. Saunders, Philadelphia, pp 52–64
67. Nanda D, de Jong M, Vogels R, Havenga M, Driesse M, Bakker W, Bijster M, Avezaat C, Cox P, Morin K, Naimi E, Knaus E, Wiebe L, Smitt PS (2002) Imaging expression of adenoviral HSV-1-*tk* suicide gene transfer using the nucleoside analogue FIRU. Eur J Nucl Med Mol Imaging 29:939–947
68. Ogawa T, Inugami A, Hatazawa J, Kanno I, Murakami M, Yasui N, Mineura K, Uemura K (1996) Clinical positron emission tomography for brain tumors: comparison of fludeoxyglucose F 18 and L-methyl-11C-methionine. AJNR Am J Neuroradiol 17: 345–353
69. Ogawa T, Shishido F, Kanno I, Inugami A, Fujita H, Murakami M, Shimosegawa E, Ito H, Hatazawa J, Okudera T (1993) Cerebral glioma: evaluation with methionine PET. Radiology 186: 45–53
70. Palu G, Cavaggioni A, Calvi P, Franchin E, Pizzato M, Boschetto R, Parolin C, Chilosi M, Ferrini S, Zanusso A, Colombo F (1999) Gene therapy of glioblastoma multiforme via combined expression of suicide and cytokine genes: a pilot study in humans. Gene Ther 6:330–337
71. Papanastassiou V, Rampling R, Fraser M, Petty R, Hadley D, Nicoll J, Harland J, Mabbs R, Brown M (2002) The potential for efficacy of the modified (ICP 34.5(-)) herpes simplex virus HSV1716 following intratumoural injection into human malignant glioma: a proof of principle study. Gene Ther 9:398–406
72. Patronas NJ, Di Chiro G, Kufta C, Bairamian D, Kornblith PL, Simon R, Larson SM (1985) Prediction of survival in glioma patients by means of positron emission tomography. J Neurosurg 62:816–822
73. Phelps ME (2000) PET: the merging of biology and imaging into molecular imaging. J Nucl Med 41:661–681
74. Price P (2001) PET as a potential tool for imaging molecular mechanisms of oncology in man. Trends Mol Med 7:442–446
75. Rainov NG (2000) A phase III clinical evaluation of herpes simplex virus type 1 thymidine kinase and ganciclovir gene therapy as an adjuvant to surgical resection and radiation in adults with previously untreated glioblastoma multiforme. Hum Gene Ther 20:2389–2401
76. Ram Z, Culver KW, Oshiro EM, Viola JJ, deVroom HL, Otto E, Long Z, Chiang Y, McGarrity GJ, Muul LM, Katz D, Blaese RM, Oldfield EH (1997) Therapy of malignant brain tumors by intratumoral implantation of retroviral vector-producing cells. Nat Med 3:1354–1361
77. Rampling R, Cruickshank G, Papanastassiou V, Nicoll J, Hadley D, Brennan D, Petty R, MacLean A, Harland J, McKie E, Mabbs R, Brown M (2000) Toxicity evaluation of replication-competent herpes simplex virus (ICP 34.5 null mutant 1716) in patients with recurrent malignant glioma. Gene Ther 7:859–866
78. Rogulski KR, Wing MS, Paielli DL, Gilbert JD, Kim JH, Freytag SO (2000) Double suicide gene therapy augments the antitumor activity of a replication-competent lytic adenovirus through enhanced cytotoxicity and radiosensitization. Hum Gene Ther 11:67–76

79. Saito Y, Price RW, Rottenberg DA, Fox JJ, Su TL, Watanabe KA, Philips FS (1982) Quantitative autoradiographic mapping of herpes simplex virus encephalitis with a radiolabeled antiviral drug. Science 217:1151–1153
80. Saito Y, Rubenstein R, Price RW, Fox JJ, Watanabe KA (1984) Diagnostic imaging of herpes simplex virus encephalitis using a radiolabeled antiviral drug: autoradiographic assessment in an animal model. Ann Neurol 15:548–558
81. Sasaki H, Zlatescu MC, Betensky RA, Johnk LB, Cutone AN, Cairncross JG, Louis DN (2002) Histopathological-molecular genetic correlations in referral pathologist-diagnosed low-grade "oligodendroglioma". J Neuropathol Exp Neurol 61:58–63
82. Sasaki M, Kuwabara Y, Yoshida T, Nakagawa M, Fukumura T, Mihara F, Morioka T, Fukui M, Masuda K (1998) A comparative study of thallium-201 SPET, carbon-11 methionine PET and fluorine-18 fluorodeoxyglucose PET for the differentiation of astrocytic tumours. Eur J Nucl Med 25:1261–1269
83. Shand N, Weber F, Mariani L, Bernstein M, Gianella-Borradori A, Long Z, Sorensen AG, Barbier N (1999) A phase 1–2 clinical trial of gene therapy for recurrent glioblastoma multiforme by tumor transduction with the herpes simplex thymidine kinase gene followed by ganciclovir. GLI328 European-Canadian Study Group. Hum Gene Ther 10:2325–2335
84. Shields AF, Grierson JR, Dohmen BM, Machulla HJ, Stayanoff JC, Lawhorn-Crews JM, Obradovich JE, Muzik O, Mangner TJ (1998) Imaging proliferation in vivo with [F-18]FLT and positron emission tomography. Nat Med 4:1334–1336
85. Sokoloff L, Reivich M, Kennedy C, des Rosiers MH, Patlak CS, Pettigrew KD, Sakurada O, Shinohara M (1977) The [14C]deoxyglucose method for the measurement of local cerebral glucose utilization: theory, procedure, and normal values in the conscious and anesthetized albino rat. J Neurochem 28: 897–916
86. Tjuvajev JG, Avril N, Oku T, Sasajima T, Miyagawa T, Joshi R, Safer M, Beattie B, DiResta G, Daghighian F, Augensen F, Koutcher J, Zweit J, Humm J, Larson SM, Finn R, Blasberg R (1998) Imaging herpes virus thymidine kinase gene transfer and expression by positron emission tomography. Cancer Res 58:4333–4341
87. Tjuvajev JG, Chen SH, Joshi A, Joshi R, Guo ZS, Balatoni J, Ballon D, Koutcher J, Finn R, Woo SL, Blasberg RG (1999) Imaging adenoviral-mediated herpes virus thymidine kinase gene transfer and expression in vivo. Cancer Res 59:5186–5193
88. Tjuvajev JG, Doubrovin M, Akhurst T, Cai S, Balatoni J, Alauddin MM, Finn R, Bornmann W, Thaler H, Conti PS, Blasberg RG (2002) Comparison of radiolabeled nucleoside probes (FIAU, FHBG, and FHPG) for PET imaging of HSV-1-*tk* gene expression. J Nucl Med 43:1072–1083
89. Tjuvajev JG, Finn R, Watanabe K, Joshi R, Oku T, Kennedy J, Beattie B, Koutcher J, Larson S, Blasberg RG (1996) Noninvasive imaging of herpes virus thymidine kinase gene transfer and expression: a potential method for monitoring clinical gene therapy. Cancer Res 56:4087–4095
90. Tjuvajev JG, Joshi A, Callegari J, Lindsley L, Joshi R, Balatoni J, Finn R, Larson SM, Sadelain M, Blasberg RG (1999) A general approach to the non-invasive imaging of transgenes using cis-linked herpes simplex virus thymidine kinase. Neoplasia 1:315–320
91. Tjuvajev JG, Stockhammer G, Desai R, Uehara H, Watanabe K, Gansbacher B, Blasberg RG (1995) Imaging the expression of transfected genes in vivo. Cancer Res 55:6126–6132
92. Todo T, Rabkin SD, Sundaresan P, Wu A, Meehan KR, Herscowitz HB, Martuza RL (1999) Systemic antitumor immunity in experimental brain tumor therapy using a multimutated, replication-competent herpes simplex virus. Hum Gene Ther 20:2741–2755
93. Voges J, Weber F, Reszka R, Sturm V, Jacobs A, Heiss WD, Wiestler O, Kapp JF (2002) Clinical protocol. Liposomal gene therapy with the herpes simplex thymidine kinase gene/ganciclovir system for the treatment of glioblastoma multiforme. Hum Gene Ther 13:675–685
94. Wiebe LI, Morin KW, Knaus EE (1997) Radiopharmaceuticals to monitor gene transfer. Q J Nucl Med 41:79–89
95. Yaghoubi S, Barrio JR, Dahlbom M, Iyer M, Namavari M, Satyamurthy N, Goldman R, Herschman HR, Phelps ME, Gambhir SS (2001) Human pharmacokinetic and dosimetry studies of [18F]FHBG: a reporter probe for imaging herpes simplex virus type-1 thymidine kinase reporter gene expression. J Nucl Med 42:1225–1234
96. Yaghoubi SS, Wu L, Liang Q, Toyokuni T, Barrio JR, Namavari M, Satyamurthy N, Phelps ME, Herschman HR, Gambhir SS (2001) Direct correlation between positron emission tomographic images of two reporter genes delivered by two distinct adenoviral vectors. Gene Ther 8:1072–1080
97. Yu Y, Annala AJ, Barrio JR, Toyokuni T, Satyamurthy N, Namavari M, Cherry SR, Phelps ME, Herschman HR, Gambhir SS (2000) Quantification of target gene expression by imaging reporter gene expression in living animals. Nat Med 6:933–937

PART III

Clinical Applications

CHAPTER 11

PET/CT: Clinical Considerations

A. Bockisch · L. Freudenberg · G. Antoch · St. Müller

11.1 Introduction

Combined positron emission tomography/computed tomography (PET/CT) scanners have recently become available commercially and are currently being evaluated at several sites. These new imaging systems are based on two mature technologies. PET is well established for quantitative imaging of the positron emitter distribution in the body. During the last 25 years, a variety of tracers have been developed, which are suitable to characterize non-invasively and in vivo a large variety of normal or pathological molecular processes (see Chap. 10) (Tewson and Krohn 1998; Varagnolo et al. 2000). Today, 2-[^{18}F]fluoro-2-deoxy-D-glucose ([^{18}F]FDG) is the dominant tracer for clinical routine applications (Ak et al. 2000; Pauwels et al. 2000; Stokkel et al. 2001; Valkema et al. 1996; van der Hiel et al. 2001; Gambhir et al. 2001; Reske and Kotzerke 2001).

Cross-sectional X-ray images (CT) became available more than 30 years ago and revolutionized non-invasive diagnostics. Since then, the performance of CT imaging systems has increased tremendously and more sophisticated contrast agent protocols have become available. However, the lack of functional information of CT imaging still limits its sensitivity and specificity in staging and clinical follow up of various malignant diseases. Also the morphology-based magnetic resonance imaging (MRI), which was introduced into clinical medicine 20 years ago, leaves diagnostic gaps to be filled by nuclear medicine imaging in general and PET in particular. Although nuclear medicine modalities deal with biomolecular imaging, it is at least helpful and often essential also to identify the anatomical structure corresponding to the functional disturbance (Akhurst and Chisin 2000; Shreve 2000; Townsend 2001; Townsend and Cherry 2001; Wahl et al. 1993).

In clinical routine, the task may be accomplished by comparing the PET emission and transmission images or by visual comparison of PET emission with CT or MR images. Assuming the availability of CT or MR images on a routine basis, this approach is straightforward and does not incur additional costs; however, the spatial accuracy of the correlation is limited. Therefore, computer-assisted approaches for retrospective image fusion have been the focus of intense research (Hutton et al. 2002). Co-registration methods relying on internal anatomical landmarks will fail, however, if the radiopharmaceutical does not provide enough anatomical detail. Approaches using external fiducial markers are successful in rigid areas in the body but are likely to be unreliable, e.g. in the abdomen, where internal structures and external markers do not correlate because of the non-rigidity of the body. Varying mobility and shifting of abdominal and thoracic organs necessitate non-linear registration algorithms of high complexity, which are far from being validated for clinical use (Hutton et al. 2002).

Furthermore, most of the computer algorithms for image fusion are only applicable to individual organs or limited whole-body areas. This, in turn, limits the localization accuracy, which increases in importance the more a diagnostic finding or therapeutic decision relies on topography. The ideal image fusion demands simultaneous data acquisition. This demand cannot be fulfilled yet, not only for technical reasons but also because the two modalities involved, e.g. PET and CT, require protocols that cannot be optimally executed simultaneously. Therefore, today, the optimal solution for aligning functional and anatomical information across extended areas (whole-body examination), overcoming the problems mentioned above, is the nearly simultaneous acquisition of functional (PET) and anatomical (CT) information using a single device, without the patient getting off the bed between scans or moving at all (Akhurst and Chisin 2000; Shreve 2000; Townsend 2001; Townsend and Cherry 2001; Wahl et al. 1993). There is much discussion about whether PET/CT is the necessary prerequisite for reaching the required accuracy in co-registration. PET/CT is the combination of well-established devices and modalities. The ease and accuracy of image fusion not only promises a higher diagnostic precision, but also has potential applications that are out of reach at the moment. In this chapter we will outline the present state of PET/CT and propose realistic developments for the future.

In summary, PET/CT resolves diagnostic problems such as unclear anatomical assignment of PET findings in normal and altered anatomy. It offers synergistic effects of PET and CT in equivocal PET and/or CT pictures. It offers metabolic-guided biopsy and guides therapy such as external radiation, chemoembolization or radiofrequency ablation. PET/CT has logistic advantages over PET, including shorter investigation times.

11.2 Present State and Use of PET/CT

Combined PET/CT devices have been commercially available since 2000/1 and have been developed for less than 10 years. Until now, only a few thousand investigations have been performed at a few sites, mostly using different protocols. Therefore, the scientific proof of the value of PET/CT must be necessarily limited, although some superiority aspects are self-evident (Fig. 1). There are only a few types of PET/CT devices available today, which are in different states of integration of the PET and CT machine. PET/CT devices operate reliably and are easy to use on a routine basis. The essential technical problems have been solved. Apart from the technical aspects, it is also important to analyze the way in which the device is operated and what degree of integration is necessary for the film reading of the two imaging modalities. There are different paradigms concerning operating the PET/CT and the power of PET/CT is applied to different extents by different users. Some users add only the morphologic information of a low-dose CT to the PET for anatomical landmarking, some acquire full-dose CT without contrast medium. Our philosophy is to combine high-quality PET with a diagnostic CT, which usually includes oral and intravenous contrast agents. Our philosophy is the joint optimization of both imaging modalities for maximum information. This mandates the use of oral and intravenous contrast agents for the CT scan and allows us to replace separate CT and PET studies with a single PET/CT scan without significant sacrifice of the diagnostic performance of either modality. We believe that otherwise some synergistic effects of PET/CT will be lost (Fig. 2).

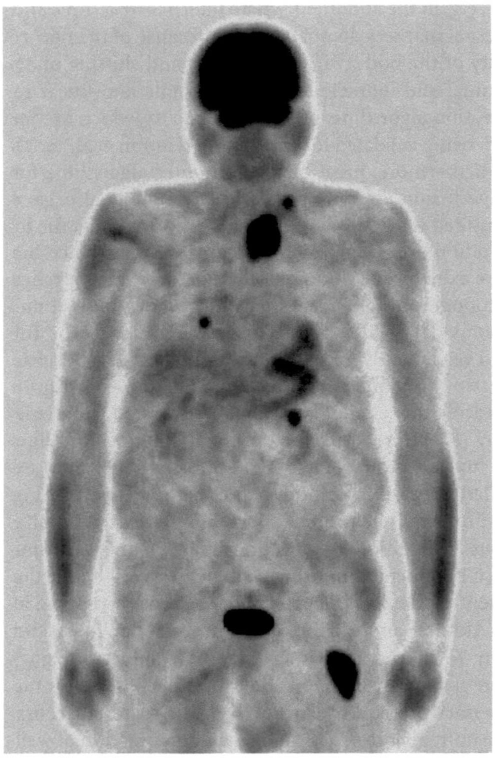

Fig. 1. A typical PET "whole" body scan using FDG for a patient suffering from non-small cell lung cancer, showing the primary, some lung metastases, as well as distant metastases likely to be in the suprarenal gland and the left femur. However, the FDG distribution provides only limited topographic information. The precise location of the metastases is not clear, especially in those cases where CT or MR images are negative. Typical questions left unanswered are the differentiation between pathological lymph node activity or unspecific intestinal activity, active urine in the ureter or a peripheral calyx, malignant lymph node involvement or metastasis in or ↔ close to the liver or suprarenal gland

11.3 Clinical Value of PET/CT at Present

There is a wide range of advantages of PET/CT over PET and CT and, at least in certain situations, over image fusion. We will discuss the known applications here; at the end of the chapter we will outline our expectations for further developments.

Using the CT data for attenuation and scatter correction (see Chap. 2) improves the image quality and also saves considerable time. Using typical protocols, a 90 cm axial field-of-view requires a 60 min scan time in the dedicated PET scanner (EXACT HR$^+$, CPS) using the 3D technique compared to 40 min in the PET/CT (Biograph, CPS). The shortened investigation time not only makes the PET investigation more cost-effective, it also – more important – reduces the time of suffering for sick patients who have problems lying motionless for so long and consequently also reduces motion artifacts.

Getting rid of the line sources, which are no longer needed, saves maintenance costs and offers a wider opening of the tunnel, which is favorable for external beam radiation planning, PET/CT-guided interventions, and reduces the likelihood of claustrophobia.

While FDG PET provides high lesion contrast in many malignant tumors, it shows only little anatomical detail in the body. The lack of specificity may introduce problems because the anatomical origin of the accumulation of activity is sometimes unclear. In some areas the diagnostic accuracy might be significantly reduced simply because of possible non-specific activity. In stand-alone PET investigations, this differentiation is performed introducing medical expert knowledge, such as anamne-

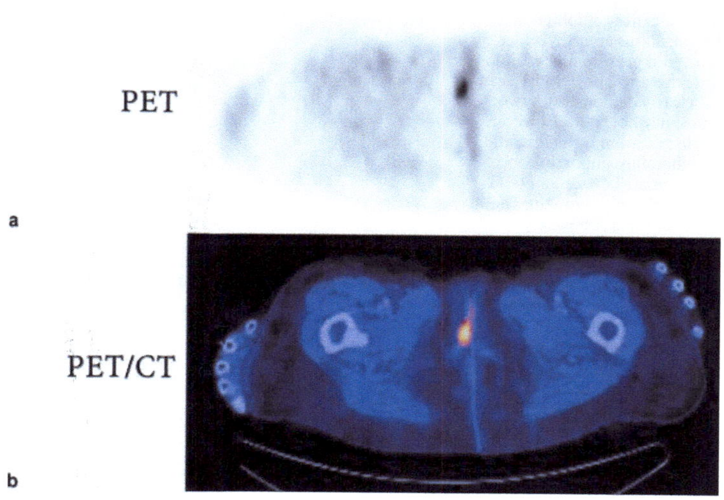

Fig. 2.
Metastasis of a sarcoma localized in the right labia. In PET (**a**) alone the FDG uptake would have been judged as contamination by urine. The location is outside of the typical CT field. The diagnosis could only be made by comparing the PET image with a diagnostic CT. The PET/CT fusion image (**b**) confirms the diagnosis

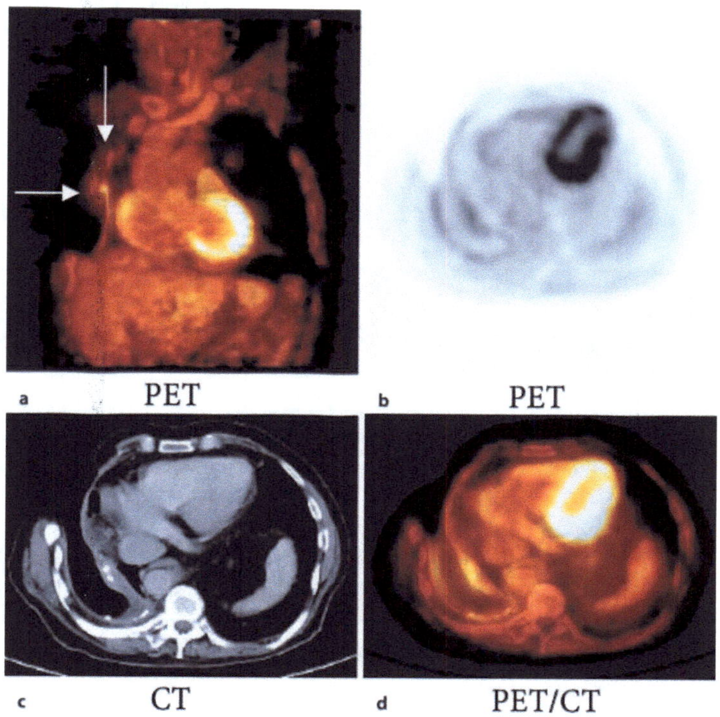

Fig. 3.
Patient with pulmonary tuberculosis 40 years ago, status post pneumothorax, chest plomb, chest wall resection and recurrent empyema, who presented with signs of infection and pericardial effusion. Conventional diagnostics did not show a conclusive focus of infection. ^{99m}Tc granulocyte scintigraphy revealed increased focal uptake in the right thorax. No topographic anatomical localization was possible because of the extensive postoperative changes of the anatomy. The PET images (**a**, **b**) show inhomogeneously increased glucose turnover, which cannot be localized because of the extensive change of anatomy. PET/CT (**d**) clearly localized an increased FDG uptake in the parietal pleura and pericardium, with accentuation in areas with calcifications (*arrows* in PET image **a**) visualized on the CT scan (**c**). Follow-up confirmed the suspicion of activated tuberculosis with perimyocarditis

sis, prevalences, image pattern, etc., ending up with a medically "reasonable" report. The use of these tools requires experience and expertise. Nevertheless they may become useless in altered anatomy, e.g. after surgery (Fig. 3).

In highly specific radiopharmaceuticals, such as [^{124}I]iodide in thyroid cancer imaging, for example, the complete lack of background information cannot be overcome by experience. Likewise, retrospective image fusion is likely to fail. This may seriously impair the diagnostic usefulness of these tracers (Fig. 4). The advent of PET/CT, therefore, may set the stage for the introduction of new highly specific radiopharmaceuticals into clinical practice.

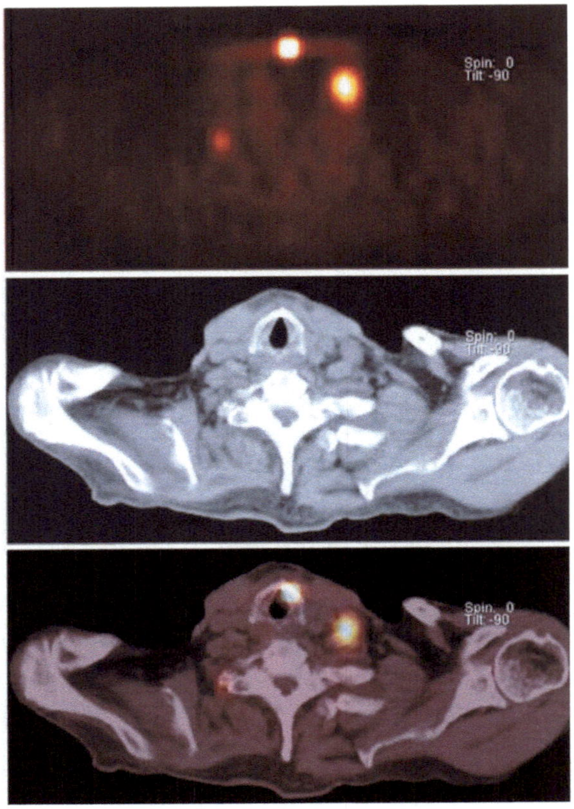

Fig. 4.
Patient with differentiated thyroid cancer of follicular origin. Status after thyroidectomy and prior to first radioiodine therapy. The ^{124}I PET scan (**a**) clearly demonstrates two extremely hot spots. However, the localization is unclear, and it is therefore impossible to differentiate between metastases and thyroid remnant. The CT scan (**b**) is completely negative. PET/CT (**c**) shows one hot spot in the typical site of the thyroid, so is interpreted as a remnant. The other is close to the trachea and even infiltrating it, being a metastasis. The functional information combined with the precise localization made the differential diagnosis

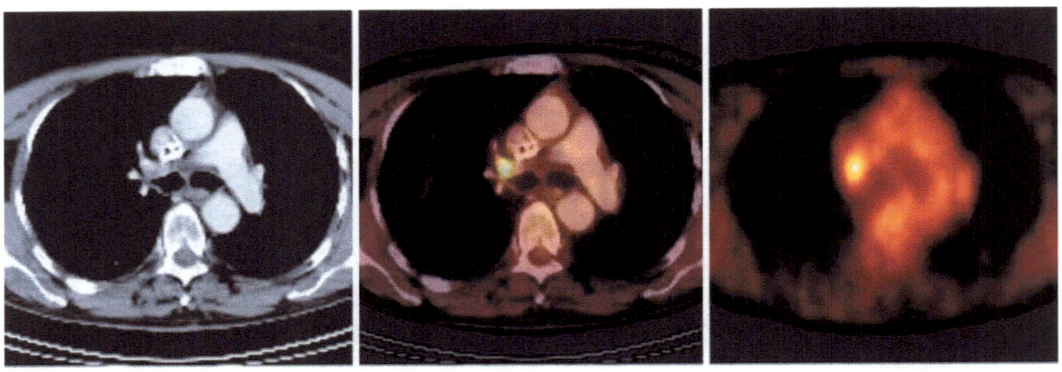

Fig. 5. FDG PET has an established role in lymph node staging of non-small cell lung cancer (Chap. 15). It is generally accepted that accurate staging requires the PET and CT images to be read together. While there is controversial evidence for improved accuracy by using fused images, PET/CT at least facilitates the diagnosis by providing PET and CT images acquired at the same time using the same slicing. This figure shows a tracheobronchial lymph node not enlarged in CT (**a**) non-enlarged with focal FDG (**c**) accumulation, indicating metastatic involvement. PET/CT (**b**) fuses the diagnosis of a metastasis from the PET investigation with the accurate localization in the CT images, resulting in the correct staging

In other applications only a precise knowledge of the anatomical correlation of the PET positive finding will answer the diagnostic question. In lung cancer the exact identification of locoregional lymph nodes determines the staging. The spatial error allowed is less than 1 cm, requiring a very precise co-registration (Fig. 5). Retrospective image fusion always has some uncertainties, when the lesion cannot be identified simultaneously in both modalities.

11.4 Patient Selection and Clinical Protocols for PET/CT Scanning

Combined PET/CT necessarily leads to radiation exposure of the patient by both the PET radiotracer and the CT X-rays. Thus the indications have to be defined under which conditions the patient will undergo the examination. The necessary prerequisite is obviously the indication for the PET scan, otherwise the standard CT would be adequate. For the CT scan, it has to be decided whether a diagnostic CT scan is performed or only a low-dose CT for landmarking plus rough image reading.

The diagnostic CT scan should be performed only if there is an indication for the CT examination by itself, and if no adequate CT has been performed previously. The CT scan may be restricted to a volume smaller than that usually investigated by PET. In this case, the missing volumes may additionally be scanned by CT in a low-dose mode for attenuation correction and landmarking.

In addition, PET/CT may be performed in those patients in whom either previous PET and/or CT scans introduced the need for the dual modality investigation to clarify uncertainties.

In order to acquire maximum information, we preferably perform the PET scan according to established rules in combination with a diagnostic CT, which usually includes oral and intravenous contrast agents. However, some compromises have to be accepted for both modalities.

The PET images are acquired and reconstructed according to the typical protocols, which depend on the radiopharmaceutical, among other factors. In PET/CT scanners without septa*, emission data have to be acquired in 3D mode. So-called whole-body scans cover the base of the skull to the pelvis. The brain is usually excluded to avoid irradiation of the lens of the eye by CT imaging. The entire head is investigated only in cases where there is a high chance of PET being required, such as positive brain metastases. The CT scan is performed first, followed by the PET scan, starting with the pelvis to minimize bladder filling between the CT and PET scans.

Computed tomography scans are acquired with a tube voltage of 130 kVp, 160 mAs, a slice width of 5 mm and a table feed of 8 mm/rotation (pitch 1.6, gantry rotation time 800 ms). To assure acquisition of a fully diagnostic CT component, intravenous and oral contrast agents are usually administered to patients (Antoch et al. 2002). The CT data are also used for PET attenuation correction (Beyer et al. 2000). Total scan time is 25–40 min depending on the number of beds scanned.

In our Biograph, the CT images are used for attenuation and scatter correction of the PET data (see Chap. 2). The application of CT contrast agents may accentuate areas in the PET images that correspond to contrast-enhancing structures on CT. This effect is most apparent in the mediastinum and must be considered in the interpretation (Antoch et al. 2002).

To minimize breathing artifacts, we have developed a breathing protocol for PET/CT. The patient is asked to perform continuous shallow breathing, and to hold his breath in an average breathing position for only approximately 20 s, while the CT scan passes the diaphragm. This protocol works well in cooperative patients and restricts misregistrations in the neighborhood of the diaphragm, which is the most sensitive location, to less than 1 cm. By excluding patient movement, we are dealing with linear shifts only, which can be easily and reliably corrected performing simple linear translation. In our experience, more than 90% of the patients follow the breathing protocol as demanded. The others show larger breathing-related misregistrations of up to 2 cm, mostly in the lower lung and upper liver, which can be corrected for as outlined above.

11.5 Clinical Impact of PET/CT

11.5.1 Primary Diagnostics

Positron emission tomography images display primarily the distribution of the applied radionuclide. Assuming a stable radiotracer or a single metabolic path, this is identical to the radiopharmaceutical distribution. For established tracers, the physiological radiopharmaceutical distribution is well known. However, this does not exclude individual activity distribution patterns, which are influenced by physiological states such as muscle tonus or insulin blood levels.

We see physiological FDG accumulation to varying extents in the intestine or in muscles, for example. Therefore, it is obvious that both the sensitivity as well as the specificity of PET interpretations (Figs. 1, 2) will be improved by correlation with morphology-based diagnostic tools, especially in situations with changed anatomy (Fig. 3), such as after surgery, where physiological variations of FDG uptake cannot easily be distinguished from pathology. In addition, in some clinical situations the PET finding may be correlated with healthy but hyperactive tissue, such as occurs in hormonal stimulation of the ovary (Fig. 6). Only precise co-registration allows the correlation of the ovary with the increased FDG uptake, which otherwise would be misinterpreted as lymph node metastasis or as unphysiological intes-

* Due to the use of the CT data for attenuation and scatter correction, the rod sources become obsolete and therefore the septa are no longer needed, offering the choice of a larger opening of the scanner. This is an important feature for radiotherapy planning.

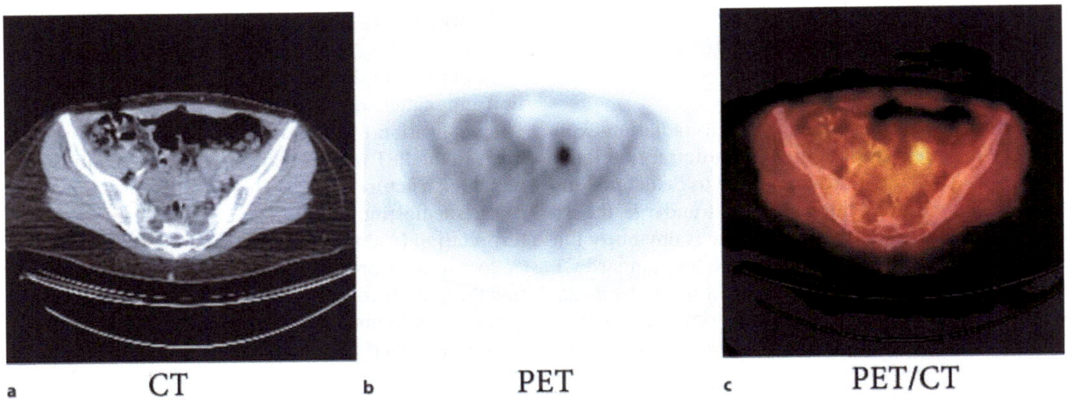

Fig. 6. In the PET hot spot in the true pelvis (**b**), the PET image suggests a metastasis and the CT image shows no pathological finding (**a**). PET/CT correlates the PET finding with the left ovary. As there was no evidence of disease and the follow-up was negative, the finding correlates with an activated ovary. This diagnosis is occasionally feasible with the help of PET/CT

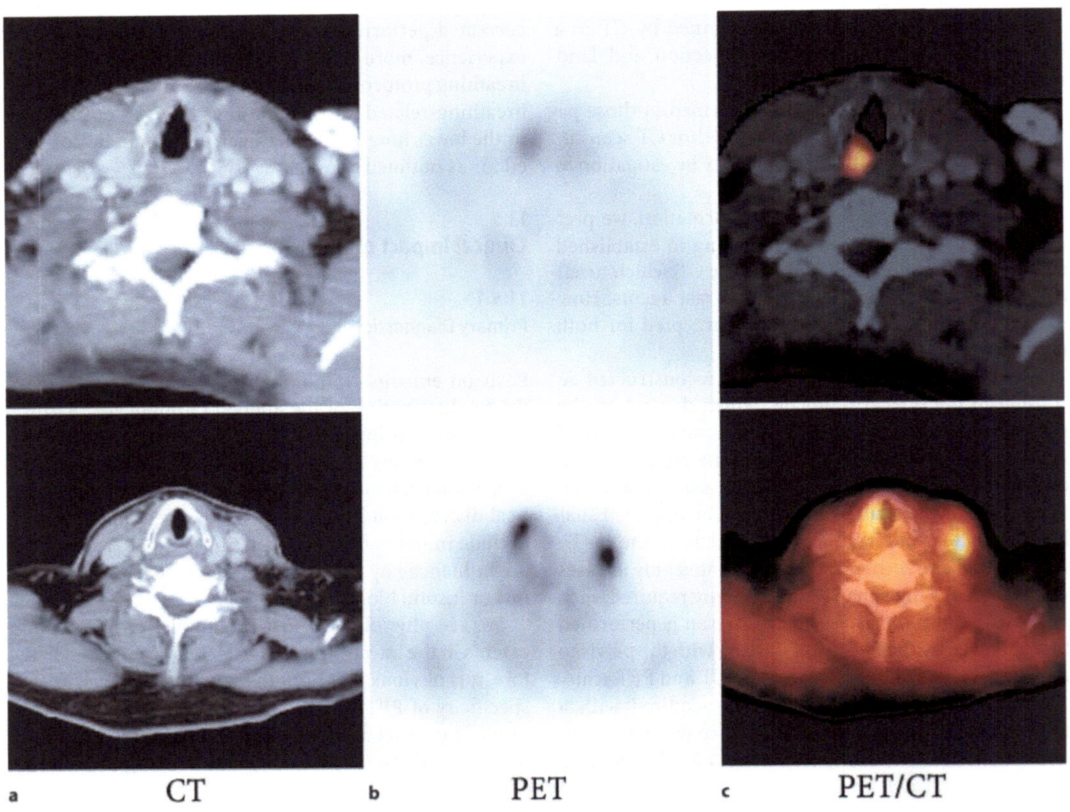

Fig. 7. *Upper row* larynx carcinoma. CT (*left*): inconclusive. PET (*middle*): increased uptake, malignant tumor or unspecific uptake in the vocal cord. PET/CT (*right*) locates the PET finding retrotracheal, therefore excluding unspecific vocal cord activity. *Lower row* similar finding, however, the activity is located in the vocal cord, which is normal. It is unspecific unilateral activity in a patient with paralysis of the left vocal cord. In addition a lymph node metastasis shows up on the left

tinal uptake. Similar situations include focal increased uptakes due to overexertion of the vocal cord contralaterally to paralysis (Fig. 7). Only the identification of the underlying structure in those examples allows the final diagnosis of physiological or pathological increased turnover to be made.

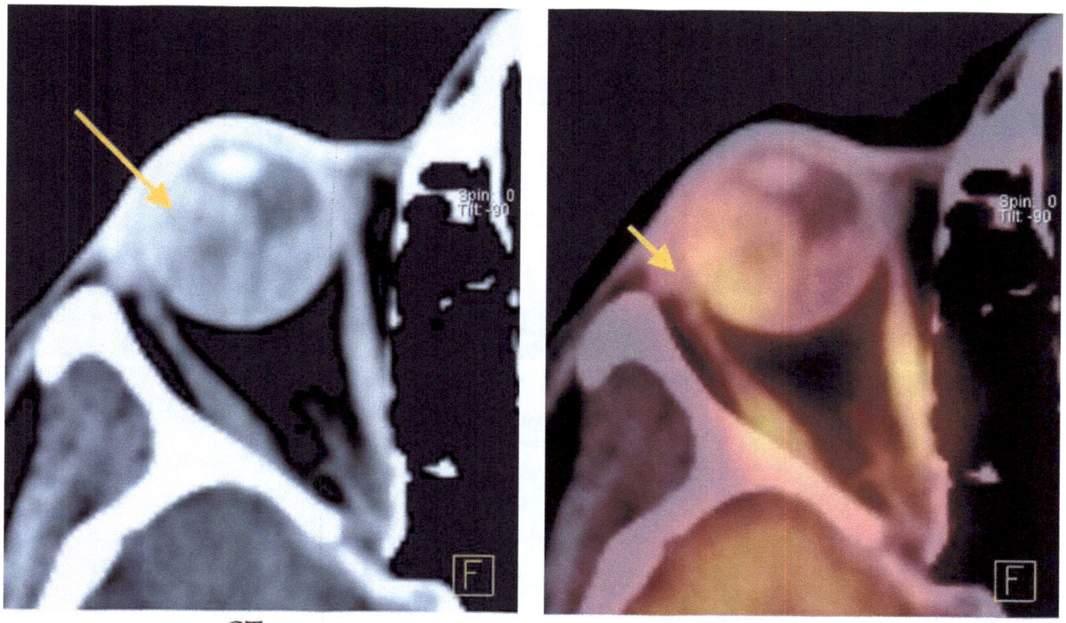

a CT b PET/CT

Fig. 8. In uveal melanoma it is crucial to determine whether the tumor is restricted to the ball of the eye. In this patient, CT (**a**) demonstrates the tumor clearly but fails to identify its limits. PET is positive, however, the spatial information of the PET cannot answer this question. The precise fusion of the PET/CT (**b**) allows the pathological uptake only inside the eye to be identified. Pathology confirmed that the tumor was restricted to the ball of the eye. Note the sharp imaging of the activity of the muscles in the PET/CT image

In many malignant diseases, PET alone has been proven to be superior to CT or MRI and to yield sensitivities and specificities of 90% or better (Gambhir et al. 2001; Reske and Kotzerke 2001). In cases of such high sensitivities for PET calculating the sensitivity and specificity for combining independent diagnostic modalities, it is far from certain a-priori that fused images from a combined PET/CT scanner will exceed the diagnostic power of separate PET and CT or MRI scans read side by side. However, the precise co-registration of PET may be of crucial clinical value, even if there is no doubt about pathological increased turnover, even if the diagnosis of malignancy is out of question. In many situations the precise knowledge of the location and the extent of the lesion is of utmost importance. Tumor staging is the basis for the selection risk-adapted therapy. This requires the exact anatomical localization of malignant tissue. Common examples are mediastinal lymph nodes in bronchial carcinoma, the decision between an infra- and supradiaphragmal location of lymphomas in non-Hodgkin's lymphoma or the restriction of uveal malignant melanoma to the eye (Fig. 8).

Of similar importance is the identification of the underlying structure when highly specific radiotracers are used. As an ideal example, we mention ^{124}I PET/CT scans in patients with newly diagnosed follicular cell-derived thyroid cancer, after surgery and prior to radioiodine therapy. High iodine uptake in the thyroid bed is normal and requires thorough local discrimination versus extrathyroidal and therefore malignant uptake (Fig. 4).

Of special interest are those constellations in which neither of the two modalities, PET or CT, can provide a probable diagnosis. A typical example is a moderately increased uptake in or around the adrenal gland, which is somewhat clumsy on CT. Only the combination of the two modalities results in suspicion of malignancy.

The investigation of the advantages of PET/CT over separate PET and CT scans has to be focused on specific circumstances, which go beyond a simple combination of decision rules.

11.5.2 Treatment Control

Combined PET/CT has an important role in follow up after treatment. Both the morphologic and the functional changes may be relevant for the judgment of treatment response. In the PET images, however, a mixture of morphologic and functional changes may be displayed. As a result of the recovery effects, shrinkage of a hot lesion may mock a decrease of uptake. Knowledge of the shape and size of the structure of interest, which

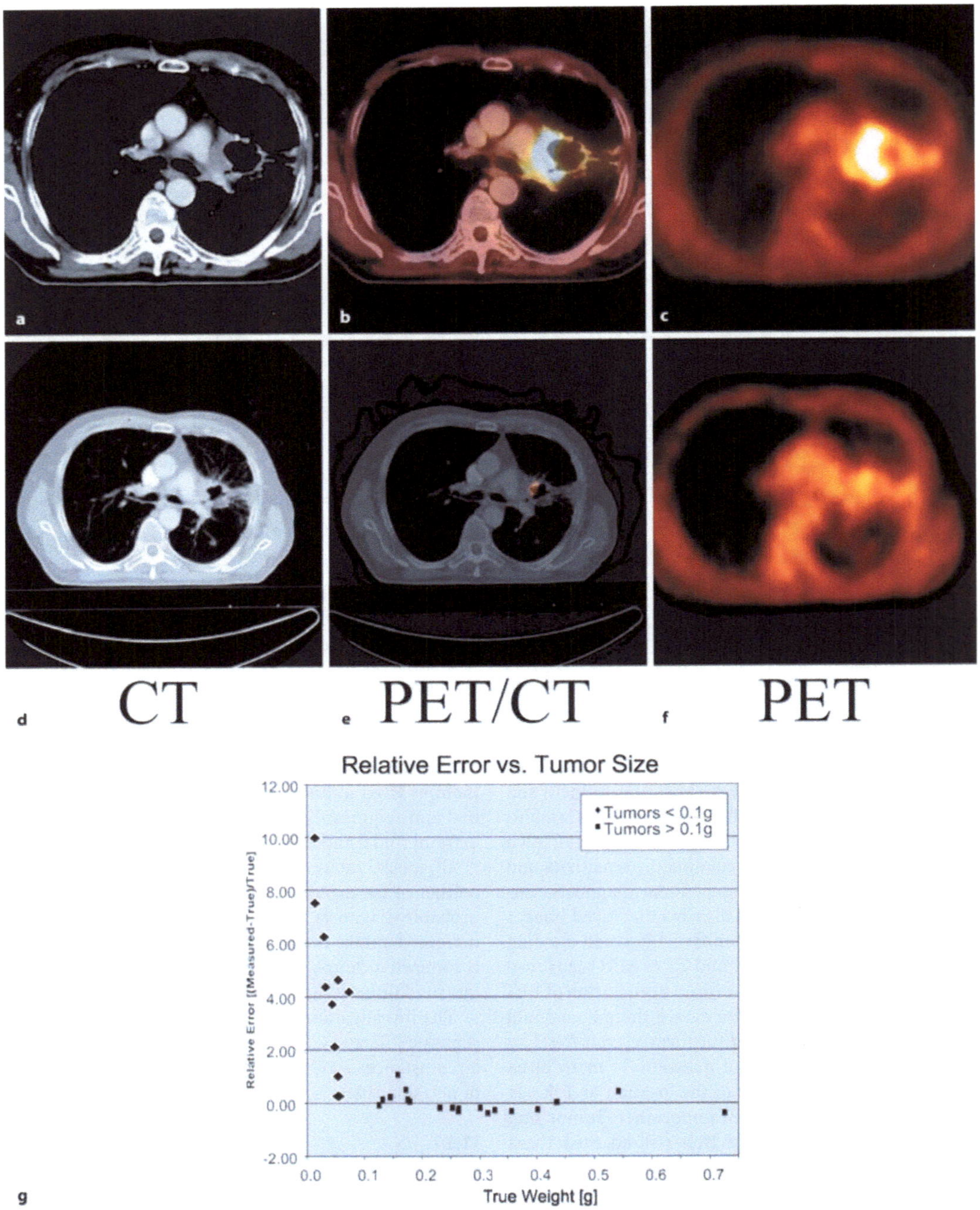
a
b
c
d
CT
e
PET/CT
f
PET
Relative Error vs. Tumor Size
Tumors < 0.1g
Tumors > 0.1g
Relative Error [(Measured-True)/True]
12.00
10.00
8.00
6.00
4.00
2.00
0.00
-2.00
0.0
0.1
0.2
0.3
0.4
0.5
0.6
0.7
True Weight [g]
g

◀ **Fig. 9.** The change in a malignant tumor under therapy is of extreme diagnostic importance. CT judges the change in volume, PET the change of turnover, e.g. represented by the standard uptake value (SUV). However, as a result of partial volume effects, the SUV is measured lower if the tumor shrinks, at least for tumor size similar to the spatial resolution of the PET scanner. The figure displays a typical example. *Upper row* mediastinal metastases prior to therapy (**a**) CT, (**b**) PET/CT, (c) PET. After therapy (*lower row*) the lesions are much smaller and the SUV is considerably reduced. The graphic (**g**) demonstrates the relation between measured SUV and true SUV depending on the size of the lesion. Thus the effect of therapy on the SUV is overestimated in shrinking tumors

is readily available from the CT data, is necessary to perform a recovery correction for accurate quantitation in small tumors. Furthermore, in longitudinal studies, PET/CT permits the unambiguous identification of marker lesions and provides more reliable information about response or progression of the disease (Fig. 9). As experience with PET/CT is limited, we are not yet in a position to present established reading rules that will predict therapy response, by judging both the PET and the CT changes. However, we are convinced that this kind of fused interpretation will improve the diagnostic precision, not only in detecting disease – which is already established – but also in the early prediction of therapy response.

11.5.3 Therapy Planning Including Percutaneous Radiation Therapy

The most convincing application of PET/CT is in directed therapeutic approaches (Kaim et al. 2001) such as minimal invasive surgery, CT-guided transcutaneous radiofrequency ablation, instillation, chemoembolization and taking biopsies. The use of PET/CT in planning percutaneous therapy promises significant improvement over present planning concepts.

Only with the aid of PET/CT, a guided intervention into a PET-positive lesion in any part of the body may be performed reliably and easily. The overlay of the PET image onto the CT allows the target to be hit precisely, even in CT-negative findings. A typical example is given in Fig. 10. After chemoembolization, the CT image of the liver is disturbed by the chemoembolizate and by therapy-induced changes. Relevant changes could not be detected for 6 months. In contrast, the PET image demonstrates two hot spots corresponding to vital tumor. PET/CT allows the aimed and localized therapy of residual or recurrent disease. More frequent applications are the guided biopsies of hyperactive lymph nodes. Likewise, FDG PET/CT may be helpful in the selective biopsy of the viable part of partially necrotic tumors. In this setting PET/CT is of special value in the presence of multiple morphologically detectable lymph nodes.

The high occurrence of recurrences within the primary target volume in some tumors, e.g., bronchial carcinoma, calls for dose escalation to improve the probability of tumor control; however, radiotoxicity to healthy tissues limits this strategy. Therefore, there is a need to increase the dose in the target volume. Because of the biological effect, this is only possible by reducing the irradiated volume. As a consequence, as safety margins are to be reduced, the extent of the disease has to be determined more precisely. PET adds valuable information in

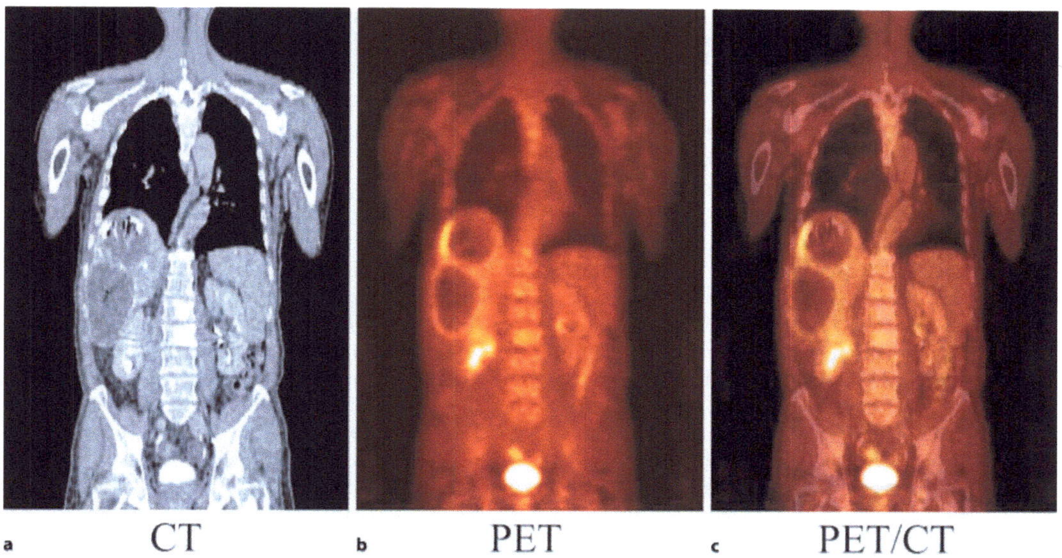

Fig. 10. Three months after chemoembolization, CT (**a**) shows no change. The reliability of CT is reduced as a result of post-therapeutic changes in chemoembolizate material. PET (**b**) shows increased glucose uptake in some spots in the lateral periphery of the tumor, proving recurrence. PET/CT (**c**) localizes the recurrence and allows a precisely guided therapy

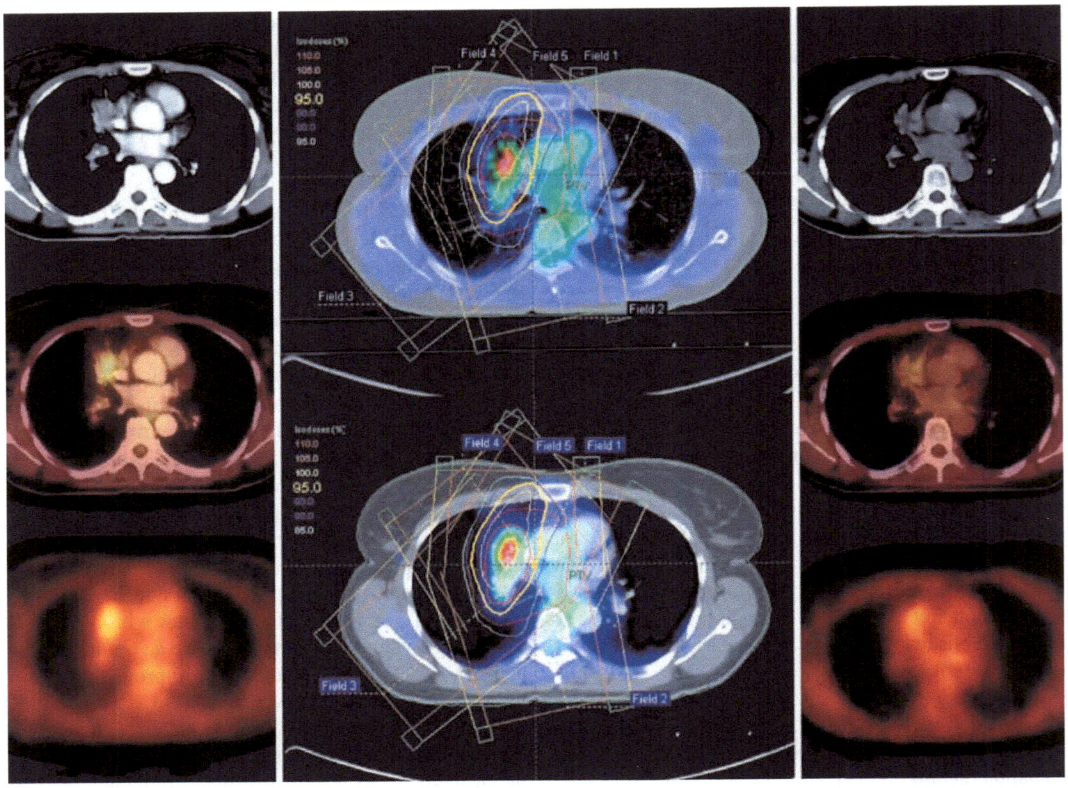

Fig. 11. Radiation planning in a patient with non-small cell lung cancer. *Left column* CT, PET/CT and PET prior to radiotherapy, *right column* after therapy. A good response of the tumor is demonstrated, as the tumor volume is reduced and the glucose uptake is close to normal after therapy. The *middle column* displays therapy planning images by fusing the PET images on the CT. The target volume planning in radiation therapy is based on a spatial coordinate system defined by the planning CT. Because of the exact co-registration of the PET data with the PET/CT metabolic information, in this figure from FDG, the image can be included in the planning process. The figure illustrates the spatial relationship between the isodose distribution, the anatomy, and the areas with increased FDG metabolism. Radiation therapy planning promises to be one of the dominant PET/CT applications. Planning image courtesy of M. Stuschke, Dept. Radiation Therapy, University Essen

this context; however, the PET findings can be translated into morphologic coordinates only by the use of PET/CT. PET data are utilized directly by mapping accurately into the spatial coordinate system of the treatment planning system. Initial data suggest a role for FDG and also more specific tracers in helping to identify areas with a high risk for tumor recurrences. This permits a risk-adapted reduction of the target volume with concomitant dose escalation by optimizing the tradeoff between out-of-field and in-field recurrences (Fig. 11) (Cai et al. 1999; Caldwell et al. 2001; Erdi et al. 2002; Graham et al. 1991; Mah et al. 2002; Munley et al. 1999; Mutic et al. 2001; Nestle et al. 1999; Rahn et al. 1998). Novel radiopharmaceuticals may play a role in further modulating the dose distribution to overcome hypoxic tumor resistance (Chao et al. 2001).

11.5.4 Practical Aspects of PET/CT

We are convinced that PET/CT will play a dominant role in the future. There is no doubt that the combination of PET and CT or MRI is superior to carrying out the film reading blinded for the other modality. The software-based fusion of PET and morphologic images may be performed easily in the future from the technical point of view. However, as a result of biological effects such as bending of the spine and the movement of internal organs, we are doubtful whether the precision of co-registration compared to PET/CT will be reached – at least in the foreseeable future. However, PET/CT offers some additional advantages, which make it superior to and preferred over separate investigations. PET/CT is much faster than PET, as the transmission measurement is performed in minimal time compared to the use of rod sources. As the patient undergoes both the PET and the

CT investigation at the same time, much logistic effort is saved, e.g. only one appointment and one transportation have to be organized. Only one report has to be written and read, which is a final report containing the conclusion of both investigations.

Often, even the widespread FDG PET images are of limited use for therapists, as they are disturbed by missing anatomical information and at the same time varying physiological activity distribution patterns. However, FDG is only one of hundreds of available tracers and one of dozens relevant for wider-spread oncologic application. Therefore, it is worthwhile to project the functional information on morphology, which is used as a kind of adapter to transfer the functional image information to the therapist, enabling him to integrate metabolic information in decision-making. Thus independently from the tracer, the referring physician only needs to be familiar with the CT image to understand the written PET report. Thus trust in the finding is created being crucial for surgeons, interventional radiologists and radiotherapists who perform invasive – potentially harmful – therapies.

11.5.5 Future Developments of PET/CT

Nowadays PET/CT must been seen as initial releases. Nevertheless, there is no doubt, that the devices already have impressively proven the basic idea of fusion machines to be successful in clinic practice. Future developments will increase the degree of integration, resulting in a single PECT emission/transmission scanner, in which dedicated PET and CT parts can no longer be identified. The data acquisition will be speeded up, resulting in shorter investigation times and subsequently less motion. Speed will also allow the use of PET/CT in cardiac diagnostics. We expect sophisticated automated software, which reliably corrects for the remaining (small and linear) displacements between emission and transmission scans. A real simultaneous emission/transmission scan may be launched in the later stages of PET/CT development. However, PET/CT imaging is much more complex than using the two modalities in a combined tomograph. The development of integrated imaging protocols will continue. Most important, a new modality such as PET/CT has to fit into established diagnostic and therapeutic strategies. Therefore, besides of the thrilling and necessary technical developments we foresee for PET/CT the definition of PET/CT indications in contrast to individual indications for PET and CT and eventually for both as today. We have no doubt that in the end PET/CT will have its evidence-based place besides PET and CT in modern non-invasive diagnostics.

References

Ak I, Stokkel MP, Pauwels EK (2000) Positron emission tomography with [18F]fluoro-2-deoxy-D-glucose in oncology, part II. The clinical value in detecting and staging primary tumours. J Cancer Res Clin Oncol 126:560–574

Akhurst T, Chisin R (2000) Hybrid PET/CT machines: optimized PET machines for the new millennium? (See comments.) J Nucl Med 41:961–963

Antoch G, Egelhof T, Korfee S, Frings M, Forsting M, Bockisch A (2002a) Recurrent schwannoma: diagnosis with PET/CT. Neurology. 59:1240

Antoch G, Freudenberg LS, Egelhof T, Stattaus J, Jentzen W, Debatin JF, Bockisch A (2002b) Focal tracer uptake: a potential artifact in contrast-enhanced dual-modality PET/CT scans. J Nucl Med 43:1339–1342

Antoch G, Freudenberg LS, Stattaus J, Jentzen W, Mueller SP, Debatin JF, Bockisch A (2002) Whole-body positron emission tomography-CT: optimized CT using oral and IV contrast materials. AJR 179:1555–1560

Becherer A, Mitterbauer M, Jaeger U, Kalhs P, Greinix HT, Karanikas G, Potzi C, Raderer M, Dudczak R, Kletter K (2002) Positron emission tomography with [18F]2-fluoro-D-2-deoxyglucose (FDG-PET) predicts relapse of malignant lymphoma after high-dose therapy with stem cell transplantation. Leukemia 16:260–267

Beyer T, Townsend DW, Brun T et al (2000) A combined PET/CT tomograph for clinical oncology. J Nucl Med 41:1369–1379

Beyer T, Watson CC, Meltzer CC et al (2001) The biograph: a premium dual-modality PET/CT tomograph for clinical oncology. Electromedica 69:120–126

Beyer T, Townsend D, Blodgett T (2002) Dual-modality PET/CT tomography for clinical oncology. Quart J Nucl Med 46:24–34

Cai J et al (1999) CT and PET lung image registration and fusion in radiotherapy treatment planning using the chamfer-matching method. Int J Radiat Oncol Biol Phys 43:883–891

Caldwell CB et al (2001) Observer variation in contouring gross tumor volume in patients with poorly defined non-small-cell lung tumors on CT: the impact of 18FDG-hybrid PET fusion. Int J Radiat Oncol Biol Phys 51:923–931

Charron M et al (2000) Image analysis in patients with cancer studied with a combined PET and CT scanner. Clin Nucl Med 25:905–910

Chao KS et al (2001) A novel approach to overcome hypoxic tumor resistance: Cu-ATSM-guided intensity-modulated radiation therapy. Int J Radiat Oncol Biol Phys 49:1171–1182

D'Amico TA et al (2002) Impact of computed tomography-positron emission tomography fusion in staging patients with thoracic malignancies. Ann Thorac Surg 74:160–163

Dizendorf EV et al (2002) Application of oral contrast media in coregistered positron emission tomography-CT. AJR Am J Roentgenol 179:477–481

Erdi YE et al (2002) Radiotherapy treatment planning for patients with non-small cell lung cancer using positron emission tomography (PET). Radiother Oncol 62:51–60

Eubank WB, Mankoff DA, Schmied IUP et al (1998) Imaging of oncologic patients: benefit of combined CT and FDG-PET in the diagnosis of malignancy. AJR 171:1101–1110

Freudenberg LS, Antoch G, Beyer T et al (2002) Erste klinische Erfahrungen mit einem kombinierten PET/CT-Tomographen an der Universität Essen. Electromedica 70:68–73

Freudenberg LS, Antoch G, Görges R et al (2002a) 124I-PET/CT in metastatic follicular thyroid carcinoma. Eur J Nucl Med 29:1106

Freudenberg LS, Antoch G, Görges R et al (2002b) Combined PET/CT with Iodine-124 in diagnosis of mediastinal micrometastases in thyroid carcinoma. Int J Radiol 2

Gambhir SS et al (2001) A tabulated summary of the FDG PET literature. J Nucl Med 42 [Suppl]

Giorgetti A, Volterrani D, Mariani G (2002) Clinical oncological applications of Positron Emission Tomography (PET) using fluorine-18-fluoro-2-deoxy-D-glucose. Radiol Med 103:293–318

Goerres GW, Kamel E, Heidelberg T-NH et al (2002a) PET-CT image co-registration in the thorax: influence of respiration. Eur J Nucl Med 29:351–360

Goerres GW, Kamel E, Seifert B, Burger C, Buck A, Hany TF, von Schulthess GK (2002b) Accuracy of image coregistration of pulmonary lesions in patients with non-small cell lung cancer using an integrated PET/CT system. J Nucl Med 43:1469–1475
Görges R, Antoch G, Brandau W et al (2002) Kombinierte PET/CT mit dem Positronenstrahler 124I bei metastasiertem follikulären Schilddrüsenkarzinom. Nuklearmedizin 5:N68–N71
Graham JD et al (1991) A non-invasive, relocatable stereotactic frame for fractionated radiotherapy and multiple imaging. Radiother Oncol 21:60–62
Hany TF, Steinert HC, Goerres GW, Buck A, von Schulthess GK (2002) PET diagnostic accuracy: improvement with in-line PET-CT system: initial results. Radiology 225:575–581
Hicks RJ, Kalff V, MacManus MP et al (2001a) The utility of (18)F-FDG-PET for suspected recurrent non-small cell lung cancer after potentially curative therapy: impact on management and prognostic stratification. J Nucl Med 42:1605–1613
Hicks RJ, Kalff V, McManus MP et al (2001b) (18)F-FDG PET provides high-impact and powerful prognostic stratification in staging newly diagnosed non-small cell lung cancer. J Nucl Med 42:1596–1604
Hoh CK, Hawkins RA, Glaspy JA et al (1993) Cancer detection with whole-body PET using 2-[18F]Fluoro-2-deoxy-D-glucose. J Comput Assist Tomogr 17:582–589
Hutton BF, Braun M, Thurfjell L et al (2002) Image registration: an essential tool for nuclear medicine. Eur J Nucl Med 29:559–577
Kaim AH et al (2001) PET-CT-guided percutaneous puncture of an infected cyst in autosomal dominant polycystic kidney disease: case report. Radiology 221:818–821
Kamel EM et al (2002) Recurrent laryngeal nerve palsy in patients with lung cancer: detection with PET-CT image fusion – report of six cases. Radiology 224:153–156
Kiffer JD et al (1998) The contribution of 18F-fluoro-2-deoxy-glucose positron emission tomographic imaging to radiotherapy planning in lung cancer. Lung Cancer 19:167–177
Kinahan PE et al (1998) Attenuation correction for a combined 3D PET/CT scanner. Med Phys 25:2046–2053
Kluetz PG, Meltzer CC, Villemagne VL et al (2000) Combined PET/CT imaging in oncology. Impact on patient management. Clin Posit Imaging 3:223–230
Mah K et al (2002) The impact of [18F]FDG-PET on target and critical organs in CT-based treatment planning of patients with poorly defined non-small-cell lung carcinoma: a prospective study. Int J Radiat Oncol Biol Phys 52:339–350
Mankoff DA, Bellon JR (2001) Positron-emission tomographic imaging of cancer: glucose metabolism and beyond. Semin Radiat Oncol 11:16–27
Munley MT et al (1999) Multimodality nuclear medicine imaging in three-dimensional radiation treatment planning for lung cancer: challenges and prospects. Lung Cancer 23:105–114
Mutic S et al (2001) Multimodality image registration quality assurance for conformal three-dimensional treatment planning. Int J Radiat Oncol Biol Phys 51:255–260
Nabi HA, Zubeldia JM (2002) Clinical applications of (18)F-FDG in oncology. J Nucl Med Technol 30:3–9
Nestle U et al (1999) 18F-deoxyglucose positron emission tomography (FDG-PET) for the planning of radiotherapy in lung cancer: high impact in patients with atelectasis. Int J Radiat Oncol Biol Phys 44:593–597
Pauwels EK et al (2000) Positron-emission tomography with [18F]fluorodeoxyglucose, part I. Biochemical uptake mechanism and its implication for clinical studies. J Cancer Res Clin Oncol 126:549–559
Phelps ME, Cherry SR (1998) The changing design of positron imaging systems. Clin Posit Imaging 1:31–45
Pietrzyk U, Herholz K, Heiss W-D (1990) Three-dimensional alignment of functional and morphological tomograms. J Comput Assist Tomogr 14:51–59
Rahn AN et al (1998) Value of 18F fluorodeoxyglucose positron emission tomography in radiotherapy planning of head-neck tumors. Strahlenther Onkol 174:358–364
Reske SN, Kotzerke J (2001) FDG-PET for clinical use. Results of the 3rd German interdisciplinary consensus conference, "Onko-PET III", 21 July and 19 Sept 2000. Eur J Nucl Med 28:1707–1723
Römer W, Hanauske AR, Ziegler S et al (1998) Positron emission tomography in Non-Hodgkin-lymphoma: assessment of chemotherapy with fluorodeoxyglucose. Blood 91:4464–4471
Shreve PD (2000) Adding structure to function. J Nucl Med 41:1380–1382
Stokkel MP, Draisma A, Pauwels EK (2001) Positron emission tomography with [18F]fluoro-2-deoxy-D-glucose in oncology, part IIIb: therapy response monitoring in colorectal and lung tumours, head and neck cancer, hepatocellular carcinoma and sarcoma. J Cancer Res Clin Oncol 127:278–285
Tai YC, Lin KP, Hoh CK et al (1997) Utilization of 3-d elastic transformation in the registration of chest x-ray CT and whole body PET. IEEE Trans Nucl Sci 44:1606–1612
Tewson TJ, Krohn KA (1998) PET radiopharmaceuticals: state-of-the-art and future prospects. Semin Nucl Med 28:221–234
Therasse P et al (2000) New guidelines to evaluate the response to treatment in solid tumors. European Organization for Research and Treatment of Cancer, National Cancer Institute of the United States, National Cancer Institute of Canada. J Natl Cancer Inst 92:205–216
Townsend DW (2001) A combined PET/CT scanner: the choices. J Nucl Med 42:533–534
Townsend DW, Cherry S (2001) Combining anatomy and function: the path to true image fusion. Eur Radiol 11:1968–1974
Valkema R et al (1996) The diagnostic utility of somatostatin receptor scintigraphy in oncology. J Cancer Res Clin Oncol 122:513–532
Van der Hiel B, Pauwels EK, Stokkel MP (2001) Positron emission tomography with [18F]fluoro-2-deoxy-D-glucose in oncology, part IIIa: therapy response monitoring in breast cancer, lymphoma and gliomas. J Cancer Res Clin Oncol 127:269–277
Vansteenkiste JF, Stroobants SG, Dupont PJ et al (1998) FDG-PET scan in potentially operable nonsmall cell lung cancer: do anatometabolic PET-CT fusion images improve the localisation of regional lymph node metastasis? Eur J Nucl Med 25:1495–1501
Vanuytsel LJ et al (2000) The impact of [18F]fluoro-2-deoxy-D-glucose positron emission tomography (FDG-PET) lymph node staging on the radiation treatment volumes in patients with non-small cell lung cancer. Radiother Oncol 55:317–324
Varagnolo L et al (2000) 18F-labeled radiopharmaceuticals for PET in oncology, excluding FDG. Nucl Med Biol 27:103–112
Von Schulthess GK (2000) Cost considerations regarding an integrated CT-PET system. Eur Radiol 10
Wahl RL, Quint LE, Cieslak RD et al (1993) Anatometabolic tumor imaging: fusion of FDG PET with CT or MRI to localize foci of increased activity. J Nucl Med 34:1190–1196
Woods RP, Cherry SR, Mazziotta JC (1992) Rapid automated algorithm for aligning and reslicing PET images. J Comput Assist Tomogr 16:620–633
Woods RP, Grafton ST, Holmes CJ et al (1998) Automated image registration. I. General methods and intrasubject, intramodality validation. J Comput Assist Tomogr 22:139–152
Young H et al (1999) Measurement of clinical and subclinical tumour response using [18F]-fluorodeoxyglucose and positron emission tomography: review and 1999 EORTC recommendations. European Organization for Research and Treatment of Cancer (EORTC) PET Study Group. Eur J Cancer 35:1773–1782
Yu JN, Fahey FH, Gage HD et al (1995) Intermodality, retrospective image registration in the thorax. J Nucl Med 36:2333–2338

CHAPTER 12

Brain Tumors

T.-Z. Wong · G.-J. van der Westhuizen · R.-E. Coleman

12.1 Incidence, Etiology, Epidemiology

An estimated 18,300 new cases of malignancy involving the brain or nervous system are projected for 2003, with 13,100 deaths attributable to these malignancies (Jemal et al. 2003). The epidemiology of primary brain tumors has recently been recently reviewed in detail (Wrensch et al. 2002). Although the incidence of brain tumors is low relative to other malignant diseases, mortality is high, and primary brain tumors account for 2% of all cancer-related deaths. Overall five-year survival has only improved slightly from 22% in 1974–1976 to 32% in 1992–1998 (Jemal et al. 2003). Although brain tumors are heterogeneous and have a wide age distribution, the average age at onset for all primary brain tumors is about 54 years. The most common primary brain tumors in adults are gliomas and meningiomas. Lower-grade gliomas, such as oligodendrogliomas tend to occur in younger patients, while higher-grade tumors such as glioblastoma multiforme (GBM) occur more frequently in older individuals. Patients with GBM have the poorest prognosis, with 2-year survival rates ranging from 30% for young patients (age <20 years) to 2% for patients older than 65 years. Meningiomas are extra-axial tumors which more frequently occur in the elderly, and have a relatively good prognosis (81% overall 5-year survival, 55% 5-year survival for malignant meningioma) (Wrensch et al. 2002). Gliomas have a slight predisposition for males, whereas meningiomas occur much more frequently in female patients. Lymphomas of the central nervous system (CNS) are also relatively common in the immunocompromised patient population (Behin et al. 2003), but will not be included in this discussion.

In children, primary malignant CNS tumors constitute approximately 16% of all malignancies, and are the most frequently occurring solid tumors. Approximately half of these tumors are astrocytomas, followed in frequency by medulloblastoma / primitive neuroectodermal tumors (PNET), other gliomas, and ependymomas. Overall prognosis is better for children with brain tumors than for adults, with an overall 5-year survival of 67%. However, local recurrence remains a long-term problem, and patients frequently suffer high morbidity as well as a high rate of late mortality (Sklar 2002).

Genetic alterations and abnormal gene expression are felt to play a major role in the development of gliomas. These include the overexpression of platelet-derived growth factor (PDGF), which promotes cellular proliferation and migration of glioma cells, and inactivation of the TP53 gene, which normally inhibits abnormal cell division (Behin et al. 2003; Wrensch et al. 2002). Patients with hereditary syndromes, such as neurofibromatosis and tuberous sclerosis, have significantly higher incidence of brain tumors. Overall, however, only 2–10% of patients with brain tumors have an identified genetic predisposition for the disease, and only approximately 5% of gliomas may be familial (Wrensch et al. 2002).

Environmental factors may play a role in the etiology of primary brain tumors (Wrensch et al. 2002). Previous radiation therapy has been shown to be a strong risk factor for development of brain tumors. Brain tumors have also been associated with other factors such as diet and chemical exposures. No definitive link between brain tumors and electromagnetic radiation or cell phone use has yet been established. Interestingly, some studies have suggested an inverse relationship between brain tumors and allergies.

In summary, a variety of genetic and environmental factors likely contribute to the development of primary brain tumors, although strong associations and direct causality are difficult to confirm. Epidemiologic studies of primary brain tumors are difficult due to the relatively low incidence, variability in case finding, and histologic heterogeneity of these tumors. In the future, molecular markers are likely to improve our understanding of the etiology of brain tumors.

12.2 Histopathological Classification

Due to the number of different cell types in the brain, the classification of brain tumors is complex. The most common brain tumors arise from neuroepithelial cells and the majority of these are glial tumors. The three major types of gliomas include astrocytomas, oligodendrogliomas, and mixed oligoastrocytomas. Currently, the most commonly used grading system for these tumors is the World Health Organization (WHO) classification (Kleihues et al. 1993). This is a four-tiered grading system, with grades I and II representing low-grade tumors, and grades III and IV considered high-grade. Low-grade tumors include pilocytic astrocytomas and well-differentiated astrocytomas or oligodendrogliomas. High-grade tumors include anaplastic astrocytoma and anaplastic oligodendroglioma, both WHO grade III. The highest-grade glioma (WHO grade IV) is the glioblastoma multiforme, which is also the most frequent subtype and has the poorest prognosis.

High-grade gliomas (anaplastic astrocytomas and glioblastoma multiforme) can classified as primary or secondary malignant astrocytomas (Behin et al. 2003). Primary malignant astrocytomas typically occur de novo in older patients, who have no history of prior low-grade tumor. These tumors are characterized by high expression of an abnormal epidermal growth factor receptor (EGFR), and do not have TP53 mutations. Secondary malignant astrocytomas usually occur in younger patients, and result from the degeneration of previously low-grade tumors. Low-grade gliomas may remain stable for years. As they degenerate, these tumors are characterized by TP53 mutations as well as other genetic alterations.

Cells within these tumors are heterogeneous, and the more malignant cells ultimately grow faster, resulting in irregularly shaped tumors containing tumor of varying grade. Over time, these degenerate into high-grade tumors. Some of the molecular factors associated with this tumor progression are beginning to be elucidated (Behin et al. 2003). For example, overexpression of platelet-derived growth factor (PDGF) causes cellular proliferation that is important in the early transformation of low-grade astrocytomas to higher grade. Genetic alterations are manifested in high-grade tumors, in particular the loss of heterozygosity on chromosome 10q.

12.3 Imaging of Brain Tumors

Currently, MRI and CT are the dominant modalities for brain tumor imaging. Advantages of MR imaging include exceptional soft tissue contrast, high spatial resolution, and excellent delineation of gray and white matter structures. Intravenous contrast plays an important role in neuroimaging both in MRI and CT, as enhancement of tumors and other pathologies can reflect disruption of the blood-brain barrier.

Standard T1 and T2-weighted MR images are highly sensitive for detecting brain tumors. High-grade tumors typically demonstrate contrast enhancement following gadolinium administration, while low-grade tumors may have low or minimal enhancement. Low-grade tumors are usually clearly depicted by increased signal on T2-weighted images. MRI is also valuable for evaluating important sequelae resulting from brain tumors, such as mass effect, edema, hemorrhage, and necrosis. In addition to the standard pulse sequences, specialized MR techniques such as MR angiography, are also available to further characterize intracranial tumors. Dynamic MR imaging following intravenous gadolinium injection can be used to estimate perfusion characteristics of tumors. Finally, MR spectroscopy may be helpful to characterize tumors (Meyerand et al. 1999) and distinguish benign from malignant lesions.

MRI and CT are very sensitive for detecting intracranial tumors and provide essential anatomic information for therapy. However, these anatomic imaging techniques cannot provide information about tumor grade. This is important, as brain tumors are frequently heterogeneous, as previously mentioned. In addition, tumors such as gliomas tend to have infiltrative borders which are not accurately defined by MRI or CT.

High-grade brain tumors demonstrate high FDG metabolism. Therefore, FDG-PET compliments MR or CT evaluation of brain tumors by providing information about tumor grade. Identifying the regions of highest grade allows biopsy targets to be defined which most accurately reflect the true tumor pathology. In addition, contrast enhancement on MRI and CT can result from post surgical changes or following radiation therapy, and this can be difficult to distinguish from recurrent tumor. The most accurate information for evaluating brain tumors is obtained by combining the anatomic and metabolic information provided by co-registered MRI and FDG-PET images. For this reason, all FDG-PET studies in patients with brain tumors are routinely co-registered with MRI at our institution. The technique used for image registration is discussed in detail in section 12.8.2.

12.4 FDG-PET Imaging of Brain Tumors

Several groups have reviewed PET imaging and have recommended that brain tumor imaging be considered a clinical indication. In 1987, the American College of Nuclear Physicians and the Society of Nuclear Medicine convened a Task Force on Clinical Positron Emission Tomography to determine the clinical status of PET. At that time, the Task Force concluded that the data in the literature supported the clinical applications of PET for the following indications: detection of coronary artery disease, determination of myocardial viability, evaluation of medically refractory epilepsy, and evaluation of brain tumors (Kuhl et al. 1988). This recommendation for the use of PET in brain tumors was based primarily on the early work of Giovanni Di Chiro and colleagues from the National Institutes of Health (Di Chiro

1987; Di Chiro et al. 1982; Patronas et al. 1985). The National Cancer Institute held a workshop entitled, "Advances in Clinical Imaging Using Positron Emission Tomography," in September 1988 (Al-Aish et al. 1990). This Workshop Panel concluded that the clinical applications of PET included the following: grading of gliomas and detection of recurrence after therapy; detection of coronary artery disease; determination of myocardial viability for selecting patients who will or will not benefit from revascularization procedures; selection of patients for surgical control of seizure disorders; and characterization of the etiology of dementia.

In 1991, the American Academy of Neurology convened a panel of experts to review the neurologic applications of PET (Mazziotta et al. 1991). This panel concluded that the data in the literature supported the following indications: presurgical evaluation of patients with refractory seizure disorders, cognitive decline in differential diagnosis of dementia, movement disorders and brain tumors. Coleman et al. (1991) published a review article summarizing the clinical applications for PET in the evaluation of brain tumors.

PET imaging of brain tumors has become a standard of care at some institutions in the United States. However, despite multiple attempts to obtain coverage by Medicare, evaluation of brain tumors is not recognized as one of the indications that is routinely covered by third party payers in the United States. In 1993, prior to the performance of whole body PET scans and before coverage policies, brain tumor indications were the primary reasons for PET scans being performed at our institution. Since that time, there has been an increase in the number of brain tumor studies performed, but the proportion of all studies performed in PET that relate to brain tumors has decreased as the number of whole body scans has increased.

Most PET centers do not perform a large number of studies in patients with brain tumors, as the prevalence of brain tumors compared to other tumors is quite low. Furthermore, because of the absence of policies for reimbursement for PET scans in brain tumors, there is a reluctance to order the scans. Duke University Medical Center (DUMC) has a large neuro-oncology program that attracts patients with primary brain tumors from throughout the world. Both conventional and experimental therapies are being used in these patients. Most of the patients have the diagnosis made by the time they arrive at our institution, and the patients are referred for therapy of the primary brain tumors. In 2002, 570 FDG-PET studies were performed at DUMC for evaluating brain tumors. The majority of these PET studies were obtained for monitoring of the effect of treatment, which include surgical resection, high-dose radiation therapy techniques, and/or chemotherapy.

12.5 Indications for FDG-PET Imaging of Brain Tumors

12.5.1 Evaluation of Primary Brain Tumors

The primary value of FDG-PET in evaluating glial and other neuroepithelial tumors is the correlation of FDG metabolism with tumor grade. Early clinical studies demonstrated that the glycolytic rate of brain tumors as determined by FDG metabolism is a more accurate reflection of tumor grade than contrast enhancement (Patronas et al. 1983). The background FDG metabolism within normal gray and white matter structures can serve as a convenient reference level. Subjectively, the FDG uptake within the tumor is compared with the metabolism in the contralateral (presumably more normal) deep white matter and contralateral cortical gray matter. Qualitatively, low-grade tumors have FDG uptake similar to or below that of normal white matter, while the FDG accumulation in high-grade tu-

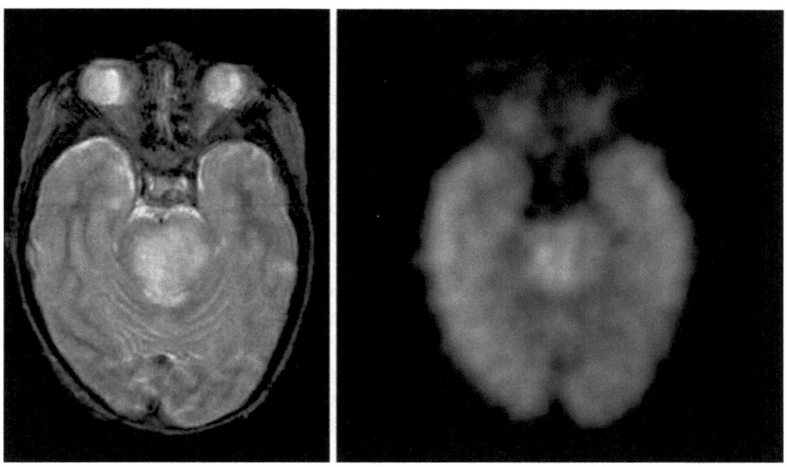

Fig. 1. High grade tumor- pontine glioma. Young child with pontine mass on MRI demonstrating high T2 signal (*left*). The degree of hypermetabolic activity on the co-registered FDG-PET image (*right*) is similar to that of cortical gray matter, and is compatible with high-grade tumor

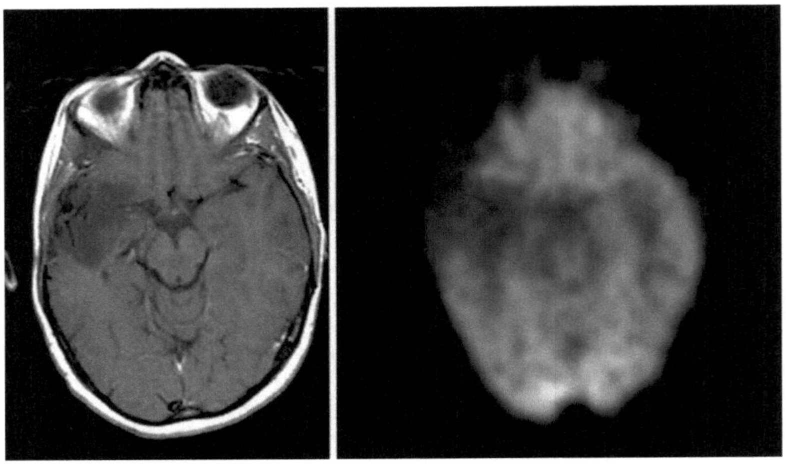

Fig. 2.
Low grade tumor. Young male with poorly-enhancing right temporal lobe tumor discovered incidentally on MRI (*left*) following trauma. Co-registered FDG-PET image (*right*) reveals metabolic activity similar to that of white matter, consistent with low grade tumor. Resection revealed well-differentiated oligodendroglioma. Reprinted from Wong and Coleman (2000), with permission

mors either approaches or exceeds that of normal gray matter. An example of a high-grade tumor (pontine glioma) is illustrated in Fig. 1. Note that the metabolic activity of the tumor generally is similar to that of cortical gray matter in the temporal lobes. An example of a low-grade tumor is shown in Fig. 2. In this example, there is no significant contrast enhancement, and the metabolic activity on FDG-PET imaging is similar to that of adjacent white matter, compatible with low tumor grade.

The FDG accumulation of low grade and high grade brain tumors relative to normal gray and white matter has also been evaluated quantitatively. Delbeke et al. (1995) studied 58 consecutive patients with histologically proven high-grade (32 patients) and low-grade (26 patients) brain tumors. These authors measured the tumor-to-white matter (T/WM) and tumor-to-gray matter (T/GM) ratios in an effort to determine the optimum cutoff values for distinguishing low-grade (WHO grades I and II) from high-grade (WHO grades III and IV) tumors. They found that T/WM ratios >1.5 and T/GM ratios >0.6 were indicative of high-grade tumors with a sensitivity of 94% and specificity of 77%. This result supports the general subjective observation that low grade tumors have metabolic activity similar to white matter, and high grade tumors have metabolic activity resembling gray matter.

As previously mentioned, an important feature of glial tumors is their heterogeneous pathology, and geographic variation of tumor grade. Paulus and Peiffer (1989), studied histologic features of 1000 samples from 50 brain tumors (20 samples per tumor to simulate biopsies). They found that different grades were detected in 82% of tumors. Moreover, a majority (62%) of the gliomas contained both high grade (III or IV) and benign (grade II) features. These findings highlight the potential for sampling errors, and provide an explanation for the growth pattern of these tumors. Focal areas having higher grade may grow faster, resulting in an irregular contour to the tumor mass. High-grade tumors, notably glioblastoma multiforme, frequently originate from malignant degeneration of lower-grade tumors. These features cannot be distinguished on conventional anatomic imaging, such as MRI. Because of this underlying cellular heterogeneity, evaluation of these tumors by stereotactic biopsy, even with MR or CT guidance, is subject to significant sampling error and potential under-staging. By mapping the metabolic pattern of these heterogeneous tumors, FDG-PET can aid in targeting for stereotactic biopsy by selecting the subregions within the tumor that are most hypermetabolic and potentially have the highest grade (Hanson et al. 1991; Pirotte et al. 1994, 1995, 1997). Metabolically-based targeting may reduce the number of tissue samples required, and may improve the accuracy of the biopsy for determining the actual tumor grade. At our institution, we can provide the neurosurgeon with co-registered MR/PET images, which enables the MRI coordinates for stereotactic biopsy to be refined based on the corresponding PET findings. In the future, the registered MRI/PET data could be integrated with the stereotactic guidance software to allow direct selection of the stereotactic biopsy coordinates based on PET-determined targets.

12.5.2
FDG-PET As an Indicator of Prognosis

In addition to providing information relative to tumor grade, the degree of FDG metabolism carries prognostic significance. In a study of 29 patients with treated and untreated primary brain tumors, Alavi et al. (1988) found that patients with hypermetabolic tumors had a significantly shorter survival than those with hypometabolic tumors. Moreover, within the subset of patients with high-grade gliomas, the patients with low tumor metabolism had a 1-year survival of 78%, while those with high tumor metabolism had a significantly poorer prognosis, with a 1-year survival of 29%. In another study involving 45 patients with high-grade tumors, Patronas et al. (1985) showed similar results. In that study, patients having tumors with high metabolic activity had a mean survival of 5 months, while those patients with less glucose metabolism had a mean survival of 19 months. The prognostic significance of FDG-PET findings in low-grade brain tumors has also been suggested. In patients with low-grade gliomas, the development of hypermetabolic features correlates with deleterious tumor evolution and poorer prognosis (DeWitte et al. 1996; Francavilla et al. 1989). These studies suggest a relationship between the metabolic activity identified on FDG-PET scan and the biologic aggressiveness of both low grade and high grade primary brain tumors, which is independent of prior therapy. There is also evidence that the prognostic information provided by FDG-PET imaging may be further improved with serial studies (Schifter et al. 1993). An example of a patient with a history of well-differentiated oligodendroglioma degenerating to high-grade tumor is shown in Fig. 4. The initial images (top row) demonstrate a surgical resection cavity with non-specific adjacent enhancement on MRI. A small only mildly enhancing focus of high FDG accumulation concerning for high-grade tumor is seen lateral to the cavity. The more prominent region of enhancement anterior to the cavity demonstrates only low FDG activity, suggesting low-grade tumor or post-therapy changes. Follow up images obtained 8 months later confirmed progression of high-grade tumor, primarily in the lateral region identified on the original PET study. The benign nature of the anterior contrast enhancement was also confirmed on the follow up study. This figure also illustrates one of the methods that can be used to evaluate co-registered images. Each axial slice can be examined over a continuum between 100% MRI and 100% PET; this technique can be particularly valuable for evaluating the metabolic activity of small foci of contrast enhancement.

12.5.3 Evaluation of Brain Tumors Following Therapy

As with newly diagnosed brain tumors, image registration of FDG-PET images with MRI is important for evaluation of recurrent tumor. Suspicious areas of enhancement must be correlated with FDG metabolism. Residual tumor and post-surgical changes can both result in abnormal enhancement and can be indistinguishable on MRI following tumor resection. Post-surgical changes do not inherently result in increased metabolic activity, and FDG-PET is relatively unaffected for evaluating the post-surgical patient for residual tumor (Hanson et al. 1990). Following surgery, a rim of contrast enhancement on MRI is typically observed surrounding the resection cavity, as illustrated in the top row of Fig. 3; note that there is no associated hypermetabolic activity at this level on the co-registered FDG-PET image. In the bottom row (b) of Fig. 3., a focal area of enhancement is identified in the same patient. The registered images demonstrate that this focus has FDG accumulation equal to that of gray matter, consistent with recurrent high-grade tumor; this was confirmed by stereotactic biopsy. Without accurate image co-registration, focal FDG activity may be difficult to distinguish from adjacent normal cortex. In the case of early recurrence, FDG-PET can help define the tumor target having the highest grade for stereotactic biopsy (Glantz et al. 1991).

Following high-dose radiation therapy, radiation necrosis is usually reflected by diminished FDG metabolism within the treated field (Di Chiro et al. 1988). However, increased FDG activity following high-dose radiation therapy can be occasionally observed. This effect is similar to hypermetabolic activity which can be seen following radiation therapy to other sites, such as the thorax. The increased FDG accumulation may be related to the metabolically active macrophages which accumulate at the therapy site. The degree of activity is usually moderate (intermediate between white and gray matter) and relatively uniform in distribution. However, in some cases the metabolic activity can be equal to or greater than gray matter activity, or may even have nodular characteristics. In these situations, radiation necrosis is indistinguishable from recurrent high-grade tumor. Barker et al. (1997) studied 55 patients with high-grade tumors treated with surgery and radiation therapy that had enlarging areas of enhancement on MRI suggesting tumor recurrence or radiation necrosis. In this study, high FDG accumulation (equal or exceeding gray matter) correlated with significantly poorer prognosis compared to patients without hypermetabolic findings. In a more recent study of 47 patients with primary and metastatic brain tumors who underwent stereotactic radiosurgery, Chao et al. (2001) reported FDG-PET to have an overall sensitivity of 75% and specificity of 81% for detecting recurrent tumor (versus radiation necrosis). In patients who received stereotactic radiosurgery for brain metastases, co-registration of the FDG-PET images with MRI improved sensitivity for detecting tumor recurrence from 65% to 86%.

High-dose brachytherapy techniques can also result in increased FDG accumulation. At our institution, one therapy under investigation involves the administration of ^{131}I-labeled monoclonal antibody, which is injected into the surgical resection cavity for treatment of primary brain tumors (Reardon et al. 2002). The beta emission from the ^{131}I results in selective high radiation dose to the tissues immediately adjacent to the surgical resection site. Following this high-dose brachytherapy, a rim of FDG accumulation and contrast enhancement is frequently observed surrounding the resection cavity. This rim of hypermetabolic activity is not generally

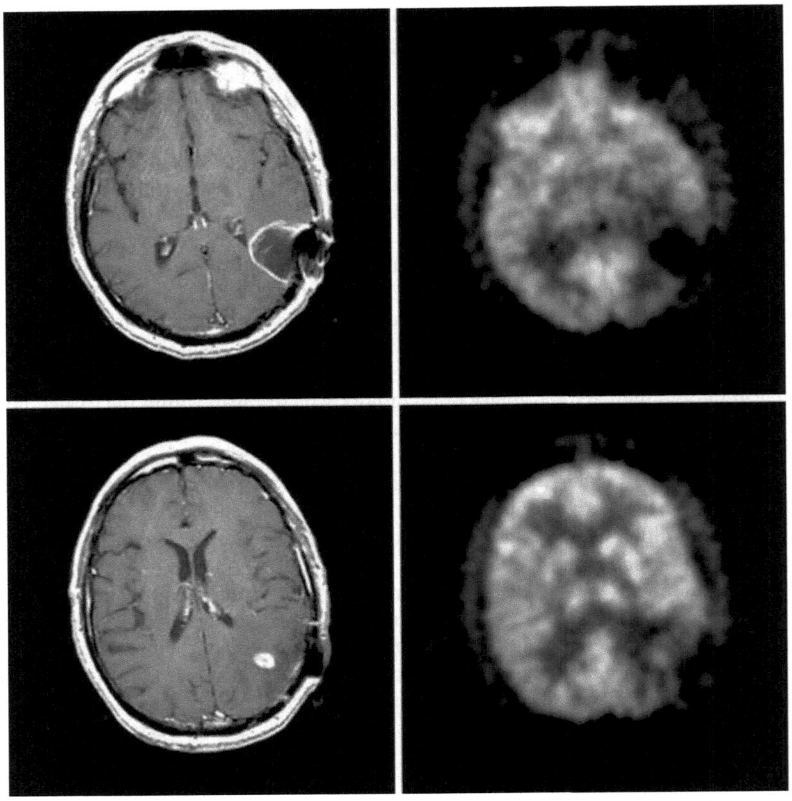

Fig. 3.
Post-surgical changes, recurrent tumor. Middle-aged patient with history of glioblastoma multiforme, status-post surgical resection and high-dose radiation therapy using I-131 labeled monoclonal antibodies. Co-registered T1-weighted MRI and FDG-PET images above reveal a thin rim of contrast enhancement surrounding the surgical resection cavity with no associated hypermetabolic activity to suggest tumor. At a different axial level, a nodular area of enhancement (*lower pair of images*) is associated with high metabolic activity (*similar to gray matter*), and represented recurrent grade IV tumor on biopsy

associated with tumor, and is more often related to radiation necrosis. Typically, the rim has low to intermediate activity (between white and gray matter) and uniform thickness. Malignant recurrence is suggested by the development of new intense nodularity within the rim of FDG accumulation (Marriott et al. 1998). Valk et al. (1988) studied 38 patients who had received interstitial brachytherapy and found that FDG-PET combined with ^{82}Rb PET (to evaluate the blood-brain barrier) was accurate in distinguishing radiation necrosis from recurrent tumor.

Patients being treated for brain tumors are frequently receiving corticosteroids, which can influence the pattern of FDG metabolism by decreasing cerebral glucose metabolism in normal brain tissue (Fulham et al. 1995). Visually, this is reflected as decreased gray/white matter differentiation on FDG-PET images. Corticosteroid-induced hyperglycemia may be a contributing factor. A study by Roelcke et al. (1998a) found that patients with brain tumors in general have decreased glucose metabolism in the contralateral cortex, and the degree of this decrease correlates with tumor size. Their study suggests that tumor size may be a more important factor than corticosteroid dose in determining the degree of decreased metabolism in the contralateral cortex. Metabolism within brain tumors, on the other hand, was not affected by corticosteroid therapy.

A false-positive diagnosis can be made on the FDG-PET scan when a patient has had a seizure close to the time of administration of the radiopharmaceutical (Coleman et al. 1991). Both clinical and subclinical seizures can result produce hypermetabolic activity. EEG monitoring during the PET study is therefore helpful in patients with suspected seizure disorders.

12.5.4 Other Primary Brain Tumors

The majority of data correlating findings on FDG-PET with tumor prognosis and grade is derived from astrocytic tumors. The correlation of high FDG metabolism with malignant behavior also generally applies to other primary brain tumors. However, there are some exceptions. Juvenile pilocytic astrocytomas may exhibit focally high FDG metabolism even though this tumor has a favorable prognosis. These tumors also show markedly increased contrast enhancement on MRI. The hypermetabolism has been explained by the presence of metabolically active fenestrated epithelial cells, which are associated with this tumor (Roelcke et al. 1998b). On the other hand, gangliogliomas are generally low-grade tumors which have been reported to be associated with low FDG accumulation (Kincaid et al. 1998). However, our experience of correlation of FDG-PET images with co-registered MRI indicates that these tumors can also contain regions of higher FDG metabolism (Provenzale et al. 1999).

Meningiomas represent 10%–15% of primary intracranial tumors, and are usually benign, curable tumors but can occasionally exhibit an aggressive behavior and recur. Di Chiro et al. (1987) found that the glucose metabolic rate of meningiomas correlates with tumor growth and aggressive behavior. In their study, an atypical meningioma had metabolic rates higher than that of the contralateral cortex.

FDG-PET is a sensitive imaging modality for evaluating both Hodgkin's lymphoma and non-Hodgkin's lymphoma in the body. Central nervous system lymphoma is also typically very metabolically active, while non-malignant etiologies such as toxoplasmosis do not show high glucose metabolism. In a study at our institution of 11 HIV-positive individuals with cerebral lesions on CT or MRI, FDG-PET accurately differentiated those patients with lymphoma from those having infectious etiologies (Hoffman et al. 1993). Other studies have supported these findings (Heald et al. 1996; Roelcke and Leenders 1999).

12.5.5 Metastatic Brain Tumors

Soft tissue metastases in the brain and elsewhere in the body generally have high glucose metabolism which renders them detectable by FDG-PET. Parenchymal brain metastases, like high-grade primary brain tumors, generally have FDG accumulation comparable to that of normal cortical gray matter. When the metabolism exceeds that of normal gray matter, metastases can be easily identified on FDG-PET imaging. However, brain metastases are frequently the result of hematogenous seeding, and often develop at the cortical gray-white junction. The high baseline glucose metabolism in the brain cortex provides a relatively low tissue-to-background environment for identifying intracranial metastases that are only mildly or moderately hypermetabolic. Small metastases adjacent to the cerebral cortex which have activity similar to that of gray matter can be impossible to detect on FDG-PET images alone. In addition, the cytotoxic edema that frequently surrounds metastatic deposits has relatively low FDG accumulation, and may decrease conspicuity of the lesions through volume averaging effects. The importance of co-registration with MRI or CT has been emphasized in the evaluation of primary brain tumors, and would appear to be equally or more important for evaluating metastatic disease. As previously mentioned, image registration may be particularly helpful in distinguishing tumor recurrence from radionecrosis in patients who have received stereotactic radiosurgery for brain metastases (Chao et al. 2001).

Larcos and Maisey (1996) reviewed FDG-PET studies on 273 patients having various primary tumors to determine the value of adding an abbreviated FDG brain scan to screen for intracranial metastases. They detected cerebral pathology in only 2% of the patients and unsuspected metastases in only 0.7%. They concluded that the addition of FDG brain scanning to routine whole-body imaging detected few clinically relevant lesions, and should therefore not be performed routinely. This low detection rate has also been our experience at Duke University Medical Center (Rohren et al. 2003); up to a few years ago, we routinely included brain imaging as part of our whole body PET studies. However, we found that the additional FDG-brain study rarely contributed to clinical management, and was less sensitive than MRI for detecting intracranial metastases. For these reasons, brain imaging is not currently included as part of our standard protocol for whole body FDG-PET studies.

12.6 Other PET Tracers

Although FDG-PET is currently the most widely used radiopharmaceutical in clinical practice, but other PET agents have been used to obtain important information about tumor physiology. These radiopharmaceuticals have allowed evaluation of other metabolic parameters for brain PET imaging including amino acid metabolism, membrane lipid synthesis, tumor blood flow, and nucleotide metabolism (Wong et al. 2002).

12.6.1 Amino Acid Metabolism

Nearly every amino acid has been radiolabeled to study potential imaging characteristics in gliomas and other brain tumors. The mechanism for imaging can be related to either amino acid metabolism or to breakdown of the blood-brain barrier. Amino acid transport is generally increased in malignant transformation (Isselbacher 1972). The amino acids that have been used most commonly in clinical PET are ^{11}C-methionine and ^{11}C-tyrosine (Jager et al. 2001). In contrast to FDG, background uptake of amino acids in normal brain tissue is low, providing good contrast with tumor uptake.

^{11}C-methionine (MET) accumulation has been shown to be 1.2 to 3.5 times greater in tumor than in normal brain. Several investigators have found MET to be superior to FDG for delineation of tumor margins and to distinguish tumor recurrence from radiation necrosis (Conti 1995; Ericson et al. 1985; Weber et al. 1999). The fact that amino acid imaging is less influenced by inflammation may be an advantage relative to F-18-FDG PET imaging, although tumor specificity is not absolute even with amino acid imaging (Jager et al. 2001).

Sasaki et al. (1998) compared ^{201}Tl SPECT (single photon emission computed tomography), FDG-PET, and MET-PET in 23 patients with astrocytic tumors. These authors found MET-PET to be more sensitive than ^{201}Tl SPECT or FDG-PET for detecting astrocytomas, particularly low-grade tumors. In this study, MET-PET was also able to distinguish low-grade (grade II) from high-grade (grades III and IV) astrocytomas. Kaschten et al. (1998) found MET to be slightly superior to FDG for predicting the histologic grade and prognosis of gliomas, in spite of the fact that the authors were unable to differentiate between Grades II and III astrocytomas with MET. Both tracers proved useful for predicting patient survival. The combination of both tracers improved the overall results compared to each tracer alone. In a recent study, Chung et al. (2002) evaluated the usefulness of MET in the evaluation of brain lesions that were hypo- or isometabolic on FDG. Thirty-one of 35 brain tumors (89% sensitivity) showed increased MET uptake despite iso- or hypometabolism on FDG-PET. By contrast, all ten benign lesions showed decreased or normal MET uptake (100% specificity). This further supports the potential advantage of MET for evaluating low grade tumors.

MET can also be used for target selection in PET-guided stereotactic brain biopsies. In a comparative study using FDG and MET to guide stereotactic biopsies, Pirotte et al. (1997) found abnormal MET uptake in all 23 tumors studied. Two non-tumorous lesions had no abnormal MET uptake. MET was used for target selection in 11 of 23 tumors in which there was no FDG uptake or where FDG uptake was equivalent to that of gray matter.

These studies all suggest that a combination of PET radiotracers may be useful to probe multiple biochemical processes in an individual tumor and thereby provide a metabolic profile of a tumor. FDG-PET can be used initially to determine the presence of hypermetabolism in a lesion. High metabolic activity on FDG-PET would confirm the presence of high-grade tumor. Low-to intermediate activity on an FDG scan is more nonspecific, and could represent a low-grade tumor, infarct, post-therapy changes, infection, or benign lesion. Regions of low FDG metabolism could be further evaluated by MET-PET to distinguish low or intermediate grade tumor from these other entities.

Amino acids other than MET could potentially be useful in the evaluation of tumor metabolism in patients, as data from experimental studies have shown the presence of altered amino acid transport and protein synthesis in malignant cells (Isselbacher 1972; Johnstone and Scholefield 1965). Derivatives of natural and synthetic amino acids being studied in patients with brain tumors include fluorotyrosine, glutamate and fluorophenylalanine (Conti 1995).

Alpha-aminoisobutyric acid (AIB), a nonmetabolized amino acid, is rapidly transported into viable cells by the A-type (or alanine-preferring) amino acid transport system. Malignant cells extract AIB to a greater extent than normal cells. Therefore, its tissue distribution reflects the relative degree of A-transport in various tissues in normal and diseased states. McConathy et al. (2002) report on two analogs of alpha-aminoisobutyric acid radiolabeled with fluorine-18: 2-amino-3-[^{18}F]fluoro-2-methylpropranoic acid and 3-[^{18}F]fluoro-2-methyl-2-(methylamino)propanoic acid. These agents have shown very high tumor accumulation relative to normal brain in a rat gliosarcoma model, and may have potential application in human brain tumors.

12.6.2 Nucleotide Metabolism

^{11}C-thymidine (dThd) has been developed for clinical use as an in vivo radiotracer of nucleotide metabolism and for use in DNA synthesis. The accumulation of radiolabeled thymidine in tumor tissue and organs having high proliferative rates is reflective of the degree of DNA synthesis and metabolic activity. Unlike other currently available PET radiotracers, thymidine uptake provides a direct in-vivo measurement of cellular proliferative activity. Eary et al. (1999) reported on a series of 13 patients who underwent contemporaneous dThd-PET, FDG-PET and MRI studies. The dThd-PET scans were qualitatively different from the other two scans in approximately 50% of the cases, suggesting that dThd-PET provided different information from FDG-PET and MRI. In two patients with less dThd uptake than FDG uptake, tumor progression was slower than in three patients with both high dThd and FDG accumulation. PET imaging with dThd can reveal the presence of viable tumor in regions where the FDG uptake is too subtle to confidently distinguish tumor from normal brain parenchyma, suggesting that tumor viability based on imaging of cell proliferation may be a more sensitive means for monitoring disease activity than FDG activity. In the future, dThd imaging may have utility in assessing tumor response to therapy.

Recently, ^{18}F-labeled thymidine analogs has been evaluated as a tumor imaging agent based on cellular proliferation. Grierson and Shields (2000) reported on the synthesis of 3'-deoxy-3'-[^{18}F]fluorothymidine (FLT), and Wang et al. (2002) studied the in-vivo distribution of 2'-fluorodeoxyuracil-beta-D-arabinofuranoside (FAU) and 2'-fluoro-5-methyldeoxyuracil-beta-D-arabinofuranoside (FMAU) as potential ^{18}F-labeled thymidine analogs. These ^{18}F-labeled analogues could have wider clinical availability by virtue of the longer half life (110 min) over the ^{11}C-labeled analogue (20 min).

12.6.3 Lipid Metabolism

Synthesis of membrane phospholipids is increased in certain malignancies, and this is reflected in choline metabolism. ^{11}C-choline has been used for PET imaging of brain tumors (Hara et al. 1997). More recently, DeGrado et al. (2001) have developed ^{18}F-labeled choline analogs for tumor imaging, which have the advantage of a longer physical half life. In particular, ^{18}F-fluorocholine (FCH) readily accumulates in brain tumors. Like ^{11}C-methionine, ^{18}F-fluorocholine has low background metabolism in normal brain. However, the relationship between the degree of FCH accumulation and tumor grade has not yet been evaluated.

12.6.4 ^{15}O tracers for PET

PET tracers with radiolabeled oxygen have been used to study cerebral blood volume (inhaled $C^{15}O$), blood flow (injected $H_2{}^{15}O$), and oxygen utilization (inhaled $O^{15}O$) (Okazawa et al. 2001; Sadato et al. 1993). Raichle et al. (1983) found excellent correlation between cerebral blood flow measured with PET and the true cerebral blood flow of anesthetized baboons. Cerebral circulation as determined by PET can be of ancillary significance in predicting the prognosis of patients with gliomas. Mineura et al. (1994) found that patients with a higher value of regional cerebral blood flow, blood volume or metabolic rates of oxygen had significantly longer survival times than those with a lower value. In addition, because the relative blood flow to the cerebral cortex is related to cortical activation, ^{15}O perfusion studies can be used to define specific functional areas. For example, $H_2{}^{15}O$ PET studies can be performed while the patient is performing prescribed tasks to localize the associated cortex, and thus identify areas to be avoided during surgical resection.

Dynamic MRI techniques are also available for estimating tumor perfusion parameters. Following bolus injection of gadolinium, dynamic susceptibility MR imaging can be performed to provide estimates of blood volume and perfusion parameters. These techniques have recently been reviewed by Aronen and Perkio (2002). In addition, functional MR imaging techniques can also be used to identify regions of cortical activation.

12.7 Summary and Outlook

FDG-PET provides unique metabolic information which can be valuable both in the initial evaluation and follow up of brain tumors. FDG-PET does not compete with MRI or CT, but rather compliments these modalities. The major advantage of FDG as a primary tracer is the correlation between glucose metabolism and tumor grade. This can have significant diagnostic, prognostic, and therapeutic implications in the management of these tumors. The major shortcomings of FDG-PET are the high background activity within the cerebral cortex and other gray matter structures, and relatively low anatomic spatial resolution. On the other hand, MRI and CT provide high spatial resolution of anatomic structures, but cannot provide information on the metabolic activity or grade of the tumor. Thus, registration of FDG-PET with MRI or CT images provides a synergism of functional/anatomic information, and is a powerful tool for brain tumor evaluation. In our experience, image registration is mandatory for accurate initial evaluation of brain tumors. In patients who have had prior PET scans, interval changes may be assessed without the necessity of formal image registration, although with some loss of sensitivity for recurrent tumor.

FDG-PET imaging can be useful for surveying patients with low-grade brain tumors for evidence of malignant degeneration. These patients are also best evaluated in combination with MRI, as illustrated in Fig. 4. When interval changes are noted on MRI, the corresponding PET studies are often valuable for guiding stereotactic biopsy and/or surgical resection.

One potential disadvantage of FDG-PET for brain tumor imaging is the low sensitivity for detecting low-grade tumors. In patients with treated low-grade tumors, evaluation with other PET tracers, such as ^{11}C-MET may be helpful to evaluate for recurrent or residual tumor. When used alone, FDG-PET imaging is not an effective screening modality for detecting intracranial metastases, which can be obscured by adjacent or involved cortex. Therefore, in our practice we do not routinely include brain imaging as part of our whole body FDG-PET studies; if brain metastases are suspected, MRI or contrast-enhanced CT is recommended.

12.8 Technical Recommendations

12.8.1 PET Imaging Protocol

Patients scheduled for brain PET studies at our institution are requested to have no caloric intake for at least 4 hours prior to the FDG-PET study, but they are encouraged to drink water. We routinely obtain a serum glucose measurement at the time of FDG injection. It is not uncommon for brain tumor patients to be on steroids, with resulting hyperglycemia. High serum glucose levels can reduce FDG accumulation by competitive inhibition, and is reflected by reduced gray-white matter differentiation on the PET images. Following intravenous injection of a standard dose of FDG (370 MBq for adults), the patient is allowed to rest quietly in a dimly-lit room for at least 30 minutes during the uptake phase. The patients are in-

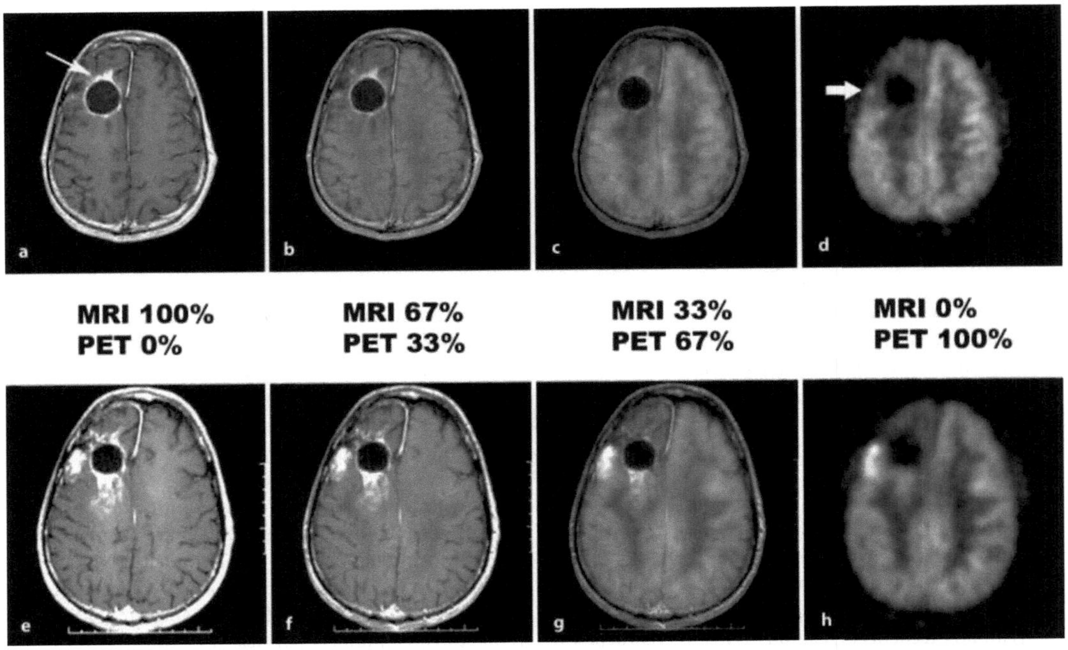

Fig. 4. Malignant degeneration from low-grade to high grade tumor. Middle-aged man with history of well-differentiated oligodendroglioma, with multiple prior therapies. On initial images (*top row*, (**a**)-(**d**)), T1-weighted MRI demonstrates non-specific contrast enhancement, particularly anterior to the surgical resection cavity (*thin arrow*); note that this region does not have high FDG metabolism. However, a mildly enhancing focus lateral to the cavity has high-grade activity (*thick arrow*). On follow-up images 8 months later (*bottom row*, (**e**)-(**h**)), there has been significant progression of the lateral focus as well as posteriorly on both MRI and FDG-PET, compatible with high-grade tumor (malignant degeneration), while the anterior margin remains stable

structed to keep their eyes open, but we do not use ear occlusion. However, auditory and visual stimulation are minimized during the uptake period to avoid extraneous cortical activation in the associated areas. Our scans are performed on a dedicated PET scanner (GE Advance, GE Medical Systems, Milwaukee, WI) using a single table position. An emission scan is obtained for 8 minutes using three-dimensional acquisition, and subsequently reconstructed using 3-D filtered backprojection. Calculated attenuation-correction is utilized, eliminating the need for a separate transmission scan. The resulting PET images have an axial slice thickness of 4.25 mm, with a 25.6 cm field-of-view represented in a 128×128 pixel matrix. The use of 3-D acquisition and calculated attenuation-correction permits brain imaging to be performed time-efficiently. The shorter acquisition time reduces the possibility of patient motion. For less cooperative patients, dynamic imaging can be performed with averaging to reduce the effects of motion.

12.8.2 Image Registration

The importance of image registration of FDG-PET with CT or MRI scans has been emphasized as a requirement for accurate evaluation of brain tumors. When the tumors have high-grade metabolic activity exceeding that of gray matter, or when high-grade tumors are located deep within the white matter, image registration may not be necessary. In most situations, however, tumors are located near cortical structures, and cannot be adequately localized on the PET images alone. Correlating axial PET images with axial MRI images side-by-side is inadequate, due to the differences in head angulation during image acquisition. Computer-based image registration can be accomplished by manually rotating and translating the 3-dimensional data sets using interactive display software. However, our experience is that a semi-automated surface-fit technique is a faster, more reliable, reproducible, and objective method for registering the images. We routinely co-register all of our brain tumor PET studies with recent MRI or CT images (in our practice, this is almost exclusively MRI). In many cases, these are transferred electronically from scanners at our institution. For patients referred for PET scanning from outside institutions, we request that they bring their films with them, and we digitize them on a high-resolution film digitizer (Vidar Systems Corporation, Herndon, VA) at the time of their PET scan. Once the digital MR or CT data are available, the entire image regis-

Fig. 5.
Image registration. Surface rendering of the axial MR images (*solid circles*) and FDG-PET data (*dots*) prior to (**a**) and following (**b**) computer-aided image registration. The 3-dimensional FDG-PET data set is iteratively rotated and shifted to minimize the error in the surface-fit. Note the difference in acquisition angle between the two imaging modalities on the co-registered image sets

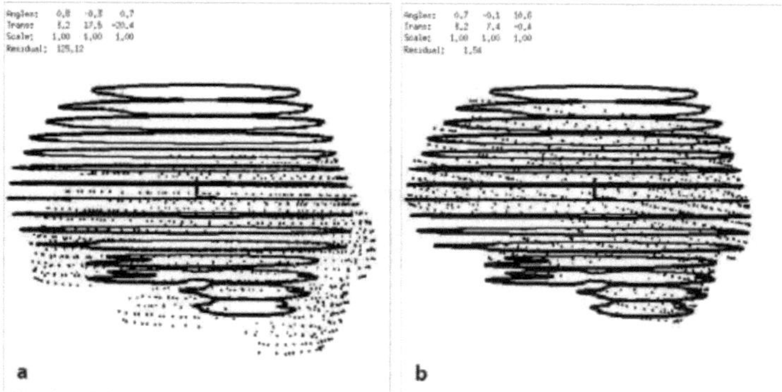

tration process takes approximately 45 minutes. Image registration is performed using an iterative surface-fit technique described by Pelizzari et al. (1989), and implemented using software which was developed and evaluated at the Duke PET facility (Turkington et al. 1993, 1995). An example of this semi-automated technique is shown in Fig. 5. The surface defined by the 3-dimensional FDG-PET data set is rotated and translated iteratively to optimize correlation with the MRI-defined surfaces.

The display software allows each axial MR image to be displayed along with the corresponding FDG-PET image. Two techniques are used to display the co-registered images. Most tumors can be evaluated by toggling between the MRI and PET images. In addition, each image can be displayed while making adjustments along a continuum between 100% MRI and 100% PET, as illustrated in Fig. 4.

In summary, primary brain tumors pose unique challenges, which include heterogeneous pathology and variable prognosis, as well as the tendency of these tumors to recur locally and to undergo malignant degeneration. The major contribution of FDG-PET imaging in brain tumor results from the relationship between FDG accumulation and tumor grade. Specific applications of FDG-PET include initial evaluation and prognosis of brain tumors, guidance for stereotactic biopsy, follow up for recurrent tumor after therapy, monitoring for malignant degeneration of low grade tumor, and treatment planning. Anatomic localization of the abnormality essential, requiring accurate image registration with MRI (or CT). These imaging modalities are complimentary, and when taken together, the combination of FDG-PET and MR imaging serves as a powerful tool for the initial evaluation and management of brain tumors.

References

Al-Aish M, Coleman RE, Larson SM et al (1990) Advances in clinical imaging using positron emission tomography. National Cancer Institute Workshop Statement. Arch Intern Med 150: 735–739

Alavi JB, Alavi A, Chawluk J et al (1988) Positron emission tomography in patients with glioma. A predictor of prognosis. Cancer 62:1074–1078

Aronen HJ, Perkio J (2002) Dynamic susceptibility contrast MRI of gliomas. Neuroimag Clin North Am 12:501–523

Barker FG 2nd, Chang SM, Valk PE et al (1997) 18-Fluorodeoxyglucose uptake and survival of patients with suspected recurrent malignant glioma. Cancer 79:115–126

Behin A, Hoang-Xuan K, Carpentier AF, Delattre JY (2003) Primary brain tumors in adults. Lancet 361:323–331

Chao ST, Suh JH, Raja S et al (2001) The sensitivity and specificity of FDG PET in distinguishing recurrent brain tumor from radionecrosis in patients treated with stereotactic radiosurgery. Int J Cancer 96:191–197

Chung JK, Kim YK, Kim SK et al (2002) Usefulness of 11C-methionine PET in the evaluation of brain lesions that are hypo- or isometabolic on 18F-FDG PET. Eur J Nucl Med Mol Imaging 29:176–182

Coleman RE, Hoffman JM, Hanson MW et al (1991) Clinical application of PET for the evaluation of brain tumors. J Nucl Med 32:616–622

Conti PS (1995) Introduction to imaging brain tumor metabolism with positron emission tomography (PET). Cancer Invest 13:244–259

DeGrado TR, Baldwin SW, Wang S et al (2001) Synthesis and evaluation of (18)F-labeled choline analogs as oncologic PET tracers. J Nucl Med 42:1805–1814

Delbeke D, Meyerowitz C, Lapidus RL et al (1995) Optimal cutoff levels of F-18 fluorodeoxyglucose uptake in the differentiation of low-grade from high-grade brain tumors with PET. Radiology 195:47–52

De Witte O, Levivier M, Violon P et al (1996) Prognostic value positron emission tomography with [18F]fluoro-2-deoxy- D-glucose in the low-grade glioma. Neurosurgery 39:470–476; discussion 476–477

Di Chiro G (1987) Positron emission tomography using [18F] fluorodeoxyglucose in brain tumors. A powerful diagnostic and prognostic tool. Invest Radiol 22:360–371

Di Chiro G, DeLaPaz RI, Brooks RA, et al (1982) Glucose utilization of cerebral gliomas measured by 18-F-2 deoxyglucose and PET. Neurology 32:1323–1329

Di Chiro G, Hatazawa J, Katz DA et al (1987) Glucose utilization by intracranial meningiomas as an index of tumor aggressivity and probability of recurrence: a PET study. Radiology 164:521–526

Di Chiro G, Oldfield E, Wright DC et al (1988) Cerebral necrosis after radiotherapy and/or intraarterial chemotherapy for brain tumors: PET and neuropathologic studies. AJR Am J Roentgenol 150:189–197

Eary JF, Mankoff DA, Spence AM et al (1999) 2-[C-11]thymidine imaging of malignant brain tumors. Cancer Res 59:615–621

Ericson K, Lilja A, Bergstrom M et al (1985) Positron emission tomography with ([11C]methyl)-L-methionine, [11C]D- glucose, and [68 Ga]EDTA in supratentorial tumors. J Comput Assist Tomogr 9:683–689

Francavilla TL, Miletich RS, Di Chiro G et al (1989) Positron emission tomography in the detection of malignant degeneration of low-grade gliomas. Neurosurgery 24:1–5

Fulham MJ, Brunetti A, Aloj L et al (1995) Decreased cerebral glucose metabolism in patients with brain tumors: an effect of corticosteroids. J Neurosurg 83:657–664

Glantz MJ, Hoffman JM, Coleman RE et al (1991) Identification of early recurrence of primary central nervous system tumors by [18F]fluorodeoxyglucose positron emission tomography. Ann Neurol 29:347–355

Grierson JR, Shields AF (2000) Radiosynthesis of 3'-deoxy-3'-[(18)F]fluorothymidine: [(18)F]FLT for imaging of cellular proliferation in vivo. Nucl Med Biol 27:143–156

Hanson MW, Hoffman JM, Glantz MJ et al (1990) FDG-PET in the early postoperative evaluation of patients with brain tumor (abstract). J Nucl Med 31:799

Hanson MW, Glantz MJ, Hoffman JM et al (1991) FDG-PET in the selection of brain lesions for biopsy. J Comput Assist Tomogr 15:796–801

Hara T, Kosaka N, Shinoura N et al (1997) PET imaging of brain tumor with [methyl-11C]choline. J Nucl Med 38:842–847

Heald AE, Hoffman JM, Bartlett JA et al (1996) Differentiation of central nervous system lesions in AIDS patients using positron emission tomography (PET). Int J STD AIDS 7:337–346

Hoffman JM, Waskin HA, Schifter T et al (1993) FDG-PET in differentiating lymphoma from nonmalignant central nervous system lesions in patients with AIDS. J Nucl Med 34:567–575

Isselbacher KJ (1972) Sugar and amino acid transport by cells in culture–differences between normal and malignant cells. N Engl J Med 286:929–933

Jager PL, Vaalburg W, Pruim J et al (2001) Radiolabeled amino acids: basic aspects and clinical applications in oncology. J Nucl Med 42:432–445

Jemal A, Murray T, Samuels A, Ghafoor A, Ward E, Thun MJ (2003) Cancer statistics, 2003. CA Cancer J Clin 53:5–26

Johnstone RM, Scholefield PG (1965) Amino acid transport in tumor cells. Adv Cancer Res 9:143–226

Kaschten B, Stevenaert A, Sadzot B et al (1998Preoperative evaluation of 54 gliomas by PET with fluorine-18- fluorodeoxyglucose and/or carbon-11-methionine. J Nucl Med 39:778–785

Kincaid PK, El-Saden SM, Park SH et al (1998Cerebral gangliogliomas: preoperative grading using FDG-PET and 201Tl- SPECT. AJNR Am J Neuroradiol 19:801–806

Kleihues P, Burger PC, Scheithauer BW (1993) Histological typing of tumours of the central nervous system. Springer, Berlin Heidelberg New York

Kuhl DE, Wagner HN, Alavi A, Coleman RE, Larson SM, Mintun MA, Siegel BA, Strudler PK (1988) Positron emission tomography (PET): clinical status in the United States in l987. J Nucl Med 29:1136–1143

Larcos G, Maisey MN (1996) FDG-PET screening for cerebral metastases in patients with suspected malignancy. Nucl Med Commun 17:197–198

Marriott CJ, Thorstad W, Akabani G et al (1998) Locally increased uptake of fluorine-18-fluorodeoxyglucose after intracavitary administration of iodine-131-labeled antibody for primary brain tumors. J Nucl Med 39:1376–1380

Mazziotta J, Coleman RE, Di Chiro G, Foster N, Fox P, Frackowiak R, Gilman S, Martin W, Raichle M, Theodore W (Panel Members) (1991) Report of the Therapeutics and Technology Assessment Subcommittee of the American Academy of Neurology Assessment: Positron emission tomography. Neurology 41:163–167

McConathy J, Martarello L, Malveaux EJ et al (2002) Radiolabeled amino acids for tumor imaging with PET: radiosynthesis and biological evaluation of 2-amino-3-[18F]fluoro-2-methylpropanoic acid and 3-[18F]fluoro-2-methyl-2-(methylamino)propanoic acid. J Med Chem 45:2240–2249

Meyerand ME, Pipas JM, Mamourian A, Tosteson TD, Dunn JF (1999) Classification of biopsy-confirmed brain tumors using single-voxel MR spectroscopy. Am J Neuroradiol 20:117–123

Mineura K, Sasajima T, Kowada M et al (1994) Perfusion and metabolism in predicting the survival of patients with cerebral gliomas. Cancer 73:2386–2394

Okazawa H, Yamauchi H, Sugimoto K et al (2001) Quantitative comparison of the bolus and steady-state methods for measurement of cerebral perfusion and oxygen metabolism: positron emission tomography study using 15O-gas and water. J Cereb Blood Flow Metab 21:793–803

Patronas NJ, Brooks RA, DeLaPaz RL et al (1983) Glycolytic rate (PET) and contrast enhancement (CT) in human cerebral gliomas. AJNR Am J Neuroradiol 4:533–535

Patronas NJ, Di Chiro G, Kufta C et al (1985) Prediction of survival in glioma patients by means of positron emission tomography. J Neurosurg 62:816–822

Paulus W, Peiffer J (1989) Intratumoral histologic heterogeneity of gliomas. A quantitative study. Cancer 64:442–447

Pelizzari CA, Chen GT, Spelbring DR et al (1989) Accurate three-dimensional registration of CT, PET, and/or MR images of the brain. J Comput Assist Tomogr 13:20–26

Pirotte B, Goldman S, Brucher JM et al (1994) PET in stereotactic conditions increases the diagnostic yield of brain biopsy. Stereotact Funct Neurosurg 63:144–149

Pirotte B, Goldman S, Bidaut LM et al (1995) Use of positron emission tomography (PET) in stereotactic conditions for brain biopsy. Acta Neurochir (Wien) 134:79–82

Pirotte B, Goldman S, David P et al (1997) Stereotactic brain biopsy guided by positron emission tomography (PET) with [F-18]fluorodeoxyglucose and [C-11]methionine. Acta Neurochir Suppl 68:133–138

Provenzale JM, Arata MA, Turkington TG et al (1999) Gangliogliomas: characterization by registered positron emission tomography-MR images. AJR Am J Roentgenol 172:1103–1107

Raichle ME, Martin WR, Herscovitch P et al (1983Brain blood flow measured with intravenous H2(15)O. II. Implementation and validation. J Nucl Med 24:790–798

Reardon DA, Akabani G, Coleman RE et al (2002) Phase II trial of murine (131)I-labeled antitenascin monoclonal antibody 81C6 administered into surgically created resection cavities of patients with newly diagnosed malignant gliomas. J Clin Oncol 20:1389–1397

Roelcke U, Leenders KL (1999) Positron emission tomography in patients with primary CNS lymphomas. J Neurooncol 43:231–236

Roelcke U, Blasberg RG, von Ammon K et al (1998a) Dexamethasone treatment and plasma glucose levels: relevance for fluorine-18-fluorodeoxyglucose uptake measurements in gliomas. J Nucl Med 39:879–884

Roelcke U, Radu EW, Hausmann O et al (1998b) Tracer transport and metabolism in a patient with juvenile pilocytic astrocytoma. A PET study. J Neurooncol 36:279–283

Rohren EM, Provenzale JM, Barboriak DB, Coleman RE (2003) Screening for cerebral metastases with FDG PET in patients undergoing whole-body staging of non-CNS malignancy. Radiology 226:181–187

Sadato N, Yonekura Y, Senda M et al (1993) PET and the autoradiographic method with continuous inhalation of oxygen-15-gas: theoretical analysis and comparison with conventional steady-state methods. J Nucl Med 34:1672–1680

Sasaki M, Kuwabara Y, Yoshida T et al (1998) A comparative study of thallium-201 SPET, carbon-11 methionine PET and fluorine-18 fluorodeoxyglucose PET for the differentiation of astrocytic tumours. Eur J Nucl Med 25:1261–1269

Schifter T, Hoffman JM, Hanson MW et al (1993) Serial FDG-PET studies in the prediction of survival in patients with primary brain tumors. J Comput Assist Tomogr 17:509–561

Sklar CA (2002) Childhood brain tumors. J Pediatr Endocrinol Metab 15:669–673

Turkington TG, Jaszczak RJ, Pelizzari CA et al (1993) Accuracy of registration of PET, SPECT and MR images of a brain phantom. J Nucl Med 34:1587–1594

Turkington TG, Hoffman JM, Jaszczak RJ et al (1995) Accuracy of surface fit registration for PET and MR brain images using full and incomplete brain surfaces. J Comput Assist Tomogr 19:117–124

Valk PE, Budinger TF, Levin VA et al (1988) PET of malignant cerebral tumors after interstitial brachytherapy. J Neuorsurg 69: 830–838

Wang H, Oliver P, Nan L et al (2002) Radiolabeled 2'-fluorodeoxyuracil-beta-D-arabinofuranoside (FAU) and 2'-fluoro-5-methyldeoxyuracil-beta-D-arabinofuranoside (FMAU) as tumor- imaging agents in mice. Cancer Chemother Pharmacol 49:419–424

Weber WA, Avril N, Schwaiger M (1999) Relevance of positron emission tomography (PET) in oncology. Strahlenther Onkol 175:356–273

Wong TZ, Coleman RE (2000) Brain tumors. In: Bender H, Palmedo H, Biersack H-J, Valk PE (eds) Atlas of clinical PET in oncology. Springer, Berlin Heidelberg New York, pp 153–170

Wong TZ, Coleman RE FDG-PET imaging of brain tumors. In: Valk PE, Bailey DL, Townsend DW et al (eds) Positron emission tomography: basic sciences and clinical practice. Springer, Berlin Heidelberg New York (in press)

Wong TZ, van der Westhuizen GJ, Coleman RE (2002) Positron emission tomography imaging of brain tumors. Neuroimag Clin North Am 12:615–626

Wrensch M, Minn Y, Chew T, Bondy M, Berger MS (2002) Epidemiology of primary brain tumors: current comcepts and review of the literature. Neurooncology 4:278–299

CHAPTER 13

Head and Neck Tumors

H. Bender · H.-J. Straehler-Pohl

13.1 Incidence, Etiology and Epidemiology

Tumors of the head and neck region (for review see [53]) involve a heterogeneous group of neoplastic processes. Because of the complicated anatomical situation, head and neck tumors (HNT) exert characteristic epidemiological, pathological and therapeutic features. Regardless of these differences, there are certain common properties concerning (a) the anatomy of the regional drainage of lymph nodes (LN) and vessels of the head and neck, (b) the pathology, (c) staging and screening, as well as (d) pertaining therapeutic approaches. Based on anatomical, clinical and therapeutic modalities, the head and neck have been subdivided into the following regions: nasal cavity, paranasal sinus, nasopharynx, oral cavity, oropharynx, hypopharynx and larynx.

The incidence of oral cancer varies greatly throughout the world and has significantly risen predominantly in females and certain ethnic groups. Overall, the incidence worldwide is around 20 in 100,000 males. Thus, 15,000 new cases are diagnosed annually in Germany and 63,000 in the United States.

In western countries, such as Europe and the United States, oral cancer accounts for 2–5% of all cancers. These numbers are low compared with a prevalence of up to 40% in Sri Lanka and 50% in India. Southeast Asian people also have a high frequency of oral cancer.

Today, oral cancer occurs twice as often in males as in females. This is considerably different from the 6:1 male to female ratio 30 years ago.

In 1994, the mortality rate was 6.3 per 100,000 males and 1.1 per 100,000 females. Interestingly, there are major regional differences (e.g. Hungary and France: ca. 14 per 100,000), with roughly one-third of patients dying as a result of the tumor. Relative survival rates are among the lowest of the major cancers. Only one-half of people diagnosed with oral cancer are alive 5 years after the diagnosis. In contrast to other cancers (e.g. breast, colorectal, and prostate cancers), the overall survival rate from oral and pharyngeal cancer has not significantly improved during the past 20 years. Survival rates for oral cancer in minorities have even decreased.

Approximately 75% of oral cavity and pharyngeal cancers are attributed to the use of smoked and smokeless tobacco. These cancers include the mouth, tongue, lips, throat, parts of the nose, and larynx. Those who chew tobacco are at high risk for gum and cheek lesions that can lead to cancer. Alcohol consumption is another risk factor. Combinations of tobacco and alcohol are believed to represent substantially greater risk factors than either substance consumed alone. Increased tobacco use (smoking and chewing) largely in women is the main reason for the change in cancer rates compared with rates in the 1950s, as well as alcohol abuse. There is a good correlation of exposure quantity and duration. Age is also a factor – 90% of oral cancers occur among persons over the age of 40 years, 60 being the average age at diagnosis, with a shift to younger age groups.

Other factors that can place a person at risk for these cancers are viral infections, poor nutrition, exposure to ultraviolet light (a major cause of cancer of the lips), and certain occupational exposures.

In tumors originating in the paranasal sinus, nasopharynx, tongue, and larynx, chronic exposure to nickel, chromium, and dust (wood, leather, synthetics, etc.) is a known risk factor.

Lately, the importance of genetic factors has been emphasized, e.g. differences in the metabolism of carcinogens or aberrant metabolic pathways of nitrosamines originating from smoke. Predominantly, females and Afro-Americans seem to be much more sensitive to assumed risk factors. An elevated incidence has been observed in chronic vitamin deficiency, Plummer-Vinson syndrome and various other genetically transmitted diseases (xeroderma pigmentosa, Fanconi anemia, etc.).

13.2 Histopathology

Most tumor lesions are histopathologically squamous cell carcinomas, which are graded depending on the degree of hornification (grade 1: well differentiated with a hornification >75%; grade 2: medium differentiated with a hornification 25–75%; grade 3: dedifferentiated with a hornification <25 %). Other variants of squamous cell carcinoma are verrucous, sarcomatous, and lymphoepithelial cancer. In addition, adenocarcinoma, lymphoma, sarcoma and metastases (kidney, thyroid, breast, lung, prostate) can be found [53].

13.3 Conventional Diagnostic Procedures

13.3.1 Tumor Detection and Primary Staging

The diagnosis of HNT is predominantly based on the physical examination, which is complemented by sonography, computed tomography (CT), magnetic resonance imaging (MRI), and biopsy. Inspection of the mucosa (with and without mechanical devices) readily provides information of the type and extension of pathological processes within the surface area. Physical palpation exerts a high specificity of pathological findings while providing information concerning structure, consistency, and a rough understanding of the relation to neighboring tissues. While clinical assessment is limited to processes comparably near to the surface, morphological imaging methods allow better evaluation of size, structure, relation to neighboring tissues, including their integrity, and the extent of the disease. The first diagnostic step is the use of ultrasound (1–30 MHz), which gives a good overview concerning soft tissues and LN status of the head and neck region. Sensitive detection of (enlarged) LN, pathological masses (e.g. presence of metastases) and differentiation between solid and cystic lesions are the stronghold of this method. Processes >1 cm can be detected with a high sensitivity (>80 %) and acceptable specificity (>65 %) [53, 60]. As ultrasound exerts no radiation hazard, it can be applied frequently, without limitations. Nevertheless, its effective use is related to the experience and ability of the investigator and documentation is only semi-standardized, complicating adequate comparison in the case of follow-up studies and between different investigators.

Introduction of CT and MRI has significantly improved the sensitivity of the overall tumor staging, associated with an objective documentation. CT is the radiological workhorse in morphological imaging of HNT. Standardized study protocols have improved the overall accuracy. As a result of their high resolution (≥1 mm), CT scans allows the detection of small pathological tissue masses and minute distortion of anatomical structures, combined with a rather precise anatomical presentation of the surrounding tissues. Thus, enlarged LN as well as pathological lesions (e.g. primary tumor) can be detected with a high sensitivity, but limited specificity (malignant versus benign processes). In addition, CT provides information concerning the structural integrity of surrounding tissues in the vicinity of a pathological mass.

Major limitations are the lack of specificity mainly in (a) small lesions without characteristic morphological changes, e.g. micrometastases, or small metastases in normal-sized LN, (b) enlarged LN lacking typical signs of malignancy, and (c) distorted anatomy caused by surgery and/or radiation therapy, which complicate differentiation between scar and tumor tissue [53, 60].

The same is true for MRI, but this is comparably rarely used for tumor evaluation and staging. MRI provides even better anatomical representation and a higher discrimination of soft tissue structures. On the other hand, MRI provides no information concerning the integrity of bony structures. Compared to CT, no significant improvement of primary tumor detection or LN assessment could be established, having sensitivities of <70 % for MRI and CT [60]. In addition, MRI is comparably time consuming and more expensive.

Primary tumor staging of HNT is focused on the primary tumor site and the cervical region, which has a direct impact on the strategy and extent of surgical intervention. Completeness of tumor resection, including all involved draining LN, is the crucial step between curative or palliative outcome. In order to exclude distant metastases (lung, liver, bone), conventional staging is completed by an X-ray of the chest, ultrasound of the liver (abdomen) and a bone scan, respectively [60].

13.3.2 Detection of Recurrence and Restaging

Follow-up of treated patients is narrowed by the therapeutic measures and the lack of specificity of the applied diagnostic strategy. The precision of palpation is restricted as a result of scarring tissue from surgical intervention and external beam radiation. Morphological imaging (ultrasound, CT and MRI) cannot differentiate between scar tissue, vital tumor remnants and/or tumor recurrence in the early stages. Repeated studies (usually at 3-monthly intervals) are necessary in order to detect tumor growth.

The same is true concerning LN involvement: while small metastases in normal-sized LN (<1–1.2 cm) cannot be identified, it is also not possible to differentiate between enlarged LN due to unspecific or chronic-inflammatory processes versus tumor infiltration.

13.3.3 Therapy Monitoring

In cases of incomplete tumor resection (R1 resection), early information concerning the response to therapy (radiation, chemotherapy), either during or shortly after completion, might have a significant impact on the overall therapy management. Until now, morphological imaging has not been able to provide these data, since most measurable changes in tumors following therapy (e.g. reduction of tumor volume) are comparably slow (weeks to months) or represent a net effect of various and somehow antagonizing mechanisms, e.g. shrinkage of vital tumor is masked by post-therapeutic edema. Thus conventional follow-up requires comparably long time-intervals (months) in order to allow clear differentiation between volume reduction (responder) or further tumor growth (non-responder).

13.4 Functional Imaging/FDG PET

While morphological imaging has limitations, it has been anticipated that application of functional imaging methods, lately also termed molecular imaging, will improve the evaluation of various tissues, e.g. by in-vivo grading (benign versus malignant; rapidly versus slowly proliferating processes) and might also offer hints concerning histology (e.g. due to expression of typical antigens). This is of major importance, as tumors exert rather typical functional patterns in the early stages and it is often a long time before morphological changes can be detected. Various tumors, including squamous cell carcinoma, exert a highly enhanced glucose utilization, which provides the basis for fluoro-2-deoxy-D-glucose positron emission tomography (FDG PET). Thus, a significantly enhanced rate of glucose utilization (>10 times) in malignant tumors as compared to normal tissues also allows the detection of smaller (<1 cm) lesions by dedicated PET scanners.

13.4.1 Physiological FDG Distribution in the Head and Neck Region

With the exception of brain (cortex, basal ganglia and cerebellum) and myocardium (postprandial), most normal tissues show minimal or moderate FDG accumulation. In our experience tracer uptake in cerebellum, mediastinum and liver is comparably constant, so they can be used as reference organs. The eyes usually present as round activity defects with V-shaped tracer uptake in the eye muscles. No uptake is observed in the eye balls or the maxillary and frontal sinuses. Maxilla and mandible show a turned-around U-shaped activity defect in the region of the dental lamina. The mucosa of the nasal and oral cavity can be delineated by a moderate and homogeneous tracer accumulation and is best seen in the sagittal views. The palatine and pharyngeal tonsils show a moderate to intense uptake and present as symmetrical (hot) spots dorsally of the maxilla/mandible.

Along the neck, in the region of the larynx, a turned-around U-shaped uptake can sometimes be observed; it has been suggested that this represents the vocal muscles as a result of speaking after tracer injection. In tense patients, cervical muscles, mainly the sternocleidomastoid muscle, show moderate to intense uptake, which can hamper interpretation of LN involvement. FDG uptake in the mediastinum is moderate and rather homogeneous, with irregular presentation of the hilum of the lungs. Depending on the fasting status, the myocardium shows intense tracer uptake after a meal as well as often after chemotherapy; in contrast, background activity is observed after a prolonged fasting period (>4 hours). The lung presents with minimal tracer accumulation and can be well differentiated from the thorax wall, mediastinum and abdominal organs (liver, stomach, spleen).

13.4.2 Primary Tumors

Histologically confirmed primary tumors show intense FDG uptake, with a rather uniform distribution, also seen in large vital tumor masses (Fig. 1). In contrast, no uptake can be observed in necrotic tissues and cysts. Overall, high sensitivities (95–100%) and specificities and an excellent grade of differentiation between malignant and benign processes have been documented [4–6, 14, 17, 20, 22, 27, 32, 34, 35, 38, 40–51, 57–59]. In our feasibility study including 50 patients, no false-negative result has been observed [5, 59], whereas false-positive findings were found in pleomorphic adenoma, Warthin's tumor and benign adenopathy due to toxoplasmosis [5, 21, 37, 40, 47, 59].

13.4.3 Lymph Node Staging

Accurate LN staging in HNT has a significant impact: (a) LN involvement is the most important prognostic factor [53]; (b) a high rate of LN involvement has to be expected at the time of primary diagnosis (Table 1); and (c) entire surgical resection of tumor-infested LN is performed as a curative measure.

According to the clinical assessment (palpation), 60% of patients present with LN involvement, but only 40% can be confirmed histologically. LN metastases exert intense FDG uptake and can be delineated with high contrast from normal surrounding tissue (Fig. 2). The lower detection limits are in the range of 5–7 mm.

The diagnostic value of FDG PET, based on histological confirmation, showed sensitivities in the range of 85% and specificities of 89%, which was better than those of CT (sensitivity 77%, specificity 87%) and MRI (sensitivity 80%, specificity 79%), as well as clinical investigation (sensitivity 71%) [1, 4, 5, 6, 11, 21, 24, 41, 43, 46, 56, 58–60].

We have prospectively studied more than 150 patients with large tumors (pT2), palpable tumors or suspected LN metastases prior to planned surgery [5, 6, 58, 59]. Our data demonstrate that FDG PET identified 13%

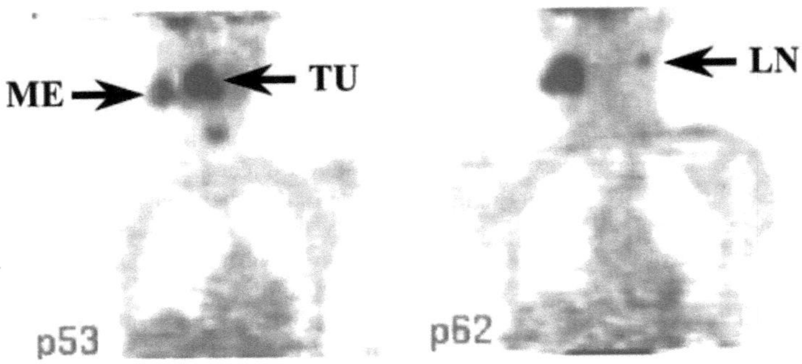

Fig. 1. Typical example of a large midline tumor (*TU*) with major palpable mass in the right neck (*ME*) exerting intense FDG uptake. An unsuspected solitary lymph node metastasis is shown on the left site (*LN*). Uptake is comparable to that of cerebellum and is thus graded as "malignancy-typical". Histology: squamous cell carcinoma

Table 1.
Incidence, gender distribution, rate of cervical metastases and prognosis of head and neck tumors as a function of their localization

Localization	Incidence/100,000	M:F	Metastases (cervical)	5-year survival
Nose/sinus	0.75	2:1	20% (clinical) 15% bilateral	I: 70% IV: 15%
Lips			<20% (late)	I: >90%
Nasopharynx	1.0	2–3:1	60–80% 53% (bilateral)	I: 60% IV: 15%
Oral cavity	13	3:1		I: 30–60% IV: <20%
Floor of the mouth	0.6	3:1	T1: 12%; T4: 50%	I: >85% IV: <30%
Tongue	3	3:1		I: >75% IV: 30%
Oropharynx	2	3–5:1	70–85%	I–II: 40–60% III–IV: 13–30%
Tonsils			T1–2: 38% T3>70%	I: >90% IV: <20%
Larynx	6	2:1		
Glottis			<10% 70%	I: >90%
Supraglottis			T1: >60% 20% bilateral	35–50%
Subglottis			20–30% IV: 20–80%	I: >80%
Hypopharynx	2		70–80%	I: 35–60% IV: <20%
Salivary glands	0.5–1	1:1	35–40%	25–80%

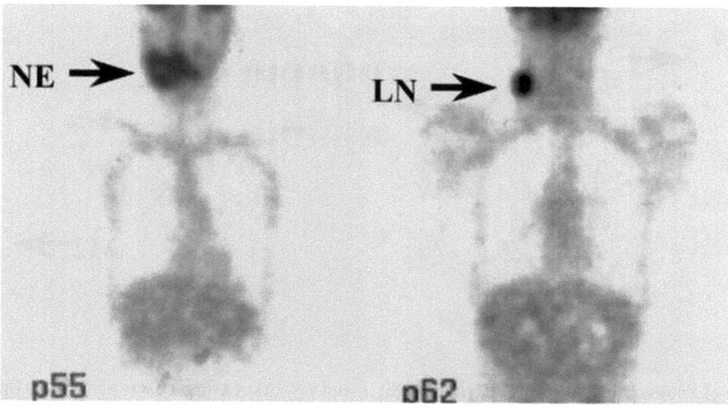

Fig. 2. Typical example of large tumor mass with central necrosis (activity defect; *NE*) and a solitary lymph node metastasis (*LN*). Because of intense FDG uptake, both tumors can be easily delineated from the normal tissue. Uptake is comparable to that of cerebellum and is thus graded as "malignancy-typical". Histology: squamous cell carcinoma

more LN metastases as compared to CT. On the other hand, 12 % of the LN graded as suspicious by CT did not show enhanced glucose uptake and were true negative, as confirmed by histology. Thus, in around 25 % of all patients, FDG PET had an influence on the final diagnosis, resulting in a 10 % improvement of the accuracy.

It is noteworthy that radiological methods are often limited in the clear differentiation of malignant versus benign LN involvement (either normal sized or borderline enlarged), while functional information (FDG PET) significantly improves the safety and accuracy of the final interpretation [58, 59].

13.4.4 Distant Metastases

Head and neck tumors predominantly show spread to local LN regions as a first step of tumor progression. Distant metastases often present as mediastinal LN metastases, while lung and bone metastases occur late in the stage of disease. Detection of distant metastases rules out curative surgery (Fig. 3).

As a result of the study mentioned above, FDG PET was able to detect mediastinal LN involvement in roughly 15 % of our patients, suffering from recurrent disease. It is noteworthy that those patients were selected for curative surgery as a result of negative conventional staging. Furthermore, in around 10 % of this patient group, FDG PET also detected distant metastases (lung, liver and/or bone) [5, 6, 20, 22, 32, 35, 41, 49, 56, 58, 59].

13.4.5 Local Recurrence/Secondary Tumors

Follow-up studies in HNT after surgery and/or radiation therapy employing physical examinations and morphological imaging modalities are not uncritical. Changes in the normal anatomy following surgery and fibrotic and sclerotic processes after radiation therapy limit their primary diagnostic value. Often only follow-up studies that present signs of volume enlargement are conclusive. Under these circumstances, the use of functional methods seems to be ideal. FDG accumulation in morphologically suspicious lesions is indicative for vital tumor tissue [18], if acute inflammatory processes have been excluded. In contrast, absent FDG uptake usually contradicts tumor remnants or recurrence [58, 59].

Our own experience [6, 58] includes more than 100 patients with suspected tumor recurrence, based on clinical examinations and CT scans. FDG PET was able to confirm the presence of tumor tissue in 90 % of the histologically proven cases, as compared to CT (86 %; statistically not significant). Interestingly, 13 % of proven local recurrences were missed by CT, but detected by FDG PET; on the other hand, 10 % of recurrent tumors were also missed by FDG PET but suspicious in CT. These false-negative findings were due to thin submucosal growth (≤2 mm), which was below the functional resolution of PET.

Published data are in accordance with these findings, demonstrating sensitivities between 70 and 90 % and specificities of 70–100 % in local recurrence; these data are somewhat better than those of CT (sensitivity 77 % and specificity 87 %, respectively).

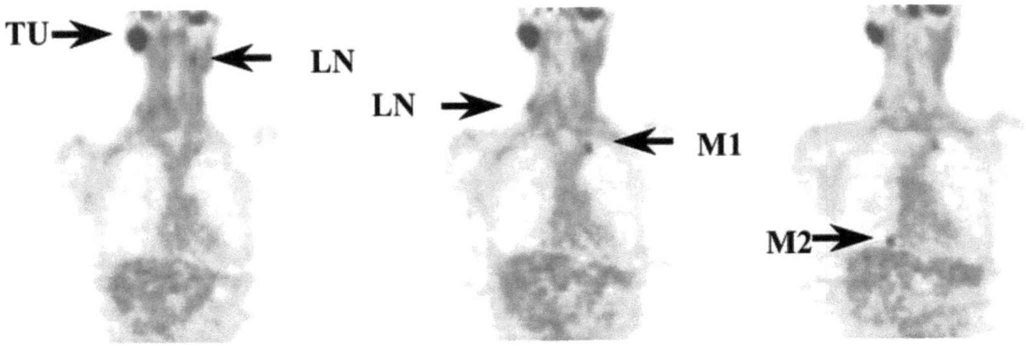

Fig. 3. Typical example of known palpable mass (*TU*) in the right upper cervical region, unsuspected normal-sized lymph node metastases (*LN*) on the left side as well as metastases in the upper left (*M1*) and lower right (*M2*) mediastine. The patient was upstaged and no curative surgery was performed. Uptake is comparable to that of cerebellum and is thus graded as "malignancy-typical". Histology: squamous cell carcinoma

On the other hand, in case of tumor recurrence, FDG PET is unquestionably superior in LN staging as compared to CT: average sensitivity 87% versus 62% and specificity 89% versus 73%, respectively [2, 5, 6, 15, 16, 29, 34, 36, 58, 59].

13.4.6
Cancer of Unknown Primary (CUP Syndrome)

Detection of a primary tumor site in patients diagnosed with cervical LN metastases is assumed to be beneficial. This effect is probably due to possible complete tumor resection and/or selection of adapted chemo- and/or radiation therapy. Published experience demonstrates that FDG PET is able to identify 20–50% of the primaries, where conventional imaging results were negative [3, 5, 9, 10, 12, 28, 31, 32, 35, 41, 43, 54, 59].

This is in good accordance with our results including 50 patients with CUP syndrome. A primary tumor was detected in 24% of the patients by FDG PET. In our patient population, more than 30% presented with distant metastases as a result of routinely applied whole-body scanning [5, 6, 58, 59].

13.4.7
Therapy Monitoring

Head and neck tumors are often diagnosed at a rather late tumor stage. Nevertheless, large primary tumors with or without locoregional LN involvement are primarily treated with a curative intention. Thus, complete tumor resection is crucial. In cases where tumor ablation cannot be performed, a combination of surgery, radiation and/or chemotherapy is applied. Assessment of the therapeutic effectiveness are (a) early proof of response, (b) evidence or exclusion of vital tumor remnants and (c) early detection of recurrence.

Previous studies indicate that diminishing glucose utilization after chemotherapy and/or radiation therapy was associated with therapy response, while unchanged glucose utilization was indicative for therapy resistance [7, 8, 13, 15, 16, 18, 19, 23, 25, 26, 30, 33, 39, 48, 55]. Interestingly, Haberkorn et al. [19] has reported that therapy effectiveness is heterogeneous in various tumor sites of a given patient. Responding and resistant tumor lesions could be identified. Nevertheless, there was a good correlation of final therapy outcome and the established effects on FDG uptake in the various lesions.

Cytotoxic effects seem to influence glucose utilization rapidly within minutes and hours, which is the basis to assume that FDG PET could be used for early prediction of therapy outcome. Thus, functional assessment of glucose utilization before and after one dose of chemotherapy might allow discrimination of responders from non-responders [7].

In the current follow-up scheme, high FDG uptake in morphologically undetermined tumor remnants or suspicious scar tissue is indicative of a vital tumor, either non-responding remnants of tumor or early recurrence.

13.4.8
Indications for FDG PET in HNT

13.4.8.1
Primary Tumor Assessment

According to the 3rd German Interdisciplinary Consensus Conference [52], the value of FDG PET in the assessment of a known primary tumor is not yet established (Table 2). Functional information of a given tumor mass (vitality, in-vivo grading) might have some prognostic impact, but has no effect on the conventional therapy management. Complementary information to morphological findings (e.g. local invasion) cannot be given.

13.4.8.2
Lymph Node Staging

The clinical value of FDG PET in LN staging has definitely been established (Table 2). While conventional imaging already has a high sensitivity and specificity, based on our extensive experience, FDG PET is especially helpful in the following settings:

(i) large primary tumors (pT>2) in order to assess LN involvement of the contralateral side and/or presence of mediastinal LN;
(ii) midline tumors in order to assess the side of LN involvement;
(iii) morphological findings are equivocal, e.g. enlarged LN without typical signs of malignancy;
(iv) equivocal clinical findings, e.g. suspicious LN with no evidence of a primary tumor or recurrence;
(v) established local recurrence without clear proof or exclusion of nodal disease, e.g. equivocal morphological and/or clinical findings.

13.4.8.3
Distant Metastases

The benefit of FDG PET in primary staging or restaging in order to assess systemic disease is still under discussion (Table 2). Nevertheless, our experience demonstrates that patients with tumor recurrence have a high risk of distant metastases (mediastinal LN >lung >bone). Thus, patients suffering from recurrence and who are designated for curative surgery, should receive a PET scan prior to surgery.

13.4.8.4
Recurrence

The clinical value of FDG PET for the diagnosis of recurrence has definitely been established (Table 2). Nevertheless, in our clinics FDG PET is only applied if clinical findings or morphological results are inconclusive or, in the case of large tumor masses, suspicion of distant metastases has arisen and the benefit of radical surgery is questionable.

Table 2. Evidence-based indications for the assessment of head and neck tumors according to the 3rd Consensus Conference (52)

Indication	Clinical value
Grading of primary tumor	Sufficient data not available
Grading of secondary tumor	Helpful in selected cases
LN staging	Proven value
M staging	Sufficient data not available
Recurrence	Proven value
Therapy monitoring	Sufficient data not available
Unknown primary (CUP)	Proven value

13.4.8.5
Therapy Monitoring

The benefit of FDG PET for therapy monitoring is still under investigation (Table 2). As only limited therapeutic options are available, therapy monitoring is currently of limited use and should be performed only in clinical studies.

13.4.8.6
Cancer of Unknown Primary

The clinical value of FDG PET in CUP has definitely been established (Table 2). In these cases, FDG PET staging should be applied routinely without exception.

13.5
Summary and Outlook

Head and neck tumors are histologically mainly squamous cell carcinomas, which exert an avid glucose utilization. On the other hand, normal tissues of the head and neck show only faint to moderate FDG uptake, providing an excellent anatomical landmarking. Thus, HNT can be delineated with high contrast from the surrounding tissues, including small lesions (>5–7 mm). Even though primary tumors exert an intense FDG uptake, FDG PET currently plays no role in their functional assessment (e.g. grading) due to a limited therapeutic impact.

Currently, the major benefit of FDG PET is established in LN staging and restaging, as well in the differentiation of scar versus tumor relapse, especially when clinical and/or morphological methods are inconclusive and surgery is planned.

In addition, when clinical and/or morphological results are inconclusive, functional information has a crucial impact on further therapeutic decisions. Our experience underscores the benefit of FDG PET in the presurgical assessment of LN status in presumably resectable primaries as well as the exclusion of distant metastases. First, FDG PET allows a better assessment of the status (malignant versus benign) of palpably or morphologically inconclusive findings; second, FDG PET is able to detect small LN metastases (0.5–1.2 cm), which are considered normal by CT criteria; and third, FDG PET is able to exclude tumor involvement in morphologically enlarged or borderline LN with a high accuracy.

Combination of both methods – morphology and function – showed further improvement of sensitivity, specificity and accuracy. It should be emphasized that the additional functional information, e.g. "malignancy-typical glucose utilization" significantly facilitates and improves the certainty of the final interpretation of the surgeons, while preoperatively reviewing the various collected results. Thus, the decision to proceed with further therapeutic measurements or to recommend "wait-and-watch" is more accurate when functional imaging results are available. Morphological imaging results, at least in our experience, often lack an unambiguous conclusion, and require a follow-up study in a few months. This not only causes significant psychological distress for the patient, but might also have an impact on tumor progression and development of metastases. Thus, FDG PET allows the missing and critical information to be obtained at an early stage.

Finally, another stronghold of FDG PET is its high sensitivity in the detection of primary tumors in CUP – syndrome; it should therefore be applied early on.

In the future, advanced assessment of various factors concerning the currently employed study techniques (head-fixation, scan times, detector resolution, etc.) might advance the detection rate of small metastases or might even allow the detection of micrometastases (>3–5 mm). In addition, automatic or semi-automatic image fusion techniques, e.g. a combination of CT and PET, should produce an almost perfect image overlay.

Generation of more data concerning therapy monitoring [7] should provide the basis to move this technique from preclinical to clinical applications. At the same time, development and availability of new tracers, e.g. amino acids and RNA/DNA precursors, might open up new options in tumor diagnostics as well as in cancer management.

13.6 Technical Recommendations

13.6.1 Patient Preparation

Patients should be fasted (>4 hours, better overnight) but well hydrated. Blood sugar values should be <120 mg%, at the time of injection. Between 185 and 740 MBq FDG are injected intravenously and patients should be kept quiet and lying in a separate room with dimmed light. In order to improve clearance from the urinary system, patients should drink up to 1 liter of water within 30 min after FDG injection, or receive an intravenous infusion.

13.6.2 Acquisition

In older software systems, a cold transmission scan (minimum from base of the skull to the lower edge of the liver), 3–10 min per bed position, depending on the age of the source (e.g. rotating Ge68/Ga68 line sources) should be performed in the supine position. If the patient is moved, the exact position has to be marked (e.g. three-point marks).

Emission scans (10 min per bed position) are started at least 45 min after injection, covering the above regions. To exclude distant metastases, short emission scans (3–5 min per bed position) of the abdomen and pelvis should be included. In the case of CUP, a complete body-trunk scan (base of the skull to pelvis) employing transmission and emission scans is recommended.

Late images (>120 min post-injection) of the head and neck region are recommended in order to exclude inflammatory processes, which are thought to show decreasing FDG uptake over time.

13.6.3 Image Reconstruction and Evaluation

Images are reconstructed either by filtered back-projection (Hanning filter; cut-off frequency 0.4/cycle; decay correction, x-y-z smoothing) or iterative reconstruction. In order to allow quantitative assessment (standard uptake value), images can be normalized for body weight (kg) or surface (m^2) and injected dose (MBq). Images are evaluated qualitatively ("hot-spot imaging") and coronal, sagittal and transverse slices are documented as black-and-white or color hardcopy. For the assessment of pathological lesions, the use of a qualitative four-point scoring system has been proven to be useful, employing individual normal organs as references: (1) uptake comparable cerebellum activity = malignancy-typical; (2) uptake comparable between liver and cerebellum activity = malignancy-suspicious; (3) uptake comparable liver activity = unspecific; (4) uptake comparable background activity (e.g. in morphologically documented lesions) = normal/no evidence of disease. In the case of quantitative assessment, standard uptake values >2.5 have been suggested to represent "malignancy-typical" uptake.

Malignant lesions typically show a high contrast compared to surrounding tissue and present with a rather round shape. Streak artifacts, e.g. due to incorrect repositioning or movements (head, arms, legs) might look like focal uptake, which are not reproducible on all three orthogonal projections. In order to minimize interpretation mistakes, use of fixed upper and lower thresholds is helpful and the cerebellum should be used as the reference for maximum activity.

These problems do not apply in the case of iterative reconstruction. Several people have reported that smaller lesions have "disappeared" in transmission-corrected images using iterative reconstruction, thus comparison with the pertaining emission scans is advisable.

13.6.4 Pitfalls

While FDG is a rather unspecific substance, proper preselection of patients by exclusion of inflammatory processes, for example, significantly enhances specificity (malignant versus benign). Detailed clinical information (surgery, radiation therapy, etc.) as well as inclusion of results of morphological diagnostics (CT, MRI) are prerequisites for final image interpretation.

FDG PET scans should not be performed <6 weeks after surgery, especially after (modified or radical) LN dissection.

References

1. Adams S, Baum RP, Stuckensen T et al (1998) Prospective comparison of 18F-FDG PET with conventional imaging modalities (CT, MRI, US) in lymph node staging of head and neck cancer. Eur J Nucl Med 25:1255–1260
2. Anzai Y, Minoshima S, Wolf GT, Wahl RL (1999) Head and neck cancer: detection of recurrence with three-dimensional principal components analysis at dynamic FDG PET. Radiology 212: 285–288
3. Assar OS, Fischbein NJ, Caputo GR et al (1999) Metastatic head and neck cancer: role and usefulness of FDG-PET in locating occult primary tumors. Radiology 210:177–181
4. Bailet JW, Abemayor E, Jabour BA et al (1992) Positron emission tomography: a new, precise imaging modality for detection of primary head and neck tumors and assessment of cervical adenopathy. Laryngoscope 102:281–288
5. Bender H, Straehler-Pohl HJ, Schomburg A et al (1997) Value of F-18-DG-PET in the assessment of head and neck tumors. J Nucl Med 38:153 (A)
6. Bender H, Straehler-Pohl HJ, Frohmann JP et al (1998) FDG-PET as a clinical routine tool for the staging of selected tumors: results and implications In: Limouris GS, Bender H, Biersack HJ (eds) Radionuclides for therapy. Mediterra Publishers, Athens
7. Bender H, Metten N, Bangard N et al (1999) Possible role of FDG-PET in the early prediction of therapy outcome in liver metastases of colorectal carcinoma. Hybridoma 18:87–91
8. Berlangieri SU, Brizel DM, Scher RL et al (1994) Pilot study of positron emission tomography in patients with advanced head and neck cancer receiving radiotherapy and chemotherapy. Head Neck 16:340–346
9. Bohuslavizki KH, Klutmann S, Buchert R et al (1999) Value of F-18-FDPET in patients with cervical lymph node metastases of unknown origin. Radiol Oncol 33:207–212
10. Bohuslavizki KH, Klutmann S, Kroger S et al (2000) FDG-PET detection of unknown primary tumors. J Nucl Med 41:816–822
11. Braams JW, Pruim J, Freling NJ et al (1995) Detection of lymph node metastases of squamous-cell cancer of the head and neck with FDG-PET and MRI. J Nucl Med 36:211–216
12. Braams JW, Pruim J, Kole AC et al (1997) Detection of unknown primary head and neck tumors by positron emission tomography. Int J Oral Maxillofac Surg 26:112–115
13. Brun E, Ohlsson T, Erlandsson K et al (1997) Early prediction of treatment outcome in head and neck cancer with 2–18FDG PET. Acta Oncol 36:741–743
14. Changlai S-P, Kao C-H, Chieng P-U (1997) 18F-2-fluoro-2-deoxy-D-glucose positron emission tomography of head and neck in patients with nasopharyngeal carcinomas. Oncol Rep 4:1331–1333
15. Farber LA, Benard F, Machtay M et al (1999) Detection of recurrent head and neck squamous cell carcinomas after radiation therapy with 2-sup(18)F-fluoro-2-deoxyD-glucose positron emission tomography. Laryngoscope 109:970–979
16. Fischbein NJ, Os AA, Caputo GR et al (1998) Clinical utility of positron emission tomography with 18F-fluorodeoxyglucose in detecting residual/recurrent squamous cell carcinoma of the head and neck. Am J Neuroradiol 19:1189–1193
17. Greven KM, McGuirt WF, Watson X et al (1995) PET in the evaluation of laryngeal carcinoma. Ann Otol Rhinol Laryngol 104: 274–278
18. Greven KM, Williams DW 3rd, Keyes JW Jr et al (1994) Positron emission tomography of patients with head and neck carcinoma before and after high dose irradiation. Cancer 74:1355–1359
19. Haberkorn U, Strauss LG, Dimitrakopoulou A et al (1993) Fluorodeoxyglucose imaging of advanced head and neck cancer after chemotherapy. J Nucl Med 34:12–17
20. Hanasono MM, Kunda LD, Segall GM, Ku GH, Terris DJ (1999) Uses and limitations of FDG positron emission tomography in patients with head and neck cancer. Laryngoscope 109:880–888
21. Horiuchi M, Yasuda S, Shohtsu A, Ide M (1998) Four cases of Warthin's tumor of the parotid gland detected with FDG PET. Ann Nucl Med 12:47–50
22. Jabour BA, Choi Y, Hoh CK et al (1993) Extracranial head and neck: PET imaging with 2-[F-18]fluoro-2-deoxy-D-glucose and MR imaging correlation. Radiology 186:27–35
23. Kao CH, ChangLai SP, Chieng PU, Yen RF, Yen TC (1998) Detection of recurrent or persistent nasopharyngeal carcinomas after radiotherapy with 18-fluoro-2-deoxyglucose positron emission tomography and comparison with computed tomography. J Clin Oncol 16:3550–3553
24. Kau RJ, Alexiou C, Laubenbacher C, Werner M, Schwaiger M, Arnold W (1999) Lymph node detection of head and neck squamous cell carcinomas by positron emission tomography with fluorodeoxyglucose F 18 in a routine clinical setting. Arch Otolaryngol Head Neck Surg 125:1322–1324
25. Kim HJ, Boyd J, Dunphy F, Lowe V (1998) F-18 FDG PET scan after radiotherapy for early-stage larynx cancer. Clin Nucl Med 23:750–753
26. Kitagawa Y, Sadato N, Azuma H et al (1999) FDG PET to evaluate combined intra-arterial chemotherapy and radiotherapy of head and neck neoplasms. J Nucl Med 40:1132–1135
27. Kitagawa Y, Nishizawa S, Sano K, Sadato N et al (2002) Whole-body (18)F-fluorodeoxyglucose positron emission tomography in patients with head and neck cancer. Oral Surg Oral Med Oral Pathol Oral Radiol Endod 93:202–207
28. Kole AC, Nieweg OE, Pruim J, et al. (1998) Detection of unknown occult primary tumors using positron emission tomography. Cancer 82:1160–1166
29. Kunkel M, Kuffner HD, Reichert TE et al (2000) (18F)-2-fluorodeoxyglucose PET. Prospects for secondary prevention of mouth cavity carcinoma. Mund Kiefer Gesichtschir 4:105–110
30. Kunkel M, Forster GJ, Reichert TE et al (2003) Radiation response non-invasively imaged by [(18)F]FDG-PET predicts local tumor control and survival in advanced oral squamous cell carcinoma. Oral Oncol 39:170–177
31. Lassen U, Daugaard G, Eigtved A, Damgaard K, Friberg L. (1999) 18F-FDG whole body positron emission tomography (PET) in patients with unknown primary tumours (UPT). Eur J Cancer 35:1076–1082
32. Laubenbacher C, Saumweber D, Wagner Manslau C et al (1995) Comparison of fluorine-18-fluorodeoxyglucose PET, MRI and endoscopy for staging head and neck squamous-cell carcinomas. J Nucl Med 36:1747–1757
33. Lowe VJ, Dunphy FR, Varvares M et al (1997) Evaluation of chemotherapy response in patients with advanced head and neck

cancer using [F-18]fluorodeoxyglucose positron emission tomography. Head Neck 19:666–669
34. Lowe VJ, Kim H, Boyd JH, Eisenbeis JF, Dunphy FR, Fletcher JW (1999) Primary and recurrent early stage laryngeal cancer: preliminary results of 2-[fluorine 18]fluoro-2-deoxy-D-glucose PET imaging. Radiology 212:799–802
35. Mancuso AA, Drane WE, Mukherji SK (1994) The promise of FDG in diagnosis and surveillance of head and neck cancer. Cancer 74:1193–1195
36. Manolidis S, Donald PJ, Volk P, Pounds TR (1998) The use of positron emission tomography scanning in occult and recurrent head and neck cancer. Acta Otolaryngol Suppl 534:1–8
37. Matsuda M, Sakamoto H, Okamura T et al (1998) Positron emission tomographic imaging of pleomorphic adenoma in the parotid gland. Acta Otolaryngol Suppl 538:214–220
38. McGuirt WF, Greven KM, Keyes JW et al (1995a) Positron emission tomography in the evaluation of laryngeal carcinoma. Ann Otol Rhinol Laryngol 104:274–278
39. McGuirt WF, Keyes JW, Greven KM et al (1995b) Preoperative identification of benign versus malignant parotid masses: a comparative study including positron emission tomography. Laryngoscope 105:579–584
40. McGuirt WF, Williams DW 3rd, Keyes JW Jr et al (1995c) A comparative diagnostic study of head and neck nodal metastases using positron emission tomography. Laryngoscope 105:373–375
41. McGuirt WF, Greven KM, Keyes JW Jr, Williams DW 3rd, Watson N (1998) Laryngeal radionecrosis versus recurrent cancer: a clinical approach. Ann Otol Rhinol Laryngol 107:293–296
42. Mendenhall WM, Manusco AA, Parsons JT et al (1998) Diagnostic evaluation of squamous cell carcinoma metastatic to cervical lymph nodes from an unknown head and neck primary site. Head Neck 20:739–744
43. Moog F, Bangerter M, Diederichs CG et al (1997) Lymphoma: role of whole-body 2-deoxy-2-[F-18]fluoro-D-glucose (FDG) PET in nodal staging. Radiology 203:795–798
44. Mukherji SK, Drane WE, Mancuso AA et al (1996) Occult primary tumors of the head and neck: detection with 2-[F-18] fluoro-2-deoxy-D-glucose SPECT. Radiology 199:761–766
45. Myers LL, Wax MK (1998) Positron emission tomography in the evaluation of the negative neck in patients with oral cavity cancer. J Otolaryngol 27:342–347
46. Nakasone Y, Inoue T, Oriuchi N et al (2001) The role of whole-body FDG-PET in preoperative assessment of tumor staging in oral cancers. Ann Nucl Med 15:505–512
47. Okamura T, Kawabe J, Koyama K et al (1998) Fluorine-18 fluorodeoxyglucose positron emission tomography imaging of parotid mass lesions. Acta Otolaryngol Suppl 538:209–213
48. Rege SD, Chaiken L, Hoh CK et al (1993) Change induced by radiation therapy in FDG uptake in normal and malignant structures of the head and neck: quantitation with PET. Radiology 189:807–812
49. Rege S, Maass A, Chaiken L et al (1994) Use of positron emission tomography with fluorodeoxyglucose in patients with extracranial head and neck cancers. Cancer 73:3047–3058
50. Reisser C, Haberkorn U, Strauss LG (1991) PET scan in tumor diagnosis in the head and neck. Laryngorhinootologie 70:214–217
51. Reisser C, Haberkorn U, Strauss LG (1993) The relevance of positron emission tomography for the diagnosis and treatment of head and neck tumors. J Otolaryngol 22:231–238
52. Reske SN, Kotzerke J (2001) FDG-PET for clinical use. Results of the 3rd German Interdisciplinary Consensus Conference. Eur J Nucl Med 28:1707–1723
53. Schantz SP, Harrison LB, Forastiere AA (1997) Tumors of the nasal cavity and paranasal sinuses, nasopharynx, oral cavity and oropharynx. In: DeVita VT, Hellman S, Rosenberg SA (eds) Cancer, principles and practice of oncology. Lippincott-Raven, New York, pp 741–801
54. Schipper JH, Schrader M, Arweiler D et al (1996) Positron emission tomography for primary tumor detection in lymph node metastases with unknown primary tumor. HNO 44:254–257
55. Seifert E, Schadel A, Haberkorn U, Strauss LG (1992) Evaluating the effectiveness of chemotherapy in patients with head-neck tumors using positron emission tomography (PET scan). HNO 40:90–93
56. Stoeckli SJ, Steinert H, Pfaltz M, Schmid S (2002) Is there a role for positron emission tomography with 18F-fluorodeoxyglucose in the initial staging of nodal negative oral and oropharyngeal squamous cell carcinoma. Head Neck 24:345–349
57. Stokkel MP, ten Broek FW, van Rijk PP (1998) The role of FDG PET in the clinical management of head and neck cancer. Oral Oncol 34:466–467
58. Straehler-Pohl HJ, Bender H, Linke D et al (1998) Value of F-18-DG-PET in the assessment of head and neck tumors: clinical experience in 152 patients. J Cancer Res Clin Oncol 124:R10
59. Straehler-Pohl HJ, Bender H, Linke D et al (1998) Value of F-18-DG-PET in the staging of head and neck tumors under clinical routine conditions. Eur J Nucl Med 25:1032(A)
60. StuckensenT,KovacsAF,AdamsS,BaumRP(2000)Stagingof the neck in patients with oral cavity squamous cell carcinomas: a prospective comparison of PET, ultrasound, CT and MRI. J Craniomaxillofac Surg 28:319–324

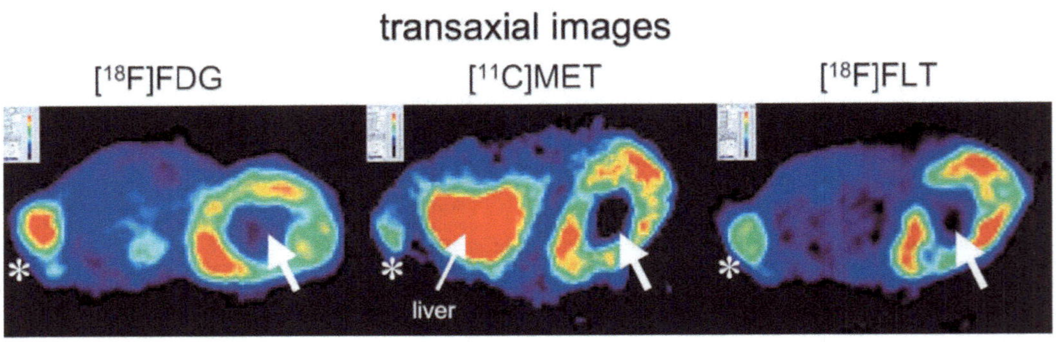

CHAPTER 14

Thyroid Carcinomas

F. Grünwald · M. Diehl

14.1 Clinical Background

The most frequent forms of thyroid cancer can be divided into two main categories: tumors with follicle cell differentiation and those with C-cell differentiation. Within the category of tumors with follicle cell differentiation, a distinction is made between papillary tumors and follicular tumors. Both undifferentiated and anaplastic tumors are also included in this category, although a clear attribution to an initial cell line is not always possible for anaplastic carcinomas. Within the largest group, the papillary carcinomas, there are several types including encapsulated, minimal invasive, diffuse sclerotic and oncocytic carcinomas. Because of their generally low iodine uptake and their high mitochondrial content, Hürthle cell carcinomas have a special position, particularly in functional imaging and with respect to therapy options. Carcinomas with C-cell differentiation are partly genetically determined, either as isolated familial medullary carcinoma or in multiple endocrine neoplasia (MEN-2a/MEN-2b). The existence of mixed follicle cell/C-cell differentiated carcinomas should be mentioned, especially in the context of radioiodine therapy, since the latter can certainly offer therapeutic options. We will not discuss the rare forms of thyroid cancer or the further subcategorization of the tumor entities described above, since this information is currently not relevant to the clinical significance of PET.

The yearly incidence of malignant thyroid tumors is approximately 4/100,000 in women and 1.5/100,000 in men. Thyroid tumors comprise approximately 1.5% of all malignant tumors in women, and approximately 0,5% in men. Incidence increases with age: in autopsy studies occult thyroid carcinomas were found in up to 35%. The basis for this observation is presumably the biological behavior of most of these malignancies, which frequently do not appear clinically for years. Exposure to ionizing radiation during childhood leads to a significant increase in the incidence of thyroid carcinomas, especially papillary carcinomas. An increase in the supply of adequate dietary iodine has led to a relative shift in histological findings involving an increase in papillary carcinoma and a decrease in follicular and anaplastic carcinomas. It is still unclear whether there is an absolute increase in the number of papillary tumors as a result of improved iodine supply.

In addition to age and sex, tumor stage and histopathological grading have the greatest prognostic significance. TNM classification according to the recommendations of the International Union Against Cancer/ Union Internationale Contre le Cancer (UICC) (Sobin and Wittekind 2002) is given in Table 1. Histopathological grading is based on the evaluation of nuclear atypia, the extent of tumor necrosis, and vascular invasion (Akslen 1993). Whereas follicular carcinomas show up more frequently with distant metastases, papillary tumors tend to exhibit lymphogenic spreading that – in

Table 1. Tumor staging

pT[a]	
pTX	Primary tumor cannot be assessed
pT0	No evidence of primary tumor
pT1	Tumor ≤2 cm, limited to the thyroid
pT2	Tumor >2 cm, ≤4 cm, limited to the thyroid
pT3	Tumor >4 cm, limited to the thyroid or any tumor with minimal extrathyroid extension (e.g. extension to sternothyroid muscle or perithyroid soft tissue)
pT4a	Tumor extends beyond the thyroid capsule and invades any of the following: subcutaneous soft tissue, larynx, trachea, esophagus, recurrent laryngeal nerve
pT4b	Tumor invades prevertebral fascia, mediastinal vessels, or encases carotid artery
pN	
pNX	Regional lymph nodes cannot be assessed
pN0	No regional lymph node metastasis
pN1a	
pN1b	
pM	
pMX	Distant metastasis cannot be assessed
pM0	No distant metastasis
pM1	Distant metastasis

[a] Multifocal tumors of all histological types should be designated (m) (the largest tumor determines the classification)

contrast to other tumors is not associated with a significantly poorer prognosis. The lungs and skeletal system are affected most frequently by distant metastases. Overall, the prognosis for differentiated thyroid carcinomas is extremely good. Encapsulated papillary tumors and minimal papillary carcinomas have a long-term survival rate of over 90%. There are different staging systems for estimating individual prognosis.

Table 2 shows a clinically suitable concept in which age is the only factor considered besides primary staging for the prognosis of life expectancy. It should be emphasized especially in comparison with other tumor entities that patients under 45 years of age enjoy the relatively favorable Stage II status even when distant metastases are present. Pulmonary metastases can be treated better with high-dose radioiodine therapy than bone metastases. Radioiodine therapy is particularly effective in diffuse pulmonary metastatic spread, which can be detected only by scintigraphy but not by chest radiography or CT (Menzel et al. 1996) The prognosis for anaplastic carcinomas is generally unfavorable; reported exceptions can generally be traced to the fact that a carcinoma was classified as anaplastic despite the presence of differentiated areas. A frequent limiting factor with anaplastic carcinomas is the invasive growth of the primary tumor or the local recurrence.

Carcinomas with C-cell differentiation occupy a midpoint between differentiated and anaplastic carcinomas with respect to the prognosis. In this regard, lymphogenic metastatic spread of C-cell carcinomas, which frequently also involves mediastinal lymph nodes, has a greater prognostic significance than in differentiated carcinomas, especially in papillary carcinomas.

Preoperative diagnostics of thyroid tumors will be described only briefly, since it is not related to the clinical application of PET. There is no indication for FDG PET as part of the preoperative status evaluation, as is explained in greater detail below. In addition to a physical exam, diagnostics includes sonography, scintigraphy, fine needle biopsy, and both morphological imaging and the analysis of thyroid-specific laboratory parameters. Recent studies increasingly recommend checking the patient's basal serum calcitonin level when there are unclear nodular changes in the thyroid (Raue and Frank-Raue 1997)

Table 2. Prognostic staging

	≤45 years of age (papillary or follicular)	Papillary or follicular >45 years of age and medullary
Stage I	Any T, any N, M0	T1, N0, M0
Stage II	Any T, any N, M1	T2, N0, M0
Stage III	–	T3,N0,M0 or T1–3, N1a, M0
Stage IVA	–	T1–3,N1b, M0 or T4a, any N, M0
Stage IVB	–	T4b, any N, M0
Stage IVC	–	Any T, Any N, M1

14.2 Therapy

Total thyroidectomy is the therapy of choice (Simon 1997) except in cases of highly differentiated encapsulated papillary carcinoma pT1a N0 M0 (in these cases, hemithyroidectomy is regarded as adequate by most authors). Total thyroidectomy removes tumor tissue, which is relevant especially because of its relatively frequent multifocal growth, although it has not yet been clarified whether an intrathyroidal metastatic spread is involved or the parallel development of several tumor clones. Furthermore, the radical removal of benign iodine-accumulating tissue is the precondition for effective radioiodine therapy. In the case of differentiated carcinomas, thyroidectomy includes lymph node dissection of the central compartment. If additional lymph node metastases are suspected, the lateral compartments (ipsilateral and also contralateral, if necessary) are dissected as well. C-cell carcinoma requires dissection of the lateral compartments: the ipsilateral compartment with the sporadic form of c-cell carcinoma and the contralateral compartment as well in patients suffering from the familial from. Surgical procedures for anaplastic carcinomas are largely determined by palliative factors.

An initial radioiodine therapy follows thyroidectomy. Exceptions include the constellation mentioned above (highly differentiated encapsulated papillary carcinoma pT1a N0 M0) and tumors that are not sufficiently operable. The isotope used is ^{131}I, which has a beta radiation energy (E_{max}) of .61 MeV and a gamma radiation energy of 364 keV. Beta radiation has a mean range of less than 1 mm and can be used therapeutically in order to achieve the highest possible dose – with minimal exposure to other tissues – in the follicle cells and their immediate environment, where iodine uptake ability has remained intact. Gamma radiation can be used for scintigraphy. Radioiodine therapy (RIT) should be performed at maximum TSH stimulation (>30 mU/l). A hormone withdrawal period of approximately four weeks usually results in maximum endogenous TSH secretion. Exceptions include cases with extended (usually pulmonary) metastatic spread, large amounts of remnant tissue in which a relevant hormone synthesis is still present, and pituitary insufficiency, which is rarely encountered. In such cases, recombinant TSH (rTSH) can be used. Studies report that the use of rTSH is equivalent to thyroid hormone withdrawal, with respect to sensitivity and specificity of whole body radioiodine scintigraphy and tumor marker levels. A combination of whole body radioiodine scintigraphy and tumor marker level after administration of rTSH detected thyroid tissue or cancer in 93 % of patients with disease in the thyroid bed and in 100 % of patients with distant metastases (Haugen et al. 1999). A comparison of rTSH versus hormone withdrawal showed a sensitivity of radioiodine scan of 69 % under rTSH versus 80 % under withdrawal and a sensitivity of tumor marker levels of 86 % and 79 %, respectively (Petrich et al. 2001). Overall increase of tumor marker levels after rTSH stimulation, compared to TSH suppression is reported to be over 30 % (Robbins et al. 2001). Indications for the use of rTSH are patients who do not tolerate thyroid hormone withdrawal due to a poor physical condition or who do not achieve sufficient TSH levels under withdrawal (Luster et al. 2000).

The first course of RIT consists of 30–100 mCi (1.1–3.7 GBq), depending on the amount of remnant tissue. Scans are made approximately three to six days after radioiodine administration, which is usually given orally. Further RITs are carried out at intervals of approximately three months. If there is no indication that any tumor tissue remains, therapy usually consists of single doses of 100 mCi (3.7 GBq), seldom reaching 200 mCi (7.4 GBq). Besides destroying any remaining malignant cells, RIT creates optimum conditions for effective follow-up by also eliminating all benign thyroid tissue (Biersack and Hotze 1991). This affects serum thyroglobulin levels, sonography of the thyroid region, and radioiodine scintigraphy.

The therapy goals are primarily a negative post-therapeutic radioiodine scan and undetectable serum thyroglobulin levels under TSH stimulation. The prognostic parameters mentioned above are the most important factor in determining to what extent one can deviate from these goals in patients in whom no remaining malignant tissue is suspected. In many cases Hürthle cell carcinomas take up radioiodine in small amounts or not at all, so that these tumors frequently evade effective therapy. But an attempt at therapy should be made in any case, especially when no other curative therapy options exist.

Suspected or detected metastatic spread or recurrence is treated with single doses of up to 300 mCi (11.1.GBq) (Grünwald et al. 1988). Pulmonary metastases respond better than bone and other metastases, especially if the spread is disseminated (Menzel et al. 1996; Reiners 1993; Georgi et al. 1992) generally decreases during the course of the disease.

In general, C-cell carcinomas do not take up radioiodine, but in the follicular type the use of radioiodine should be tried. The thyroglobulin immunohistochemistry of the primary tumor and of metastases, where applicable, can provide clinically useful information. Therapeutic options for C-cell carcinomas are the use of ^{131}I-metaiodobenzylguanidine (MIBG) or the somatostatin analog ^{90}Y-tetra-azacyclododecan-tricarboxymethyl-acetyl (DOTATOC) (Clarke 1991; Waldherr et al. 2001). Anaplastic carcinomas seldom take up radioiodine, and RIT rarely results in an appreciable effect on tumor growth even when tumors are radioiodine-positive.

Surgical intervention is a curative option for single metastases and can be used in multiple metastases for the purpose of reducing tumor size (to optimize the radioiodine effect before RIT). Percutaneous radiation is used less often in therapy for thyroid carcinoma than it was in the past. It is indicated for inoperable tumors, local tumor compression, and skeletal metastases, particularly in cases with risk of a fracture. There is still disagreement concerning the prophylactic radiation therapy of the lymph vessels with respect to the prognosis for all pT_4 tumors.

Chemotherapeutic agents can be used in certain circumstances for undifferentiated carcinomas and the progression of multiple metastases of differentiated carcinomas. Studies with 13-cis retinoic acid – a substance that has already been used widely in the field of hematooncology – show that its use can induce radioiodine uptake in negative tumor localizations in some patients (Grünwald et al. 1998; Simon et al. 1996; van Herle et al. 1990; Boerner et al. 1997, 2002). This is particularly interesting with respect to FDG PET, since PET can be used here to test whether radioiodine uptake was induced in all tumor sites.

14.3 Use of FDG PET

There are no preoperative indications (evaluation of unclear lesions) for FDG PET in thyroid tumors, in contrast to other tumor entities. Increased FDG uptake in malignant thyroid tumors has often been observed incidentally, and some authors also describe a differentiation between malignant and benign tumors based on semiquantitative data. But the specificity of FDG PET is too low to insist on its use for malignant thyroid tumors, since even benign adenomas frequently show an increased tracer uptake and some carcinomas (particularly those with papillary growth patterns) take up no FDG at all (Feine et al. 1996; Joensuu and Ahonen 1987; Sisson et al. 1993; Adler and Bloom 1993).

The sensitivity and specificity of FDG PET increase if the scan is performed postoperatively when no large amounts of thyroid remnant tissue remain. Therefore, the scan should generally not be done earlier than approximately two months after the first RIT. At that time the rate of false positive findings due to unspecific postoperative changes is also significantly lower.

Studies on the value of FDG PET for differentiated thyroid carcinoma have often focused in part on the situation involving a negative radioiodine scan with the suspicion of metastatic spread (based on an increase in the serum thyroglobulin value or unclear morphological findings) (Feine et al. 1996; Baqai et al. 1994; Messa et al. 1996; Easton et al. 1995; Grünwald et al. 1996, 1997; Tatsch et al. 1996; Conti et al. 1996; Platz et al. 1995). Morphological imaging methods (sonography, CT, MRI) can be used to detect radioiodine-negative tissue. But they have the disadvantage that only limited areas can be studied and that their specificity is extremely limited in patients with altered anatomical conditions (for example, after neck dissection) (Schober et al. 1986). The value of CT is also reduced by the fact that with respect to further RIT, no iodine-containing contrast medium may be used. The specificity of CT in particular is comparatively low in these cases. This necessitates the use of tumor-seeking tracers. Thallium-201 (Tl), technetium-99m-methoxyisobutylisonitrile (^{99m}Tc-MIBI), and technetium-99m 1,2-bis [bis(2-ethoxyethyl)phosphino]ethane(tetrofosmin) have emerged as suitable, single pho-

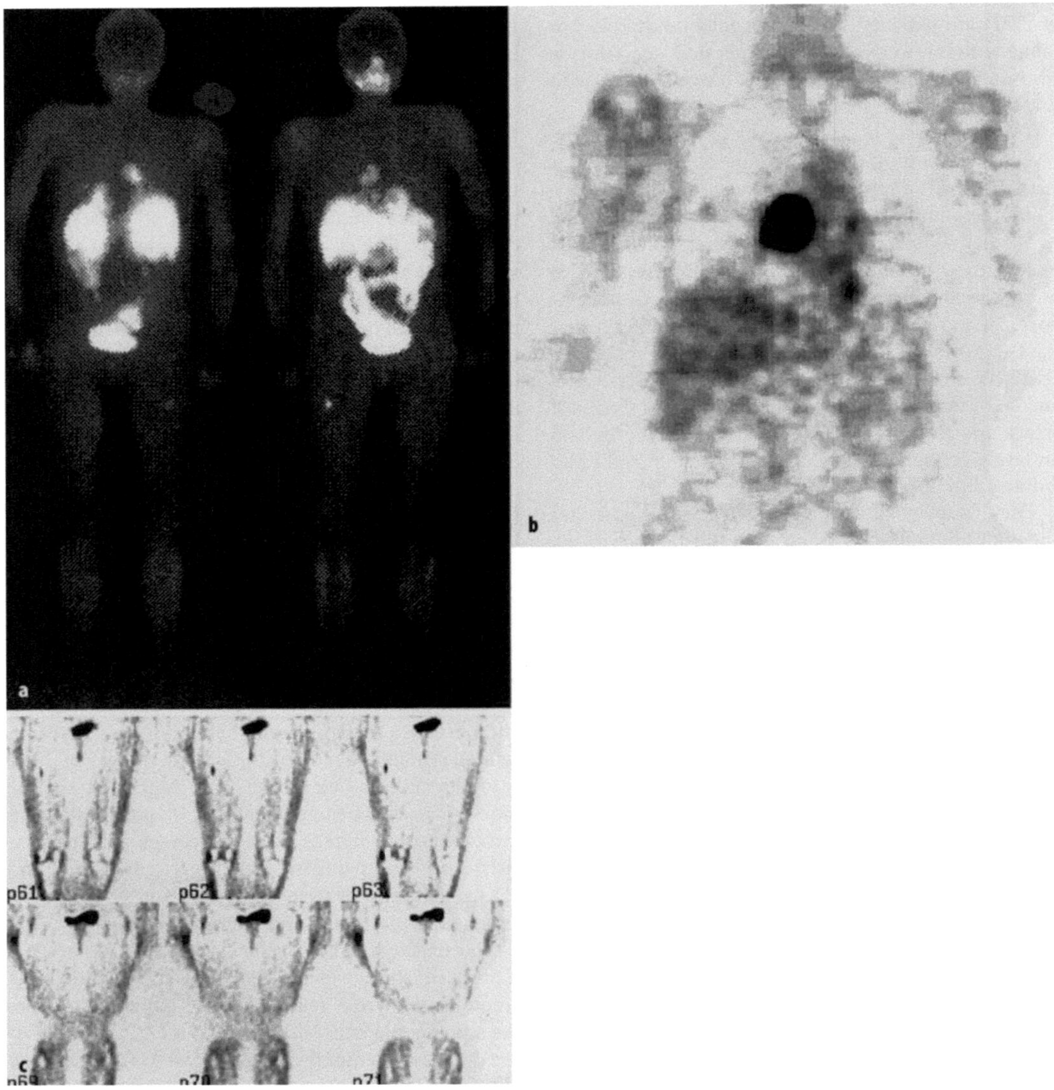

Fig. 1a–c. Huethle cell follicular thyroid carcinoma (pT4NxM1) with pulmonary and bone metastases; serum thyroglobulin: >10,000 μg/l. MIBI scintigraphy (**a**: dorsal projection on the *left*, ventral projection on the *right*) showed pathological accumulations in the mediastinum (right paramedian) and in the right femur. FDG PET shows a clearly positive finding in the mediastinum (right paramedian), a small nodule left paramedian, a suspicious finding right pulmonary (**b**), which was confirmed as positive during subsequent follow-up, and a metastasis in the right femur (**c**). In the radioiodine scan, the localizations were partly positive and partly negative

ton-emitting tracers (Dadparvar et al. 1995; Briele et al. 1991; Gallowitsch et al. 1996; Nemec et al. 1996). MIBI exhibits a sensitivity of approximately 80–90% and is especially well suited for imaging tumor tissue in Hürthle cell carcinoma. Whereas most authors describe a high sensitivity in local recurrence, Nemec et al. (1996) report that MIBI is especially sensitive in distant metastases, particularly in bone metastases.

Many studies dealing with groups of approximately 50 patients each have shown that FDG PET has a sensitivity of over 90% in cases with a negative radioiodine scintiscan (Feine et al. 1996; Grünwald et al. 1997; Dietlein et al. 1997). It has been found that tumor localizations very often take up either only radioiodine or only FDG (Figs. 1–5). This holds true for both the interindividual comparison of patients with a single tumor site and for cases with several localizations, some of which are radioiodine-positive and some FDG-positive. The reason for this alternating uptake behavior is presumably a varying degree of differentiation in the tumor clone. Like other tumor entities (especially neuroendocrine tumors), poorly differentiated tumors take up FDG to a great extent, while well differentiated tumors prefer the organ-specific tracer radioiodine, which indicates that the Na/I symporter is still present. A significant correlation has been demonstrated between primary tumor grading and differences in sensitivity for radioiodine and FDG PET (Grünwald et al. 1996).

A number of studies show that FDG-PET is a sensitive method for detection of metastases or recurrence of

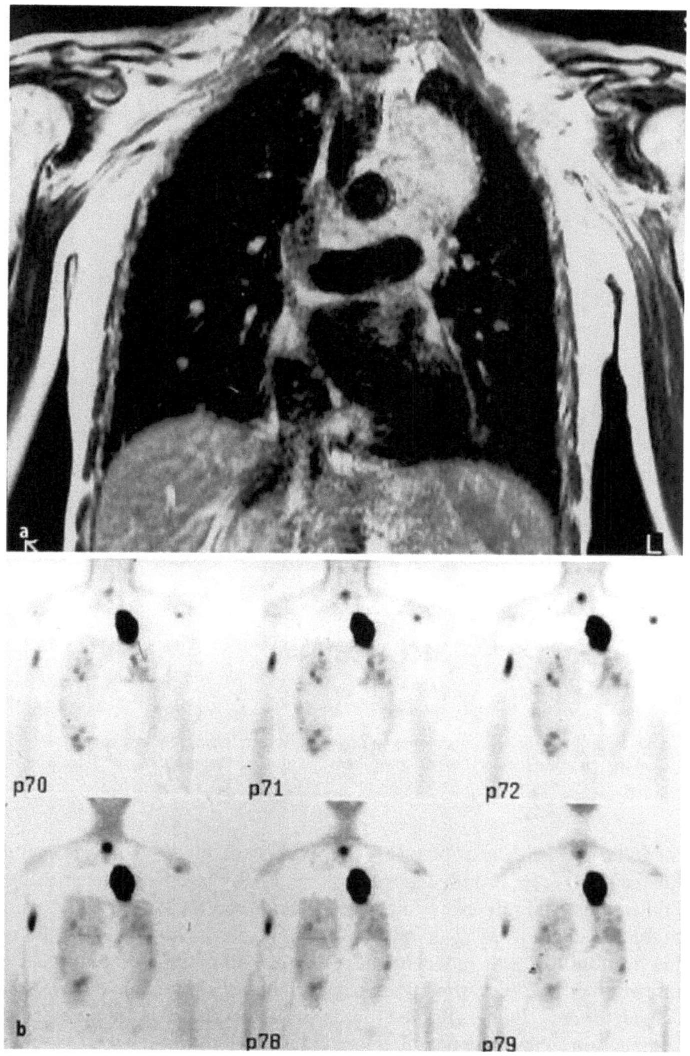

Fig. 2a,b. Papillary thyroid carcinoma (pTxN1M1) with metastases in the lymph nodes, lung, bone, liver, spleen, and kidneys. Serum thyroglobulin: 134 μg/l. **a** MRI shows a large mediastinal metastasis as well as multiple pulmonary metastases. **b** with FDG PET, metastases can be detected in the jugulum, mediastinum, lung, right humerus, left shoulder joint, liver, spleen and kidneys. Only a small percentage of the tumor localizations showed any radioiodine uptake

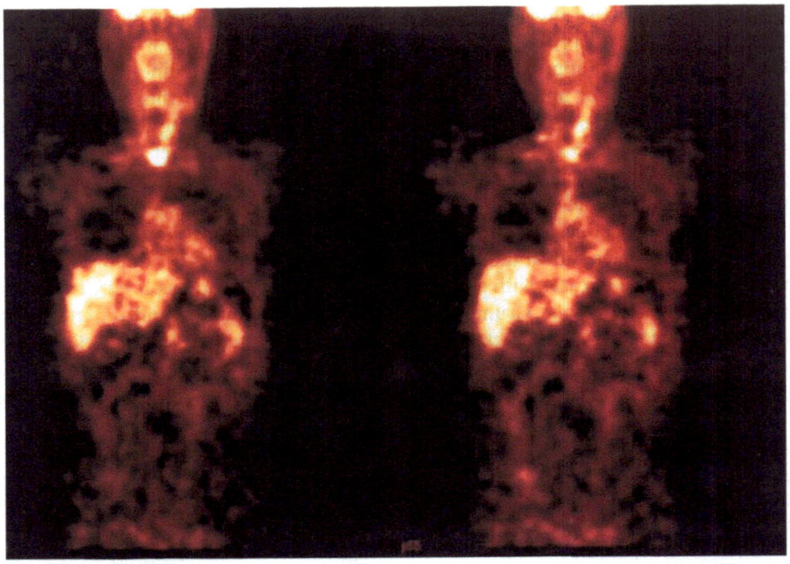

Fig. 3. Follicular thyroid carcinoma (pT4N1Mx). Serum thyroglobulin: 850 μg/l. Local recurrence (median) and cervical lymph node metastases on both sides were detectable using FDG PET

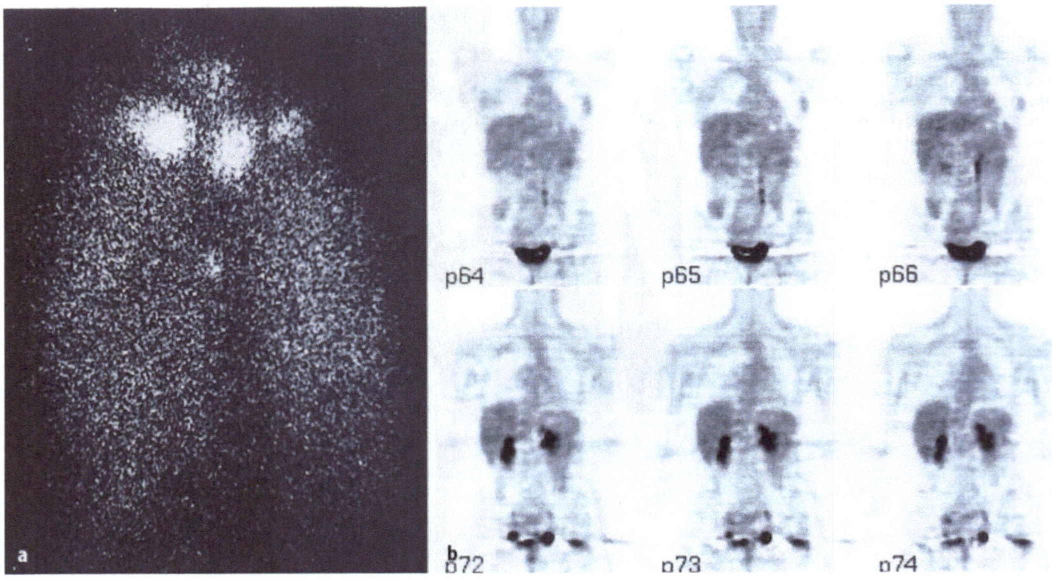

Fig. 4a,b. Papillary thyroid carcinoma (pT4N1M1). Serum thyroglobulin: 334 μg/l. Radioiodine-positive disseminated pulmonary and regional lymph node metastases (**a**). No increase in glucose metabolism was detectable with FDG PET (**b**)

medullary thyroid carcinoma (MTC) (Simon et al. 1996; Köster et al. 1999; Brandt-Mainz et al. 2000). A recent multicenter study describes a sensitivity and specificity for FDG PET in MTC of 78% and 79% respectively. In addition, PET was independent of the extend of tumor marker hCT elevation, presenting a high sensitivity even for only slightly elevated tumor marker levels. In comparison to imaging techniques using single photon emitters as well as CT and MRI PET appeared as the superior method (Diehl et al. 2001).

At this point we will present a detailed comparison of FDG PET and scintigraphy using tumor-seeking radiopharmaceuticals (specifically MIBI) with respect to an optimal diagnostic process. The following aspects should be considered.

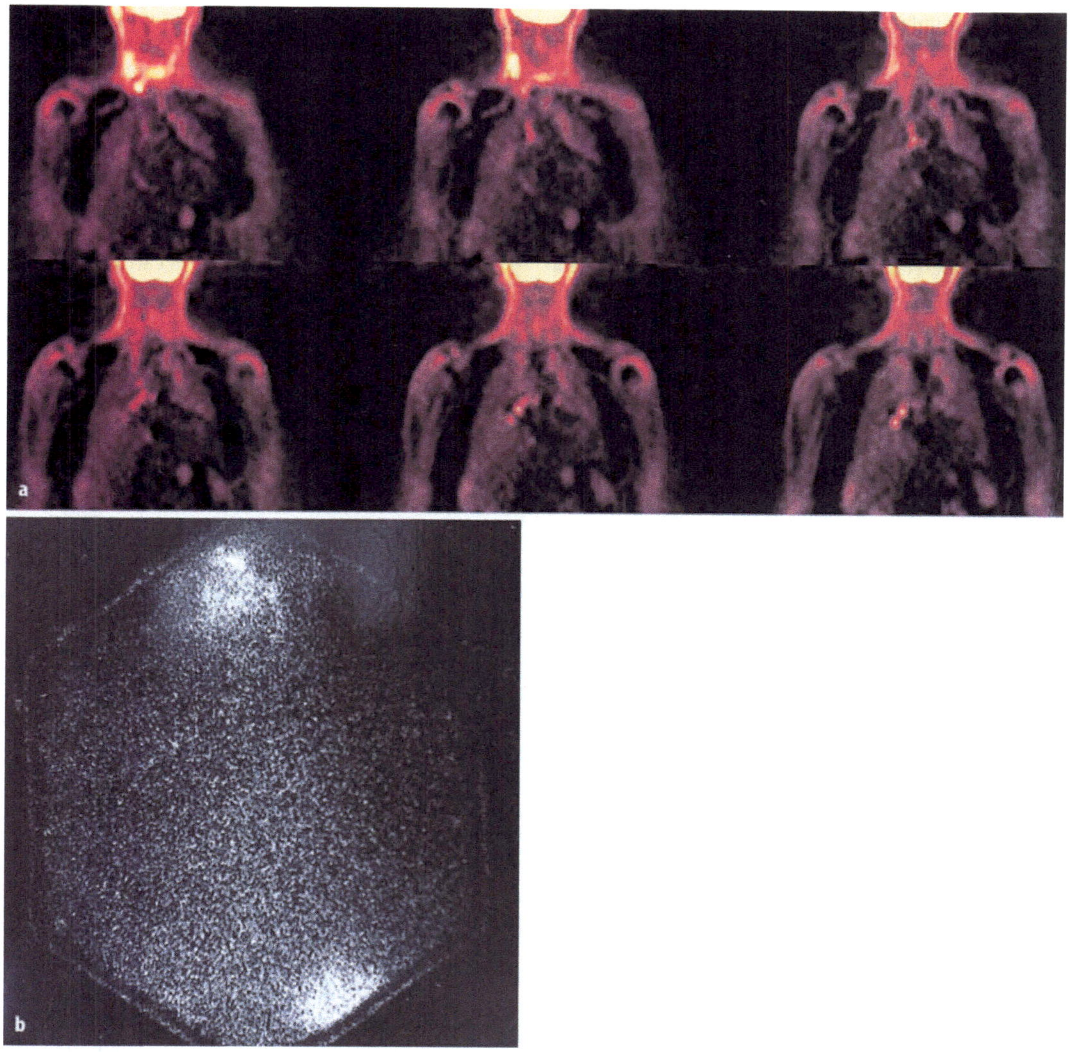

Fig. 5a,b. Papillary thyroid carcinoma (pT4N1M1). Serum thyroglobulin: . 10,000 μg/l. Using FDG PET (**a**) pulmonary and bilateral cervical lymph node metastases were detected; radioiodine scintigraphy showed no pathological findings (**b**)

14.3.1 Spatial Resolution

Spatial resolution is approximately 5 mm for PET under clinical conditions, while SPECT with a dual head camera achieves a maximum resolution of approximately 10 mm. Thus PET should be preferred for any problem requiring tomographic examination. In regions where planar imaging usually suffices (for example, superficially located cervical lymph node metastases), the difference between PET and SPECT due to varying tomographic resolution is not so significant. In contrast, there are definite advantages in using PET for mediastinal and pulmonary processes.

14.3.2 Tumor Tracer Uptake Mechanisms

FDG uptake correlates frequently with proliferative activity and is determined by glucose metabolism in both the tumor cells and the macrophages associated with tumors, among others (Kubota et al. 1994, 1995). Quickly growing tumors therefore usually exhibit a higher sensitivity with FDG PET. Yoshioka et al. (1994) demonstrated that FDG uptake in various gastrointestinal tumors increases with the loss of differentiation. Most differentiated thyroid carcinomas, especially G1 tumors, are relatively slow-growing and are therefore frequently FDG-negative, whereas they can be detected in a radioiodine scan because of their intact Na/I symporters (Dai et al. 1996). MIBI uptake is, above all, a function of mitochondrial potential. More than 90 % of the tracer is taken up in the inner mitochondrial matrix (Piwinica-Worms et al. 1990). Therefore mitochondrial content and metabolic requirements, which determine potential, have a significant influence on the sensitivity of MIBI scintigraphy. This would lead to the expectation that Hürthle cell carcinomas in particular (which are frequently radioiodine-negative) would show a pronounced MIBI uptake (Balone et al. 1992). However, MIBI scintigraphy has not been proven to be clinically superior to FDG PET in Hürthle cell carcinomas.

14.3.3 Tracer Uptake in Other Organs

Physiological accumulation of both FDG and MIBI is very low in the neck and upper mediastinum, so that clinical evaluation of local recurrences and regional lymph node metastases is not significantly affected by high levels of background activity (with the exception of the problems described below). In other organs where FDG PET and MIBI scintigraphy can be used for detecting distant metastases, physiological tracer uptake is extremely variable. MIBI uptake in the myocardium is high, with the result that pericardial pulmonary metastases can be detected with an inferior sensitivity. In this situation it is especially important that FDG is administered in a fasted state, so that predominantly free fatty acids will be metabolized in the myocardium and FDG uptake will be minimized. In contrast, FDG uptake is always very high in the brain, so that sensitivity (with respect to hot lesions) is very low for distant metastases, whereas MIBI accumulation in the brain is low (with the exception of the choroid plexus), making scintigraphy with tumor-seeking single-photon-emitters clearly superior for detecting cerebral metastases. The detection of distant metastases in the kidneys and lower urinary tract is made difficult by renal excretion of FDG, but this plays a smaller role with thyroid carcinomas than with other tumors since metastases of differentiated thyroid carcinomas seldom appear at this particular localization. MIBI uptake is extremely high in the liver. FDG uptake, on the other hand, is relatively low (especially with late acquisition of emission images), so that FDG PET is superior for this localization (Briele et al. 1991; Dietlein et al. 1997; Pirro et al. 1994).

Radioiodine uptake has a significant prognostic relevance, with the result that a prognostic statement can be made on the basis of the detection of radioiodine-negative and FDG-positive tumor localizations. Even though a current radioiodine scan is essential for therapy planning, information about FDG-positive and radioiodine-negative tumor cells is extremely important, since we must consider a selection pressure on the different clones that favors the poorly differentiated FDG-positive cells, while the well differentiated are exposed to a higher radiation effect.

Serum calcitonin and CEA levels are the most important parameters in the follow-up of carcinomas with C-cell differentiation (Becker et al. 1986). It has been shown that for these tumors FDG PET can detect tumor tissue with approximately the same sensitivity as MRI (Köster et al. 1996). FDG PET findings and the «tissue-specific» methods – somatostatin receptor scintigraphy and scintigraphy with pentavalent DMSA (Adams et al. 1998) – provide an indication of the current degree of differentiation in C-cell carcinomas just as they do in carcinomas with follicle cell differentiation. It has been demonstrated through correlation with Ki-67 antigens associated with cell cycles that tumors with a high proliferation tendency tend to be FDG-positive. In addition, MIBI scintigraphy offers an alternative scintigraphic method for these tumors as well.

Nothing has been published yet regarding experiences with FDG PET for anaplastic carcinoma. However, this method does not yet seem to have any appreciable significance for either prognosis or changes in procedure.

14.4 Indications

Indications for clinical use were evaluated at the consensus conference in September 2000 (Reske and Kotzerke 2001, Table 3). Of note is the highest classification – 1a – for differentiated thyroid carcinomas when radioiodine scintigraphy is negative and there is an indication of recurrence due to an increase in serum thyroglobulin

Table 3. Indications for FDG PET in differentiated thyroid carcinomas

Differentiated thyroid carcinoma	
Differential diagnosis (benign/malignant) of the primary tumor	4
Therapy control	3
Restaging in radioiodine-negative lesions	1a
Radioiodine-positive lesions	1b
Medullary thyroid carcinoma	3

1a: established clinical use
1b: clinical use probable
3: not yet assessable owing to missing or incomplete data
4: clinical use rare (as inferred from theoretical considerations or as demonstrated by published studies)

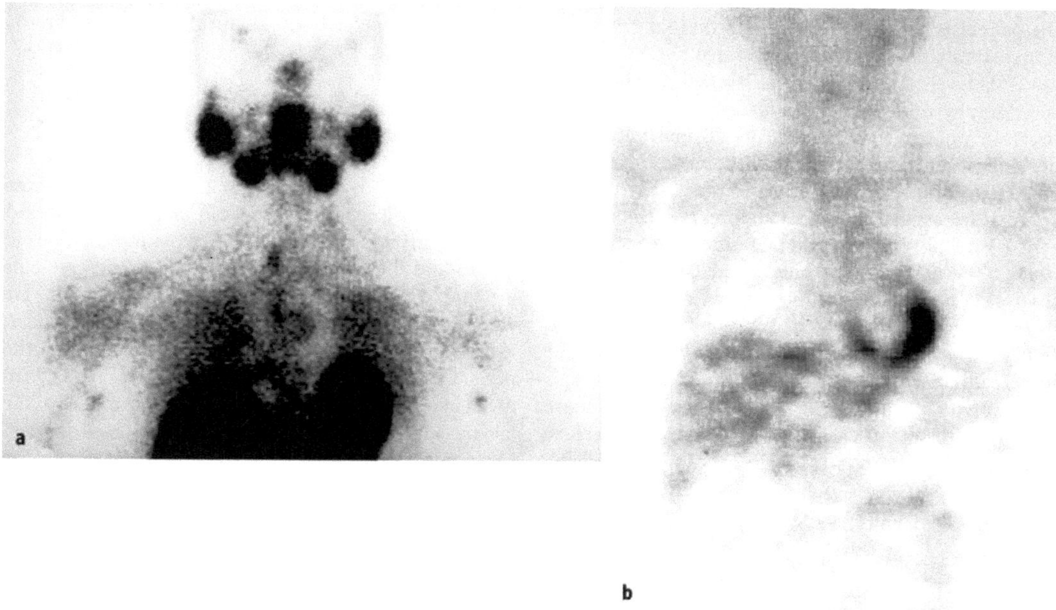

Fig. 6a,b. Suspected local recurrence after thyroidectomy and multiple radioiodine therapy for papillary thyroid carcinoma (pT2N1M0) and known tubercular lymph node changes right cervical; serum thyroglobulin: 2 μg/l. **a** A positive finding is visible right paratracheal in MIBI scintigraphy. **b** FDG PET shows negative findings (confirmed as correct in subsequent follow-up)

and/or unclear morphological findings (Figs. 5, 6). Cases with a positive radioiodine scintiscan are also an indication for FDG PET – in spite of the 1b rating (Figs. 1, 2) – since it is crucial to the further course of treatment to know whether there are poorly differentiated tumor cell clones, which are frequently only detectable with FDG, in addition to well differentiated cells. The indications for C-cell carcinoma are both preoperative and postoperative in connection with staging or when recurrence or metastases are suspected during follow-up (Fig. 7). In particular, changes in the calcitonin level (basal and after pentagastrin stimulation) and serum CEA level are decisive. FDG PET is especially sensitive in cases with a rapidly rising CEA level, which indicates a high proliferation tendency (Adams et al. 1998).

14.5 Results and Interpretation

The results of clinical studies are described in detail above. The information shown in Table 4 is important for interpreting FDG PET findings in carcinoma with follicle cell differentiation and should therefore be available. Evaluation of PET findings in the thyroid region and lymph node compartments requires a great deal of experience, particularly in view of the limitations mentioned below. For this reason, PET results should in principle only be evaluated by a practiced well trained physician. While TSH stimulation is essential for radioiodine scintigraphy, FDG PET (and also MIBI scintigraphy or thallium scintigraphy) can be performed while

Table 4. Test results that should be available for diagnosis and the evaluation of an FDG PET scan in cases of differentiated thyroid carcinoma

Obligate	Facultative
Serum thyroglobulin level (with recovery and recovery testing)	Neck / chest CT (without contrast medium!)
Sonography of the thyroid bed and associated lymph node compartments	MRI of the neck
Radioiodine scan (with therapeutic doses, if possible)	MIBI-/tetrofosmin-/thallium scintigraphy, including SPECT of the neck and chest
Chest X-ray	Bone scintigraphy
	Morphological imaging of other organ systems if metastases e.g. are suspected

the patient is being medicated with thyroid hormones. It appears that PET has a higher sensitivity even with low TSH levels, in direct comparison with radioiodine scintigraphy under TSH stimulation (Grünwald et al. 1997). In 3 out of 10 patients, FDG PET performed under TSH stimulation detected additional lesions or classified FDG uptake pattern as typical for malignancy in contrast to results under TSH suppression (Moog et al. 2000). Van Tol et al. reported in 2002 one out of five patients to be FDG positive only under TSH stimulation. If we assume that metabolism is TSH-dependent even in malignant follicle cells and that the functional activity of glucose transport is increased in hypothyroidism (Matthaei et al. 1995), then we would expect a higher sensitivity during TSH stimulation. But what is more decisive with hypothyroidism is the absolute decrease in glucose transporters (Matthaei et al. 1995) and the generally reduced metabolic requirement of all tissues, which also affects tumor cell and consequently their detectability by FDG. Tatsch et al. (1996) observed a somewhat higher detectability of papillary tumors in comparison with follicular tumors in a small collective of radioiodine-negative and MIBI-negative cases. But in larger patient groups this trend could not be confirmed, so that there is no significant difference between papillary and follicular tumors with respect to sensitivity and specificity.

14.6 Limits of Interpretation

As explained above, the evaluation of regions with high physiological tracer uptake (brain, salivary glands, kidneys, bladder) is limited. When evaluating the thyroid region and the associated lymph node compartments, we should also consider unspecific uptake in the larynx, the neck muscles and occasionally the thymus. It is therefore important during the examination that the patient does not talk after the tracer injection has been given in order to avoid activating the musculature of the larynx (Fig. 8) and that the patient is as relaxed as possible to minimize glucose utilization by the neck muscles. Beyond this, the general guidelines for whole-body FDG PET should of course be followed.

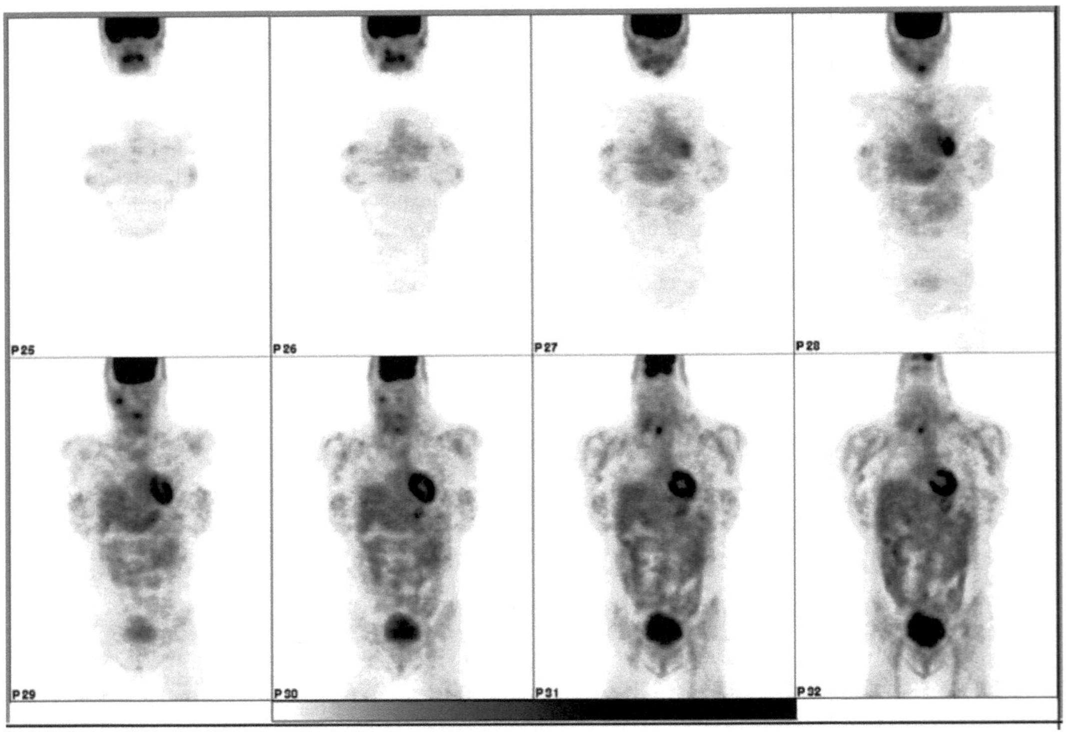

Fig. 7. 37-year-old patient with MTC (pT2) with an elevated hCT level. PET images show cervical lymph nodes metastases on the right side

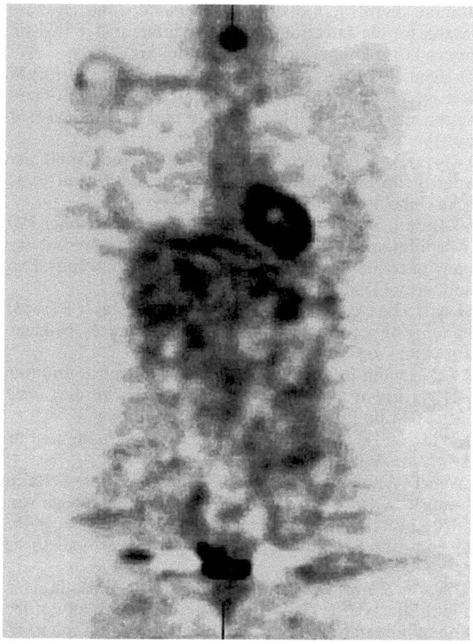

Fig. 8. Pitfall in the thyroid region: intensive accumulation in the larynx due to speaking after tracer injection

References

Adams S, Baum R, Rink T, Schumm-Dräger PM, Usadel KH, Hör G (1998) Limited value of fluorine-18 fluorodeoxyglucose positron emission tomography for the imaging of neuroendocrine tumours. Eur J Nucl Med 25:79–83

Adler LP, Bloom AD (1993) Positron emission tomography of thyroid masses. Thyroid 3:195–200

Akslen LA (1993) Prognostic importance of histological grading in papillary carcinoma. Cancer 72:2680–2685

Balone HR, Fing-Bennett D, Stoffer SS (1992) 99mTc-sestamibi uptake by recurrent Hürthle cell carcinoma of the thyroid. J Nucl Med 33:1393–1395

Baqai FH, Conti PS, Singer PA, Spencer CA, Wang CC, Nicoloff JT (1994) 18 F-FDG-PET scanning – a diagnostic tool for detection of recurrent and metastatic differentiated thyroid cancers. Abstract, 68th annual meeting of the American Thyroid Association, Chicago, p 9

Becker W, Spiegel W, Reiners C, Börner W (1986) Besonderheiten bei der Nachsorge des C-Zell-Karzinoms. Nuklearmediziner 9:167–181

Biersack HJ, Hotze A (1991) The clinician and the thyroid. Eur J Nucl Med 18:761–778

Boerner AR, Simon D, Mueller-Gaertner HW (1997) Isotretinoin therapy in oxyphilic follicular thyroid cancer. Ann Intern Med 127:146

Boerner AR, Petrich T, Weckesser E, Fricke H, Hofmann M, Otto D, Weckesser M, Langen KJ, Knapp WH (2002) Monitoring isotretinoin therapy in thyroid cancer using 18F-FDG PET. Eur J Nuck Med Mol Imaging 29:231–236

Brandt-Mainz K, Muller SP, Gorges R, Saller B, Bockisch A (2000) The value of fluorine-18 fluorodeoxyglucose PET in patients with medullary thyroid cancer. Eur J Nucl Med 27:490–496

Briele B, Hotze AL, Kropp J et al (1991) A comparison of 201 Tl and 99mTc-MIBI in the follow-up of differentiated thyroid carcinoma. Nucl Med 30:115–124

Clark SE (1991) 131J-metaiodobenzylguanidine therapy in medullary thyroid cancer: Guy´s Hospital experience. J Nucl Biol Med 35:323–326

Conti PS, Durski JM, Grafton ST, Singer PA (1996) PET imaging of locally recurrent and metastatic thyroid cancer. J Nucl Med 37:135P

Dadparvar S, Chevres A, Tulchinsky M, Krishna-Badrinath L, Khan AS, Slizofski WJ (1995) Clinical utility of technetium-99m methoxyisobutylisonitrile imaging in differentiated thyroid carcinoma: comparison with thallium-201 and iodine-131 Na scintigraphy, and serum thyroglobulin quantitation. Eur J Nucl Med 22:1330–1338

Dai G, Levy O, Carrasco N (1996) Cloning and characterization of the thyroid iodide transporter. Nature 379:458–460

Diehl M, Risse JH, Brandt-Mainz K, Dietlein M, Bohuslavizki KH, Matheja P, Lange H, Bredow J, Körber C, Grünwald F (2001) Fluorine-18 fluorodeoxyglucose positron emission tomography in medullary thyroid cancer: results of a multicentre study. Eur J Nucl Med 28:1671–1676

Dietlein M, Scheidhauer K, Voth E, Theissen P, Schicha H (1997) Fluorine-18 fluorodeoxyglucose positron emission tomography and iodine-131 whole-body scintigraphy in the follow-up of differentiated thyroid cancer. Eur J Nucl Med 24:1342–1348

Easton E, Coates D, McKusick A, Borchert R, Zuger J (1995) Concurrent FDG F-18 thyroid PET imaging in J-131 therapy patients. J Nucl Med 36:197

Feine U, Lietzenmayer R, Hanke JP, Held J, Wöhrle H, Müller-Schauenburg W (1996) Fluorine-18-FDG and iodine-131-iodide uptake in thyroid cancer. J Nucl Med 37:1468–1472

Gallowitsch HJ, Kresnik E, Mikosch P, Pipam W, Gomez I, Lind P (1996) Tc-99m tetrofosmin scintigraphy: an alternative scintigraphy method for following up differentiated thyroid carcinoma – preliminary results. Nucl Med 35:230–235

Georgi P, Emrich D, Heidenreich P, Moser E, Reiners C, Schicha H (1992) Radiojodtherapie des differenzierten Schilddrüsenkarzinoms. Empfehlungen der Arbeitsgemeinschaft Therapie der Deutschen Gesellschaft für Nuklearmedizin. Nuklearmedizin 31:151–153

Grünwald F, Ruhlmann J, Ammari B, Knopp R, Hotze A, Biersack HJ (1988) Experience with a high-dose concept of differentiated metastatic thyroid cancer therapy. Nucl Med 27:266–271

Grünwald F, Schomburg A, Bender H et al (1996) Fluorine-18 fluorodeoxyglucose positron emission tomography in the follow-up of differentiated thyroid cancer. Eur J Nucl Med 23:312–319

Grünwald F, Menzel C, Bender H et al (1997) Comparison of 18-FDG-PET with 131-Iodine and 99mTc-sestamibi scintigraphy in differentiated thyroid cancer. Thyroid 7:327–335

Grünwald F, Menzel C, Bender H et al (1998) Redifferentiation induced radioiodine uptake in thyroid cancer. J Nucl Med 39: 1903–1906

Haugen BR, Pacini F, Reiners C, Schlumberger M, Ladenson PW, Sherman SI, Cooper DS, Graham KE, Braverman LE, Skarulis MC, Davies TF, de Groot LJ, Mazzaferri EL, Daniels GH, Ross DS, Luster M, Samuels MH, Becker DV, Maxon HR 3rd, Cavalieri RR, Spencer CA, McEllin K, Weintraub BD, Ridgway EC (1999) A comparison of recombinant human thyrotropin and thyroid hormone withdrawal for the detection of thyroid remnant or cancer. J Clin Endocrinol Metab 84:3877–3885

Joensuu H, Ahonen A (1987) Imaging of metastases of thyroid carcinoma with fluorine-18 fluorodeoxyglucose. J Nucl Med 28: 910–914

Köster C, Ehrenheim C, Burchert W, Oetting G, Hundeshagen H (1996) F-18-FDG-PET, MRT und CT in der Nachsorge des medullären Schilddrüsenkarzinoms. Nuklearmedizin 35:A60

Kubota R, Kubota K, Yamada S, Tada M, Ido T, Tamahashi N (1994) Microautoradiographic study for the differentiation of intratumoral macrophages, granulation tissues and cancer cells by the dynamics of fluorine-18-fluorodeoxyglucose uptake. J Nucl Med 35:104–112

Kubota R, Kubota K, Yamada S, Tada M, Takahashi T, Iwata R, Tamahashi N (1995) Methionine uptake by tumor tissue: a microautoradiographic comparison with FDG. J Nucl Med 36: 484–492

Luster M, Lassmann M, Haenscheid H, Michalowski U, Incerti C, Reiners C (2000) Use of recombinant human thyrotropin before radioiodine therapy in patients with advanced differentiated thyroid carcinoma. J Clin Endocrinol Metab 85:3640–3645

Matthaei S, Trost B, Hamann A et al (1995) Effect of in vivo thyroid hormone status on insuline signalling and GLUT1 and GLUT4 glucose transport systems in rat adipocytes. J Endocrinol 144:347–357

Menzel C, Grünwald F, Schomburg A, Palmedo H, Bender H, Späth G, Biersack HJ (1996) "High-dose" radioiodine therapy in advanced differentiated thyroid carcinoma. J Nucl Med 37:1496–1503

Messa C, Landoni C, Fridrich L, Lucignani G, Striano G, Riccabona G, Fazio F (1996) F-18-FDG uptake in metastatic thyroid carcinoma prior and after J-131 therapy. Eur J Nucl Med 23:1097

Moog F, Linke R, Manthey N, Tiling R, Knesewitsch P, Tatsch K, Hahn K (2000) Influence of thyroid-stimulating hormone levels on uptake of FDG in recurrent and metastatic differentiated thyroid carcinoma. J Nucl Med 41:1996–1998

Nemec J, Nyvltova O, Blazek Tb et al (1996) Positive thyroid cancer scintigraphy using technetium-99m methoxyisobutylisonitrile. Eur J Nucl Med 23:69–71

Petrich T, Börner AR, Weckesser E, Soudah B, Otto D, Widjaja A, Hofmann M, Kreipe HH, Knapp WH (2001) Nachsorge des differenzierten Schilddrüsenkarzinoms unter Verwendung von rhTSH – vorläufige Ergebnisse. Nuklearmedizin 40:7–14

Pirro JP, di Rocco RJ, Narra RK, Nunn AD (1994) Relationship between in vitro transendothelial permeability and in vivo single-pass brain extraction. J Nucl Med 35:1514–1519

Piwinica-Worms D, Kronauge JF, Chiu ML (1990) Uptake and retention of hexakis (2-methoxyisobutyl-isonitrile) technetium (I) in cultured chick myocardial cells, mitochondrial and plasma membrane potential dependence. Circulation 82:1826–1838

Platz D, Lübeck M, Beyer W, Grimm C, Beuthin-Baumann B, Gratz KF, Hotze LA (1995) Einsatz der 18-F-deoxyglucose-PET (FDG-PET) in der Nachsorge von Patienten mit differenziertem und medullärem Schilddrüsenkarcinom. Nucl Med 34:152

Raue F (1997) Chemotherapie bei Schilddrüsenkarzinomen: Indikation und Ergebnisse. Onkologe 3:55–58

Raue F, Frank-Raue K (1997) Gehört die Calcitoninbestimmung zur Abklärung der Struma nodosa? Dtsch Ärztebl 94:855–856

Reiners C (1993) Radiojodtherapie – Indikation, Durchführung und Risiken. Dtsch Ärztebl 90:2217–2221

Reske SN, Kotzerke J (2001) FDG-PET for clinical use. Results of the 3rd German Interdisciplinary Consensus Conference, „Onko-PET III“, 21 July and 19 Sept 2000. Eur J Nucl Med 28: 1707–1723

Robbins RJ, Tuttle RM, Sharaf RN, Larson SM, Robbins HK, Ghossein RA, Smith A, Drucker WD (2001) Preparation by recombinant human thyrotropin or thyroid hormone withdrawal are comparable for the detection of residual differentiated thyroid carcinoma. J Clin Endocrinol Metab 86:619–625

Schober O, Heintz P, Schwarzrock R, Dralle H, Gratz KF, Döhring W, Hundeshagen H (1986) Schilddrüsen-Carcinom: Rezidiv- und Metastasensuche; Sonographie, Röntgen und CT. Nuklearmediziner 9:139–148

Simon D (1997) Von limitierter bis erweiterter Radikalität der Operation beim Schilddrüsenkarzinom. In: Roth et al (eds) Klinische Onkologie. Huber, Bern, pp 347–357

Simon D, Köhrle J, Schmutzler C, Mainz K, Reiners C, Röher HD (1996) Redifferentiation therapy of differentiated thyroid carcinoma with retinoic acid: basics and first clinical results. Exp Clin Endocrinol Diabetes 104 [Suppl 4]:13–15

Simon GH, Nitzsche EU, Laubenberger JJ, Einert A, Moser E (1996) PET imaging of recurrent medullary thyroid cancer. Nuklearmedizin 35:102–104

Sisson JC, Ackermann RJ, Meyer MA (1993) Uptake of 18-fluoro-2-deoxy-D-glucose by thyroid cancer: implications for diagnosis and therapy. J Clin Endocrinol Metab 77:1090–1094

Sobin LH, Wittekind C (2002) TNM classification of malignant tumours, 6th edn. Wiley, New York, p 52

Tatsch K, Weber W, Rossmüller B, Langhammer H, Ziegler S, Hahn K, Schwaiger M (1996) F-18 FDG-PET in der Nachsorge von Schilddrüsencarcinom-Patienten mit hTg-Anstieg aber fehlender Jod- und Sestamibi-Speicherung. Nuklearmedizin 35: A34

Van Herle AJ, Agatep M, Padua DN 3rd, van Herle HML, Juillard GJF (1990) Effects of 13 cis-retinoic acid on growth and differentiation of human follicular carcinoma cells (UCLA RO 82 W-1) in vitro. J Clin Endocrinol Metab 71:755–763

Van Tol KM, Jager PL, Piers DA, Pruim J, de Vries EG, Dullaart RP, Links TP (2002) Better yield of 18-fluorodeoxyglucose-positron emission tomography in patients with metastatic differentiated thyroid carcinoma during thyrotropin-stimulation. Thyroid 12:381–387

Waldherr C, Schumacher T, Pless M, Crazzolara A, Maecke HR, Nitz Mueller-Brand J (2001) Radiopeptide transmitted internal irradiation of non-iodophil thyroid cancer and conventionally untreatable medullary thyroid cancer using 90Y-DOTATOC. Nucl Med Commun 22:673–678

Yoshioka T, Takahashi H, Oikawa H et al (1994) Accumulation of 2-deoxy-2-18F-fluoro-D-glucose in human cancer heterotransplanted in nude mice: comparison between histology and glycolytic status. J Nucl Med 35:97–103

CHAPTER 15

Lung Cancer

J.F. Vansteenkiste · S.S. Stroobants

15.1 Incidence, Etiology and Epidemiology

Lung cancer is the most common cause of cancer-related death in the western world, with approximately 3 million new cases per year world-wide, of which more than 200,000 are in the European Union. In men, mortality from lung cancer is much higher than from the second in rank, prostate cancer. In women, breast cancer is the leading cause of cancer death in many countries, but lung cancer also accounts for 10 %.

Cigarette smoking is responsible for approximately 90 % of lung cancers. The association between smoking and lung cancer arose from epidemiological studies in the 1950s [1], but the direct link between tobacco smoke and lung cancer has been shown recently: metabolites of benzopyrene, a chemical component of tobacco smoke, damage three specific loci on the p53 suppressor gene, an abnormality present in 50 % of non-small cell lung cancers (NSCLCs) and 70 % of small cell lung cancers (SCLCs) [2]. In 2002, the World Health Organization (WHO) also declared passive smoking to be carcinogenic to humans.

Common environmental causes are exposure to asbestos fibers and radon. Until recent years, asbestos was a very commonly used insulation agent, e.g. in shipyards. Radon is a gaseous decay product from uranium 228 and radium 226, responsible for a high incidence of lung cancer in uranium miners, but also for a small but significantly raised risk to people exposed to increased levels of indoor radon [3].

Despite advances in treatment, mainly by multimodality approaches, the death rate remains high, because of the late stage of presentation in many cases.

Reducing the prevalence of smoking, especially in teenagers, and modern screening studies by low-dose spiral computed tomography (CT) [4] and perhaps positron emission tomography (PET), in order to detect lung cancer at an earlier stage, are the main hopes for future improvement.

Table 1. Histopathological classification of lung cancer (adapted and shortened from [6])

Benign epithelial tumors
Preinvasive lesions
Malignant epithelial lesions
Squamous cell carcinoma (and variants)
Small cell carcinoma (and variant)
Adenocarcinoma
acinar
papillary
bronchioloalveolar cell carcinoma
solid adenocarcinoma with mucin
adenocarcinoma with mixed subtypes
variants
Large cell carcinoma (and variants, including large cell neuroendocrine carcinoma)
Adenosquamous carcinoma
Carcinoma with pleomorphic sarcomatoid or sarcomatous elements
Carcinoid tumors
Carcinoma of salivary-gland type
Unclassified carcinoma
Soft tissue tumors

15.2 Histopathological Classification

The 1981 edition of the WHO classification of lung tumors [5] underwent a revision, based on more recent insights, by a joint WHO and IASLC (International Association for the Study of Lung Cancer) panel, and was published in 1999 [6] (Table 1).

Most important for daily clinical practice remains the distinction, based on light microscopic criteria, between NSCLC, comprising nearly 80 % of all patients, and SCLC, accounting for nearly 20 %. These two categories of malignant epithelial tumors thus represent most of the patients, and benign, other epithelial, or non-epithelial tumors are all far less frequent.

The NSCLC group comprises the tumors with squamous cell differentiation, with adenocarcinomatous differentiation and the poorly or non-differentiated large cell cancers. These three types are brought together under the clinical heading of NSCLC, because most of these tumors have a less aggressive behavior than SCLC, which often is a very rapidly growing and disseminating cancer.

Two specific pathological entities deserve mentioning in the light of their behavior on fluoro-2-deoxy-D-glucose (FDG) PET. Bronchioloalveolar cell carcinoma (BAC), previously a type of adenocarcinoma, now has a restrictive definition of a non-invasive tumor with growth along existent alveolar septa. If invasion is seen, the tumor is classified as adenocarcinoma. This implies that most BACs present as solitary masses smaller than 3 cm with a rather low number of tumor cells, with the possibility of false-negative FDG PET findings. The second category comprises the typical carcinoid tumors. These are very slowly growing neoplasms arising from pulmonary neuro-endocrine cells, with low metabolic activity, and therefore often not FDG avid on PET.

15.3 Conventional Diagnostic Procedures

Imaging techniques such as chest X-ray, CT, ultrasonography, and magnetic resonance imaging (MRI) are essential in the diagnosis, staging, and follow-up of patients with lung cancer. These imaging tests are based on differences in the structure of tissues. Their current technology allows exquisite anatomic detail, but differences in structure often do not allow a definitive histopathological assessment, so that invasive tests with tissue sampling are required.

15.3.1 Diagnosis of Lung Nodules

While tumors located in the central airways can usually be diagnosed by bronchoscopic biopsy, peripheral solitary pulmonary nodules (SPNs) represent a diagnostic challenge, especially if they are non-calcified [7]. Absence of growth over a 2-year period is highly suggestive of a benign lesion, but many patients do not have comparative chest X-rays [8]. Bronchoscopic samples from patients with a peripheral nodule of less than 3 cm yield a pathologic diagnosis in only 20% of the cases [9], a figure that can be improved by using fluoroscopic guidance. A transthoracic needle aspiration biopsy has a much better diagnostic yield, but can be complicated by a pneumothorax, requiring drainage in 5–10% of the procedures [10]. Moreover, the aspiration can be false negative, leading to unacceptable expectation in early-stage lung cancer [11, 12]. Often more invasive procedures such as thoracoscopy or thoracotomy are needed for a final diagnosis.

15.3.2 Staging

Accurate staging is essential to make estimates of prognosis, and to choose the best combination of treatment modalities such as surgery, radiation and chemotherapy, in an attempt to improve survival.

The latest revision of the tumor-node-metastasis (TNM) system for lung cancer is listed in abbreviated form in Table 2. The T-factor describes the primary tumor, going from T1 (less than 3 cm and entirely surrounded by lung tissue) to T4 (invading critical organs, e.g. the aorta; for more details, see [13]). The N-factor describes the locoregional lymph node (LN) spread, either no metastatic nodes (N0), only intrapulmonary or hilar ones (N1), ipsilateral mediastinal ones (N2), or contralateral mediastinal or supraclavicular ones (N3). The M-factor points at absence (M0) or presence (M1) of distant metastasis.

Patients are then grouped in stages with more or less homogeneous prognosis. For practical clinical considerations, patients with stage I and II are often referred to as "early stages", for whom the standard of care is local treatment, preferably resection, or radical radiotherapy in cases of poor cardiopulmonary function. Stage III patients have "locally advanced disease", either IIIA (N2: LN spread in the ipsilateral mediastinal nodes only) or IIIB (N3: LN spread in the contralateral mediastinal or supraclavicular nodes). The best prospects for remission, or sometimes cure, can be offered if they are treated by a combination of local and systemic treatment. In North America, this will often be concurrent chemoradiotherapy [14], while many European centers will offer these patients induction chemotherapy followed by attempted complete resection [15, 16]. Stage IV patients have "advanced or metastatic" disease and are no longer amenable to cure. Chemotherapy can result in a moderate improvement of the median survival, and subjective clinical benefit [17] or quality-of-life improvement [18].

15.3.2.1 *The Primary Tumor (T-factor)*

Extension of the primary tumor is usually assessed by thoracic CT, occasionally complemented by MRI, e.g. in situations where superior sulcus extension or relationship with the heart or large vessels is of importance [19]. With their exquisite anatomical detail, modern CT and MRI are the preferred tests to evaluate the T-factor.

15.3.2.2 *Locoregional Lymph Nodes (N-factor)*

Computed tomography is the most commonly used non-invasive staging method, but is far from satisfactory and less accurate than invasive surgical staging [20, 21]. In prospective data from the Radiological Diagnostic Oncology Group, the sensitivity and specificity of thoracic CT in detecting mediastinal LN involvement were only 52% and 69% [22]. In our group [23], CT had a sensitivity of 69% and a specificity of 71% when mediastinal lymph nodes ≥1.5 cm in the long axis were considered to be abnormal. Size is a relative criterion, since lymph

Table 2.
TNM descriptors and stage grouping of TNM subsets in lung cancer (adapted from [13])

Primary tumor (T)	
Tx	Primary tumor cannot be assessed
T0	No evidence of primary tumor
T1	Tumor <3 cm in greatest dimension, surrounded by lung or visceral pleura, without bronchoscopic evidence of invasion more proximal than the lobar bronchus (i.e., not in the main bronchus)
T2	Tumor with any of the following features of size or extent: >3 cm in greatest dimension Involves main bronchus, >2 cm distal to the carina Invades the visceral pleura Associated with atelectasis or obstructive pneumonitis that extends to the hilar region but does not involve the entire lung
T3	Tumor of any size that directly invades any of the following: chest wall (including superior sulcus tumors), diaphragm, mediastinal pleura, parietal pericardium; or tumor in the main bronchus <2 cm distal to the carina, but without involvement of the carina; or associated atelectasis or obstructive pneumonitis of the entire lung
T4	Tumor of any size that invades any of the following: mediastinum, heart, great vessels, trachea, esophagus, vertebral body, carina; or tumor with a malignant pleural or pericardial effusion, or with satellite tumor nodule(s) within the ipsilateral primary-tumor lobe of the lung

Regional lymph nodes (N)	
NX	Regional lymph nodes cannot be assessed
N0	No regional lymph node metastasis
N1	Metastasis to ipsilateral peribronchial and/or ipsilateral hilar lymph nodes, and intrapulmonary nodes involved by direct extension of the primary tumor
N2	Metastasis to ipsilateral mediastinal and/or subcarinal lymph node(s)
N3	Metastasis to contralateral mediastinal, contralateral hilar, ipsilateral or contralateral scalene, or supraclavicular lymph node(s)

Distant metastasis (M)	
MX	Presence of distant metastasis cannot be assessed
M0	No distant metastasis
M1	Distant metastasis present

Stage	TNM Subset	5-year survival (clinical stage)	5-year survival (pathological stage)
0	Carcinoma in situ	?	?
IA	T1N0M0	61 %	67 %
IB	T2N0M0	38 %	57 %
IIA	T1N1M0	34 %	55 %
IIB	T2N1M0	24 %	39 %
	T3N0M0	22 %	38 %
IIIA	T3N1M0	9 %	25 %
	T1–3N2M0	13 %	23 %
IIIB	T4N0–2M0	7 %	Not applicable
	T1–4N3M0	3 %	Not applicable
IV	Any T Any N M1	1 %	Not applicable

nodes can be enlarged as a result of infectious or inflammatory causes, and small-sized nodes can nonetheless harbor metastases. Given this very moderate level of accuracy of CT, invasive surgical staging was the only adequate conventional tool for LN staging. A detailed map to describe locoregional LN involvement at surgical staging has been developed (Fig. 1), but this tool can likewise be of value for those interpreting CT or PET scans [24]. At cervical mediastinoscopy, the highest mediastinal nodes (level 1), left and right upper paratracheal nodes (levels 2L and 2R), left and right lower paratracheal nodes (levels 4L and 4R) and subcarinal nodes (level 7) can be sampled. For left upper lobe tumors, left anterior mediastinotomy may be indicated, with sampling of the subaortic (level 5) and para-aortic nodes (level 6).

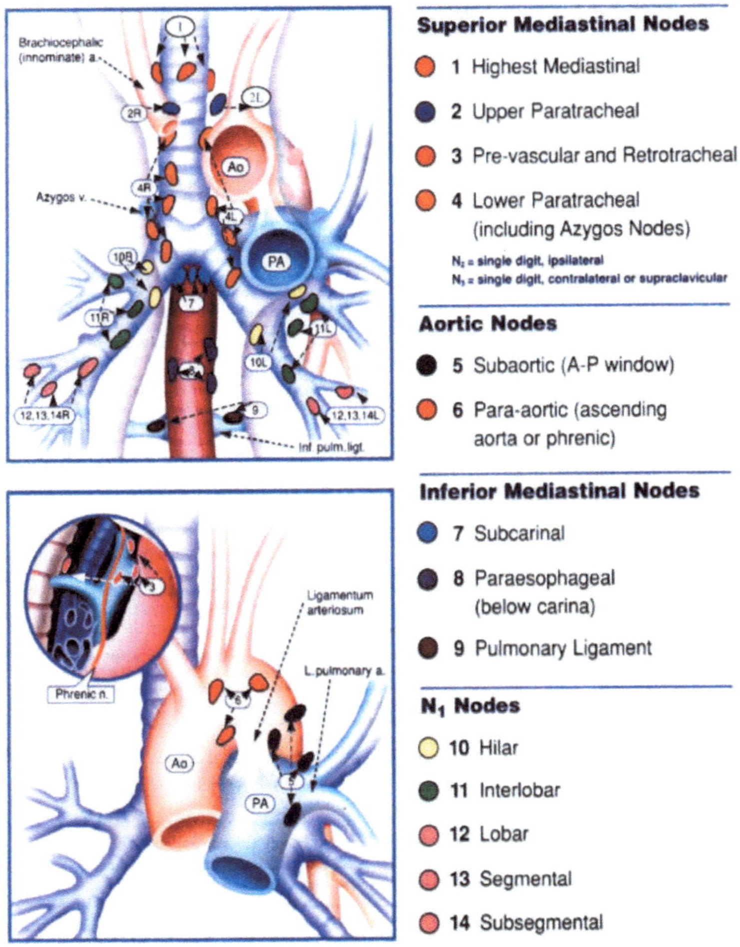

Fig. 1.
Regional lymph node map for lung cancer staging, according to the 1997 revision (by Mountain and Dresler [24], may be reproduced for educational purposes without permission; numbers and arrows have been added for clarity)

15.3.2.3
Extrathoracic Metastases (M-factor)

The finding of extrathoracic metastases implies that a patient can no longer be cured. The most common sites of metastasis are the adrenal glands, bones, brain, and liver [25]. Up to 35–45 % of the patients will have detectable distant disease at presentation [26]. Standard staging for extrathoracic disease is based on clinical and biological factors, and imaging tests, such as CT or ultrasound of the abdomen, CT or MRI of the brain, and bone scintigraphy. Whether these examinations need to be performed in every patient remains controversial. This issue is beyond this review, and we only want to refer to some recent guidelines [27–29].

Overall, we should realize that our current staging tools are far from perfect, and that we are not able to detect micrometastases already present at the time of diagnosis [30]. After radical treatment for apparently localized disease, an important proportion of patients, ranging from 20 [31] to 22 % [32, 33], will therefore experience an early distant relapse.

15.3.2.4
Small Cell Lung Cancer: Limited Versus Extensive Disease

Because of the aggressive spread of SCLC, only very few patients with this tumor need a detailed TNM staging in the light of potential resectability. Many teams therefore use the classification of limited versus extensive disease. This practical classification results from the fact that patients with limited disease are optimally treated with combined chemoradiotherapy [34]. Therefore, limited disease is defined as tumor spread that can be irradiated within a reasonable radiation port: according to the IASLC consensus definition, this comprises all tumor within one hemi-thorax, and ipsi- and contralateral hilar, mediastinal and supraclavicular LN spread [35]. All other patients with further disease spread have extensive disease, and are usually treated with chemotherapy alone.

15.3.3 Assessment of Response to Treatment

Response to radiotherapy is usually evaluated by comparing tumor diameters [36] or surfaces [37] on chest X-rays or CT images pre- and post-therapy. An important limitation of this method is the difficulty in distinguishing post-radiotherapy inflammatory or fibrotic changes from residual tumor, and the fact that changes in tumor viability (essential for the outcome) do not necessarily correlate with changes in dimension.

Correct assessment of response to chemotherapy is especially important in patients with "locally advanced" stage IIIA-N2 NSCLC treated with induction chemotherapy. Resection after induction will be a rewarding option, particularly in patients who achieve downstaging, either clearance of viable tumor cells in the diseased LNs [38–40], or, even better, pathological complete response [41]. Comparison of CT scans before and after treatment is the classical, but very moderately adequate, tool to evaluate downstaging after induction chemotherapy. Patients with little decrease in measurements on CT can nonetheless have mediastinal LN downstaging, while those with a significant decrease can still have viable tumor in their mediastinal nodes.

15.3.4 Follow-up, Detection of Recurrence

After treatment for local or locally advanced disease, lung cancer patients will usually be followed by routine clinical examination and chest X-ray every 3–6 months, with further imaging tests being performed on indication. The interpretation of a post-treatment chest X-ray, or even CT, can be hampered by treatment-related anatomic changes such as distortion of bronchi, infiltration of the lung parenchyma or mediastinum, or fibrotic changes, which may be difficult to distinguish from tumor relapse. The exact differential diagnosis can be of importance, especially in the light of the expanding possibilities for second-line treatment [42, 43].

15.4 PET

15.4.1 Differential Diagnosis of Lung Nodules

The earliest clinical PET studies have concentrated on the evaluation of indeterminate SPNs or pulmonary masses (Fig. 2). Prospective studies with at least 50 patients [44–50] are listed in Table 3. Sensitivity ranges from 89 to 100%, specificity from 52 to 100%, and accuracy from 89 to 96%. The different results can be explained by the prevalence of malignancy in the study population, which is the result of the varying epidemiology of SPNs in different areas of the world (e.g. more histoplasmosis in North America than in Europe). Another factor is the inclusion criteria of the different se-

Fig. 2. A 74-year-old male with an indeterminate nodule in the left upper lobe on CT (**a**). Whole-body PET (**b, c**) shows intense FDG uptake in the nodule. Pathology of the resection specimen: undifferentiated large cell carcinoma. Note false-positive FDG uptake in the pelvis caused by a dysplastic colon polyp (**c**, *arrow*)

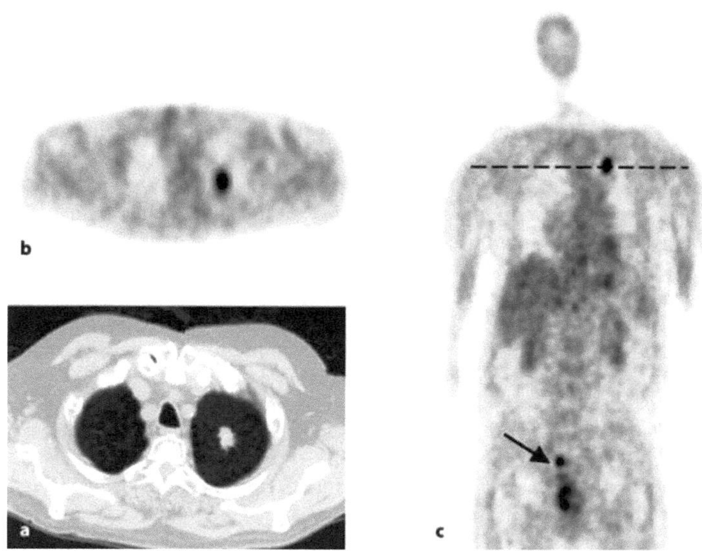

Table 3.
Prospective series on the use of PET in the differential diagnosis of lung nodules or masses reporting on at least 50 patients

First author	N	Method of analysis[a]	Sensitivity	Specificity	Accuracy	Prevalence[b]
Sazon [44]	107	Visual	100 %	52 %	89 %	77 %
Lowe [45]	89	Visual	98 %	69 %	89 %	67 %
		Semiquantitative	92 %	90 %	91 %	
Duhaylongsod [46]	87	Semiquantitative	97 %	82 %	92 %	68 %
Gupta [47]	61	Semiquantitative	93 %	88 %	92 %	74 %
Nackaerts [48]	52	Semiquantitative	94 %	82 %	90 %	67 %
Patz [49]	51	Semiquantitative	89 %	100 %	92 %	65 %
Bury [50]	50	Visual	100 %	88 %	96 %	66 %

[a] *Method of analysis* visual = visual interpretation on whole-body images; semiquantitative = using a threshold of a semiquantitative measure of FDG uptake (e.g. SUV)
[b] *Prevalence* proportion of malignant cases in the total group of studied nodules

ries (e.g. a lower sensitivity can be expected in series on very small nodules). The technique is accurate in differentiating benign from malignant lesions in SPNs as small as 1 cm. There is no significant difference in accuracy when a visual analysis of whole-body images and a semi-quantitative approach using a threshold standard uptake value (SUV) of 2.5 are compared [45, 51, 52]. Based on the available experience, a meta-analysis has been reported [53].

A critical mass of metabolically active malignant cells is required for PET diagnosis. False-negative findings can occur in lesions smaller than 1 cm [46, 48, 54–56], in tumors with low metabolic activity, e.g. carcinoid tumors [48, 57], or in BAC [54, 58, 59]. Sensitivity of PET is probably slightly less in the lower lung fields, due to respiratory motion.

Fluoro-2-deoxy-D-glucose uptake is not specific for malignancy, and false-positive findings can occur in inflammatory conditions, such as bacterial pneumonia [60], pyogenic abscess or aspergillosis, granulomatous diseases, such as active sarcoidosis [61], tuberculosis, histoplasmosis, coccidiomycosis, Wegener's disease and coal miner's lung. In these lesions, the FDG uptake has been attributed to an increase in granulocyte and/or macrophage activity [62].

For some lesions with equivocal findings on whole-body images or with a SUV between 2 and 3, the use of dynamic measurement of FDG uptake can be of additional benefit to discriminate inflammatory from malignant lesions [52]. Matthies et al. described distinct time-activity curve patterns with continuous uptake in malignant lesions and a rapid uptake followed by a fast and then gradual washout in benign masses [63]. Based on this difference in tracer kinetics, dual time-point imaging has also proved beneficiary. With a threshold value of 10 % increase in uptake between a PET scan performed after 1 hour (scan 1) and 2 hours after injection (scan 2), a sensitivity of 100 % and a specificity of 89 % was obtained, compared to only 80 % and 94 %, respectively, if the standard threshold SUV of 2.5 was used on scan 1.

In North-American series, it was shown that PET reduced the number of patients with an indeterminate SPN undergoing unnecessary resection of a benign lesion by 15 %. This resulted in a decrease in cost of $ 1,192 per patient [64, 65]. It is not yet clear whether this cost saving will also be present in Europe. In a Japanese study, the use of PET was unlikely to be cost-effective, maybe because of the different prevalence of malignancy in patients with an SPN in Japan and the differences in costs of surgical procedures [66].

15.4.2 PET in Lung Cancer Staging

15.4.2.1 *The Primary Tumor (T-factor)*

The spatial resolution and anatomical detail of PET are inferior to CT or MRI. Therefore, PET is not expected to offer extra benefit in assessing local invasion by the primary tumor. A few small studies have reported on the assessment of pleural involvement (T4-disease), but these suffered from a lack of specificity because only a few patients with benign pleural disease were studied [67, 68]. One more recent study in 35 lung cancer patients compared the results of PET versus CT in distinguishing benign from malignant pleural disease [69]. PET correctly detected the presence of malignant pleural involvement in 16 of 18 patients and excluded malignant effusion in 16 of 17 patients (sensitivity 89 %, specificity 94 %, accuracy 91 %).

15.4.2.2 *Locoregional Lymph Nodes (N-factor)*

The most documented step forward in NSCLC staging by PET is the assessment of mediastinal LNs in potentially operable NSCLC. Prospective studies specifically addressing this issue are listed in Table 4 [70–77]. When the results of Table 4 are put together, an overall sensitivity of 89 % (range 67–93), specificity of 92 % (range

Table 4.
Prospective comparative studies on locoregional lymph node staging of NSCLC by PET versus CT reporting on at least 50 patients

First author	N	Method of analysis[a]	Sensitivity	Specificity	Accuracy	Prevalence[b]	P
Saunders [70]	84	Independent	71%	97%	92%	18%	NR
		CT	20%	90%	77%		
Valk [71]	76	Complementary	83%	94%	91%	32%	<0.01
		CT	63%	73%	70%		
Vansteenkiste [72]	68	Complementary	93%	95%	94%	41%	0.0004
		CT	75%	63%	68%		
Kerstine [73]	64	Independent	70%	86%	84%	25%	<0.001
		CT	65%	79%	76%		
Vansteenkiste [74]	56	Fusion images	89%	82%	86%	50%	0.04
		Complementary	89%	82%	86%		
		CT	86%	43%	64%		
Vansteenkiste [75]	50	Independent	67%	97%	88%	30%	0.004
		Complementary	93%	97%	96%		
		CT	67%	59%	64%		
Bury [76]	50	Independent	90%	86%	NR	32%	<0.05
		CT	72%	81%	NR		
Weng [77]	50	Independent	73%	94%	87%	38%	0.03
		Complementary	82%	96%	91%		
		CT	73%	77%	76%		

N number of patients, *P* significance of the difference in performance between CT and PET, usually examined with a McNemar test

[a] *Method of analysis* independent = interpretation of PET without CT; complementary = interpretation with aid of CT

[b] *Prevalence* proportion of cases with diseased mediastinal lymph nodes in the total group of studied patients

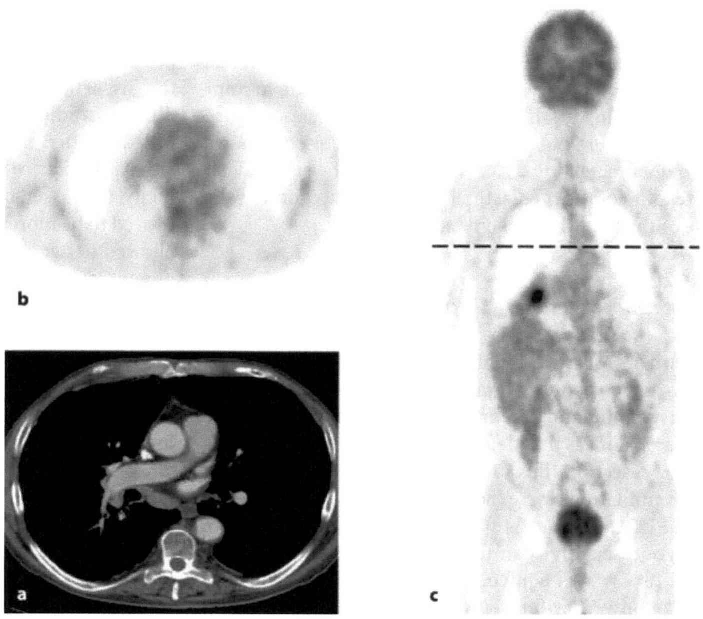

Fig. 3.
A 70-year-old male with a large cell carcinoma of the right lower lobe with suspected mediastinal involvement in the subcarinal nodes on CT (**a**). Whole-body PET shows elevated FDG uptake in the primary tumor (C), but not in the subcarinal region (**b, c**). The patient was referred for thoracotomy without prior mediastinoscopy. Final histology of the radical lymph node dissection specimen confirmed absence of lymph node involvement as predicted by PET

82–97), and accuracy of 90% (range 84–94) are obtained for PET. For CT, the results are: sensitivity 65% (range 20–86), specificity 80% (range 43–90), and accuracy 75% (range 64–77). PET performed significantly better than CT in nearly all of the adequately powered studies. As could be expected, this was confirmed in a meta-analysis [78]. The superiority of PET can be explained by the more frequent correct identification of "small malignant nodes" and "large benign nodes" (Fig. 3). From previous data, it is well known that size on CT is a relative criterion, since LNs can be enlarged due to infectious or inflammatory causes, and small-sized nodes can nonetheless harbor metastases [20, 22, 23], resulting in overstaging as well as understaging. False-negative findings can occur when the tumor deposit in the mediastinal nodes is small. In our experience, this was mainly the case in some patients with minimal areas of metastatic cells in LNs, with a maximal diameter rarely exceeding 2.5 mm. False-positive images are possible in LNs containing inflammatory or granulomatous tissue with high metabolic activity [50, 61].

Regarding the methods of acquisition and analysis, two studies specifically compared the interpretation of PET images with the aid of CT (complementary) or without it (independently). A gain in sensitivity was noted from 67 to 93% [75] in one study, and from 73 to 82% in the other [77]. This difference is the expression of the fact that the precise anatomic information on CT is complementary to the metabolic information images of PET, which lack precise anatomical detail. Therefore, the correlative interpretation will help in the distinction between e.g. central tumors and adjacent LNs, or between adjacent LN stations. This difference can be of clinical relevance, e.g. when the distinction of hilar (N1, operable) and adjacent subaortic nodes (N2, locally advanced) is to be made. A prospective study in our group addressed the question of whether digitally fused CT and PET images (so-called anatometabolic fusion images) could further increase the accuracy of non-invasive LN staging [74]. It was found that, for an experienced reader, the gain in accuracy compared to visual correlation was very small, since the errors due to minimal tumor load (false negatives) or inflammation (false positives) were not corrected. In one of our studies, we also documented that, just as for SPNs, the simple visual reading of the mediastinal images was as good as the use of the SUV threshold of 4.4 for LNs [72].

15.4.2.3
Extrathoracic Metastases (M-factor)

Up to 20% of NSCLC patients may have adrenal masses at diagnosis [79–81], and up to two-thirds of these are asymptomatic adrenal adenomas [79, 82]. An isolated adrenal mass that determines the indication for lung tumor resection thus often deserves further (pathologic) examination by e.g. puncture or biopsy of the lesion [82]. PET can be a useful tool in this assessment. There is a good sensitivity in the detection of adrenal metastases [83–85]. An equivocal lesion on CT without FDG uptake on PET will usually not be metastatic. Interpretation should be careful in small adrenal lesions, since very few of these were present in the prospective series. Specificity is between 80 and 100% [83], since FDG uptake is also described in adrenal adenomas. To increase specificity, FDG uptake in the adrenal lesion can be compared to the liver uptake as suggested by Yun et al. [86]. Adenomas usually have faint uptake, less than or equal to liver uptake, whereas metastases show intense FDG uptake. But even in the latter case, the isolated FDG-positive adrenal lesion should have pathologic verification before a patient is excluded from radical treatment.

The evaluation of the liver is usually less difficult, because the liver is less frequently an isolated site of disease, and because the combination of ultrasound and/or CT can solve most cases [87]. There are no specific series on evaluation of the liver in NSCLC, but data from NSCLC staging in general suggest that PET is more accurate than CT, mainly because of a better specificity [88, 89]. A series in patients with different primary tumors reported a sensitivity of 97% and a specificity of 88% for PET, in comparison to 93% and 75% for CT (non-significant difference) [90]. False-positive findings have been described in some liver abscesses [91]. The most useful aspect of PET is its ability to differentiate hepatic lesions that remain indeterminate by conventional studies: in one such study, PET accurately indicated liver metastases in 11 patients, of whom two had a negative and nine had an equivocal conventional imaging. PET could also exclude metastasis in four cases with suspect conventional imaging [90].

99m Technetium methylene diphosphonate bone scintigraphy is considered to be the standard technique in the search for bone metastases. Bone scintigraphy has a reasonable sensitivity of about 90%, but the interpretation is hampered by false-positive findings in arthrosis, arthritis, post-traumatic abnormalities, etc. Additional studies such as bone X-rays, bone CT, or bone MRI are often indicated. In one study, PET had a sensitivity similar to bone scintigraphy, but a better specificity (98% versus 61%) [92]. In another series, PET proved to be more sensitive than bone scintigraphy, and allowed better differentiation between benign and malignant lesions [93]. Only one lesion in the distal femur, correctly identified as metastasis on bone scan, was missed on PET because the lesion was situated outside the standard field-of-view of PET imaging. Indeed, an important difference is that bone scan images the entire skeleton, while PET only views from the head to just below the pelvis.

Positron emission tomography can also detect metastases that otherwise might escape our attention, e.g. small nodules in the other lung, soft tissue lesions, retroperitoneal LNs or hardly palpable supraclavicular LNs.

Positron emission tomography is not suited for the detection of brain metastases. The sensitivity of PET in the detection of brain lesions is low, because the surrounding normal brain tissue has a high glucose uptake. CT and/or MRI remain the standard imaging tests to stage the brain.

15.4.2.4
Small Cell Lung Cancer: Limited Versus Extensive Disease

In contrast to the rapidly evolving data on the role of PET in NSCLC, there are only a few anecdotal reports [94–96], one retrospective [97], and one prospective series [98] on SCLC. In the last one, as few as 18 patients were studied, and it was reported that PET stage agreed with conventional staging in 15 of 18 patients (eight extensive, seven limited), while PET showed more extensive disease in two of three patients for whom PET and conventional staging disagreed.

15.4.3
Assessment of Response to Treatment

The data on the possible extra value of PET in assessing response to radiotherapy in NSCLC are still limited. In one study, tumors with a high FDG uptake responded better to radiotherapy than those with a low uptake [99]. A correlation between volume changes on CT and decrease of FDG uptake on PET has been described, but a persistently elevated FDG uptake after radiotherapy predicted an early relapse, irrespective of the volume changes on CT [99, 100].

The first prospective feasibility study on the value of PET in response evaluation after induction chemotherapy was carried out in our group [101]. PET proved to be more accurate than CT in the evaluation of downstaging. There also proved to be a prognostic value: patients achieving "PET-response" after induction (defined as mediastinal clearance and at least 50% decrease in primary tumor SUV on the post-induction scan) had a significantly better treatment outcome after the entire combined modality treatment (Fig. 4). An interim report on an ongoing larger prospective multi-center trial also suggested that PET might be a useful non-invasive tool to select patients for intensive locoregional treatment after induction chemotherapy [102], and the final results of this analysis are awaited. One retrospective study looked at the correlation between histopathology and PET findings after induction chemoradiotherapy [103]. SUV-based analysis had a high sensitivity (88%) but limited specificity (67%) for the detection of residual disease in the primary tumor, but in contrast a high specificity (93%) and limited sensitivity (58%) in restaging of the mediastinal LNs. In another retrospective experience, it was reported that PET imaging after induction therapy (mainly chemotherapy) overstaged nodal status in 33% of patients, understaged nodal status in 15%, and was correct in only 52% [104].

15.4.4
Follow-up, Detection of Recurrence and Prognosis

Studies in patients with CT images suspect for recurrence have pointed at the possible distinction between post-therapy scarring and new viable tumor with a sensitivity for PET of 97–100%, a specificity of 62–100%, and an accuracy of 78–98% [105–111]. False-positive findings, due to radiation pneumonitis or macrophage glycolysis in tumor necrosis, may occur if the PET is performed shortly after radiotherapy [108]. An interval of 4–6 months after therapy is recommended to allow correct assessment of tumor viability. In one study, both the presence and extent of relapse on PET were of prognostic value [111]. One series also pointed at a correct positive result in 16 indeterminate lung lesions after previous surgical treatment [46].

Some studies reported an independent prognostic value of assessing the glucose metabolism in NSCLC in vivo by means of PET. Part of the explanation may be

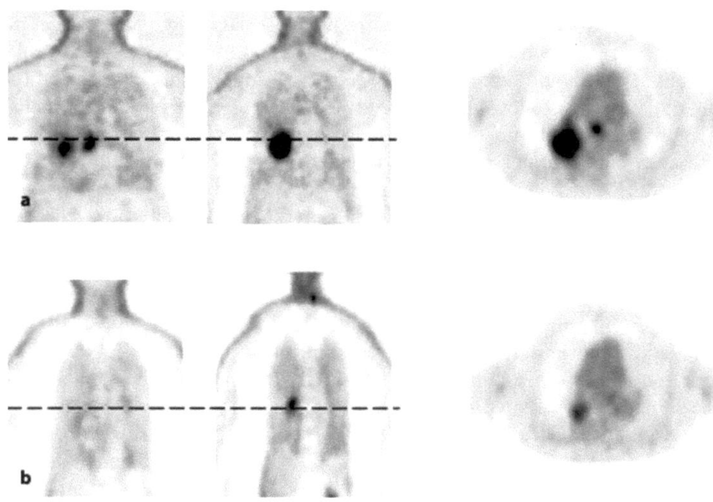

Fig. 4. A 56-year-old male with squamous cell carcinoma of the right lower lobe, stage IIIA-N2. High FDG uptake is seen in the primary tumor (SUVmax: 10.6) and in a subcarinal lymph node prior to the start of induction chemotherapy (**a**). After three cycles of chemotherapy, a major response was noted on CT, whereas PET showed persistent high FDG uptake in the primary tumor (SUVmax: 6) (**b**). The patient underwent radical surgery but died 15 months later of carcinomatous lymphangitis

that FDG uptake in NSCLC is correlated with growth rate and proliferation capacity [112]. One study in 125 NSCLC patients found that an SUV of the primary tumor of more than 7 had independent prognostic value, apart from the performance status and stage. In patients with a resected T1 tumor, the 2-year survival was 86% if the SUV was below 7, and 60% if above 7 [113]. Similar findings, based on a cut-off SUV of 10, were reported by another group [114].

It has also been reported that PET might have prognostic value after treatment [115]. Patients with a positive PET after initial treatment had a median survival of 12 months, in contrast with those with a negative PET, of whom 85% were still alive at the time of analysis, after a median follow-up of 34 months ($P=0.002$).

15.5 Indications for PET – Practical Clinical Guidelines

15.5.1 Differential Diagnosis of Lung Nodules

The key question for the clinician in this setting is not "can I be sure about malignancy?" but rather "based on what test result can an SPN be considered benign, and will the ensuing conservative approach not lead to unjustifiable expectation in a curatively resectable patient?" Therefore, one should be aware of the possibilities and limitations of PET in the patient with an SPN. An SPN with low or absent uptake on whole-body images is likely to be benign. With its sensitivity of 96%, PET will indeed have a very good negative predictive value, and will be able to exclude malignancy correctly in the vast majority of cases. In these patients, a thoracotomy can be avoided, and a repeat chest X-ray or CT at 6 months or a year can be used to confirm the absence of growth. Tricky situations, where a false-negative test result may be present, are: (a) lesions smaller than 1 cm, where other clinical (age, smoking history) and radiological factors (e.g. irregular margins) determining the likelihood of malignancy should be considered. Specific CT study [116,117], very close follow-up, or more invasive tests can be appropriate; (b) tumors with low metabolic activity, such as carcinoid tumors, but these usually have a central location, amenable to bronchoscopic biopsy [118]; and (c) BAC, where CT features will often help obtain a correct diagnosis [119]. With its specificity of 79%, PET will also have a good positive predictive value, but not as good as its negative one. A positive scan is possible in different inflammatory conditions, which should be excluded by appropriate tests in cases of clinical suspicion. In doubtful cases, lesions with increased FDG uptake should be considered malignant until proven otherwise, and managed accordingly.

15.5.2 Staging of NSCLC

As for locoregional LN staging, our group suggested in 1997 that, based on the high negative predictive value of PET, mediastinoscopy could be omitted in patients with normal mediastinal PET readings [75]. This strategy has gradually gained widespread acceptance, and is now implemented in e.g. the recent Lung Cancer Guidelines of the American College of Chest Physicians (ACCP) [29], with a grade B recommendation, and adopted in many other countries. This implementation should be handled with care in patients with central tumors or with central hilar N1-disease (since adherent N2 can be missed in these instances), and in those with BAC (because of its low FDG avidity). Occasionally, a patient with a false-negative mediastinal PET proceeds to straightforward thoracotomy, but in these cases "minimal N2" is found, where a reasonable prognosis after surgical resection can be expected [120]. If the PET images suggest mediastinal LN disease, mediastinoscopy cannot be left out, because LN mapping is justified before the start of an induction protocol, and is needed to avoid denial of direct surgical resection based on a false-positive mediastinal PET reading. This strategy of histological confirmation also has a grade B recommendation in the ACCP guidelines. Overall, this results in a decrease of the number of invasive procedures, which has been shown to be cost-effective in a US setting [65,121].

As for extrathoracic staging, PET improves the conventional imaging for two reasons. First, it is able to detect metastatic lesions that would have been missed by conventional methods, or located in clinically hidden or difficult areas (bone (Fig. 5), liver, soft tissue, some LNs, etc.). As most of the organ-specific literature series are still based on small numbers of patients and contain some false-positive findings, verification by other imaging techniques or by tissue sampling is mandatory in the case of an isolated PET-positive finding that determines resectability. Second, PET is able to evaluate the likelihood of malignancy in lesions that are equivocal on conventional imaging (Fig. 6). Malignancy should be excluded with caution by PET in cases of small lesions (e.g. adrenal nodules of less than 1 cm).

Because PET is able to stage both intra- and extrathoracic sites in one examination, and because of its greater accuracy than conventional imaging, this technique is reported to change patient management in 19% [89], 20% [88], 30% [71], 31% [122], or even 41% of patients [123]. Although numerous data indicate that PET complements conventional imaging, we do not (yet) have enough data to accept that PET can replace it. In contrast with the large amount of data on locoregional staging, most of the organ-specific studies are small, and do not include an adequate number of small lesions,

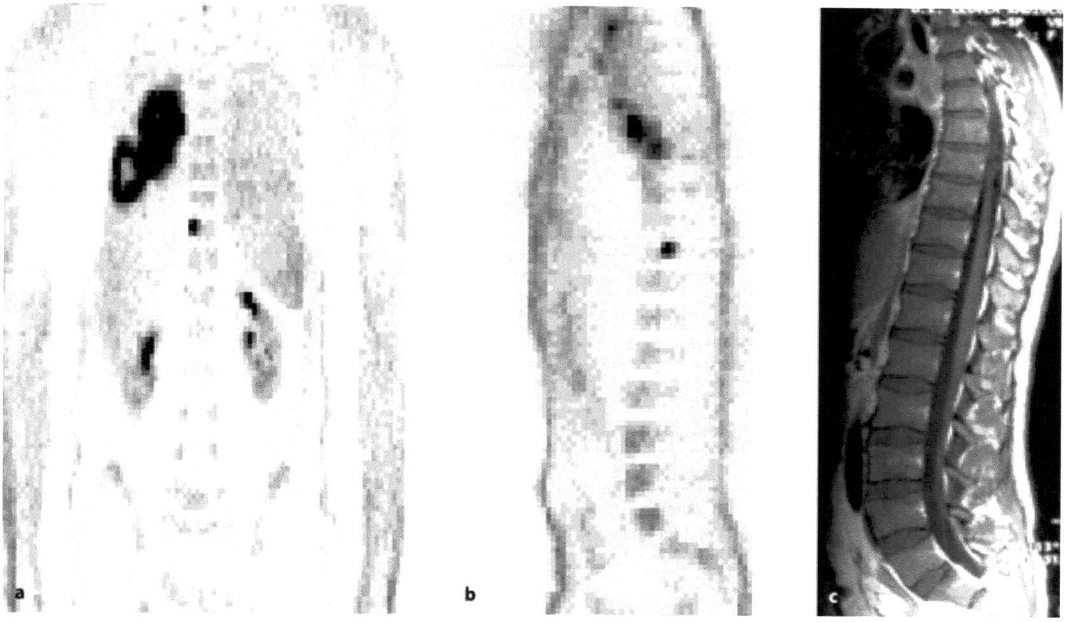

Fig. 5. Patient with right lower lobe adenocarcinoma and ipsilateral mediastinal lymph node metastases. Conventional staging for distant metastases, including bone scintigraphy, was negative. WB-PET (**a, b**) reveals suspect lesion in the lower dorsal spine. Since MRI (**c**) could not confirm bone invasion, the patient was regarded as having no metastases and treated with induction chemotherapy. Restaging after induction chemotherapy revealed diffuse overt bone metastases on planar X-rays and bone scintigraphy, confirming the bone involvement initially only seen on PET

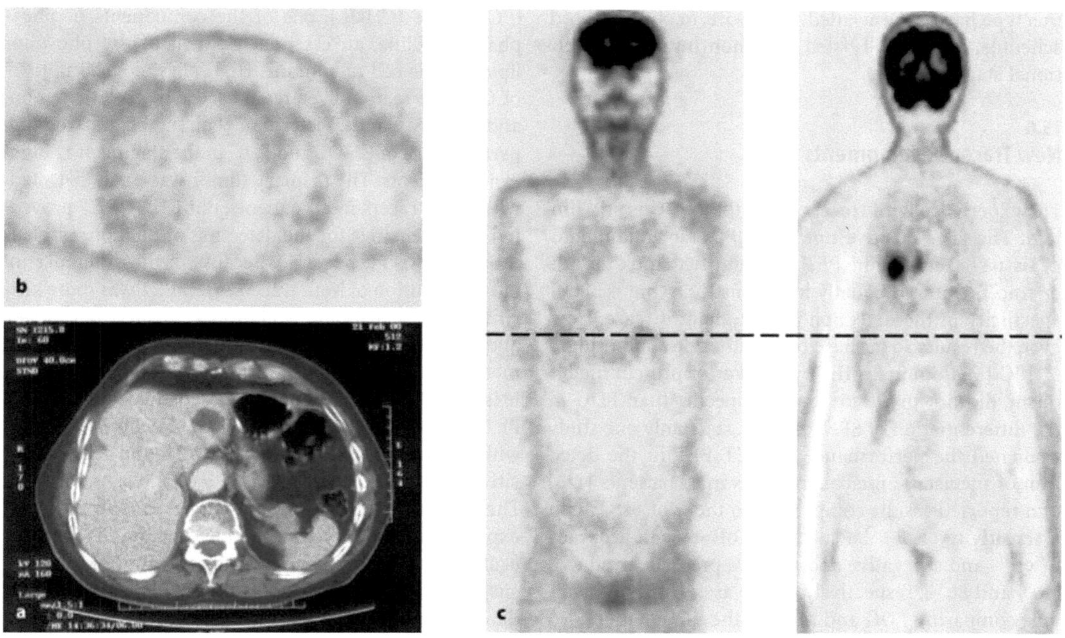

Fig. 6. Equivocal lesion in the left hepatic lobe on CT (**a**). Whole-body PET demonstrates enhanced FDG uptake in the primary squamous cell carcinoma in the right lung, but no abnormalities are present in the liver area (**b, c**). The patient underwent induction chemotherapy followed by radical resection but died of diffuse pulmonary involvement 15 months after surgery. During this follow-up the liver lesion remained unchanged, confirming its benign nature, probably hemangioma

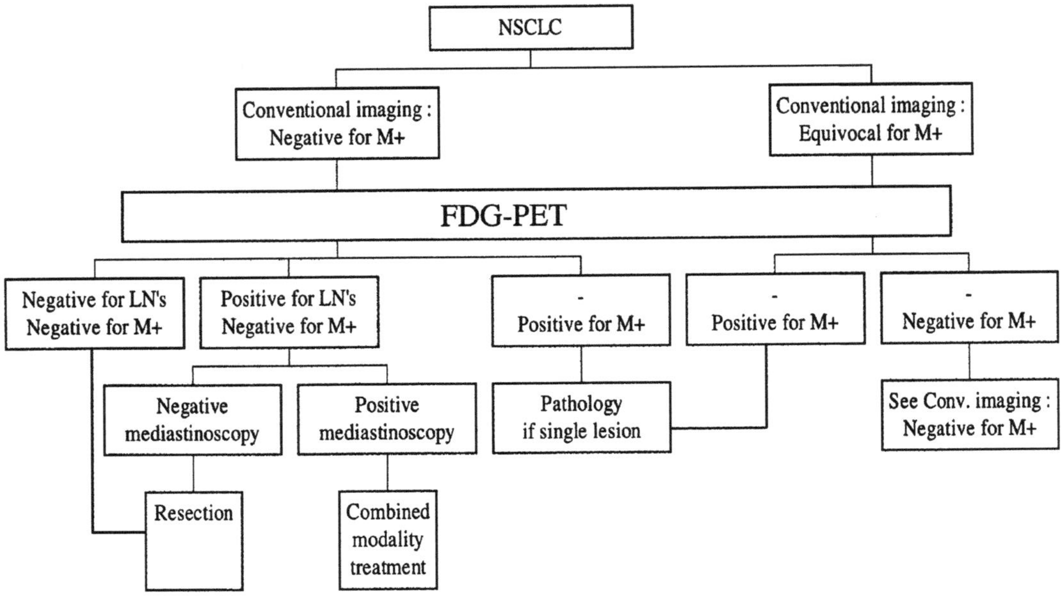

Fig. 7. Possible implementation of PET in the staging of NSCLC, as an adjunct to conventional staging

which truly challenge the technique. Further studies of this type have to be awaited. Therefore, in our proposed schedule, PET is still listed after non-invasive conventional staging (Fig. 7).

15.6 New Tracer Developments

The experience with tracers other than FDG is still limited. The false-positive uptake of FDG in inflammatory tissue has forced the PET community to look for other tracers with an equally high sensitivity but a better specificity in the detection of malignant disease. However, the results so far have been rather disappointing.

[^{11}C]Methionine (MET), a marker of protein metabolism, did not prove to be more specific than FDG in the differentiation of SPNs [55, 124, 125]. Only one study evaluated the performance of MET PET in the detection of metastatic mediastinal LNs in 41 patients [126] and reported results comparable to those of FDG, with a sensitivity of 86%, a specificity of 91%, an accuracy of 90% and a negative and positive predictive value of 94% and 80%, respectively. There are no studies available comparing FDG and MET in the same patient. No data are available yet for the detection of distant metastasis, but it is very unlikely that MET PET will be better than FDG PET given its high physiological uptake in liver, pancreatic region and gut.

Tumor cells also show an increased uptake of [^{11}C]choline (CHOL), one of the components of phosphatidylcholine, an essential element of the phospholipids in the cell membrane. High physiological uptake of CHOL is seen in liver, renal cortex, pancreatic region and salivary glands. Pieterman et al. [127] compared the performance of CHOL and FDG in the staging of 17 lung cancer patients. The primary tumor was easily detected with both tracers in all patients, but CHOL PET proved to be less sensitive for the detection of pulmonary/pleural metastasis (57 vs 98%). Because of the difference in bio-distribution of both tracers, FDG PET was more sensitive in the detection of abdominal spread (100 vs 57%) and CHOL PET was superior for the detection of brain metastasis (100 vs 13%). For the detection of metastatic LNs, FDG PET proved to be more sensitive than CHOL – PET, with a sensitivity of 95 vs 67%. This is in contrast with the study of Hara et al. [128] who found a 100% sensitivity for CHOL, and a sensitivity of only 75% for FDG. The discrepancy between both studies can probably be explained by the difference in image analysis. Pieterman et al. analyzed their images visually and any hot spot was suspected for metastatic spread. Hara et al. used a semiquantitative scale making any hot spot with an SUV similar to that of the primary tumor ±40% positive. Since the SUVs of the primary tumor were lower for CHOL than for FDG, this led to a more sensitive cut-off for CHOL, maybe explaining its higher sensitivity.

Probably the most interesting new tracer is [^{18}F]fluoro-thymidine (FLT), a marker of cell proliferation [129]. Accumulation of FLT is dependent on cellular thymidine kinase-1 (TK-1) activity, the key enzyme of the pyrimidine salvage pathway of DNA synthesis. Although FLT is not incorporated into the DNA, FLT uptake is correlated with DNA synthesis, since TK-1 is only functional in the S-phase of the cell cycle. Initial experience in lung cancer patients confirmed the high correlation between FLT uptake and proliferation rate as measured by Ki-67 immunohistochemistry and DNA flow cytometry [130]. In the differentiation of SPNs, FLT proved to be highly specific for malignancy, with none of the eight benign lesions showing elevated FLT uptake [131]. The sensitivity in this study was only 86% with false-negative results in tumors with low Ki-67 index. Therefore FDG and FLT are probably complementary in the diagnostic work-up of SPNs. Given its close relationship to cell proliferation, FLT is potentially the best tracer to measure response to treatment, and results in this setting are eagerly awaited.

15.7 Summary and Outlook

Positron emission tomography as a complementary tool to CT is useful in the diagnosis and staging of NSCLC, and is now reimbursed for these indications in many western countries. When more commercial isotope distributors are able to deliver FDG, so that an on-site cyclotron is no longer a prerequisite, the technique will become accessible to larger parts of the medical community. FDG has a half-life of 110 minutes, so a practical distribution radius of 200–300 kilometers should be feasible.

The current use of PET in lung cancer now needs further validation in multi-center large-scale randomized studies, focusing mainly on treatment outcome parameters, and on the question of whether PET actually decreases the number of needless surgical procedures, improves choices of therapy or survival prospects, and reduces cost of lung cancer care. On such recent study looked at the effectiveness of PET in reducing the number of "futile" thoracotomies for (suspected) NSCLC [132]. After conventional staging, 188 patients were randomly assigned to operation after conventional staging alone, or the same plus PET. A thoracotomy was considered futile in cases of benign disease, exploration only, pathologic stage IIIA-N2 or IIIB, or postoperative relapse or death within 1 year. The addition of PET to conventional staging reduced the number of futile thoracotomies from 39 (41%) to 19 (21%) patients ($P=0.003$). This corresponded to avoidance of unnecessary surgery in one of five patients. However, not all thoracotomies for benign disease can be considered "futile" (some are essential for certainty of diagnosis and avoiding long-term uncertainty for the patient), and surgery is not necessarily futile in cases of stage IIIA-N2 disease, especially in a combined modality treatment setting [15].

Finally, a whole new field using PET in molecular applications is under exploration. FDG, which enables tumor glucose metabolism to be studied, has paved the way for PET in clinical oncology. Several other radiopharmaceuticals can also be used to study processes such as blood flow ([^{15}O]H_2O), protein metabolism ([^{11}C]MET, [^{11}C]CHOL) and carbohydrate metabolism ([^{11}C]acetate) [133]. One step further is the study by PET of cellular functions such as receptors, transport proteins or intracellular enzymes. The use of PET to study the efficacy of gene therapy in cancer is one example [134, 135]. Another example is how we could use PET as a guide in the selection or early assessment of anti-cancer therapy, e.g. with thymidine analogues. If this concept could be brought into broader practice, it would enable us to tailor therapy for a specific patient, and to progress faster in testing new drugs in phase I and II clinical studies, by using the endpoint of subclinical PET response [136].

15.8 Technical Recommendations

For a more comprehensive overview, we refer to the guidelines for tumor imaging with FDG of the Society of Nuclear Medicine (www.snm.org). An overview of possible pitfalls in interpretation can be found in the paper by Shreve et al. [137]. Here we only focus on the more specific requirements for lung cancer imaging.

15.8.1 Patient Preparation

Since FDG uptake in lung cancers is reduced in the hyperglycemic state [138], blood glucose levels should be checked prior to tracer injection. To reduce the chance of a false-negative PET result, it is advised to proceed only if the glucose level is within a normal range. Although diabetic patients were often excluded in the prospective studies, FDG uptake is probably not significantly influenced in these patients if the blood glucose levels are reasonably controlled [139].

15.8.2 Data Acquisition

Since tumors show a steady increase in FDG uptake over time, tumor to background ratios (and thus lesion detection) improve over time. Therefore, it is advised to wait at least 60 min after tracer injection (and preferably even longer) before starting the acquisition.

In most cases, a whole-body acquisition is preferred to survey the entire body for areas of abnormal FDG accumulation. Whole-body imaging can be limited to the trunk (from the base of the skull to the pelvis), as metastasis to the lower limbs is rare.

With the introduction of post-injection transmission on recent PET systems, attenuation-corrected whole-body scans became the standard procedure in oncology. Compared to non-attenuation-corrected scans, anatomical detail is improved, which simplifies the localization of hot spots, and quantification with SUV measurements becomes possible, which is essential if one wants to use PET as a prognostic parameter or for treatment-response assessment. However, if the aim of the study is just to stage the patient, non-attenuation-corrected images are probably as good, as has been pointed out by different prospective studies.

If FDG PET is used for response assessment, a quantitative assessment of the FDG uptake is essential. The different analytical methods have been reviewed by Hoekstra et al. [140]. Dynamic imaging with full kinetic modeling is accepted as the method of reference, but it is time consuming and can only be performed in one bed position. Semi-quantitative analysis based on SUV measurements is the most frequently used method in clinical oncology, but is hampered by the fact that important errors can be introduced, since several factors, like the time between tracer injection and PET scanning (uptake period) and plasma glucose levels, are not taken into account. In a study comparing full kinetic modeling with different simplified methods in lung cancer patients [141], the SUV value that correlated best with the reference method was the one corrected for body surface area and plasma glucose.

15.8.3 Image Reconstruction

There is no evidence that a particular reconstruction algorithm is superior to any other. Therefore, images can be reconstructed using the reconstruction algorithms available at each center. Although iterative reconstruction algorithms give "nicer" images (fewer streak artifacts) compared to filtered back projection and make the interpretation easier, the diagnostic accuracy for both reconstruction algorithms for experienced readers is comparable. If an iterative reconstruction algorithm is used, the number of iterations should be sufficient, as convergence is dependent on image content. To reduce the noise propagated into the reconstructed image, a three-dimensional post-smooth can be applied.

15.8.4 Image Interpretation

For the discrimination of SPNs [53] and the evaluation of mediastinal involvement [72], quantification did not prove to be superior to visual analysis (i.e. any hot spot higher than background activity is regarded positive for tumor).

As attenuation correction can induce different artifacts (e.g. motion artifacts, segmentation errors, noise), attenuation-corrected images should be viewed together with non-attenuation-corrected images.

For the evaluation of the mediastinum, one should try to localize the hot spots according to a standard lymph node map (Fig. 1) so that invasive surgical staging for confirmation of nodal involvement can be optimized (e.g. suspected nodes in the sub-aortic or para-aortic region require a left anterior mediastinotomy). Localization of hot spots can be facilitated by correlating PET with CT images or by projecting the hot spots onto the reconstructed transmission scan on which the main bronchi are often visible.

References

1. Doll R, Peto R (1978) Cigarette smoking and bronchial carcinoma: dose and time relationships among regular smokers and lifelong non-smokers. J Epidemiol Commun Health 32: 303–313
2. Denissenko MF, Pao A, Tang M et al (1996) Preferential formation of benzo[a]pyrene adducts at lung cancer mutational hotspots in P53. Science 274:430–432
3. Darby S, Hill D, Doll R (2001) Radon: a likely carcinogen at all exposures. Ann Oncol 12:1341–1351
4. Swensen SJ, Jett JR, Sloan JA et al (2002) Screening for lung cancer with low-dose spiral computed tomography. Am J Respir Crit Care Med 165:508–513
5. World Health Organization (1982) Histological typing of lung tumors, 2nd edn. Am J Clin Pathol 77:123–136
6. Travis WD, Colby TV, Corrin B et al (1999) Histological typing of lung and pleural tumours. WHO international classification of lung tumours, 3rd edn. Springer, Berlin Heidelberg New York
7. Cummings SR, Lillington GA, Richard RJ (1986) Managing solitary pulmonary nodules. The choice of strategy is a "close call". Am Rev Respir Dis 134:453–460
8. Yankelevitz DF, Henschke CI (1997) Does 2-year stability imply that pulmonary nodules are benign? AJR Am J Roentgenol 168:325–328
9. Arroliga AC, Matthay RA (1993) The role of bronchoscopy in lung cancer. Clin Chest Med 14:87–98
10. Santambrogio L, Nosotti M, Bellaviti N et al (1997) CT-guided fine-needle aspiration cytology of solitary pulmonary nodules: a prospective, randomized study of immediate cytologic evaluation. Chest 112:423–425
11. Larscheid RC, Thorpe PE, Scott WJ (1998) Percutaneous transthoracic needle aspiration biopsy: a comprehensive review of its current role in the diagnosis and treatment of lung tumors. Chest 114:704–709
12. Michiels E, Demedts M (1991) Pitfalls of transthoracic needle aspiration biopsy. Acta Clin Belg 46:359–363
13. Mountain CF (1997) Revisions in the international system for staging lung cancer. Chest 111:1710–1717
14. Jett JR, Scott WJ, Rivera MP et al (2003) Guidelines on treatment of stage IIIB non-small cell lung cancer. Chest 123 [Suppl 1]:221S–225S
15. Vansteenkiste J, De Leyn P, Deneffe G et al (1998) Present status of induction treatment for N2 non-small cell lung cancer: a review. Eur J Cardiothorac Surg 13:1–12
16. Rosell R, Gomez Codina J, Camps C et al (1994) A randomized trial comparing preoperative chemotherapy plus surgery with surgery alone in patients with non-small-cell lung cancer. N Engl J Med 330:153–158
17. Vansteenkiste JF, Vandebroek JE, Nackaerts KL et al (2001) Clinical benefit response in advanced non-small cell lung can-

cer. A multicenter prospective randomized phase III study of single agent gemcitabine versus cisplatin-vindesine. Ann Oncol 12:1221–1230
18. Numico G, Russi E, Merlano M (2001) Best supportive care in non-small cell lung cancer: is there a role for radiotherapy and chemotherapy? Lung Cancer 32:213–226
19. Bittner RC, Felix R (1998) Magnetic resonance (MR) imaging of the chest: state-of-the-art. Eur Respir J 11:1392–1404
20. McLoud TC, Bourgouin PM, Greenberg RW et al (1992) Bronchogenic carcinoma: analysis of staging in the mediastinum with CT by correlative lymph node mapping and sampling. Radiology 182:319–323
21. Staples CA, Miller RR, Evans KG et al (1988) Mediastinal nodes in bronchogenic carcinoma: comparison between CT and mediastinoscopy. Radiology 167:367–372
22. Webb WR, Gatsouris S, Zerhouni EA et al (1991) CT and MR imaging in staging non-small cell bronchogenic carcinoma: report of the Radiology Diagnostic Oncology Group. Radiology 178:705–713
23. Dillemans B, Deneffe G, Verschakelen J et al (1994) Value of computed tomography and mediastinoscopy in preoperative evaluation of mediastinal nodes in non-small cell lung cancer. Eur J Cardiothorac Surg 8:37–42
24. Mountain CF, Dresler CM (1997) Regional lymph node classification for lung cancer staging. Chest 111:1718–1723
25. Quint LE, Tummala S, Brisson LJ et al (1996) Distribution of distant metastases from newly diagnosed non-small cell lung cancer. Ann Thorac Surg 62:246–250
26. Parker SL, Tong T, Bolden S et al (1997) Cancer statistics 1997. CA Cancer J Clin 47:5–27
27. American Thoracic Society (ATS), European Respiratory Society (ERS) (1997) Pretreatment evaluation of non-small cell lung cancer. Am J Respir Crit Care Med 156:320–332
28. Goldstraw P, Rocmans P, Ball D et al (1994) Pretreatment minimal staging for non-small cell lung cancer: an updated consensus report. Lung Cancer 11 [Suppl 3]:1–4
29. Silvestri GA, Tanoue LT, Margolis ML et al (2003) The noninvasive staging of non-small cell lung cancer: the guidelines. Chest 123 [Suppl 1]:147S–156S
30. Pantel K, Izbicki J, Passlick B et al (1996) Frequency and prognostic significance of isolated tumour cells in bone marrow of patients with non-small cell lung cancer without overt metastases. Lancet 347:649–653
31. Martini N, Bains MS, Burt ME et al (1995) Incidence of local recurrence and second primary tumors in resected stage I lung cancer. J Thorac Cardiovasc Surg 109:120–129
32. Pairolero PC, Williams DE, Bergstralh EJ et al (1984) Postsurgical stage I bronchogenic carcinoma: morbid implications of recurrent disease. Ann Thorac Surg 38:331–338
33. Yano T, Yokoyama H, Inoue T et al (1994) The first site of recurrence after complete resection in non-small cell carcinoma of the lung. Comparison between pN0 disease and pN2 disease. J Thorac Cardiovasc Surg 108:680–683
34. De Ruysscher D, Vansteenkiste J (2000) Chest radiotherapy in limited stage small cell lung cancer: facts, questions, prospects. Radiother Oncol 55:1–9
35. Micke P, Faldum A, Metz T et al (2002) Staging small cell lung cancer: Veterans Administration Lung Study Group versus International Association for the Study of Lung Cancer – what limits limited disease? Lung Cancer 37:271–276
36. Therasse P, Arbuck SG, Eisenhauer EA et al (2000) New guidelines to evaluate the response to treatment in solid tumors. J Natl Cancer Inst 92:205–216
37. Miller AB, Hoogstraten B, Staquet M et al (1981) Reporting results of cancer treatment. Cancer 47:207–214
38. Martini N, Kris MG, Flehinger B et al (1993) Preoperative chemotherapy for stage IIIa (N2) lung cancer: the Sloan-Kettering experience with 136 patients. Ann Thorac Surg 55:1365–1374
39. Strauss GM, Herndon JE, Sherman DD et al (1992) Neoadjuvant chemotherapy and radiotherapy followed by surgery in stage IIIA non-small-cell carcinoma of the lung: report of a Cancer and Leukemia Group B phase II study. J Clin Oncol 10:1237–1244
40. Choi NC, Carey RW, Daly W et al (1997) Potential impact on survival of improved tumor downstaging and resection rate by preoperative twice-daily radiation and concurrent chemotherapy in stage IIIA non-small-cell lung cancer. J Clin Oncol 15:712–722
41. Pisters KM, Kris MG, Gralla RJ et al (1993) Pathologic complete response in advanced non-small-cell lung cancer following preoperative chemotherapy: implications for the design of future non-small-cell lung cancer combined modality trials. J Clin Oncol 11:1757–1762
42. Crino L, Mosconi AM, Scagliotti GV et al (1999) Gemcitabine as second-line treatment for advanced non-small cell lung cancer: a phase II trial. J Clin Oncol 17:2081–2085
43. Shepherd FA, Dancey J, Ramlau R et al (2000) Prospective randomized trial of docetaxel versus best supportive care in patients with non-small cell lung cancer previously treated with platinum-based chemotherapy. J Clin Oncol 18:2095–2103
44. Sazon DA, Santiago SM, Soo Hoo GW et al (1996) Fluorodeoxyglucose-positron emission tomography in the detection and staging of lung cancer. Am J Respir Crit Care Med 153:417–421
45. Lowe VJ, Fletcher JW, Gobar L et al (1998) Prospective investigation of positron emission tomography in lung nodules. J Clin Oncol 16:1075–1084
46. Duhaylongsod FG, Lowe VJ, Patz EF et al (1995) Detection of primary and recurrent lung cancer by means of F-18 fluorodeoxyglucose positron emission tomography (FDG PET). J Thorac Cardiovasc Surg 110:130–139
47. Gupta NC, Maloof J, Gunel E (1996) Probability of malignancy in solitary pulmonary nodules using fluorine-18-FDG and PET. J Nucl Med 37:943–948
48. Nackaerts K, Stroobants S, Vansteenkiste J et al (1997) The use of positron emission tomography (PET) in the differential diagnosis of indeterminate solitary pulmonary lesions, 10th edn.
49. Patz EF, Lowe VJ, Hoffman JM et al (1993) Focal pulmonary abnormalities: evaluation with F-18 fluorodeoxyglucose PET scanning. Radiology 188:487–490
50. Bury T, Dowlati A, Paulus P et al (1996) Evaluation of the solitary pulmonary nodule by positron emission tomography imaging. Eur Respir J 9:410–414
51. Lowe VJ, Hoffman JM, DeLong DM et al (1994) Semiquantitative and visual analysis of FDG-PET images in pulmonary abnormalities. J Nucl Med 35:1771–1776
52. Gupta N, Gill H, Graeber G et al (1998) Dynamic positron emission tomography with F-18 fluorodeoxyglucose imaging in differentiation of benign from malignant lung/mediastinal lesions. Chest 114:1105–1111
53. Gould MK, Maclean CC, Kuschner WG et al (2001) Accuracy of positron emission tomography for diagnosis of pulmonary nodules and mass lesions: a meta-analysis. JAMA 285:914–924
54. Scott WJ, Schwabe JL, Gupta NC et al (1994) Positron emission tomography of lung tumors and mediastinal lymph nodes using [18F]fluorodeoxyglucose. The Members of the PET-Lung Tumor Study Group. Ann Thorac Surg 58:698–703
55. Kubota K, Matsuzawa T, Fujiwara T et al (1990) Differential diagnosis of lung tumor with positron emission tomography: a prospective study. J Nucl Med 31:1927–1932
56. Dewan NA, Gupta NC, Redepenning LS et al (1993) Diagnostic efficacy of PET-FDG imaging in solitary pulmonary nodules. Potential role in evaluation and management. Chest 104: 997–1002
57. Erasmus JJ, McAdams HP, Patz EF et al (1998) Evaluation of primary pulmonary carcinoid tumors using FDG PET. AJR Am J Roentgenol 170:1369–1373
58. Higashi K, Ueda Y, Seki H et al (1998) Fluorine-18-FDG PET imaging is negative in bronchioloalveolar lung carcinoma. J Nucl Med 39:1016–1020
59. Kim BT, Kim Y, Lee KS et al (1998) Localized form of bronchioloalveolar carcinoma: FDG PET findings. AJR Am J Roentgenol 170:935–939
60. Kapucu LO, Meltzer CC, Townsend DW et al (1998) Fluorine-18-fluorodeoxyglucose uptake in pneumonia. J Nucl Med 39: 1267–1269

61. Brudin LH, Valind SO, Rhodes CG et al (1994) Fluorine-18 deoxyglucose uptake in sarcoidosis measured with positron emission tomography. Eur J Nucl Med 21:297–305
62. Bakheet SM, Saleem M, Powe J et al (2000) F-18 fluorodeoxyglucose chest uptake in lung inflammation and infection. Clin Nucl Med 25:273–278
63. Matthies A, Hickeson M, Cuchiara A et al (2002) Dual time point 18F-FDG PET for the evaluation of pulmonary nodules. J Nucl Med 43:871–875
64. Gambhir SS, Shepherd JE, Shah BD et al (1998) Analytical decision model for the cost-effective management of solitary pulmonary nodules. J Clin Oncol 16:2113–2125
65. Scott WJ, Shepherd J, Gambhir SS (1998) Cost-effectiveness of FDG-PET for staging non-small cell lung cancer: a decision analysis. Ann Thorac Surg 66:1876–1883
66. Kosuda S, Ichihara K, Watanabe M et al (2000) Decision-tree sensitivity analysis for cost-effectiveness of chest 2-fluoro-2-D-[(18)F]fluorodeoxyglucose positron emission tomography in patients with pulmonary nodules (non-small cell lung carcinoma) in Japan. Chest 117:346–353
67. Carretta A, Landoni C, Melloni G et al (2000) 18-FDG positron emission tomography in the evaluation of malignant pleural diseases – a pilot study. Eur J Cardiothorac Surg 17:377–383
68. Erasmus JJ, McAdams HP, Rossi SE et al (2000) FDG PET of pleural effusions in patients with non-small cell lung cancer. AJR Am J Roentgenol 175:245–249
69. Gupta NC, Rogers JS, Graeber GM et al (2002) Clinical role of F-18 fluorodeoxyglucose positron emission tomography imaging in patients with lung cancer and suspected malignant pleural effusion. Chest 122:1918–1924
70. Saunders CA, Dussek JE, O'Doherty MJ et al (1999) Evaluation of fluorine-18-fluorodeoxyglucose whole body positron emission tomography imaging in the staging of lung cancer. Ann Thorac Surg 67:790–797
71. Valk PE, Pounds TR, Hopkins DM et al (1995) Staging non-small cell lung cancer by whole-body positron emission tomographic imaging. Ann Thorac Surg 60:1573–1581
72. Vansteenkiste JF, Stroobants SG, de Leyn PR et al (1998) Lymph node staging in non-small cell lung cancer with FDG-PET scan: a prospective study on 690 lymph node stations from 68 patients. J Clin Oncol 16:2142–2149
73. Kernstine KH, Stanford W, Mullan BF et al (1999) PET, CT, and MRI with Combidex for mediastinal staging in non-small cell lung carcinoma. Ann Thorac Surg 68:1022–1028
74. Vansteenkiste JF, Stroobants SG, Dupont PJ et al (1998) FDG-PET scan in potentially operable non-small cell lung cancer: do anatometabolic PET-CT fusion images improve the localisation of regional lymph node metastases? Eur J Nucl Med 25: 1495–1501
75. Vansteenkiste JF, Stroobants SG, de Leyn PR et al (1997) Mediastinal lymph node staging with FDG-PET scan in patients with potentially operable non-small cell lung cancer: a prospective analysis of 50 cases. Chest 112:1480–1486
76. Bury T, Paulus P, Dowlati A et al (1996) Staging of the mediastinum: value of positron emission tomography imaging in non-small cell lung cancer. Eur Respir J 9:2560–2564
77. Weng E, Tran L, Rege S et al (2000) Accuracy and clinical impact of mediastinal lymph node staging with FDG-PET imaging in potentially resectable lung cancer. Am J Clin Oncol 23: 47–52
78. Dwamena BA, Sonnad SS, Angobaldo JO et al (1999) Metastases from non-small cell lung cancer: mediastinal staging in the 1990s. Meta-analytic comparison of PET and CT. Radiology 213:530–536
79. Oliver TW, Bernardino ME, Miller JI et al (1984) Isolated adrenal masses in non-small cell bronchogenic carcinoma. Radiology 153:217–218
80. Nielsen ME, Heaston DK, Dunnick NR et al (1982) Preoperative CT evaluation of adrenal glands in non-small cell bronchogenic carcinoma. AJR Am J Roentgenol 139:317–320
81. Pagani JJ (1984) Non-small cell lung carcinoma adrenal metastases. Computed tomography and percutaneous needle biopsy in their diagnosis. Cancer 53:1058–1060
82. Ettinghausen SE, Burt ME (1991) Prospective evaluation of unilateral adrenal masses in patients with operable non-small cell lung cancer. J Clin Oncol 9:1462–1466
83. Erasmus JJ, Patz EF, McAdams HP et al (1997) Evaluation of adrenal masses in patients with bronchogenic carcinoma using 18F-fluorodeoxyglucose positron emission tomography. AJR Am J Roentgenol 168:1357–1360
84. Boland GW, Goldberg MA, Lee MJ et al (1995) Indeterminate adrenal mass in patients with cancer: evaluation at PET with 2-[F-18]-fluoro-2-deoxy-D-glucose. Radiology 194:131–134
85. Maurea S, Mainolfi C, Bazzicalupo L et al (1999) Imaging of adrenal tumors using FDG PET: comparison of benign and malignant lesions. AJR Am J Roentgenol 173:25–29
86. Yun M, Kim W, Alnafisi N et al (2001) 18F-FDG PET in characterizing adrenal lesions detected on CT or MRI. J Nucl Med 42: 1795–1797
87. Patz EF, Erasmus JJ, McAdams HP et al (1999) Lung cancer staging and management: comparison of contrast-enhanced and nonenhanced helical CT of the thorax. Radiology 212:56–60
88. Weder W, Schmid RA, Bruchhaus H et al (1998) Detection of extrathoracic metastases by positron emission tomography in lung cancer. Ann Thorac Surg 66:886–892
89. Marom EM, McAdams HP, Erasmus JJ et al (1999) Staging non-small cell lung cancer with whole-body PET. Radiology 212: 803–809
90. Hustinx R, Paulus P, Jacquet N et al (1998) Clinical evaluation of whole-body 18F-fluorodeoxyglucose positron emission tomography in the detection of liver metastases. Ann Oncol 9: 397–401
91. Delbeke D, Martin WH, Sandler MP et al (1998) Evaluation of benign vs malignant hepatic lesions with positron emission tomography. Arch Surg 133:510–515
92. Bury T, Barreto A, Daenen F et al (1998) Fluorine-18 deoxyglucose positron emission tomography for the detection of bone metastases in patients with non-small cell lung cancer. Eur J Nucl Med 25:1244–1247
93. Schirrmeister H, Guhlmann A, Elsner K et al (1999) Sensitivity in detecting osseous lesions depends on anatomic localization: planar bone scintigraphy versus 18F-PET. J Nucl Med 40: 1623–1629
94. Lassen U, Andersen P, Daugaard G et al (1998) Metabolic and hemodynamic evaluation of brain metastases from small cell lung cancer with positron emission tomography. Clin Cancer Res 4:2591–2597
95. Shuke N, Tonami N, Shintani H et al (1999) Differential uptake of TI-201 by small cell lung cancer in a patient with pneumoconiosis-related pulmonary nodules. Clin Nucl Med 24:687–690
96. Hauber HP, Bohuslavizki KH, Lund CH et al (2001) Positron emission tomography in the staging of small cell lung cancer: a preliminary study. Chest 119:950–954
97. Shen YY, Shiau YC, Wang JJ et al (2002) Whole-body 18F-2-deoxyglucose positron emission tomography in primary staging small cell lung cancer. Anticancer Res 22:1257–1264
98. Chin R, McCain TW, Miller AA et al (2002) Whole body FDG-PET for the evaluation and staging of small cell lung cancer: a preliminary study. Lung Cancer 37:1–6
99. Ichiya Y, Kuwabara Y, Sasaki M et al (1996) A clinical evaluation of FDG-PET to assess the response in radiation therapy for bronchogenic carcinoma. Ann Nucl Med 10:193–200
100. Kubota K, Yamada S, Ishiwata K et al (1993) Evaluation of the treatment response of lung cancer with positron emission tomography and L-[methyl-11C]methionine: a preliminary study. Eur J Nucl Med 20:495–501
101. Vansteenkiste JF, Stroobants SG, de Leyn PR et al (1998) Potential use of FDG-PET scan after induction chemotherapy in surgically staged IIIA-N2 non-small cell lung cancer: a prospective pilot study. Ann Oncol 9:1193–1198
102. Vansteenkiste J, Stroobants S, Hoekstra C et al (2001) 18fluoro-2-deoxyglucose positron emission tomography (PET) in the assessment of induction chemotherapy (IC) in stage IIIA-N2 NSCLC: a multi-center prospective study, 20th edn.

103. Ryu JS, Choi NC, Fischman AJ et al (2002) FDG-PET in staging and restaging non-small cell lung cancer after neoadjuvant chemoradiotherapy: correlation with histopathology. Lung Cancer 35:179–187
104. Akhurst T, Downey RJ, Ginsberg MS et al (2002) An initial experience with FDG-PET in the imaging of residual disease after induction therapy for lung cancer. Ann Thorac Surg 73:259–266
105. Kubota K, Yamada S, Ishiwata K et al (1992) Positron emission tomography for treatment evaluation and recurrence detection compared with CT in long-term follow-up cases of lung cancer. Clin Nucl Med 17:877–881
106. Inoue T, Kim EE, Komaki R et al (1995) Detecting recurrent or residual lung cancer with FDG-PET. J Nucl Med 36:788–793
107. Patz EF, Lowe VJ, Hoffman JM et al (1994) Persistent or recurrent bronchogenic carcinoma: detection with PET and 2-[F-18]-2-deoxy-D-glucose. Radiology 191:379–382
108. Frank A, Lefkowitz D, Jaeger S et al (1995) Decision logic for retreatment of asymptomatic lung cancer recurrence based on positron emission tomography findings. Int J Radiat Oncol Biol Phys 32:1495–1512
109. Hebert ME, Lowe VJ, Hoffman JM et al (1996) Positron emission tomography in the pretreatment evaluation and follow-up of non-small cell lung cancer patients treated with radiotherapy: preliminary findings. Am J Clin Oncol 19:416–421
110. Bury T, Corhay JL, Duysinx B et al (1999) Value of FDG-PET in detecting residual or recurrent non-small cell lung cancer. Eur Respir J 14:1376–1380
111. Hicks RJ, Kalff V, Mac Manus MP et al (2001) The utility of (18)F-FDG PET for suspected recurrent non-small cell lung cancer after potentially curative therapy: impact on management and prognostic stratification. J Nucl Med 42:1605–1613
112. Duhaylongsod FG, Lowe VJ, Patz EF et al (1995) Lung tumor growth correlates with glucose metabolism measured by fluoride-18 fluorodeoxyglucose positron emission tomography. Ann Thorac Surg 60:1348–1352
113. Vansteenkiste JF, Stroobants SG, de Leyn PR et al (1999) Prognostic importance of the Standardized Uptake Value on FDG-PET-scan in non-small cell lung cancer: an analysis of 125 cases. J Clin Oncol 17:3201–3206
114. Ahuja V, Coleman RE, Herndon J et al (1998) The prognostic significance of fluorodeoxyglucose positron emission tomography imaging for patients with nonsmall cell lung carcinoma. Cancer 83:918–924
115. Patz EF, Connolly J, Herndon J (2000) Prognostic value of thoracic FDG PET imaging after treatment for non-small cell lung cancer. AJR Am J Roentgenol 174:769–774
116. Swensen SJ, Brown LR, Colby TV et al (1996) Lung nodule enhancement at CT: prospective findings. Radiology 201:447–455
117. Seemann MD, Seemann O, Luboldt W et al (2000) Differentiation of malignant from benign solitary pulmonary lesions using chest radiography, spiral CT and HRCT. Lung Cancer 29: 105–124
118. Schreurs AJ, Westermann CJ, van den Bosch JM et al (1992) A twenty-five-year follow-up of ninety-three resected typical carcinoid tumors of the lung. J Thorac Cardiovasc Surg 104: 1470–1475
119. Jang HJ, Lee KS, Kwon OJ et al (1996) Bronchioloalveolar carcinoma: focal area of ground-glass attenuation at thin-section CT as an early sign. Radiology 199:485–488
120. Vansteenkiste JF, de Leyn PR, Deneffe GJ et al (1997) Survival and prognostic factors in resected N2 non-small cell lung cancer: a study of 140 cases. The Leuven Lung Cancer Group. Ann Thorac Surg 63:1441–1450
121. Gambhir SS, Hoh CK, Phelps ME et al (1996) Decision tree sensitivity analysis for cost-effectiveness of FDG- PET in the staging and management of non-small cell lung carcinoma. J Nucl Med 37:1428–1436
122. Bury T, Dowlati A, Paulus P et al (1996) Staging of non-small cell lung cancer by whole-body fluorine-18 deoxyglucose positron emission tomography. Eur J Nucl Med 23:204–206
123. Lewis P, Griffin S, Marsden P et al (1994) Whole-body 18F-fluorodeoxyglucose positron emission tomography in preoperative evaluation of lung cancer. Lancet 344:1265–1266
124. Nettelbladt OS, Sundin AE, Valind SO et al (1998) Combined fluorine-18-FDG and carbon-11-methionine PET for diagnosis of tumors in lung and mediastinum. J Nucl Med 39:640–647
125. Sasaki M, Kuwabara Y, Yoshida T et al (2001) Comparison of MET-PET and FDG-PET for differentiation between benign lesions and malignant tumors of the lung. Ann Nucl Med 15: 425–431
126. Yasukawa T, Yoshikawa K, Aoyagi H et al (2000) Usefulness of PET with 11C-methionine for the detection of hilar and mediastinal lymph node metastasis in lung cancer. J Nucl Med 41: 283–290
127. Pieterman RM, Que TH, Elsinga PH et al (2002) Comparison of (11)C-choline and (18)F-FDG PET in primary diagnosis and staging of patients with thoracic cancer. J Nucl Med 43:167–172
128. Hara T, Inagaki K, Kosaka N et al (2000) Sensitive detection of mediastinal lymph node metastasis of lung cancer with 11C-choline PET. J Nucl Med 41:1507–1513
129. Shields AF, Grierson JR, Dohmen BM et al (1998) Imaging proliferation in vivo with [F-18]FLT and positron emission tomography. Nat Med 4:1334–1336
130. Vesselle H, Grierson J, Muzi M et al (2002) In vivo validation of 3'deoxy-3'-[(18)F]fluorothymidine (18F-FLT) as a proliferation imaging tracer in humans: correlation of 18F-FLT uptake by positron emission tomography with Ki-67 immunohistochemistry and flow cytometry in human lung tumors. Clin Cancer Res 8:3315–3323
131. Buck AK, Schirrmeister H, Hetzel M et al (2002) 3-deoxy-3-[(18)F]fluorothymidine-positron emission tomography for noninvasive assessment of proliferation in pulmonary nodules. Cancer Res 62:3331–3334
132. Van Tinteren H, Hoekstra OS, Smit EF et al (2002) Effectiveness of positron emission tomography in the preoperative assessment of patients with suspected non-small cell lung cancer: the PLUS multicentre randomised trial. Lancet 359:1388–1393
133. Tewson TJ, Krohn KA (1998) PET radiopharmaceuticals: state-of-the-art and future prospects. Semin Nucl Med 28:221–234
134. Alauddin MM, Shahinian A, Kundu RK et al (1999) Evaluation of 9-[(3–18F-fluoro-1-hydroxy-2-propoxy)methyl]guanine ([18F]-FHPG) in vitro and in vivo as a probe for PET imaging of gene incorporation and expression in tumors. Nucl Med Biol 26:371–376
135. Alauddin MM, Conti PS (1998) Synthesis and preliminary evaluation of 9-(4-[18F]-fluoro-3-hydroxymethylbutyl)guanine ([18F]FHBG): a new potential imaging agent for viral infection and gene therapy using PET. Nucl Med Biol 25:175–180
136. Price P, Jones T (1995) Can positron emission tomography (PET) be used to detect subclinical response to cancer therapy? The EC PET Oncology Concerted Action and the EORTC PET Study Group. Eur J Cancer 31A:1924–1927
137. Shreve PD, Anzai Y, Wahl RL (1999) Pitfalls in oncologic diagnosis with FDG PET imaging: physiologic and benign variants. Radiographics 19:61–77
138. Langen KJ, Braun U, Rota Kops E et al (1993) The influence of plasma glucose levels on fluorine-18-fluorodeoxyglucose uptake in bronchial carcinomas. J Nucl Med 34:355–359
139. Gorenberg M, Hallett WA, O'Doherty MJ (2002) Does diabetes affect (18)F-FDG standardised uptake values in lung cancer? Eur J Nucl Med Mol Imaging 29:1324–1327
140. Hoekstra CJ, Paglianiti I, Hoekstra OS et al (2000) Monitoring response to therapy in cancer using [18F]-2-fluoro-2-deoxy-D-glucose and positron emission tomography: an overview of different analytical methods. Eur J Nucl Med 27:731–743
141. Hoekstra CJ, Hoekstra OS, Stroobants SG et al (2002) Methods to monitor response to chemotherapy in non-small cell lung cancer with 18F-FDG PET. J Nucl Med 43:1304–1309

CHAPTER 16

Breast Cancer

H. Palmedo

16.1 Incidence and Epidemiology

Breast cancer is one of the biggest challenges for medical care in the modern industrial countries. It is the most frequent cancer disease in women and the second leading cause of cancer-related death. In the USA, about 180,000 new cases are diagnosed annually and approximately 13 out of 100 women will develop breast cancer during their lifetime [1]. As millions of women are at risk, this disease is responsible for a considerable amount of patient anxiety as well as medical cost.

The incidence of breast cancer has increased over recent decades but mortality has been stabilizing over the past few years [2]. Generally, the risk for having breast cancer increases during a lifetime, reaching a maximum incidence between the fifth and sixth decades. Breast cancer is uncommon in women under the age of 30 years. However, if a woman is a carrier of the BRCA gene 1 or 2, development of breast cancer early during her lifetime is probable [3, 4].

16.2 Histopathological Classification, Pathology and Prognosis of Breast Cancer

The mammary gland consists of 16–20 lobes, which are embedded in the dense fibroareolar stroma [5]. Each lobe is composed of multiple ducts branching to the terminal ducts, which are followed by the lobules, the exocrine-active tissue. Most breast cancers develop in this terminal duct lobular area.

Generally, tumors are classified into invasive and non-invasive carcinomas and, additionally, subdivided into ductal and lobular types. The ductal carcinomas are diagnosed most frequently, comprising approximately 80 % of all invasive breast cancers [6]. Invasive lobular carcinomas account for about 10 % and medullary carcinomas for 5 % of malignant breast tumors. Tumors such as tubular and papillary carcinomas are less common and often have a better prognosis.

Non-invasive breast cancer is divided into two subgroups, ductal (DCIS) and lobular (LCIS) carcinoma in situ [5]. The growth pattern of these tumors is characterized by intraductal tumor extension without invasion of the basement membrane. Tumor cell masses fill in the terminal duct lobular unit and the adjacent ducts. Malignant cells may then break through the basement membrane and the tumor becomes invasive. DCIS is traditionally considered a pre-cancer stage that can convert into invasive cancer after a certain time. It has been recognized recently that LCIS is also a significant risk factor for developing breast cancer. Multicentric and bilateral growth of LCIS is responsible for the high breast cancer risk. LCIS does not present as a palpable tumor and is often diagnosed incidentally in breast biopsies. DCIS produces microcalcification in about 50 % of cases and can, therefore, be diagnosed on mammograms. In comparison to LCIS, tumor growth of DCIS is more often confined to one breast or even one quadrant, but both types of CIS frequently occur bilaterally.

Invasive breast cancers can also present more than one solid tumor. Multifocal tumor growth is defined as one quadrant of the breast with at least two different tumor sites, multicentric growth as two different quadrants of the same breast revealing tumor tissue. It has been found that about 60 % of tumors with a diameter of up to 4 cm have satellites around the main focus [7]. Most breast cancers are found in the upper outer quadrant of the breast. All malignant breast tumors are classified following the tumor–node–metastasis (TNM) classification of the American Joint Committee on Cancer (AJCC) and the Union Internationale Contre le Cancer (UICC), summarized in Table 1. Classification of the primary tumor includes carcinomas in situ and that of the tumor size only relates to the invasive component of the cancer. If multiple tumors are present at the same time in one breast, the tumor with the largest dimension is taken into account for T-staging. In the case of bilateral tumor growth, each cancer is staged separately. T1 tumors are subdivided into four subgroups.

Most breast carcinomas first metastasize in the locoregional lymph nodes. In over 90 % of cases, lymph node metastases develop in the axillary region. If the carcinoma is located in the medial part of the breast (upper or lower medial quadrant), lymph node metastases of the internal mammary chain will be present in up to 10 % of the axilla-negative patients. If the axilla is

Table 1. Pathologic TNM classification of breast cancer

Primary tumor (T)	
Tx	Primary tumor cannot be assessed
T0	No evidence of primary tumor
Tis	Carcinoma in situ
T1	Tumor 2 cm or less in greatest dimension
T1mic	Microinvasion 0.1 cm or less in greatest dimension
T1a	Tumor more than 0.1 cm but not more than 0.5 cm in greatest dimension
T1b	Tumor more than 0.5 cm but not more than 1 cm in greatest dimension
T1c	Tumor more than 1 cm but not more than 2 cm in greatest dimension
T2	Tumor more than 2 cm but not more than 5 cm in greatest dimension
T3	Tumor more than 5 cm in greatest dimension
T4	Tumor of any size with direct extension to
T4a	– the chest wall (does not include the pectoral muscle)
T4b	– the skin
T4c	– the chest wall and the skin
T4d	Inflammatory carcinoma
Regional lymph nodes (N)	
Nx	Regional lymph nodes cannot be assessed
N0	No regional lymph node metastasis
N1	Metastasis to movable ipsilateral axillary lymph node(s)
N1a	Only micrometastases (none larger than 0.2 cm)
N1b	Metastasis to lymph node(s), any larger than 0.2 cm
N1bi	Metastasis in 1–3 lymph nodes, any more than 0.2 cm but less than 2 cm
N1bii	Metastasis to 4 or more lymph nodes, any more than 0.2 cm but less than 2 cm
N1biii	Extension beyond the capsule of a lymph node less than 2 cm in diameter
N1biv	Metastasis to a lymph node 2 cm or more in greatest dimension
N2	Metastasis to ipsilateral axillary lymph nodes that are fixed
N3	Metastasis to ipsilateral internal mammary lymph node(s)
Distant metastasis (M)	
Mx	Distant metastasis cannot be assessed
M0	No distant metastasis
M1	Distant metastasis[a]

[a] Supraclavicular lymph nodes are considered distant metastases

positive, it will be in up to 30 % of the cases. In 80 % of breast cancer patients, the axilla is the only site of metastatic disease. The axillary lymph nodes are divided into three different groups depending on their anatomical location: level I marking the lymphatic region located laterally from the minor pectoralis muscle; level II indicating all lymph nodes that are located between the large and small pectoralis muscles; level III lymph nodes lying medially from the minor pectoralis muscle. Generally, tumor cells start metastasizing in level I followed by the next higher level. In about 1 % of cases, so-called skip metastases can be found, meaning that a higher level presents metastatic disease while level I is free of lymph node metastases [8]. The principle of sentinel node biopsy is based on the theory that one or more specific lymph node(s) in the local lymphatic basin drains the tumor. These node(s) should then be the first site of lymph node metastases.

There is a clear correlation between the tumor size and the frequency of axillary lymph node metastases [9]. However, about 30 % of large tumors never develop lymphatic disease (and 10 % never develop distant metastases) and approximately 15 % of small tumors less than 1 cm have deposited axillary and distant metastases. This shows that, apart from tumor size, the biological behavior determines the time point of metastasizing. Traditionally, it was thought that breast carcinoma cells first entered the locoregional lymph nodes. These diseased nodes could then be the origin of distant metastases. Recent data have led us to understand breast cancer as a systemic disease. Therefore, it is likely that in a certain percentage of cases, distant metastases will develop even if axillary lymph nodes do not reveal metastatic disease. Distant metastases are frequently located in the bone and bone marrow, the lung, the liver and the brain.

The size of the tumor and the number of lymph node metastases also correlate with the frequency of distant metastatic disease and, therefore, with the prognosis of the patient [10, 11]. The most important factors predicting survival of breast cancer patients are tumor size, tumor differentiation (grade 1 well differentiated, grade 2 moderately differentiated, grade 3 poorly differentiated, grade 4 undifferentiated), lymph node and distant metastases, and expression of progesterone and estrogen receptors.

16.3 Conventional Diagnostic Procedures and Treatment Strategies

Over 80 % of breast tumors are detected by the woman herself or by a routine breast examination. This fact clearly emphasizes the importance of self-examination. Generally, each newly detected breast mass is considered suspicious and needs further examination. Typical clinical signs indicating malignancy are retraction of the skin, peau d'orange, deviation of the nipple and ulceration of the skin. However, these are signs of a late stage cancer. Depending on the size and tissue density of the breast as well as the location of the tumor, cancers can be palpable down to a size of 1 cm. In women with large breasts or dense tissue, breast cancer may have grown much bigger before it can be detected by palpation. This problem also exists in patients with fibrocystic disease, who often present with multiple palpable breast masses. Breast cancers are frequently described as painless, irregularly defined, not removable nodules or masses of augmented consistency. However, there are no criteria that allow clear differentiation between malignant and non-malignant lesions. Additionally, tumors with a diffuse growth pattern may not be palpable at all.

To increase the sensitivity and specificity of physical examination, further diagnostic methods are necessary. In the diagnostic work-up of patients with a suspicious breast mass, mammography plays a major role. Mammography is needed to localize and assess the extent of a suspicious tumor. In the case of a breast carcinoma, mammography typically reveals an ill-defined opacity with stellar extensions that is identified on a lateral and craniocaudal view of the compressed breasts. Microcalcification of a polymorph pattern may be present and indicates malignancy with high accuracy. Moreover, non-palpable intraductally growing parts of the tumor can be diagnosed mammographically, allowing optimization of the therapeutic management of the patient. In about 25% of all invasive breast cancers, intraductal tumor growth is present in addition to a solid tumor mass. Finally, mammography is used to examine the asymptomatic breast of the patient because breast cancer may appear bilaterally. If the described mammographic signs for malignancy are present, the sensitivity of mammography is approximately 90% [12]. However, mammography has some important shortcomings that make further diagnostic tools necessary, including its low positive predictive value. Also regularly shaped opacities can be generated by cancers and many suspicious microcalcifications are benign, resulting in a low specificity. Diagnosis of malignant tumor will be confirmed by histopathology in only about three of ten patients with suspected breast cancer [13]. This means that many patients with benign breast lesions must undergo surgery because differentiation between malignant and benign lesions is often impossible by mammography. Furthermore, the cancer disease in the breast will be missed by mammography in about 10% of cases, even if the carcinoma is palpable.

Mammography is the only imaging modality in breast cancer patients that has been proven to be useful as a screening tool in asymptomatic women [14–16]. In women older than 50 years, several studies have provided evidence that mammography decreases mortality from breast cancer by approximately 30%. In this context, it is important that mammography is not only able to detect the smallest cancers, but also pre-malignant lesions and carcinomas in situ (DCIS and LCIS), being mainly diagnosed by microcalcifications. Although mammography does not have all the properties of an ideal screening method (high sensitivity, high specificity, high availability, low costs, non-invasive and harmless), the benefit is clearly high enough to recommend it to all women over 49 years. Countries that perform a mammographic screening program generally advise women to have one screening mammogram per year, including a physical examination.

Sonography of the breasts is widely used as an adjunct to mammography because it can increase specificity during the diagnostic work-up of a palpable breast lesion. Ultrasound is able to differentiate between cystic and solid tumors [12]. Normally, a cystic lesion has a sharply delineated borderline surrounding an echo-free area and induces strengthening of the echo signal behind the cyst, resulting in an hyperechogenic area. If a lesion is malignant, typically an irregularly shaped and hypoechogenic mass with posterior shadowing phenomenon is found. Limitations of sonography are that microcalcifications are not detectable and that interobserver variability is high because the clinician's experience significantly influences the diagnostic accuracy. Although specificity of sonography is higher than that of mammography, biopsy of the lesion is still indispensable for most patients. Sonography is used to help localize the lesion before fine needle aspiration, core needle biopsy or placing of a preoperative wire is performed. Sonography of the breast is not recommended as a screening method for breast cancer.

Magnetic resonance imaging (MRI) of the breast has gained interest due to its high sensitivity for the detection of breast cancer [17]. MRI is performed after injection of the contrast agent gadolinium, positioning the patient's breasts in a special table device with a breast coil. The intensity and velocity of gadolinium enhancement in breast lesions is used for diagnosis of breast disease. It has been shown that most breast cancers can be detected because of their contrast agent enhancement mirroring neovascularization of the tumor. Sensitivity of MRI for invasive breast cancer was calculated between 90 and 95% in several studies. There is no negative impact of breast density on tumor detection by MRI but medication with estrogens and the hormonal status during the first part of the cycle can result in a diffuse uptake pattern of gadolinium in normal breast tissue and mask breast cancer or mimic multifocal cancer disease. MRI of the breast is often recommended if mammography is not diagnostic in patients with dense breast tissue or with unclear findings. Furthermore, MRI can be used to exclude preoperatively multifocal or multicentric disease and to explore breast prostheses suspected for recurrent breast cancer. However, MRI is not able to detect microcalcifications and has a low sensitivity for diagnosing carcinoma in situ. Specificity of MRI is markedly lower than sensitivity, so that biopsy is still necessary in most patients. MRI cannot replace mammography.

As a result of the above limitations of the imaging modalities, in most patients, fine needle aspiration, core needle or open biopsy of the tumor will be necessary to find the final diagnosis.

If breast cancer has been diagnosed, the tumor is removed surgically. For many years, radical mastectomy has been the treatment of choice in this patient group, as first proposed by Halsted [18]. During the past few decades, modified mastectomy was the main operation used to eliminate tumor tissue. However, the esthetic results of mastectomy are generally not well accepted by the woman. Studies have shown that breast-conserving surgery, e.g. lumpectomy, is an effective treatment option if the tumor-to-breast relation allows an adequate tumor resection [19]. In many centers, breast-conserving surgery is confined to patients with tumors of a maximum size between 2 and 3 cm, provided their breast size is 'normal'. Patients with bigger tumors, multifocal/multicentric disease or small breasts often still have to undergo mastectomy. If breast-conserving surgery is performed, external beam irradiation of the breast is mandatory to avoid a higher risk of local recurrence compared to mastectomy. If locally advanced breast cancer is present, generally, preoperative chemotherapy will be performed. After reduction of tumor masses by chemotherapy, surgical resection of the remaining cancer cells is feasible.

Axillary lymph node dissection is performed in all breast cancer patients who undergo breast surgery due to primary invasive breast cancer. At least ten lymph nodes (for levels I and II; only six for level III) have to be sampled and histopathologically examined to stage the axilla. Axillary staging is dependent on macroscopic criteria (N1 = movable, N2 = fixed lymph node metastasis), the number and the size of lymph node metastases (N1a–N1biv). Operative lymph node sampling is necessary to obtain sufficient prognostic information about the patient and to be able to choose the optimal treatment procedure after surgery. It is known that patients with axillary lymph node metastases have a significantly lower survival rate compared with lymph node negative patients. Traditionally, the prognosis becomes worse with the following three groups: patients with no axillary lymph node metastases; those with -one to three axillary lymph node metastases; those with more than three axillary lymph node metastases [20]. The likelihood of developing distant metastases increases from group to group. The axillary lymph node status is still one of the most important factors for predicting the survival rate. The internal mammary lymph nodes (N3-metastases) are not principally investigated. Supraclavicular lymph node metastases are considered as distant metastases. With the more widespread use of screening mammography, the amount of breast cancers detected at an earlier stage is increasing and consequently, axillary lymph node metastases are present in only one-third of patients. Axillary dissection will, however, cause side effects of lymphedema and movement disorders in up to 30 % of these patients. One effort to optimize the benefit for patients with smaller breast cancer is the strategy of sentinel node biopsy (SNB). The principle of SNB is to mark the sentinel lymph node (see Chap. 2) using radioactively labeled colloid or blue dye and to localize it for operative resection. Using the radioactive labeling method, the sentinel node can be identified preoperatively by scintigraphy and by a hand-held gamma probe. The probe also helps the surgeon to localize the sentinel node intraoperatively and to reduce the operating time. When the surgeon has removed the sentinel node, it is examined by the pathologist. As only one to three lymph node(s) have to be examined, histopathological examination is not confined to conventional hematoxylin and eosin (HE) staining. Furthermore, the thin-layer technique and immunohistochemical tests can be applied, often detecting micrometastases that would have been missed by conventional HE staining. If histopathological examination shows that the sentinel node is not diseased, the patient would be considered as lymph node metastases negative. The results of ongoing studies will determine whether SNB can replace standard axillary lymph node dissection in breast cancer patients. The advantage of this new method is a significant reduction of operation-related morbidity because the surgeon only has to resect one to three lymph nodes.

Preoperative staging of breast cancer patients should comprise X-ray of the thorax, sonography of the liver and bone scintigraphy. In symptomatic patients, imaging modalities such as computed tomography (CT) and MRI will also be performed.

Depending on the results of the preoperative and the operative staging procedures, an adjuvant treatment will be chosen. Generally, the oncologist has to decide if no further treatment is necessary or if adjuvant chemotherapy and/or hormonal therapy must be performed. The prognostic factors that are taken into account for this decision-making are expression of estrogens and progesterone receptors, tumor size and differentiation, axillary lymph node status, distant metastases and the menopausal status of the patient. In Europe, new treatment recommendations are regularly elaborated for breast cancer patients at the St. Gallen consensus meeting [21]. The last conference proposed to divide patients with primary breast cancer into three groups (low, intermediate and high risk), depending on the aforementioned predictive parameters. For each group, an adjuvant treatment scheme is recommended to increase the survival rate of patients.

If distant metastases are diagnosed, a palliative treatment option (chemotherapy, bisphosphonates, radiotherapy) is initiated in symptomatic patients.

16.4 PET in Breast Cancer

16.4.1 Methodological Aspects of PET Imaging

The standard protocol used for fluoro-2-deoxy-D-glucose (FDG) positron emission tomography (PET) imaging in oncologic patients is also applied for breast cancer imaging. The patient is advised to fast for at least 6 hours before the FDG injection. This procedure stabilizes the plasma glucose and plasma insulin level. It has been demonstrated that glucose levels correlate inversely with FDG uptake in tumors and the brain [22]. Therefore, FDG uptake in breast cancers will be inhibited in hyperglycemic patients. A high plasma glucose level also induces insulin secretion, which mediates glucose transport in many tissue such as muscles. Thus monitoring of the blood sugar level is mandatory before the FDG injection and the glucose concentration should be below 150 mg/100 ml. Acute normalization of high glucose levels by injection of insulin is not advisable because this procedure leads to increased background activity (e.g. muscle), resulting in a high risk of false-negative PET images. Generally, it is recommended to inject intravenously 370 MBq (10 mCi) [^{18}F]FDG using a two-dimensional (2D) acquisition mode. Also normal lymph nodes are frequently visualized if FDG is injected subcutaneously by paravasation. For this purpose, the injection should be performed into an arm vein contralateral to the suspected breast or (if both breasts are affected) into a foot vein. When the breasts are examined, the patient must be positioned in a prone position with raised arms. A special table device allowing the breasts to hang freely is necessary to avoid breast compression and imaging artifacts. For whole-body imaging, the patient is normally studied in the supine position. Acquisition should be started 60 minutes after the FDG injection. Delayed scans (90–120 min) are possible and seem to reduce background activity; however, the loss of image quality due to the physical decay has to be taken into account. Acquisition time of emission scans should be at least 10 minutes using the 2D mode. Scanning time can be reduced if the 3D mode is used because the sensitivity is much higher compared to the 2D mode. With whole-body imaging, the patient is advised to void the bladder before the start of imaging to avoid artifacts caused by bladder activity. Data acquisition should begin at the proximal femora and the pelvic region and then move on up to the head and neck. Iterative reconstruction algorithms are preferred to filtered back projection [23]. Attenuation correction is essential to guarantee optimal diagnostic accuracy. Tumors that are located in deeper regions in comparison to the body surface may be missed without attenuation correction. However, pulmonary lesions are often better visualized in non-corrected images. Thus, it is advisable to read corrected as well as non-corrected PET images to yield the most accurate results. All lesions should be quantified by determining standard uptake values (SUV) of the suspicious region. This can be helpful in differentiating and characterizing malignant and benign lesions. Calculating SUV by normalization of injected dose and body weight is the most common method for tumor quantification. SUV correction for partial volume effects and normalization to glucose concentration can furthermore enhance the diagnostic power of PET. Breast cancer typically presents with one or more areas of focally increased FDG uptake and benign tumors show no or faint tracer accumulation. Benign proliferative breast tissue may demonstrate diffuse and moderately augmented FDG uptake. When evaluating whole-body images, FDG uptake of suspicious lesions can be compared to the physiologic uptake intensity of other organs, e.g. the liver, to build a score.

16.4.2 Imaging of the Breast

Several studies have investigated PET in primary breast carcinoma with a total of more than 450 patients [24–35]. Data are summarized in Table 2. The first reports of FDG PET imaging of the breast included patients with locally advanced breast cancer and metastatic disease that had already been diagnosed by other techniques. Nevertheless, sensitivity was high, approaching 100%. Later studies with larger patient groups generally confirmed the good results, with sensitivities and specificities ranging between 67 and 95%, and 70 and 90%, respectively.

One important limitation demonstrated by various investigators is a low detection rate of small breast cancers. A sharp decline of sensitivity has been noted if the maximum tumor diameter is below 1 cm. In a larger study of 185 breast tumors [32], Avril et al. found a sensitivity of 68% in stage pT1 cancers (<2 cm) compared

Table 2. FDG PET for imaging of the breasts

Authors	Patients (n)	Sensitivity (%)	Specificity (%)
Wahl et al. [26]	10	100	–
Tse et al. [27]	10	86	100
Adler et al. [28]	28	96	100
Hoh et al. [29]	20	88	33[a]
Avril et al. [32]	51	68–83[b]	84–97[b]
Scheidhauer et al. [33]	30	91b	86b
Palmedo et al. [34]	20	92	86
Avril et al. [35]	144	64–80	75–94
Schirrmeister et al. [44]	117	93	75

[a] Only three patients with benign tumors were studied;
[b] range due to sensitive vs normal image reading

to a sensitivity of 92% in stage pT2 cancers (2–5 cm). The same group evaluated the impact of sensitive image reading in contrast to conventional image reading on diagnostic accuracy. Sensitive (also suspicious FDG uptake regarded as positive) reading was able to increase overall sensitivity from 64 to 80% but decreased specificity from 94 to 75%. Our experience in a smaller group of patients undergoing scintimammography with Tc-99m MIBI and FDG PET of the breasts, did not show a difference in palpable cancers; however, both techniques missed an 8 mm malignant tumor (Fig. 1) [34].

The spatial resolution of PET systems, which ranges between 6 and 8 mm in most scanners, significantly influences the detection rate of breast cancer. Partial volume effects cause a small cancer to appear larger and less intensive. This means that small tumors have to accumulate proportionally more radioactivity than bigger tumors to be detectable. Besides the technical parameters already mentioned, the tumor-to-background ratio has a major impact on detectability of the lesion. It has been found that the phosphorylation rate of FDG by the enzyme hexokinase is much lower in breast cancer cells compared to lung cancer tissue, resulting in a lower FDG uptake in breast carcinomas. FDG uptake in breast cancer is influenced by several factors, such as the microvasculature, glucose-1 transporter expression, hexokinase activity, the number of tumor cells per volume and the proliferation rate [36]. It is likely that glucose utilization increases exponentially with tumor growth and that only bigger cancers (>1 cm) are mainly composed of less oxygen-dependent cell clones, which have a high rate of anaerobic glycolysis. Moreover, normal breast tissue frequently shows a certain physiological FDG uptake, decreasing the image contrast. Investigations with animal breast cancer models have demonstrated that FDG uptake reflects predominantly the proliferating activity of the tumor [37]. Our own experience from a breast cancer model is that FDG has nevertheless favorable characteristics for breast cancer imaging due to its trapping mechanism and low uptake in muscles [38].

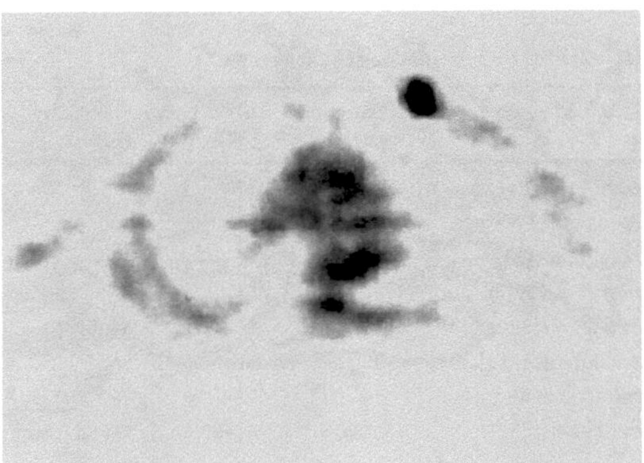

Fig. 1. Transverse FDG PET slice with focal accumulation in an invasive ductal carcinoma of the left breast (pT2N0)

It is of relevance that the histological tumor type influences the diagnostic accuracy of PET breast imaging. Studies have reported that invasive lobular carcinomas have lower SUV and sensitivities than invasive ductal carcinomas. Avril et al. found a rate of false-negative findings of 65% in lobular cancers compared to 24% in ductal cancers. Invasive lobular carcinomas of the breast are also more difficult to diagnose by conventional imaging methods such as mammography due to the diffuse growth pattern.

Before breast-conserving surgery is performed, multifocal and multicentric breast disease must be excluded. Avril et al. found a sensitivity of 50% for the detection of multifocal or multicentric disease in 18 patients. Since multifocally growing tumor sites are often small, the limitations of PET mentioned previously also apply to this clinical situation.

There are only few data on PET and the detection of carcinomas in situ. So far only larger in situ cancers have been detected by PET. It is likely that PET imaging cannot improve diagnosis of this tumor group, which is increasingly detected by mammography.

Generally, FDG uptake in benign lesions of the breast is low [28, 32, 34]. In our patient group, we found one fibroadenoma demonstrating a moderate FDG accumulation. Other authors have also reported false-positive findings in fibroplastic or dysplastic tissue, ductal and fibroadenoma. Inflammatory processes such as an abscess can result in significant FDG uptake but they principally do not represent a diagnostic problem for conventional breast imaging. Avril et al. reported three false-positive findings out of 53 benign breast masses demonstrating focally increased accumulation. Although the number of benign breast lesions investigated is lower than the number of cancers, intense FDG accumulation in these lesions is not common. The SUV has been studied in breast lesions by several authors, who have tried to use it to differentiate malignant from benign masses. Generally, most cancers reveal a SUV higher than 2.5 [32] and most benign tumors are below this level. However, there is a significant overlap between the two groups that does not allow them to be separated clearly. Correction for partial volume effect delivers most accurate results for quantitation.

16.4.3
Locoregional Lymph Node Involvement

Although various predictive factors for survival of breast cancer patients have been found, axillary lymph node involvement is still one of the most important predictors and needs to be available to help the clinician choose the right adjuvant therapy. So far no non-invasive imaging method has revealed a diagnostic accuracy high enough to replace surgical removal of axillary lymph nodes. More than 600 patients have been studied and showed sensitivities and specificities ranging between 73 and 100%, and 93 and 100%, respectively (Table 3, Fig. 2) [28, 33, 39–42]. It seems that due to the spatial resolution, small lymph node metastases are frequently missed. Therefore, FDG PET cannot be used to diagnose the exact number of affected lymph nodes, which needs to be known for subsequent therapy recommendations. Avril et al. observed six patients with pT1 tumors (<2 cm) and axillary micrometastases. In only two of the six patients with micrometastases, PET was able to detect lymph node involvement resulting in a sensitivity of 33%. In contrast, in patients with primaries larger than 2 cm (>pT1), FDG PET achieved a sensitivity of 94%. Utech et al., however, studied patients with primaries bigger than 1 cm and found a high sensitivity (100%) and a low specificity (69%; 20 of 64 false-positive lymph nodes). We studied 63 patients suspected to have recurrent breast carcinoma and compared FDG PET findings with those of CT and MRI [43]. Sensitivity of PET for the detection of lymph node metastases was 97%. Overall, 17 of a total of 25 (68%) identified lymph nodes were true-positive by PET and CT/MRI. Additionally, five true-positive lesions (20%) were only identified by FDG PET but no lesion was identified by CT/MRI alone. Other authors have also observed that PET imaging provided additional diagnostic information in about 30% of the breast cancer patients studied, mainly due to diagnosis of axillary involvement at level III, of periclavicular or of retrosternal lymph node metastases [39, 42].

The data indicate that FDG PET is a very sensitive imaging modality to detect lymph node metastases. It can be particularly helpful in the evaluation of parasternal/mediastinal lymph nodes if the tumor is located in the inner quadrants of the breast.

Table 3. FDG PET for assessment of lymph node metastases

Authors	Patients (*n*)	Sensitivity (%)	Specificity (%)
Adler et al. [28]	10	90	100
Avril et al. [32]	51	79	96
Scheidhauer et al. [33]	18	100	89
Utech et al. [53]	124	100	75
Adler et al. [28]	50	95	66
Bender et al. [43]	75	97	91
Crippa et al. [54]	68	85	91
Smith et al. [51]	50	90	97
Greco et al. [41]	167	94	86
Eubank et al. [42]	73	85	90

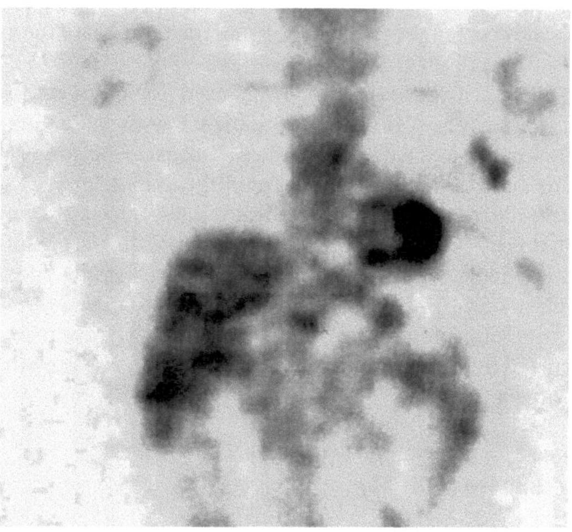

Fig. 2. Coronal slice of FDG PET of a patient with breast cancer pT1c and axillary disease demonstrating axillary uptake in lymph node metastases

16.4.4 Distant Metastases

There is evidence that treatment of relapsed breast cancer does not prolong survival of patients. This fact has led to a change of the traditional follow-up scheme recommending that imaging modalities such as bone scintigraphy are performed at defined time intervals. Since there is no treatment option increasing survival for asymptomatic patients with recurrent disease that has been detected early, the follow-up program has been confined to mammography and a clinical examination. However, when the patient becomes symptomatic or tumor markers begin to rise further, imaging will be initiated. If recurrent disease has been diagnosed, palliative treatment will be started to improve quality of life.

One major advantage of PET imaging is the ability to use this method for whole-body staging. Some studies report high sensitivities and specificities for the detection of distant metastases at different sites [43–45]. In our study group, consisting of 75 patients suspected of recurrent or metastatic disease, whole-body PET findings were compared with those of CT/MRI. PET imaging correctly identified 28 (97%) out of 29 cases with lymph node involvement (Fig. 3), 15 (100%) of 15 patients with bone metastases, five (83%) of six with lung and two patients with liver metastases. Interestingly, PET diagnosed seven bone metastases that were not detected by CT or MRI. In a study with a similar patient group, Moon et al. [46] observed a sensitivity and specificity of whole-body PET imaging of 85 and 79%, respectively, if calculated on a per-lesion basis. On a per-patient basis, the sensitivity increased to 93% with identical specificity. In contrast to our findings, the authors report a relatively high number of false-negative bone metastases. It has been shown that osteolytic metastases accu-

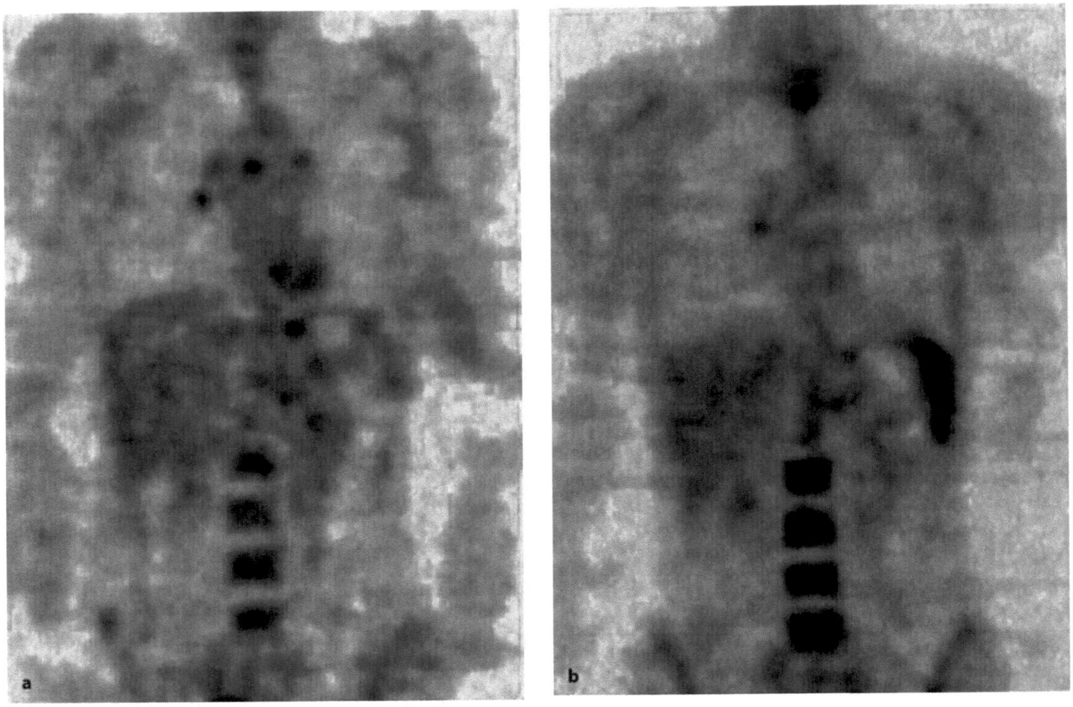

Fig. 3. a Coronal FDG PET slice demonstrates metastatic disease of breast cancer to the mediastinal lymph nodes. **b** After chemotherapy, FDG accumulation has almost completely disappeared, indicating good response to treatment

mulate FDG with much higher intensity than osteosclerotic lesions. In a study comparing conventional bone scintigraphy with FDG PET, PET identified more lesions than bone scintigraphy [47]. However, in the subgroup of osteosclerotic disease, osseous metastases were often missed by FDG PET. The data indicate that bone scintigraphy cannot simply be replaced by FDG PET without further evaluation. Schirrmeister et al. found that FDG PET is more accurate than standard staging procedures (X-ray, sonography, bone scintigraphy) in the preoperative staging of breast cancer patients [44].

In comparison to conventional imaging, there is evidence that FDG PET is able to detect additional metastatic lesions. Therefore, PET can be useful if identifying metastatic disease is of therapeutic relevance and if conventional imaging is non-diagnostic but tumor markers are rising.

16.4.5 Local Recurrence

In approximately 80 % of cases, local recurrence appears within the 5 years following breast surgery. The risk of developing local recurrence correlates with the same factors that predict distant metastases: tumor size and differentiation, axillary lymph node status and disease-free interval. The risk for local recurrence of a node-negative woman is about 5–9 % and increases to 20–28 % if axillary nodes are positive. Most local recurrences are localized in the direct vicinity of the primary tumor. Local recurrence is the only site of tumor manifestation in about half of patients; the remainder present distant metastases at the time of diagnosis of local recurrence or within a few months later. In general, all patients with local recurrence will develop distant metastases, so the 5-year overall survival ranges between 0 and 50 %.

Primarily, mammography is used to diagnose local recurrence. However, in patients with augmentation mammoplasties or after breast-conserving surgery and radiation therapy, it is often difficult to diagnose local recurrence mammographically. Studies have shown that FDG PET can detect local recurrence. In a group of 20 patients, we found a sensitivity of 80 % and a specificity of 96 % for FDG PET compared to 93 and 98 % for MR imaging of the breast. False-negative results occurred in tumors with small diameter or diffuse growth pattern (<7 mm).

16.4.6 Monitoring of Therapy

In locally advanced breast cancer, preoperative chemotherapy is increasingly used to increase the rate of breast-conserving surgery. Moreover, neoadjuvant che-

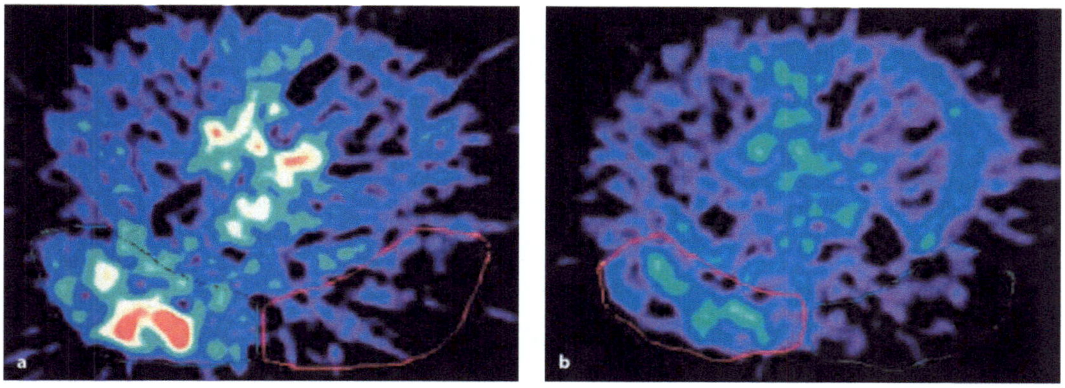

Fig. 4. a Transverse FDG PET slice of a patient with locally advanced breast carcinoma before chemotherapy. **b** One week after the first cycle of treatment, FDG PET clearly demonstrates decrease of FDG accumulation, indicating good response to chemotherapy. The clinical course of the disease thereafter confirmed this finding

motherapy may improve the patient's survival. It offers the clinician the possibility to change the chemotherapeutic regimen if there is no response to treatment. There is evidence that tumor response to preoperative chemotherapy correlates strongly with disease-free and overall survival [48, 49]. Clinical response criteria are frequently insufficient to define the effect of chemotherapy on the tumor prior to definitive breast surgery. In these cases, it would be helpful to use an imaging modality indicating tumor response with the same high accuracy that histopathology offers. In patients with distant metastases, therapeutic monitoring is also important; however, it is more difficult because no histopathological results are available routinely. As a compromise, anatomical imaging is performed to determine therapeutic success by comparing the tumor size of repeated scans. The disadvantage of this procedure is that scar tissue frequently cannot be differentiated from tumor. An imaging approach such as FDG PET visualizing tumor viability offers the chance of predicting early whether the patient is responding or not.

Several studies have demonstrated that FDG PET can predict therapeutic outcome very early and with high accuracy (Fig. 4) [50, 51]. Recent studies examined patients with locally advanced breast cancer receiving preoperative chemotherapy and correlated the results of FDG PET with the histopathologic findings after surgery. For this purpose, quantification of local tumor glucose metabolism has been shown to be very helpful for monitoring early effects of chemotherapy. Smith et al. investigated 30 patients with locally advanced breast cancer and performed a dynamic PET before and several times after different cycles of chemotherapy. They measured uptake ratios in primary tumors and axillary lymph node metastases and calculated the glucose influx constant. It was found that FDG PET after the first pulse of chemotherapy could predict complete pathological remission with a sensitivity and specificity of 90 and 74%, respectively. Also in lymph node metastases, the mean change in uptake ratios and the influx constant were significantly greater in responding patients. Schelling et al. studied 22 patients with locally advanced breast cancer undergoing dose-intense preoperative chemotherapy and compared a baseline FDG PET with that after the first and second course of chemotherapy. Tracer uptake was measured by the assessment of SUV and was correlated to histopathology findings classifying patients as having gross residual disease or minimal residual disease. As early as after the first cycle of chemotherapy, responders could be identified with a sensitivity and specificity of 100 and 85% using a decrease of tracer uptake of 55% or more in comparison to the baseline uptake as a response criterion. This means that all responders could be revealed and, moreover, that a missing FDG decrease always indicated a non-response to chemotherapy. The authors of these studies found FDG PET helpful in deciding whether or not a chemotherapeutic regimen should be continued. Larger patient series still have to be studied before FDG PET can be considered as a standard therapy-monitoring procedure in breast cancer patients.

16.5 Indications

According to the 3rd German Consensus Conference on clinical indications of FDG PET in oncology in 2000 [52], the indications for PET are graded into: 1a = established clinical use, 1b = clinical use probable, 2 = useful in individual cases, 3 = not yet assessable because of missing or incomplete data and 4 = clinical use rare. For breast cancer, the Consensus Conference classified the N-staging as 1b indication provided that the primary tumor is of a sufficient size that lymph node metastases can be frequently expected. The available data indicate that FDG PET cannot replace axillary lymph node dissection or sentinel node biopsy. Therefore, the performance of a FDG PET scan seems more adequate to diagnose lymph node metastases in the internal mammaria region or in the mediastinum. This is important in patients with breast carcinoma located in the inner quadrants of the breast. If lymphatic disease in the parasternal nodes is apparent, radiotherapy of this region might be initiated.

The M-staging of breast cancer patients is considered a type 2 indication. In patients demonstrating elevated tumor markers and unsuspicious findings in conventional imaging modalities, FDG PET can be used as a whole-body imaging method and to help find the site of tumor recurrence and to confirm diagnosis.

FDG PET can also be helpful in differentiating benign from malignant breast tumor in selected patients (type 2 indication). Because small tumors are frequently missed there is only a minor role for FDG PET in this group.

The use of PET to monitor chemotherapy is still under investigation (type 3 indication). The first encouraging results have to be confirmed by larger patient series before further evaluation is possible.

16.6 Technical Recommendations

16.6.1 Patient Preparation

Patients should be fasted for at least 6 h.

16.6.2 Positioning

For breast imaging, the patient should be in a prone position with raised arms and breasts hanging freely.

For whole-body imaging, the patient should be in the supine position.

16.6.3 Radiopharmaceutical

The radiopharmaceutical is 300–400 MBq (ca. 10 mCi) FDG in the contralateral arm vein.

16.6.4 Data Acquisition

Acquisition times are 10–15 min for emission scans using the 2D mode, 5–10 min for emission scans using the 3D mode, 3–5 min for transmission scan or CT-corrected attenuation.

16.6.5 Reconstruction

Iterative reconstruction.

16.6.6 Image Evaluation

Visual analysis (focally increased activity), quantification of regional tracer uptake (e.g. standard uptake value).

16.6.7 Pitfalls

Pitfalls include tracer uptake in muscles of the neck and axillary uptake following paravasation.

References

1. Yim JH, Barton P, Weber B et al (1996) Mammographically detected breast cancer. Ann Surg 223:688–700
2. Levi F, La Vecchia C, Lucchini F, Negri E (1995) Cancer mortality in Europe 1990–92. Eur J Cancer Prev 4:389–417
3. Healy B (1997) BRCA genes – bookmaking, fortune telling, and medical care. N Engl J Med 336:1448–1449
4. Couch FJ, DeShano ML, Blackwood MA, Calzone K, Stopfer J, Campeau L, Ganguly A, Rebbeck T, Weber BL (1997) BRCA1 mutations in women attending clinics that evaluate the risk of breast cancer. N Engl J Med 336:1409–1415
5. Meuret G (1995) Grundlagen. In: Meuret G (ed) Mammakarzinom. Thieme, Stuttgart, pp 1–21
6. Masood S, Chiao J (1998) Pathology of breast cancer. In: Taillefer R, Khalkhali I, Waxman AD, Biersack HJ (eds) Radionuclide imaging of the breast. Dekker, New York
7. Holland R, Veling SH, Mravunac M, Hendriks JH (1985) Histologic multifocality of Tis, T1–2 breast carcinomas. Implications for clinical trials of breast-conserving surgery. Cancer 56:979–990
8. Veronesi U, Rilke F, Luini A, Sacchini V, Galimberti V, Campa T, Dei Bei E, Greco M, Magni A, Merson M et al (1987) Distribution of axillary node metastases by level of invasion. An analysis of 539 cases. Cancer 59:682–687
9. Smart CR, Myers MH, Gloeckler LA (1978) Implications from SEER data on breast cancer management. Cancer 41:787
10. Fisher B, Redmond C, Fisher ER et al (1985) Ten-year result of randomized clinical trial comparing radical mastectomy and total mastectomy with or without radiation. N Engl J Med 312:674
11. Koscielny S, Tubiana M, Le MG, Valleron AJ, Mouriesse H, Contesso G, Sarrazin D (1984) Breast cancer: relationship between the size of the primary tumour and the probability of metastatic dissemination. Br J Cancer 49:709–715
12. Meuret G (1995) Diagnostik, Krankheitsstadien und Prognose. In: Meuret G (ed) Mammakarzinom. Thieme, Stuttgart, pp 26–36
13. Kopans DB (1992) Positive predictive value of mammography. AJR 158:521–526
14. Andersson I (1988) Mammographic screening and mortality from breast cancer: Malmö mammographic screening trial. Br J Med 297:943–948
15. Frisell J, Eklund G, Hellström L et al (1991) Randomized study of mammography screening – preliminary report on mortality in the Stockholm trial. Breast Cancer Res Treat 18:49–56
16. Miller AB, Baines CJ, To T et al (1992) Canada national breast screening study. Can Med Assoc J 147:1459–1488
17. Kuhl CK, Bieling HB, Gieseke J, Kreft BP, Sommer T, Lutterbey G, Schild HH (1997) Healthy premenopausal breast parenchy-

ma in dynamic contrast-enhanced MR imaging of the breast: normal contrast medium enhancement and cyclical-phase dependency. Radiology 203:137–144
18. Laffer U (1995) Chirurgische Therapie. In: Meuret G (ed) Mammakarzinom. Thieme, Stuttgart, pp 40–43
19. Fisher B, Redmond C, Poisson R, Margolese R, Wolmark N, Wickerham L, Fisher E, Deutsch M, Caplan R, Pilch Y et al (1989) Eight-year results of a randomized clinical trial comparing total mastectomy and lumpectomy with or without irradiation in the treatment of breast cancer. N Engl J Med 320: 822–828
20. Carter CL, Allen C, Henson DE (1989) Relation of tumor size, lymph node status and survival in 2474 breast cancer patients. Cancer 63:181
21. Thuerlimann B (2001) International consensus meeting on the treatment of primary breast cancer 2001, St Gallen, Switzerland. Breast Cancer 8:294–297
22. Wahl RL, Henry CA, Ethier SP (1992) Serum glucose: effects on tumor and normal tissue accumulation of 2-[F-18]-fluoro-2-deoxy-D-glucose in rodents with mammary carcinoma. Radiology 183:643–647
23. Riddell C, Carson RE, Carrasquillo JA, Libutti SK, Danforth DN, Whatley M, Bacharach SL (2001) Noise reduction in oncology FDG PET images by iterative reconstruction: a quantitative assessment. J Nucl Med 42:1316–1323
24. Wahl RL, Cody RL, Hutchins GD, Kuhl DE (1989) Primary and metastatic breast carcinoma: initial clinical evaluation with PET imaging of breast cancer with 18FDG. Radiology 173:419
25. Kubota K, Matsuzawa T, Amemiya A, Kondo M, Fujiwara T, Watanuki S, Ito M, Ido T (1989) Imaging of breast cancer with FDG and positron emission tomography. J Comput Assist Tomogr 13:1097–1098
26. Wahl RL, Cody RL, Hutchins GD, Mudgett EE (1991) Primary and metastatic breast carcinoma: initial clinical evaluation with PET with the radiolabeled glucose analogue F-18 fluoro-2-deoxy-D-glucose. Radiology 179:765–770
27. Tse NY, Hoh CK, Hawkins RH, Zinner MJ, Dahlbom M, Choi Y, Maddahi J, Brunicardi FC, Phelps ME, Glaspy JA (1992) The application of positron emission tomographic imaging with FDG to the evaluation of breast disease. Ann Surg 216:27–34
28. Adler LP, Crowe JP, Al Kaisi NK, Sunshine JL (1993) Evaluation of breast masses and axillary lymph nodes with F-18 deoxy-2-fluoro-D-glucose PET. Radiology 187:743–750
29. Hoh CK, Hawkins RH, Glaspy JA, Dahlbom M, Tse NY, Hoffmann EJ, Schiepers C, Choi Y, Rege S, Nitzsche E (1993) Cancer detection with whole body PET using 18F-deoxyglucose. J Comput Assist Tomogr 17:582–589
30. Nieweg OE, Kim EE, Wong WH, Broussard WF, Singletary SE, Hortobagyi GN, Tilbury RS (1993) Positron emission tomography with FDG in the detection and staging of breast cancer. Cancer 71:3920–3925
31. Crowe JP, Adler LP, Shenk RR, Sunshine J (1994) Positron emission tomography and breast masses: comparison with clinical, mammographic, and pathological findings. Ann Surg Oncol 1: 132–140
32. Avril N, Dose J, Jänicke F et al (1996) Metabolic characterization of breasts tumors with PET using F-18 fluorodeoxyglucose. J Clin Oncol 14:1848–1856
33. Scheidhauer K, Scharl A, Pietrzyk U et al (1996) Qualitative F-18 FDG positron emission tomography in primary breast cancer: clinical relevance and practicability. Eur J Nucl Med 23:618–623
34. Palmedo H, Bender H, Grünwald F et al (1997) FDG-PET and scintimammography with Tc-99m MIBI in breast tumors. Eur J Nucl Med 24:1138–1145
35. Avril N, Rose CA, Schelling M, Dose J, Kuhn W, Bense S, Weber W, Ziegler S, Graeff H, Schwaiger M (2000) Breast imaging with positron emission tomography and fluorine-18 fluorodeoxyglucose: use and limitations. J Clin Oncol 18:3495–3502
36. Bos R, van Der Hoeven JJ, van Der Wall E, van Der Groep P, van Diest PJ, Comans EF, Joshi U, Semenza GL, Hoekstra OS, Lammertsma AA, Molthoff CF (2002) Biologic correlates of (18)fluorodeoxyglucose uptake in human breast cancer measured by positron emission tomography. J Clin Oncol 20:379–387
37. Brown RS, Leung JY, Fisher SJ, Frey KA, Ethier SP, Wahl RL (1995) Intratumoral distribution of tritiated fluorodeoxyglucose in breast carcinoma: I. Are inflammatory cells important? J Nucl Med 36:1854–1861
38. Palmedo H, Hensel J, Reinhardt M, von Mallek D, Matthies A, Biersack HJ (2002) Breast cancer imaging with PET and SPECT agents: an in vivo comparison. Nucl Med Biol 29:809–815
39. Avril N, Dose J, Janicke F, Ziegler S, Romer W, Weber W, Herz M, Nathrath W, Graeff H, Schwaiger M (1996) Assessment of axillary lymph node involvement in breast cancer patients with positron emission tomography using radiolabeled 2-(fluorine-18)-fluoro-2-deoxy-D-glucose. J Natl Cancer Inst 88: 1204–1209
40. Van der Hoeven JJ, Hoekstra OS, Comans EF, Pijpers R, Boom RP, van Geldere D, Meijer S, Lammertsma AA, Teule GJ (2002) Determinants of diagnostic performance of [F-18]fluorodeoxyglucose positron emission tomography for axillary staging in breast cancer. Ann Surg 236:619–624
41. Greco M, Crippa F, Agresti R, Seregni E, Gerali A, Giovanazzi R, Micheli A, Asero S, Ferraris C, Gennaro M, Bombardieri E, Cascinelli N (2001) Axillary lymph node staging in breast cancer by 2-fluoro-2-deoxy-D-glucose-positron emission tomography: clinical evaluation and alternative management. J Natl Cancer Inst 93:630–635
42. Eubank WB, Mankoff DA, Takasugi J, Vesselle H, Eary JF, Shanley TJ, Gralow JR, Charlop A, Ellis GK, Lindsley KL, Austin-Seymour MM, Funkhouser CP, Livingston RB (2001) 18Fluorodeoxyglucose positron emission tomography to detect mediastinal or internal mammary metastases in breast cancer. J Clin Oncol 19:3516–3523
43. Bender H, Kirst J, Palmedo H, Schomburg A, Wagner U, Ruhlmann J, Biersack HJ (1997) Value of 18fluoro-deoxyglucose positron emission tomography in the staging of recurrent breast carcinoma. Anticancer Res 17:1687–1692
44. Schirrmeister H, Kuhn T, Guhlmann A, Santjohanser C, Horster T, Nussle K, Koretz K, Glatting G, Rieber A, Kreienberg R, Buck AC, Reske SN (2001) Fluorine-18 2-deoxy-2-fluoro-D-glucose PET in the preoperative staging of breast cancer: comparison with the standard staging procedures. Eur J Nucl Med 28: 351–358
45. Kim TS, Moon WK, Lee DS, Chung JK, Lee MC, Youn YK, Oh SK, Choe KJ, Noh DY (2001) Fluorodeoxyglucose positron emission tomography for detection of recurrent or metastatic breast cancer. World J Surg 25:829–834
46. Moon DH, Maddahi J, Silverman DH, Glaspy JA, Phelps ME, Hoh CK (1998) Accuracy of whole-body fluorine-18-FDG PET for the detection of recurrent or metastatic breast carcinoma. J Nucl Med 39:431–435
47. Cook GJ, Houston S, Rubens R, Maisey MN, Fogelman I (1998) Detection of bone metastases in breast cancer by 18FDG PET: differing metabolic activity in osteoblastic and osteolytic lesions. J Clin Oncol 16:3375–3379
48. Fisher B, Bryant J, Wolmark N et al (1998) Effect of preoperative chemotherapy on the outcome of women with operable breast cancer. J Clin Oncol 16:2672–2685
49. Kuerer HM, Newman LA, Smith TL et al (1999) Clinical course of breast cancer patients with complete pathologic primary tumor and axillary lymph node response to doxorubicin-based neoadjuvant chemotherapy. J Clin Oncol 17:460–469
50. Schelling M, Avril N, Nahrig J, Kuhn W, Romer W, Sattler D, Werner M, Dose J, Janicke F, Graeff H, Schwaiger M (2000) Positron emission tomography using [(18)F]Fluorodeoxyglucose for monitoring primary chemotherapy in breast cancer. J Clin Oncol 18:1689–1695
51. Smith IC, Welch AE, Hutcheon AW et al (2000) Positron emission tomography using [(18)F]-fluorodeoxy-D-glucose to predict the pathologic response of breast cancer to primary chemotherapy. J Clin Oncol 18:1676–1688
52. Reske SN, Kotzerke J (2001) FDG-PET for clinical use. Results of the 3rd German Interdisciplinary Consensus Conference, "Onko-PET III", 21 July and 19 Sept 2000. Eur J Nucl Med 28: 1707–1723
53. Utech CI, Young CS, Winter PF (1996) Prospecive evaluation of fluorine-18 fluorodeoxyclucose positron emission tomography

in breast cancer for staging of the axilla related to surgery and immunocytochemistry. Eur J Nucl Med 23(12):1588-93
54. Crippa F, Agresti R, Seregni E, Greco M, Pascali C, Bogni A, Chiesa C, De Sanctis V, Delledonne V, Salvadori B, Leutner M, Bombardieri E (1998) Prospective evaluation of fluorine-18-FDG PET in presurgical staging of the axilla in breast cancer. J Nucl Med 39(1):4–8

CHAPTER 17

Pancreatic Cancer

D. Delbeke

17.1 Epidemiology and Histopathological Types

The focus of this chapter is on pancreatic ductal adenocarcinoma because it represents 80–90% of pancreatic malignancy and has a poor prognosis. It occurs in the head of the pancreas in about two-thirds of patients and in the body and the tail in the other third. When located in the head of the pancreas, patients present with jaundice and pain due to obstruction of the extrahepatic bile ducts. Extrapancreatic extension is common at the time of diagnosis. Pancreatic ductal adenocarcinoma commonly spreads to peripancreatic lymph nodes and distant metastases are often found in the liver and lungs. Tumors from the body and tail of the pancreas grow more insidiously and can be widely metastatic at the time of diagnosis. In 2001, 29,200 new cases of pancreatic cancer were diagnosed and there were an estimated 28,900 deaths. For all stages combined, the survival at 1 and 5 years respectively is 20% and 4% of newly diagnosed cases. Pancreaticoduodenectomy improves the 5-year survival to over 20% but with a 2–3% mortality rate. The preoperative diagnosis, staging, and treatment of pancreatic cancer remain challenging.

Carcinomas of the periampullary region are much less frequent than in the pancreas but they are important because they are much more curable. They are usually diagnosed earlier and less than 50% are associated with lymph node metastases at the time of diagnosis. The 5-year survival rate is in the 20–30% range.

Acinar cell carcinomas comprise no more than 1–2% of all pancreatic cancer and the prognosis is as poor as for ductal cell carcinoma.

Cystic neoplasms can arise in the pancreas and differentiation of benign from malignant is critical. Benign cystadenoma (also called microcystic or glycogen-rich adenomas) are usually large and the cells lining the cysts are flat or cuboidal and contain abundant glycogen. Malignant cystadenocarcinoma (mucinous cystic tumors) are usually large and multilocular, and are lined by mucin-producing cells, often forming papillae.

Islet cell tumors and other endocrine tumors make up a small fraction of all pancreatic neoplasms and are most often located in the body and tail of the pancreas. They are usually slow-growing tumors and are associated with endocrine abnormalities.

17.2 Conventional Diagnostic Imaging Modalities

The suspicion for pancreatic cancer is often raised by sonographic or computed tomography (CT) findings, including the presence of a low-attenuation pancreatic mass and dilatation of the pancreatic duct and/or biliary tree. CT is the most common diagnostic imaging modality utilized in the preoperative diagnosis of pancreatic cancer. In a multicenter trial [1] the diagnostic accuracy of CT for staging and resectability was 73%, with a positive predictive value for non-resectability of 90%, but more recent studies have reported accuracies of 85–95%, likely related to improvements in CT technology [2, 3]. Unfortunately, interpretation of the CT scan is sometimes difficult in the setting of mass-forming pancreatitis or questionable findings such as enlargement of the pancreatic head without definite signs of malignancy or discrete mass [4, 5]. The diagnosis of locoregional lymph node metastases is also difficult with CT, because they are often small. In addition, small hepatic metastases (<1 cm) cannot reliably be differentiated from cysts [6]. Therefore, the reported negative predictive value for non-resectability is less than 30%. However, recent technical advancement of CT with the multidetector technology allows the entire pancreas to be imaged by 1 mm slices in under 20 seconds, volume acquisitions and 3D arterial and venous-phase mapping [7]. Despite recent technical improvements in magnetic resonance imaging (MRI), including MR cholangiopancreatography (MRCP), the diagnostic performance of MRI remains similar to CT [8–11]. Endoscopic ultrasound (EUS) offers the possibility of tissue diagnosis with fine needle aspiration (FNA), but the field-of-view is limited [12–14]. The accuracy of endoscopic retrograde cholangiopancreatography (ERCP) is 80–90% to differentiate benign from malignant pancreatic mass, including differentiation of tumor from chronic pancreatitis because of the high degree of resolution of ductal structures. The limitations include false-negative findings when the tumor does not originate from the main duct, a 10% rate of technical failure, and up to 8% morbidity due to iatrogenic pancreatitis. The main advantages are the possibilities of interventional procedures and FNA, although this technique suffers from significant sampling error [15, 16] with a false-negative incidence of 8–17%.

The difficulty in making a preoperative diagnosis is associated with two types of adverse outcomes. First, less aggressive surgeons may abort attempted resection due to a lack of tissue diagnosis. This is borne out by the significant rate of "reoperative" pancreaticoduodenectomy performed at major referral centers [17–19]. A second type of adverse outcome generated by failure to obtain a preoperative diagnosis occurs when more aggressive surgeons inadvertently resect benign disease. This is particularly notable in those patients who present with suspected malignancy without an associated mass on CT scan. This has been reported to occur in up to 55% of patients in some series [20].

17.3 FDG PET Imaging

In order to avoid these adverse outcomes, metabolic imaging with fluoro-2-deoxy-D-glucose (FDG) positron emission tomography (PET) has been used to improve the accuracy of the preoperative diagnosis of pancreatic carcinoma. Most malignancies, including pancreatic carcinoma, demonstrate increased glucose utilization due to an increased number of glucose transporter proteins and increased hexokinase and phosphofructokinase activity [21, 22]. There is recent evidence that the over-expression of glucose transporters by malignant pancreatic cells contributes to the increased uptake of FDG by these neoplasms [22, 23, 24]. Basically, high-resolution FDG PET emission scans provide high-resolution images of the distribution of FDG in the body, reflecting tissue metabolism at the time of the study. However, interpretation of these emission scans is often complicated by the absence of detailed anatomy in the emission data. The problem of anatomical localization of the foci of abnormal uptake and differentiation of physiologic from pathologic foci of uptake is compounded by lower resolution and increased noise in the images of some of the systems at the low end of the spectrum. Close correlation of FDG studies with conventional CT scans helps to minimize these difficulties. In practice, interpretation is accomplished by visually comparing the emission scans with high-quality anatomical maps such as those provided by clinical CT scanners. The interpreting physician visually integrates the two image sets in order to locate precisely a region of increased uptake on the CT scan that was identified on the PET scan. To aid in image interpretation, several techniques have been developed to co-register the FDG PET emission scans with the high-resolution anatomical maps provided by CT [25]. Co-registration can be obtained using methods such as fitting techniques and image alignment using co-registration software. These methods offer acceptable fusion images for the brain, which is surrounded by a rigid structure, the skull. For the body, co-registration of two images, often obtained at different points in time, is much more difficult. Identical positioning of the patient on the imaging table is critical and internal organ peristalsis and motion add to the problem. The recent technical developments of integrated PET-CT systems provide CT and FDG PET images obtained in a single imaging setting, allowing optimal co-registration of images. The fusion images provided by these systems allow the most accurate interpretation of both CT and FDG PET studies, which can be integrated for optimal patient care. For patients with suspected pancreatic carcinoma, precise localization of foci of FDG uptake in the pancreas allows differentiation of physiologic uptake in the adjacent bowel from pathologic uptake in the pancreas.

17.3.1 FDG PET Imaging in the Preoperative Diagnosis of Pancreatic Carcinoma

In 12 studies [26–37] the performance of FDG PET to differentiate benign from malignant lesions ranged from 85 to 100% for sensitivity, 67 to 99% for specificity, and 85 to 93% for accuracy. In the majority of these studies the accuracy of FDG PET imaging was superior to that of CT. For example, in the study of Delbeke et al. [37] the sensitivity and specificity of FDG PET imaging was 92 and 85% respectively, compared with 65 and 62% for CT. In addition, the sensitivity of CT imaging improves with the size of the lesion, but the sensitivity of FDG PET is not as dependent on lesion size [38]. In a study of 35 patients comparing EUS, PET and CT, the sensitivity for detection of pancreatic cancer was higher for EUS (93%) and FDG PET (87%) than for CT (53%) [14].

Serti et al. [39] have reviewed the performance of FDG PET in 56 patients with a suspected cystic tumor of the pancreas. They concluded that FDG PET was more accurate than CT and tumor markers to differentiate malignant from benign lesions. The sensitivity and specificity of FDG PET were 94 and 97% respectively, compared with 65 and 87% for CT. A comprehensive tabulated review of the PET literature (387 patient studies) has reported weighted averages for FDG PET sensitivity and specificity of 94 and 90% respectively, compared with 82 and 75% for CT [40]. Together, these series support the conclusion that FDG PET imaging may represent a useful adjunctive study in the evaluation of patients with suspected pancreatic cancer.

Preliminary reports suggest that the degree of FDG uptake has a prognostic value. The degree of uptake can be measured with the standard uptake value (SUV), that is, the radioactivity in a region of interest normalized for the dose administered and the body weight. Nakata et al. [41] noted a correlation between SUV and survival in 14 patients with pancreatic adenocarcinoma. Patients with an SUV over 3.0 had a mean survival of 5 months compared with 14 months in those with an SUV less than 3.0. In a multivariate analysis of 52 patients with pancreatic carcinoma, the median survival of patients with an SUV over 6.1 was 5 months compared with 9 months for patients with an SUV less than 6.1 [42].

17.3.2 FDG PET for Staging Pancreatic Carcinoma

Stage II disease is characterized by extrapancreatic extension (T-stage), stage III by lymph node involvement (N-stage), and stage IV by distant metastases (M-stage). T-staging can only be evaluated with anatomical imaging modalities that demonstrate the relationship between the tumor, adjacent organs and vascular structures. EUS appears more sensitive than CT for evaluation of vascular invasion of the portal and superior mesenteric veins [14]. Functional imaging modalities cannot replace anatomical imaging in the assessment of local tumor resectability.

Both FDG PET and CT are poor for N-staging, probably due to the proximity of regional lymph nodes to the primary tumor [27, 33, 37]. However, FDG PET is more accurate than CT for M-staging. In the study of Delbeke et al. [37], metastases were diagnosed both on CT and PET in 10/21 patients with stage IV disease, but PET demonstrated hepatic metastases not identified or equivocal on CT and/or distant metastases unsuspected clinically in seven additional patients (33%). In four patients (19%), neither CT nor PET imaging showed evidence of metastases, but surgical exploration revealed miliary carcinomatosis in three and a small liver metastasis in one patient. FDG PET is sensitive for detection of hepatic metastases but false-positive findings have been reported in the liver of patients with dilated bile ducts and inflammatory granulomas [43].

The tabulated review of the PET literature has reported weighted averages for FDG PET sensitivity and specificity of 83 and 82% respectively, compared with 65 and 61% for CT for staging pancreatic carcinoma (461 patient studies) [40].

17.3.3 Impact of FDG PET on the Management of Patients with Pancreatic Carcinoma

The rate at which FDG PET may lead to alterations in clinical management clearly depends on the specific therapeutic philosophy employed by the evaluating surgeon. In the study of Delbeke et al. [37], the surgeons advocate pancreaticoduodenectomy only for those patients with potentially curable pancreatic cancer, and take an aggressive approach to resection including en bloc retroperitoneal lymphadenectomy and selective resection of the superior mesenteric–portal vein confluence when necessary, while the majority of patients with non-malignant biliary strictures are managed without resection. In that series of 65 patients, the application of FDG PET imaging in addition to CT altered the surgical management in 41% of the patients, 27% by detecting CT-occult pancreatic carcinoma and 14% by identifying unsuspected distant metastases, or by clarifying the benign nature of lesions equivocal on CT [37].

17.3.4 FDG PET for Monitoring Therapy and Detection of Recurrent Pancreatic Carcinoma

Preliminary studies suggest that neo-adjuvant chemoradiation improves the resectability rate and survival of patients with pancreatic carcinoma [44, 45]. A pilot study determined that FDG PET imaging may be useful for the assessment of tumor response to neo-adjuvant therapy and the evaluation of suspected recurrent disease following resection [38]. Nine patients underwent FDG PET imaging before and after neo-adjuvant chemoradiation therapy. FDG PET successfully predicted histological evidence of chemoradiation-induced tumor necrosis in all four patients who demonstrated at least a 50% reduction in tumor SUV following chemoradiation. Among these patients, none showed a measurable reduction in tumor diameter as assessed by CT. The four patients who had FDG PET evidence of tumor response went on to successful resection, all showing 20–80% tumor necrosis in the resected specimen. Three patients showed stable FDG uptake and two showed increasing FDG uptake indicative of tumor progression. Among the two patients with progressive disease demonstrated by FDG PET, one showed tumor progression on CT, and the other demonstrated stable disease. Among the five patients who showed no response by FDG PET, the disease could be subsequently resected in only two, and only one patient who underwent resection showed evidence of chemoradiation-induced necrosis in the resected specimen. Another pilot study suggests that the absence of FDG uptake at 1 month following chemotherapy is an indicator of improved survival [46]. Definitive conclusions regarding the role of FDG PET in assessing treatment response will obviously require evaluation in a larger population of patients. However, given the poor track record of CT in assessing histological response to neo-adjuvant chemoradiation, the potential utility of FDG PET in this capacity deserves further investigation.

The majority of reports concerning the clinical utilization of FDG PET imaging for pancreatic malignancy have emphasized the identification of recurrent nod-

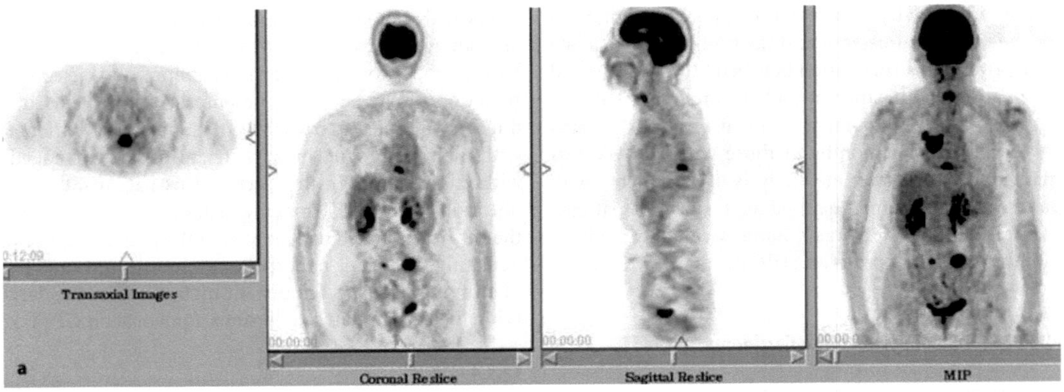

Fig. 1a,b.
A 79-year-old male with a history of Whipple procedure for pancreatic carcinoma 2 years earlier presented a pulmonary nodule on CT. **a** The FDG PET images demonstrated marked FDG uptake in the pulmonary nodule consistent with a metastasis. In addition, there are foci of uptake in the sacrum bilaterally, in T9 and the right upper cervical spine consistent with skeletal metastases. **b** The findings on PET triggered an MRI scan of the spine, showing erosive enhancing processes in T9, L1, L2 and S1. A biopsy of the lesion in the left sacrum confirmed metastatic adenocarcinoma of the pancreas

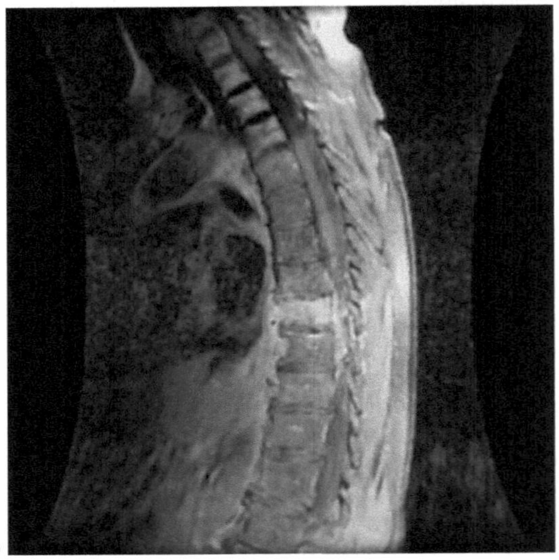

al or distant metastatic disease. In a preliminary study [38], eight patients were evaluated for possible recurrence because of either indeterminate CT findings or a rise in serum tumor marker levels. All were noted to have significant new regions of FDG uptake, four in the surgical bed and four in new hepatic metastases. In all patients, metastasis or local recurrence was confirmed pathologically or clinically. Another study of 19 patients concluded that FDG PET added important incremental information in 50% of the patients, resulting in a change of therapeutic procedure [47]. This included patients with elevated serum tumor marker levels but no findings on anatomical imaging. An example of a patient with widely metastatic recurrent adenocarcinoma of the pancreas is shown in Fig. 1.

Therefore, FDG PET may be particularly useful (1) when CT identifies an indistinct region of change in the bed of the resected pancreas that is difficult to differentiate from post-operative or post-radiation fibrosis, (2) for the evaluation of new hepatic lesions that may be too small to biopsy, and (3) in patients with rising serum tumor marker levels and a negative conventional work-up.

17.3.5
Limitations of FDG PET Imaging

The high incidence of glucose intolerance and diabetes exhibited by patients with pancreatic pathology represents a potential limitation of this modality in the diagnosis of pancreatic cancer. Elevated serum glucose levels result in decreased FDG uptake in tumors by up to 50% due to competitive inhibition. Several studies have reported a lower sensitivity in hyperglycemic compared with euglycemic patients [29, 34, 37]. For example, in a study of 106 patients with a disease prevalence of 70% [34], FDG PET had a sensitivity of 98% in a subgroup of euglycemic patients versus 63% in hyperglycemic patients. This has led some investigators to suggest that the SUV be corrected according to serum glucose level [48–51]. In the studies of Delbeke et al. [37] and Diederichs et al. [51], the presence of elevated serum glucose levels and/or diabetes mellitus may have contributed to false-negative interpretations; but correction of the SUV for serum glucose level has not significantly improved the sensitivity of FDG PET in the diagnosis of pancreatic carcinoma. The true impact of serum glucose levels on the accuracy of FDG PET in pancreatic cancer and other neoplasms remains controversial.

False-negative studies may also occur when the tumor diameter is <1 cm (i.e., small ampullary carcinoma). Ampullary carcinomas arise from the ampulla of Vater and have a better prognosis than pancreatic carcinoma because they cause biliary obstruction and are diagnosed earlier in the course of the disease. A recent study evaluating 44 patients with suspected periampullary neoplasms demonstrated a sensitivity of 90% (37/41) patients, but the authors concluded that FDG PET did not change the clinical management of these patients [52].

Both glucose and FDG are substrates for cellular mediators of inflammation. Some benign inflammatory lesions, including chronic and acute pancreatitis with or without abscess formation, can accumulate FDG and result in false-positive interpretations on PET images [29, 32, 53, 54]. In addition, post-stenotic pancreatitis can obscure FDG uptake in the tumor itself. False-positive studies are more frequent in patients with elevated C-reactive protein and/or acute pancreatitis with a specificity as low as 50% [54, 55]. Therefore, screening for acute inflammatory disease with serum C-reactive protein has been recommended.

More recent data suggest that delayed scanning (2 hours after FDG administration) may help differentiate malignant from benign pancreatic lesions [56]. Other preliminary findings suggest that the retention index (the ratio of the difference between the SUV at 2 hours and the SUV at 1 hour divided by the SUV at 1 hour) obtained from dual-phase FDG PET can predict hexokinase II expression and that the SUV (at 1 hour) has a positive correlation with the glucose transporter protein (GLUT-1) expression but not with hexokinase II expression [57].

Another recent study suggests that non-invasive differentiation between pancreatic cancer and chronic pancreatitis may best be achieved based on a dynamic FDG PET study including kinetic analysis. This approach yields results superior to those obtained from a semi-quantitative analysis of pancreatic lesions [58].

17.4 FDG PET for Evaluation of Islet Cells and Other Endocrine Tumors of the Pancreas

Most neuroendocrine tumors, including carcinoid, paraganglioma, and islet cell tumors, express somatostatin receptors (SSR) and can, therefore, be imaged effectively with somatostatin analogs such as [^{111}In]octreotide. This modality has been reported to be more sensitive than CT for defining the extent of metastatic disease, especially in extrahepatic and extra-abdominal sites. However, there may be significant heterogeneity with regards to SSR expression, even in the same patient in adjacent sites, probably related to dedifferentiation of the tumor. Absence of SSR positivity is reported to be a poor prognostic sign, but virtually all of these SSR-negative neuroendocrine tumors will accumulate FDG and can therefore be imaged with PET [59]. More differentiated SSR-positive tumors do not reliably accumulate significant FDG and may, therefore, be false negative with FDG PET imaging [60]. Both techniques may detect the primary gastrointestinal or islet cell tumor in a minority of cases. FDG PET imaging is ideally suited to monitoring the success of locally directed therapy such as chemoembolization, alcohol instillation, and radiofrequency ablation. An example of an incidental finding of neuroendocrine tumor of the pancreas is shown in Fig. 2.

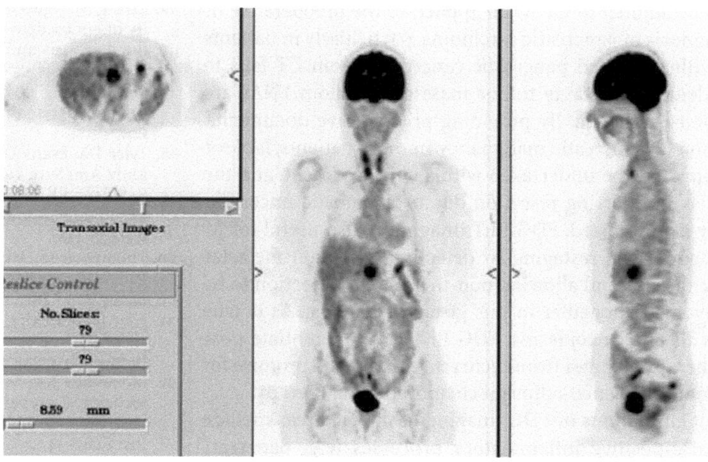

Fig. 2. A 64-year-old female presented for evaluation of abdominal aortic aneurysm. An ultrasound of the abdomen demonstrated a 3 cm mass in the head of the pancreas (not shown). FDG PET images was performed and demonstrated a focus of uptake in the region of the pancreatic mass. In addition, heterogeneous uptake is seen in the thyroid gland, consistent with multinodular goiter. A biopsy of the pancreatic lesion revealed a neuroendocrine tumor

There is controversy in the literature about the sensitivity of FDG imaging for detection of carcinoid tumors [61, 62] but at least in some reports, [^{111}In]octreotide scintigraphy is more sensitive than FDG PET imaging; FDG-positive/octreotide-negative tumors tend to be less differentiated and may have a less favorable prognosis.

Other positron emitter tracers seem to be more promising. A serotonin precursor 5-hydroxytryptophan labeled with ^{11}C has shown an increased uptake in carcinoids. This uptake seems to be selective and some clinical evidence has demonstrated that it allows the detection of more lesions with PET than with CT or octreotide scintigraphy. Another radiopharmaceutical in development for PET is [^{11}C] L-DOPA, which seems to be useful in visualizing endocrine pancreatic tumors [63, 64].

[^{111}In]Octreotide was developed for imaging somatostatin-receptor-positive tumors using conventional scintigraphy and single photon emission computed tomography (SPECT). An octreotide derivative can be labeled with ^{64}Cu (half-life 12.7 h; beta$^+$ 0.653 MeV [17.4 %]; beta$^-$ 0.579 MeV [39 %]) and has shown potential as a radiopharmaceutical for PET imaging and radiotherapy. A pilot study in humans has demonstrated that [^{64}Cu]TETA-octreotide (where TETA is 1,4,8,11-tetraazacyclotetradecane-N,N',N",N'"-tetraacetic acid) and PET can be used to detect somatostatin-receptor-positive tumors in humans. The high rate of lesion detection, sensitivity, and favorable dosimetry and pharmacokinetics of [^{64}Cu]TETA- octreotide indicated that it was a promising radiopharmaceutical for PET imaging of patients with neuroendocrine tumors [65].

17.5 Summary

Imaging with FDG PET does not replace but is complementary to morphological imaging with CT; therefore, integrated PET–CT imaging provides optimal images for interpretation. FDG PET imaging is a sensitive and specific adjunct to CT when applied to the preoperative diagnosis of pancreatic carcinoma, particularly in patients with suspected pancreatic cancer in whom CT fails to identify a discrete tumor mass or in whom FNAs are non-diagnostic. By providing preoperative documentation of pancreatic malignancy in these patients, laparotomy may be undertaken with a curative intent, and the risk of aborting resection due to diagnostic uncertainty is minimized. FDG PET imaging is also useful for M-staging and restaging by detecting CT-occult metastatic disease, and allowing non-therapeutic resection to be avoided altogether in this group of patients. As is true with other neoplasms, FDG PET can differentiate post-therapy changes from recurrence and holds promise for monitoring neo-adjuvant chemoradiation therapy.

Limitations of FDG imaging of the pancreas include false-positive inflammatory processes (e.g. pancreatitis, stent, cholangitis) and false-negative findings in patients with diabetes and hyperglycemia and in patients with differentiated neuroendocrine tumors.

References

1. Megibow AJ, Zhou XH, Rotterdam H et al (1995) Pancreatic adenocarcinoma: CT versus MR imaging in the evaluation of resectability – report of the Radiology Diagnostic Oncology Group. Radiology 195:327–332
2. Diehl SJ, Lehman KJ, Sadick M, Lachman R, Georgi M (1998) Pancreatic cancer: value of dual-phase helical CT in assessing resectability. Radiology 206:373–378
3. Lu DSK, Reber HA, Krasny RM, Sayre J (1997) Local staging of pancreatic cancer: criteria for unresectability of major vessels as revealed by pancreatic-phase, thin section helical CT. Am J Radiol 168:1439–1444
4. Johnson PT, Outwater EK (1999) Pancreatic carcinoma versus chronic pancreatitis: dynamic MR imaging. Radiology 212:213–218
5. Lammer J, Herlinger H, Zalaudek G, Hofler H (1995) Pseudotumorous pancreatitis. Gastrointest Radiol 10:59–67
6. Bluemke DA, Cameron IL, Hurban RH et al (1995) Potentially resectable pancreatic adenocarcinoma: spiral CT assessment with surgical and pathologic correlation. Radiology 197:381–385
7. Fishman EK, Horton KM (2001) Imaging pancreatic cancer: the role of multidetector CT with three dimensional CT angiography. Pancreatology 1:610–624
8. Bluemke DA, Fishman EK (1998) CT and MR evaluation of pancreatic cancer. Surg Oncol Clin North Am 7:103–124
9. Catalano C, Pavone P, Laghi A et al (1998) Pancreatic adenocarcinoma: combination of MR angiography and MR cholangiopancreatography for the diagnosis and assessment of resectability. Eur Radiol 8:428–434
10. Irie H, Honda H, Kaneko K et al (1997) Comparison of helical CT and MR imaging in detecting and staging small pancreatic adenocarcinoma. Abdom Imag 22:429–433
11. Trede M, Rumstadt B, Wendl et al (1997) Ultrafast magnetic resonance imaging improves the staging of pancreatic tumors. Ann Surg 226:393–405
12. Hawes RH, Zaidi S (1995) Endoscopic ultrasonography of the pancreas. Gastrointest Endosc Clin North Am 5:61–80
13. Legmann P, Vignaux O, Dousset B et al (1998) Pancreatic tumors: comparison of dual-phase helical CT and endoscopic sonography. Am J Roentgenol 170:1315–1322
14. Mertz HR, Sechopoulos P, Delbeke D, Leach SD (2000) EUS, PET, and CT scanning for evaluation of pancreatic adenocarcinoma. Gastrointest Endosc 52:367–371
15. Brandt KR, Charboneau JW, Stephens DH, Welch TJ, Goellner JR (1993) CT- and US-guided biopsy of the pancreas. Radiology 187:99–104
16. Chang KJ, Nguyen P, Erickson RA et al (1997) The clinical utility of endoscopic ultrasound-guided fine-needle aspiration in the diagnosis and staging of pancreatic carcinoma. Gastrointest Endosc 45:387–393
17. McGuire GE, Pitt HA, Lillemoe KD et al (1991) Reoperative surgery for periampullary adenocarcinoma. Arch Surg 126:1205–1212
18. Tyler DS, Evans DB (1994) Reoperative pancreaticoduodenectomy. Ann Surg 219:211–221
19. Robinson EK, Lee JE, Lowy AM et al (1996) Reoperative pancreaticoduodenectomy for periampullary carcinoma. Am J Surg 172:432–438
20. Thompson JS, Murayama KM, Edney JA, Rikkers LF (1994) Pancreaticoduodenectomy for suspected but unproven malignancy. Am J Surg 169:571–575
21. Flier JS, Mueckler MM, Usher P, Lodish HF (1987) Elevated levels of glucose transport and transporter messenger RNA are induced by ras or src oncogenes. Science 235:1492–1495
22. Monakhov NK, Neistadt EL, Shavlovskil MM et al (1978) Physiochemical properties and isoenzyme composition of hexokinase from normal and malignant human tissues. J Natl Cancer Inst 61:27–34

23. Higashi T, Tamaki N, Honda T et al (1997) Expression of glucose transporters in human pancreatic tumors compared with increased F-18 FDG accumulation in PET study. J Nucl Med 38: 1337–1344
24. Reske S, Grillenberger KG, Glatting G et al (1997) Overexpression of glucose transporter 1 and increased F-18 FDG uptake in pancreatic carcinoma. J Nucl Med 38:1344–1348
25. Berger C, Berthold T (2000) Image fusion. In: Von Schulthess GK (ed) Clinical positron emission tomography (PET). Lippincott Williams and Wilkins, Philadelphia PA, pp 41–48
26. Bares R, Klever P, Hellwig D et al (1993) Pancreatic cancer detected by positron emission tomography with 18F-labelled deoxyglucose: method and first results. Nucl Med Commun 14: 596–601
27. Bares R, Klever P, Hauptmann S et al (1994) F-18-fluorodeoxyglucose PET in vivo evaluation of pancreatic glucose metabolism for detection of pancreatic cancer. Radiology 192:79–86
28. Stollfuss JC, Glatting G, Friess H, Kocher F, Berger HG, Reske SN (1995) 2-(Fluorine-18)-fluoro-2-deoxy-D-glucose PET in detection of pancreatic cancer: value of quantitative image interpretation. Radiology 195:339–344
29. Inokuma T, Tamaki N, Torizuka T et al (1995) Evaluation of pancreatic tumors with positron emission tomography and F-18 fluorodeoxyglucose: comparison with CT and US. Radiology 195:345–352
30. Kato T, Fukatsu H, Ito K et al (1995) Fluorodeoxyglucose positron emission tomography in pancreatic cancer: an unsolved problem. Eur J Nucl Med 22:32–39
31. Friess H, Langhans J, Ebert M et al (1995) Diagnosis of pancreatic cancer by 2[F-18]-fluoro-2-deoxy-D-glucose positron emission tomography. Gut 36:771–777
32. Ho CL, Dehdashti F, Griffeth LK et al (1996) FDG PET evaluation of indeterminate pancreatic masses. Comput Assist Tomogr 20:363–369
33. Bares R, Dohmen B, Cremerius U et al (1996) Results of positron emission tomography with fluorine-18-labeled fluorodeoxyglucose in differential diagnosis and staging of pancreatic carcinoma. Radiologe 36:435–440
34. Zimny M, Bares R, Fass J et al (1997) Fluorine-18 fluorodeoxyglucose positron emission tomography in the differential diagnosis of pancreatic carcinoma: a report of 106 cases. Eur J Nucl Med 24:678–682
35. Keogan MT, Tyler D, Clark L, Branch MS, McDermott VG, DeLong DM, Coleman RE (1998) Diagnosis of pancreatic carcinoma: role of FDG PET. Am J Roentgenol 171:1565–1570
36. Imdahl SA, Nitzsche E, Krautmann F et al (1999) Evaluation of positron emission tomography with 2-[18F]fluoro-2-deoxy-D-glucose for the differentiation of chronic pancreatitis and pancreatic cancer. Br J Surg 86:194–199
37. Delbeke D, Chapman WC, Pinson CW, Martin WH, Beauchamp DR, Leach S (1999) F-18 fluorodeoxyglucose imaging with positron emission tomography (FDG PET) has a significant impact on diagnosis and management of pancreatic ductal adenocarcinoma. J Nucl Med 40:1784–1792
38. Rose DM, Delbeke D, Beauchamp RD et al (1998) 18Fluorodeoxyglucose – positron emission tomography (18FDG – PET) in the management of patients with suspected pancreatic cancer. Ann Surg 229:729–738
39. Sperti C, Pasquali C, Chierichetti F et al (2001) Value of 18-fluorodeoxyglucose positron emission tomography in the management of patients with cystic tumors of the pancreas. Ann Surg 234:675–680
40. Gambhir SS, Czernin J, Schimmer J, Silverman DHS, Coleman RE, Phelps ME (2001) A tabulated review of the literature. J Nucl Med 42 [Suppl]:9S–12S
41. Nakata B, Chung YS, Nishimura S et al (1997) 18F-fluorodeoxyglucose positron emission tomography and the prognosis of patients with pancreatic carcinoma. Cancer 79:695–699
42. Zimny M, Fass J, Bares R et al (2000) Fluorodeoxyglucose positron emission tomography and the prognosis of pancreatic carcinoma. Scand J Gastroenterol 35:883–888
43. Frolich A, Diederichs CG, Staib L et al (1999) Detection of liver metastases from pancreatic cancer using FDG PET. J Nucl Med 40:250–255
44. Yeung RS, Weese JL, Hoffman JP et al (1993) Neoadjuvant chemoradiation in pancreatic and duodenal carcinoma. A phase II study. Cancer 72:2124–2133
45. Jessup JM, Steele G Jr, Mayer RJ et al (1993) Neoadjuvant therapy for unresectable pancreatic adenocarcinoma. Arch Surg 128: 559–564
46. Maisey NR, Webb A, Flux GD, Padhani A, Cunningham DC, Ott RJ, Norman A (2000) FDG PET in the prediction of survival of patients with cancer of the pancreas: a pilot study. Br J Cancer 83:287–293
47. Franke C, Klapdor R, Meyerhoff K, Schauman M (1999) 18-F positron emission tomography of the pancreas: diagnostic benefit in the follow-up of pancreatic carcinoma. Anticancer Res 19:2437–2442
48. Wahl RL, Henry CA, Ethrer SP (1992) Serum glucose: effects on tumor and normal tissue accumulation of 2-[F-18]-fluoro-2-deoxy-D-glucose in rodents with mammary carcinoma. Radiology 183:643–647
49. Lindholm P, Minn H, Leskinen-Kallio S et al (1993) Influence of the blood glucose concentration on FDG uptake in cancer – a PET study. J Nucl Med 34:1–6
50. Diederichs CG, Staib L, Glatting G, Beger HG, Reske SN (1998) FDG PET: elevated plasma glucose reduces both uptake and detection rate of pancreatic malignancies. J Nucl Med 39:1030–1033
51. Diederichs CG, Staib L, Vogel J et al (2000) Values and limitations of FDG PET with preoperative evaluations of patients with pancreatic masses. Pancreas 20:109–116
52. Kalady MF, Clary BM, Clark LA et al (2002) Clinical utility of positron emission tomography in the diagnosis and management of periampullary neoplasms. Ann Surg Oncol 9:799–806
53. Zimny M, Buell U, Diederichs CG, Reske SN (1998) False positive FDG PET in patients with pancreatic masses: an issue of proper patient selection? Eur J Nucl Med 25:1352
54. Shreve PD (1998) Focal fluorine-18-fluorodeoxyglucose accumulation in inflammatory pancreatic disease. Eur J Nucl Med 25:259–264
55. Diederichs CG, Staib L, Glasbrenner B et al (1999) F-18 fluorodeoxyglucose (FDG) and C-reactive protein (CRP). Clin Pos Imaging 2:131–136
56. Nakamoto Y, Higashi T, Sakahara H et al (2000) Delayed (18)F-fluoro-2-deoxy-D-glucose positron emission tomography scan for differentiation between malignant and benign lesions in the pancreas. Cancer 89:2547–2554
57. Higashi T, Saga T, Nakamoto Y et al (2002) Relationship between retention index in dual-phase (18)F-FDG PET and hexokinase II and glucose transporter-1 expression in pancreatic cancer. J Nucl Med 43:173–180
58. Nitzsche EU, Hoegerle S, Mix M et al (2002) Non-invasive differentiation of pancreatic lesions: is analysis of kinetics superior to semiquantitative uptake value analysis. Eur J Nucl Med Mol Imaging 29:237–242
59. Adams S, Baum R, Rink T, Schumm-Drager PM, Usadel KH, Hor G (1998) Limited value of fluorine-18 fluorodeoxyglucose positron emission tomography for the imaging of neuroendocrine tumors. Eur J Nucl Med 25:79–83
60. Jadvar H, Segall GM (1997) False-negative fluorine-18-FDG PET in metastatic carcinoid. J Nucl Med 38:1382–1383
61. Foidart-Willems J, Depas G, Vivegnis D et al (1995) Positron emission tomography and radiolabeled octreotide scintigraphy in carcinoid tumors. Eur J Nucl Med 22:635
62. Jadvar H, Segall GM (1997) False-negative fluorine-18-FDG-PET in metastatic carcinoid. J Nucl Med 38:1382–1383
63. Eriksson B, Bergstrom M, Sundin A et al (2002) The role of PET in localization of neuroendocrine and adrenocortical tumors. Ann NY Acad Sci 970:159–169
64. Bombardieri E, Maccauro M, de Deckere E et al (2001) Nuclear medicine imaging of neuroendocrine tumours. Ann Oncol 12 [Suppl 2]:S51–S61
65. Anderson CJ, Dehdashti F, Cutler PD et al (2001) 64Cu-TETA-octreotide as a PET imaging agent for patients with neuroendocrine tumors. J Nucl Med 42:213–221

CHAPTER 18

Gastro-Esophageal Cancer

P. Flamen · L. Mortelmans

18.1 Introduction

18.1.1 Incidence, Etiology, Epidemiology, Histopathology

Esophageal cancer (EC) represents the third most common gastrointestinal cancer and has been reported as the ninth most common malignancy in the world. The incidence shows a remarkably strong regional variation, with extremes ranging from 5 cases per 100,000 (USA, whites) to more than 100 cases per 100,000 (e.g. China, Iran). The majority of epidemiologic studies suggest that these cancers arise from chronic irritation of esophageal mucosa. The most common agents or conditions associated with EC include tobacco and alcohol use, ingestions, esophageal dysfunction, and dietary deficiencies [1].

Squamous cell carcinoma is historically the most common cancer of the esophagus. This type of tumor is most commonly found in the proximal two-thirds of the esophagus. Esophageal adenocarcinomas, on the other hand, typically arise in the distal esophagus. Considerable data indicate that esophageal adenocarcinomas result from chronic gastro-esophageal reflux, often in the context of hiatal hernia. A marked increase in the incidence of esophageal adenocarcinoma has been noted in white men in western countries since the early 1970s, to the extent that the incidence rates of this disease in younger white men were equaling or exceeding those of squamous cell carcinoma in the same population. Importantly, no significant survival differences have been noted in adenocarcinoma patients compared with similarly staged individuals with squamous cell cancers [2].

The number of newly diagnosed patients with cancer of the proximal stomach and gastro-esophageal junction (GEJ) has increased markedly since the mid-80s. These tumors are thought to be more aggressive than distal esophageal tumors and more complex to treat. Two distinct histopathologic types have been described: intestinal (arising from precancerous areas such as intestinal metaplasia) and diffuse (less related to precancerous conditions; more genetic etiology; little tumor cell cohesion). Although the diffuse-type cancers are generally associated with a worse outcome than the intestinal type, this finding is not independent of tumor-node-metastasis (TNM) stage.

18.1.2 Conventional Diagnostic Procedures in Relation to Treatment Modalities

18.1.2.1 *Pretreatment Staging*

Pretreatment assessment and classification of disease extent is essential in the management of cancer of the esophagus or of the GEJ [3, 4]. The TNM-based tumor stage is the major determinant of prognosis and provides the basis for selection of the most appropriate therapeutic strategy. The therapeutic options in EC management include radical esophagectomy in early disease, multimodal treatment schemes combining neo-adjuvant chemotherapy and radiotherapy followed by surgery in locoregional advanced disease, and palliative schemes in cases of distant metastatic disease. The current staging system for EC is entirely TNM based as codified in the almost identical staging systems of the American Joint Committee on Cancer (AJCC) and the International Union Against Cancer (UICC) [5, 6]. The pivotal variables of this stage system are the depth of wall penetration of the primary tumor (T-stage), the presence of locoregional lymph node metastasis (stage IIb and stage III), and of distant lymph node or organ metastasis (stage IV).

18.1.2.2 *T-stage*

Trans-esophageal endoscopic ultrasound (EUS) has recently emerged as an important tool for the evaluation of the T-stage. EC is visualized as hypoechoic areas with the typical five-layer ultrasound stratification of the esophageal wall. Depth of invasion within these five layers corresponds to T-stage in the TNM staging system. T1 lesions are characterized by invasion within the first three layers (mucosa and submucosa), T2 lesions are contained within the fourth layer (muscularis propria), T3 lesions penetrate layer 5 (adventitia), and T4 disease is indicated by the invasion of adjacent organs. The accuracy of T-staging by EUS is 79–92% [7]. EUS understages the primary tumor about 5% of the time and overstages 6–11% of the time [8].

Computed tomography (CT) remains unreliable in determining the depth of tumor invasion in the esophageal wall. A T4-stage can be diagnosed with moderate accuracy by indicating invasion of the peri-esophageal fat and adjacent structures (i.e. aorta and tracheobronchial tree). Magnetic resonance imaging (MRI) does not seem to increase the diagnostic accuracy of determining the T-stage.

18.1.2.3 *NM-stage*

In patients with metastatic EC (M_1 disease: presence of distant lymph node involvement or organ metastasis), first-line surgery with a curative intent is contraindicated. The prognosis for these patients is too short to justify a curative surgical approach with all the induced morbidity and loss of quality of life. Palliative approaches (stenting, radiotherapy, palliative surgery, chemotherapy) are preferred. In non-metastatic EC ($T_{<4}N_{1 \text{ or } 2}M_0$), locoregional lymph node involvement is the most important prognostic factor, with a dramatic fall in the cure rate in patients with positive nodes. Even in early T_{1b}/T_2 tumors, nodal involvement is common (30–50% of patients). Esophageal cancer is characterized by an excessive and chaotic lymphatic spread. This was most impressively illustrated by the results from three-field lymphadenectomy (i.e. extensive lymphadenectomy comprising upper abdominal, mediastinal and cervical lymph nodes), as has been reported mainly by Japanese investigators. Akiyama et al. studied the lymph node metastasis pattern in a series of 200 patients [9]. The frequency of nodal metastasis was related to the location of the primary tumor and each of the three dissected fields. According to the location of the tumor (upper, middle, or distal third), cervical lymph node involvement was seen in 46, 29, and 27% of patients; the corresponding incidence of abdominal lymph nodes was 12, 40, and 74%. Moreover, the involvement of distant lymph nodes was unpredictable regardless of tumor location.

Current NM-staging modalities include CT and EUS. Although these methods provide a combined accuracy of 70–90% in the preoperative identification of metastatic (M_1) disease, in many patients advanced disease is detected only during surgery or after minimally invasive surgical staging by both laparoscopy and thoracoscopy. The standard non-invasive staging modalities are CT of the chest and abdomen for the detection of distant metastases, and trans-esophageal EUS for the evaluation of locoregional lymph node staging in non-obstructing EC [10–14]. However, these techniques entirely depend on structural characteristics for diagnosis. This inevitably causes limitations in diagnostic specificity (false-positive findings in enlarged inflammatory lymph node) and sensitivity (false-negative findings in non-enlarged invaded lymph node). An illustrative example of the inherent inaccuracy of CT for defining lymph node involvement is provided by a study by McLoud et al. He reported that, in lung cancer, nearly 40% of enlarged mediastinal lymph nodes of 2–4 cm do not harbor tumor cells, whereas smaller nodes may still contain metastatic cells [15]. Some centers have, therefore, propagated the routine use of the minimally invasive surgical staging procedures, consisting of a thoracoscopy combined with a staging abdominal laparoscopy, thus aiming at a greater accuracy in the evaluation of regional and celiac lymph node, and allowing the detection of unimaged pleural or peritoneal disease [16–18]. However, the long surgery and hospitalization times, and the high costs of these invasive procedures strongly limit their routine implementation.

18.1.2.4 *Diagnosis and Staging of Recurrent Disease*

The disease-free survival of cancer of the esophagus remains poor despite significant advances in surgical techniques and perioperative management [19–21]. Even after apparently curative surgery, the overall 5-year survival is only 30–50%. The available therapeutic modalities in recurrent cancer are radical re-resection, palliative resection and bypass, laser thermocoagulation, stenting, chemotherapy, brachytherapy, and radiotherapy, alone or in combination. The choice of a specific therapeutic modality depends on the localization and extent of the recurrence. In approximately one-third of patients, the recurrence is located in the operation field. The lesions are usually seen in regional lymph nodes, or as a mass originating in the mediastinum and infiltrating the gastric pull up from outside. The majority of the recurrences, however, are distant metastases, indicating the systemic character of the disease [22–24]. Two-thirds of patients present with recurrence within 1 year, and nearly all within 2 years after primary surgery [25]. Some reports suggested that early detection of recurrent disease is desirable, as aggressive treatment may result in prolonged tumor-free survival or occasional cure [26]. The conventional diagnostic work-up currently available for the postoperative diagnosis and staging of recurrent disease includes endoscopy, trans-esophageal EUS, and CT. A fundamental limitation of these techniques is that they entirely depend on anatomical and/or structural criteria for diagnosis. Therefore, in this particular diagnostic setting, their specificity is severely hampered by therapy-induced changes of the tissue characteristics at the operation site [27]. Moreover, strictures at the esophagogastric anastomosis often preclude full passage of the endoscope, resulting in incomplete diagnosis in one-third of the patients [28].

18.1.2.5
Assessing the Response to Neo-adjuvant Treatment

The prognosis of locally advanced cancer of the esophagus or GEJ, i.e. tumors clinically staged as T_4 without evidence of organ metastases, remains poor (median survival 3–5 months) [29]. Preoperative downstaging of these patients by multimodality treatment that combines chemotherapy and radiotherapy before esophagectomy holds promise [30, 31]. The radiotherapy aims to improve local resectability by reducing the primary tumor extension and to reduce local recurrences. The chemotherapy is based on the rationale that subclinical distant metastatic disease is present in the majority of these patients at diagnosis. Most centers prefer concurrent treatment schemes exploiting the radiation-enhancing effects of chemotherapy. Several reports indicate that after surgery, the patients who respond to the neo-adjuvant treatment have a better prognosis than those who do not respond [32, 33]. In 10–20% of patients, such therapy results in a pathologic complete response ($pT_0N_0M_0$), in which no residual tumor is found at surgery. The patients achieving such a response have the best outcome [34]. On the other hand, about 50% of the patients will not respond to neo-adjuvant chemoradiation therapy (CRT) and carry the risk for the progression of disease beyond resectability and for the distant spread of therapy-resistant disease. Much futile treatment would be avoided if these patients could be identified before or early after initiating CRT. Accurate non-invasive pre- and post-CRT staging and response assessment, differentiating responders from non-responders, would thus contribute to optimal patient management. The conventional structure-based imaging techniques (CT, endoscopy, EUS) are generally considered as inaccurate in this setting [35, 36]. These techniques are severely hampered by their inability to distinguish treatment-induced fibrosis and inflammation from residual viable tumor tissue. CT is not useful because it cannot evaluate response at the primary tumor site and has too low an accuracy for detection of lymph node metastases. EUS staging criteria cannot reliably determine T-stage nor N-stage after preoperative CRT. The reported accuracy of post-CRT EUS for pathological T-stage was 37%, and its sensitivity for N_1 disease was only 37% [35]. Moreover, EUS suffers from inter- and intraobserver variability, rendering the comparisons between tests, patients and institutions difficult. Another drawback of these techniques is their limited field-of-view. The responsiveness of the lesions to chemotherapy or radiotherapy of the primary tumor and the metastatic lesions may differ, which then gives rise to a variable response in different tumor sites. Therefore, a whole-body response assessment is preferable.

18.2
PET: Current Status

18.2.1
Metabolic Evaluation of the Primary Tumor

Several pilot studies have reported a high sensitivity of fluoro-2-deoxy-D-glucose (FDG) positron emission tomography (PET) for primary squamous cell carcinoma of the esophagus. False-negative FDG PET findings are always related to small-volume (T_{is} or T_1) tumors, suggesting that a limitation in the spatial resolution of the PET imaging device, currently around 5–8 mm, is the only cause for non-visualization of primary spinocellular EC. Choi et al. performed dynamic quantitative FDG PET in eight patients with squamous cell carcinoma and reported that five of the patients showed increasing FDG accumulation until 90 minutes after FDG injection. This indicates the need for standardization of imaging timing when using standard uptake value (SUV) or tumor-to-normal tissue uptake ratios as the semiquantitative parameter in serial PET studies [37].

Adenocarcinomas of the esophagus and GEJ, on the other hand, can sometimes show a limited or absent FDG accumulation regardless of tumor volume (FDG non-avidity). In our experience, this is found in 10–15% of these patients, and FDG non-avidity is almost uniquely (ca. 90% of the non-avid tumors) found in strongly undifferentiated adenocarcinomas, often with a signet ring cell characteristic. We observed that around 50% of the undifferentiated adenocarcinomas of the distal esophagus and proximal stomach did not accumulate FDG (unpublished results). Whether this is correlated with the lack of expression of GLUT-1 or GLUT-3 in these tumors and whether this has a prognostic importance is currently the subject of further research. In our experience, the non-avidity for FDG is also constantly present in all metastases of the primary non-avid gastro-esophageal tumor. Therefore, in these patients, the result of the PET scan cannot be taken into account for staging or restaging purposes. An example of a non-FDG-accumulating junctional adenocarcinoma and the resulting FDG PET false-negativity in multiple bony metastases is shown in Fig. 5. Similar observations have been made in gastric adenocarcinoma. Stahl et al. attributed "false-negative" FDG PET findings to a frequent FDG non-avidity found in signet ring cell and mucinous gastric carcinomas [38]. In that study, only two of eight (25%) of the signet ring cell carcinomas and four of six (67%) of the mucinous carcinomas were visualized by FDG PET, whereas all other types of primary gastric cancer were detected, regardless of tumor grade or growth type. It was postulated that the false-negative PET findings in signet cell cancers resulted from the high content of metabolically inert mucus, leading to a reduced FDG concentration falling below the detection limits of the PET camera. Another reason might be the lack of expression of the glucose transporter GLUT-1 on the cell membrane of most of the signet ring cell carcinoma and mucinous adenocarcinoma, as was recently reported by Kawamra et al. [39] Research performed in human pancreatic tumors has indeed shown a correlation between the FDG-uptake intensity and the expression of GLUT-1 [40].

Flamen et al. did not find a significant relationship between the primary tumor SUV and the depth of tumor invasion (pT-stage), nor with the extent of lymph node metastasis (N-stage) [41]. These results are in conformity with an earlier report by Fukunaga et al. who, moreover, demonstrated that the uptake was not related to clinicopathological tumor grading [42]. The latter report, however, indicated a faint correlation between the degree of FDG accumulation, as expressed by SUV, and the prognosis.

18.2.2 Preoperative TNM-staging

18.2.2.1 *Detection of Distant Lymph Node or Organ Metastasis*

One of the first reports suggesting a promising role of FDG PET for preoperative staging was performed by Flanagan et al. [43] In a series of 36 patients, FDG PET and CT were performed. The imaging results were compared with pathologic findings. EUS, however, was not performed. PET revealed CT-negative metastatic disease in five patients (14%), all of whom avoided needless surgery. This was the first study to indicate the potential cost-effectiveness of FDG PET by decreasing the number of unnecessary surgeries in patients with unresectable tumors. In a similar study design, Block et al. compared FDG PET to CT in 58 patients. PET identified the M_1 disease in more patients than CT (sensitivity: 100% for PET; 29% for CT) [44]. Luketich et al. studied 91 patients with PET and CT. In that study, CT was only 63% accurate compared to 84% for PET for detecting distant metastases. False-negative PET lesions were all less than 10 mm in size and occurred typically in the lung or liver. The same study also assessed the prognostic relevance of PET in the patient population: the 30-month survival rate was 60% in patients with only local disease and 20% in patients with distant disease demonstrated by FDG PET [45].

Flamen et al. performed a prospective study on the use of FDG PET for preoperative evaluation of 74 patients with EC (50%) or cancer of the GEJ (50%) compared to the standard combined use of spiral CT and an EUS [46]. FDG PET had a higher accuracy compared with the combined use of CT and EUS (82 vs 64%, respectively; $p=0.004$), mainly by virtue of a superior sensitivity (74 vs 47%, respectively) (Fig. 1). In that study a concordance analysis between FDG PET and the combination of CT and EUS for the diagnosis of M_1 disease indicated a diagnostic discordance in 24% of the cases. FDG PET was correct in 16 (89%) of these, which resulted in the upstaging of 11 patients (15%) from M_0 to M_1 disease, and in the downstaging of five patients (7%) from M_1 to M_0 disease. The FDG PET lesions responsible for the upstaging were located in distant lymph nodes located at the supraclavicular and retroperitoneal region, the liver, the pleura, the chest wall, and in bone. One of these patients is shown in Fig. 2. In one patient, PET detected a second primary carcinoma of the glottis. Interestingly, in the 11 patients upstaged by FDG PET, EUS and CT reported a T_3 classification in ten patients and a T_2-stage in one patient. It is known that the frequency of lymphatic metastases, and therefore the probability of an unsuspected positive PET finding, is related to increasing depth of tumor invasion [47]. FDG PET for detection of unsuspected M_1 disease in early-stage EC (T_{is} and T_1) is very low, questioning the value of FDG PET as a routine procedure in these patients. In two patients, FDG PET falsely understaged the M-stage because of 'false-negative' PET findings in two involved supradiaphragmatic lymph nodes in two patients with cancer of the GEJ. Using PET in these tumors it is often impossible to locate exactly the lymph node in relation to the diaphragm. The consequence of this is important, as if it is located above the diaphragm, the positive lymph node categorizes the patient to an M_1-stage, but if it is below the diaphragm, it is only an N_1-stage. Moreover, these lymph nodes are often located in the close vicinity of the primary cancer of the GEJ. In the same study of Flamen et al., a subanalysis was performed assessing the sensitivity for detection of M_1 disease of EUS and FDG PET in the subset of patients in whom CT did not indicate organ metastatic disease. The sensitivity of EUS in this subgroup (including the three patients in whom endoscopy was inconclusive due to an incomplete passage of the scope) was only 3/20 (15%), in contrast to 12/20 (60%) of FDG PET, confirming the superiority of the latter technique in this regard.

18.2.2.2 *Diagnosis of Lymph Node Involvement*

An illustration of the high sensitivity of FDG PET for diagnosis of small distant lymph metastasis and the need for correlative imaging with CT is given in Fig. 1. Several studies assessed the accuracy of FDG PET for assessment of the lymph node involvement in EC. Some methodological issues have to be taken into account when

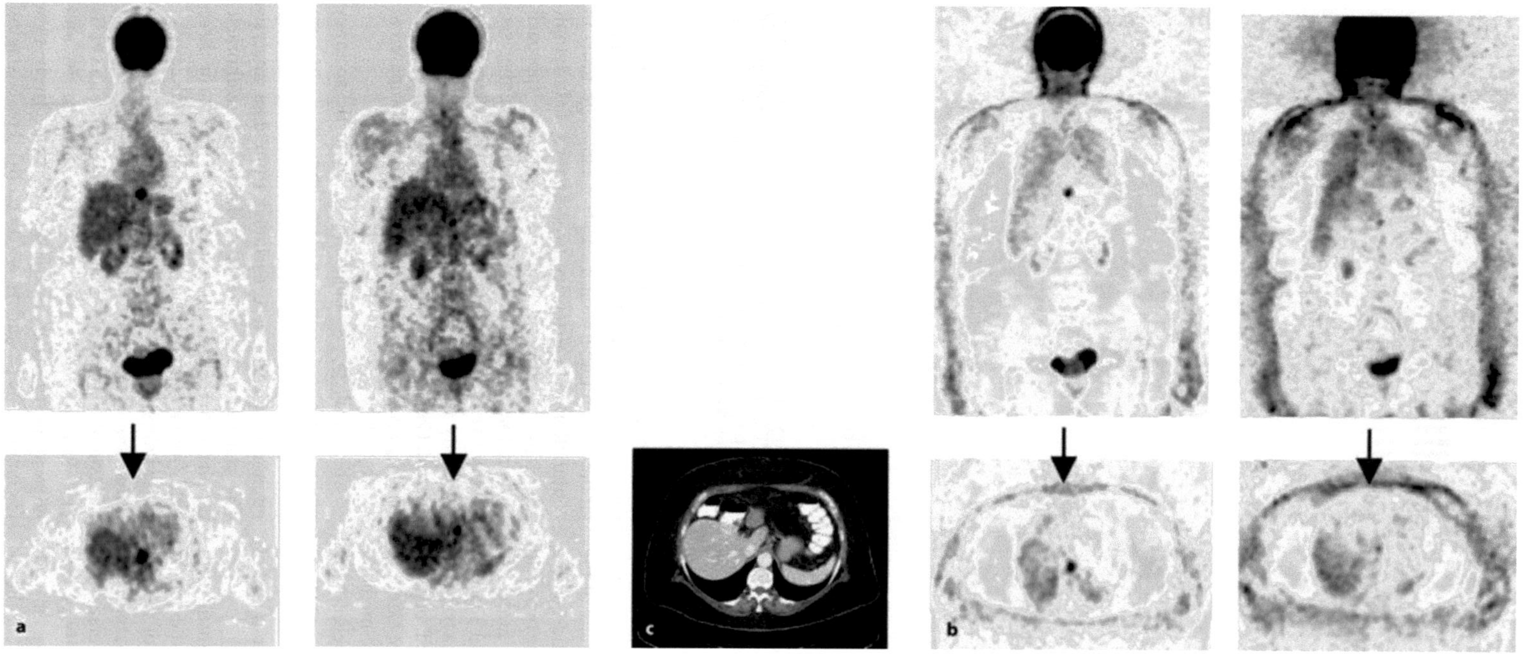

Fig. 1. Attenuation-corrected (**a**) and non-corrected (**b**) FDG PET for primary, preoperative staging of a distal esophageal adenocarcinoma. FDG PET shows the FDG-avid primary tumor and a small hyperactive focus in the upper retroperitoneal space. The contrast of the small spot was similar for both attenuation-corrected and non-corrected images. Correlative CT imaging (**c**) indicated that the hot spot on PET corresponded to a lymph node at the truncus coeliacus (diameter 12 mm). PET upstaged the patient to a M_{1a} stage

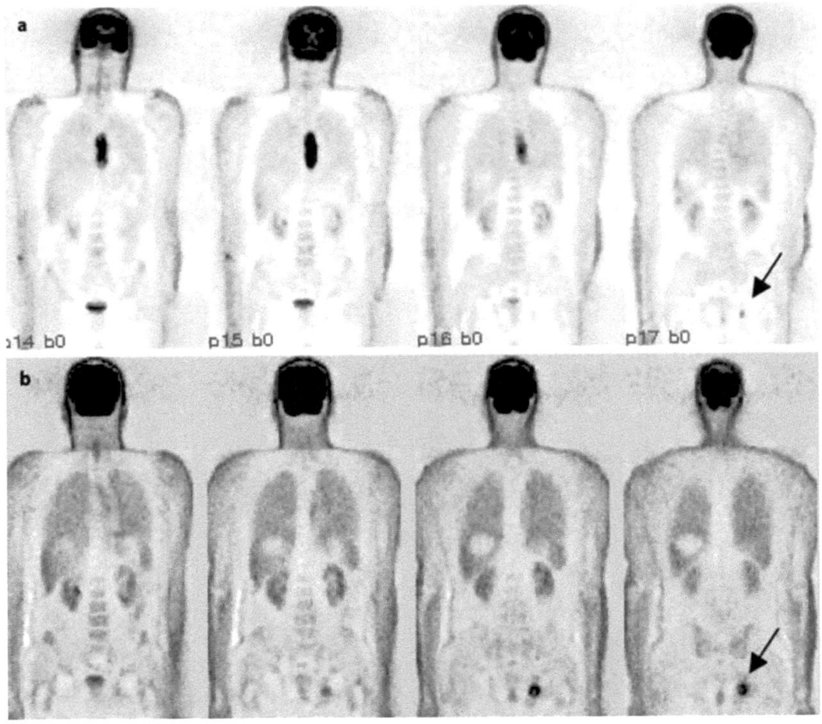

Fig. 2. FDG PET at initial diagnosis (**a**) showed a large primary tumor, and a small focus located in the left ischium. Radiology of the ischium was negative, further dedicated examinations were not performed, and the patient underwent induction chemoradiation therapy. Four weeks after the end of chemoradiation therapy (**b**) FDG PET showed a major response of the primary tumor load, but clear progression of the bony lesions. MRI of the ischium at that time revealed a bone metastasis

evaluating the scientific value of these studies. One of the major methodological requisites of such research is that FDG PET is compared to a correct estimate of the true lymph node status. For this, in conjunction with a radical esophagectomy, extensive peroperative two-field (mediastinum and upper abdominal lymph nodes) or, preferably, three-field (also including cervical) lymphadenectomies have to be performed. For this, a transthoracic surgical approach is certainly preferred, because a transhiatal approach can underestimate the extent of lymph node involvement, as sampling of the mediastinal lymph nodes is incomplete. A second methodological prerequisite of these studies is that PET must be compared to the combined use of EUS and CT, as this combination is currently considered as the standard of staging EC nowadays.

Three early studies indicated the diagnostic utility of FDG PET for assessing the presence and extent of lymph node involvement in EC and cancer of the GEJ. Flanagan et al., [43] in a retrospective study, found an accuracy for lymph node staging of 76% (versus 45% by CT); Block et al. [44] reported a sensitivity of 52%, and Kole et al. [48] a sensitivity of 92%. Kim et al. compared the diagnostic accuracy of FDG PET in the detection of lymph node metastasis to spiral CT prospectively in 50 patients with esophageal squamous cell carcinomas who underwent a curative esophagectomy in conjunction with extensive two- or three-field lymphadenectomy and performing a transthoracic approach [49]. In that study, PET had a significantly higher sensitivity (42 vs 15%, respectively) than CT, whereas the specificity was similar (94 vs 97%). EUS was not performed. Considering only distant lymph node metastasis (M_{1a}-stage), PET had a 69% sensitivity compared to 15% by CT.

Choi et al. [37] evaluated the diagnostic accuracy of FDG PET in 61 consecutive patients. PET was compared to CT and EUS. Thirteen patients who were treated non-surgically were excluded from data analysis. The remaining 48 patients underwent transthoracic esophagectomy with either a two-field ($n=35$) or three-field ($n=13$) lymph node dissection. Histopathology of these lymph nodes served as gold standard. Of the 382 lymph nodes dissected, 100 (in 32 patients) were malignant on histologic examination. On a lymph node basis, FDG PET showed 57% sensitivity, 97% specificity, and 86% accuracy, whereas CT showed respectively 18% ($p<0.0001$), 99%, and 78% ($p=0.003$). For N-staging (diagnostic categories: N_0 and N_1), FDG PET was correct in 83% of the patients, whereas CT and EUS were correct in 60% ($p=0.006$) and 58% ($p=0.003$), respectively. The authors reported that the sensitivity for detecting local lymph node involvement (i.e. less than 3 cm from the primary tumor) is low due to the limited resolution of the PET apparatus and scatter effects coming from the intense radioactivity accumulation in the primary EC tumor. They also reported a lower sensitivity for cervical and abdominal lymph node involvement than for thoracic lymph nodes. However, in that study, correction for tissue attenuation was not performed in all patients, probably partially accounting for this observation. Because the regional lymph nodes involved in EC are usually located in the highly attenuated parts of the body (upper abdominal area, posterior mediastinum), and are often smaller than 2 cm in diameter, accurate attenuation correction is important for correct assessment of lymph nodes with FDG PET. Lerut et al. performed a similar study on the use of FDG PET for assessing lymph node involvement in EC [50]. Forty-two patients were included prospectively. All patients underwent whole-body attenuation-corrected FDG PET imaging, a spiral CT of thorax and abdomen, and EUS. The gold standard consisted exclusively of histology. Histological diagnosis was available in 224 lymph node regions. The accuracy for distant lymph node metastasis (M_1) was significantly higher for FDG PET compared to the combined use of CT and EUS (86 vs 62%, $p=0.0094$). This was based on both a higher sensitivity (77 vs 46%) and a higher specificity (90 vs 69%, $p=0.04$) of FDG PET. Considering the diagnosis of M_{1a} disease, the result of FDG PET was discordant compared to the combination of EUS and CT in 12/42 patients (29%). In these patients FDG PET was correct in 11/12 patients: five patients were correctly upstaged from M_0-stage to M_{1a}-stage, and six patients were correctly downstaged from M_{1a}-stage to M_0-stage.

For the diagnosis of locoregional lymph node (N-stage 1 or 2), FDG PET was not found useful because of a lack of sensitivity compared to EUS and CT (22 vs 83%, $p=0.0026$). The low sensitivity of FDG PET for locoregional lymph node staging was explained by the difficulty in discriminating the primary tumor from local,

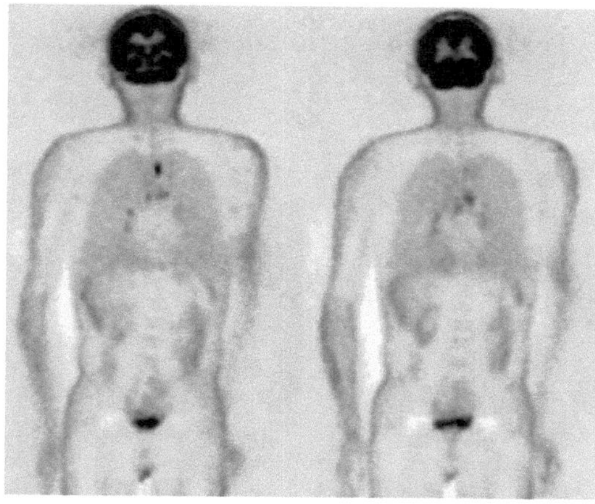

Fig. 3. False-positive FDG PET. Non-attenuation-corrected FDG PET for primary, preoperative staging of a proximal esophageal squamous cell carcinoma in a patient with chronic obstructive pulmonary disease. FDG PET shows the FDG-avid primary tumor and multiple hyperactive lymph nodes at the mediastinum and both lung hili. CT also showed multiple enlarged lymph nodes. The distribution of the PET lesions suggested inflammatory disease; however, formal exclusion of lymph node metastasis is not possible in this setting. Esophagectomy and lymphadenectomy were performed. Histopathology showed a $pT_2N_0M_0$-stage

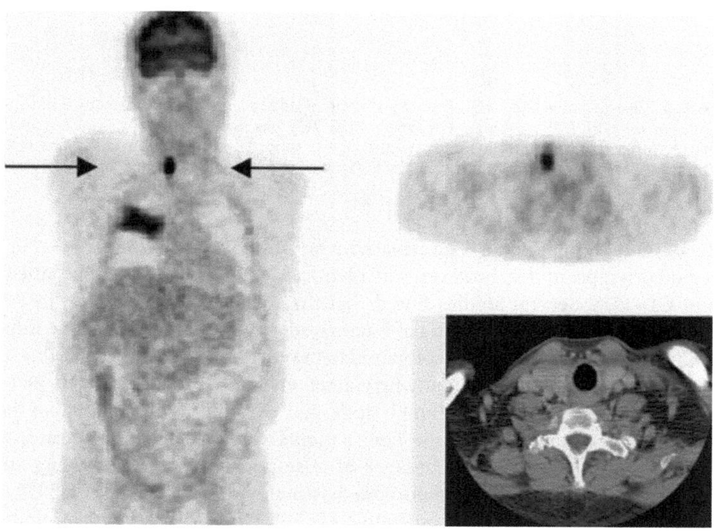

Fig. 4. False-positive FDG PET. Primary staging of adenocarcinoma of the GEJ. The primary tumor was not visualized because of a small tumor volume (EUS: T_1). FDG PET indicated a large hyperactive nodule located at the right paratracheal area. Correlative imaging with CT indicated that the PET lesion corresponded with a nodule in the thyroid gland. Intense lobar FDG uptake is seen in the right lung, indicating active pneumonia. Postoperative histopathology staging: $pT_1N_0M_0$. Histopathology of the thyroid (partially resected during esophagectomy): benign nodular hyperplasia

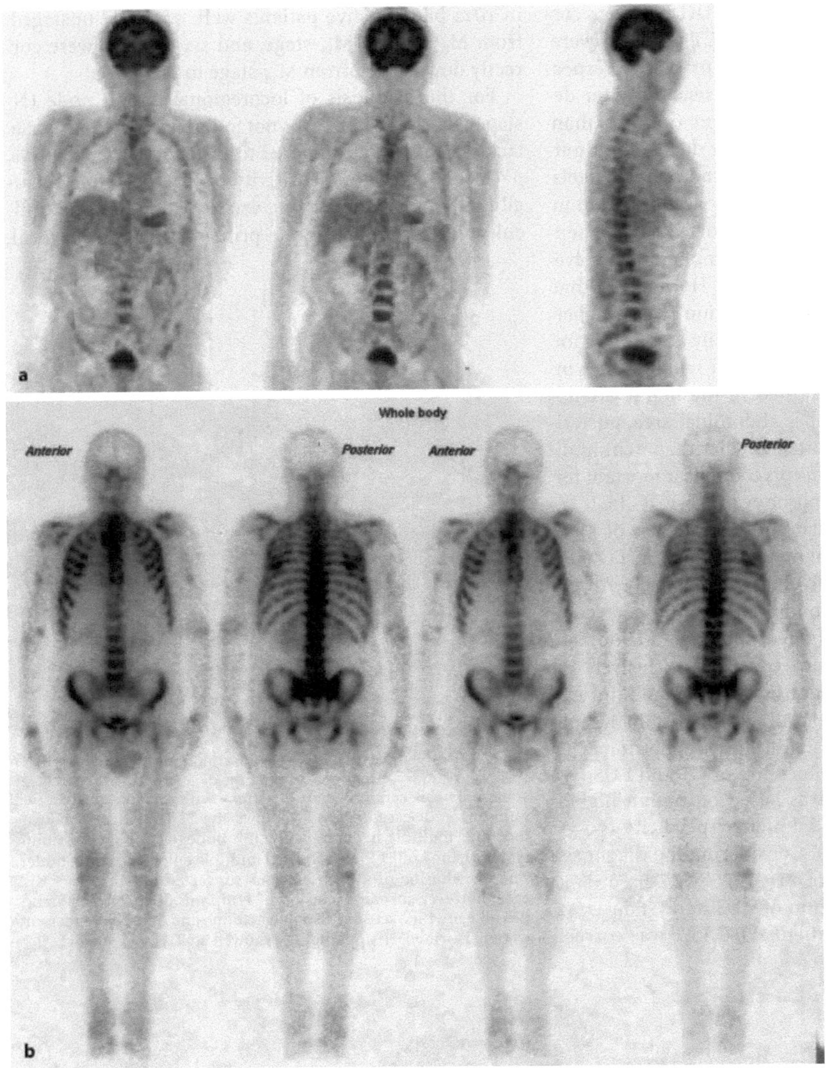

Fig. 5. a False-negative FDG PET. Primary staging of adenocarcinoma of the GEJ. EUS showed a T_3N_1-stage. FDG PET was negative. A diffusely increased bone marrow uptake was reported. As tumor load was significant (as indicated by EUS), it was concluded that the tumor did not have enough FDG avidity and that, therefore, PET was not useful as a staging modality in this patient. **b** One week later, a bone scan (Tc-99m MDP) showed multiple bone metastases, not seen on the FDG PET

peritumoral lymph nodes. The sensitivity for non-local, regional lymph nodes, however, was identical for PET and CT+EUS. Several studies found that the specificity of FDG PET for the diagnosis of lymph node involvement was significantly higher compared to the currently standard modalities. In the study by Flamen et al., PET specificity was 89 % for local lymph node, and 98 % for regional and distant lymph node. Four patients were incorrectly overstaged by PET because of false-positive FDG accumulation in inflammatory mediastinal lymph nodes. Some examples of false-positive FDG PET findings are shown in Figs. 3, 4 and 5. In the study of Choi et al., eight patients had false-positive thoracic lymph node groups by FDG PET [37]. Six of these were proven to have active inflammatory pulmonary disease. Therefore, even if the specificity and the positive predictive value of FDG PET seem very high, we still recommend confirmation of the malignant nature of the PET lesions that could lead to a change in therapeutic management.

Considering all available staging modalities together, including PET, a considerable staging inaccuracy still persists. The underlying major type of staging inaccuracy, however, depends on the modality under consideration. Flamen et al. reported that PET understaged the extent of lymph node involvement in 19/39 (49%) patients, whereas the combination of CT and EUS overstaged the lymph node extent in 14/39 (36%) patients [46].

18.2.2.3
Diagnosis and Staging of Recurrent Disease

Generally speaking, the diagnostic superiority of metabolism-based methods such as FDG PET should be most pronounced during follow-up because aspecific sequels of surgery, radio- or chemotherapy render the conventional, anatomy-based modalities far less accurate. An example of the successful use of FDG PET in this setting is shown in Fig. 6. One study specifically addressed the use of FDG PET for the diagnosis and staging of symptomatic recurrent cancer after a presumably curative resection of cancer of the esophagus or GEJ [51]. In that study, 41 symptomatic patients underwent conventional diagnostic work-up (CDW) and a whole-body FDG PET. Forty recurrences were found in 33 patients. The lesions were located at peri-anastomotic ($n=9$), regional ($n=12$), and distant sites ($n=19$). For the diagnosis of a peri-anastomotic recurrence, the sensitivity and specificity of FDG PET were 100 and 57%, versus 100 and 93% for CDW, respectively. For the diagnosis of a regional and distant recurrence, the sensitivity and specificity of PET were 94 and 82%, versus 81 and 82% for CDW. PET provided additional information in 11/41 (27%) patients: a major impact on diagnosis was found in five patients with equivocal or negative CDW findings in whom PET provided a true-positive diagnosis. Five other patients were upstaged from localized to extended recurrent disease; and in one patient with an equivocal CDW lesion, PET correctly excluded malignancy.

These results suggest that FDG PET provides a highly sensitive diagnosis of recurrent disease, both locoregionally and at distant sites. This supports the hypothesis that PET could allow an earlier and presumably preclinical diagnosis of EC recurrence, and certainly justifies further prospective studies in this respect. A second noteworthy finding in that study was the high incidence of false-positive PET findings at the peri-anastomotic region. An example is shown in Fig. 7. By reviewing the patients' records, it was found that those with intense false-positive FDG uptake had all undergone an endoscopic dilatation of a benign anastomotic stricture as long as 55 days before the PET scan. The dilatation had probably induced trauma, resulting in an inflammatory reaction. Three other patients had only moderate uptake at the anastomosis. In two of these, a non-tumoral stricture was found endoscopically. However, a dilatation had not been performed, and it can be hypothesized that the accumulation of FDG is due to proliferating fibroblastic and/or granulomatous tissue at the anastomosis. The other patient was scanned less than 2 months after primary surgery. The FDG uptake in this patient probably reflected a normal inflammatory healing process. This means that interpretation of the PET scan at the anastomotic site needs careful correlation with clinical and radiological data. The specificity of PET at the regional and distant sites is clearly higher, though certainly not perfect. Multidisciplinary con-

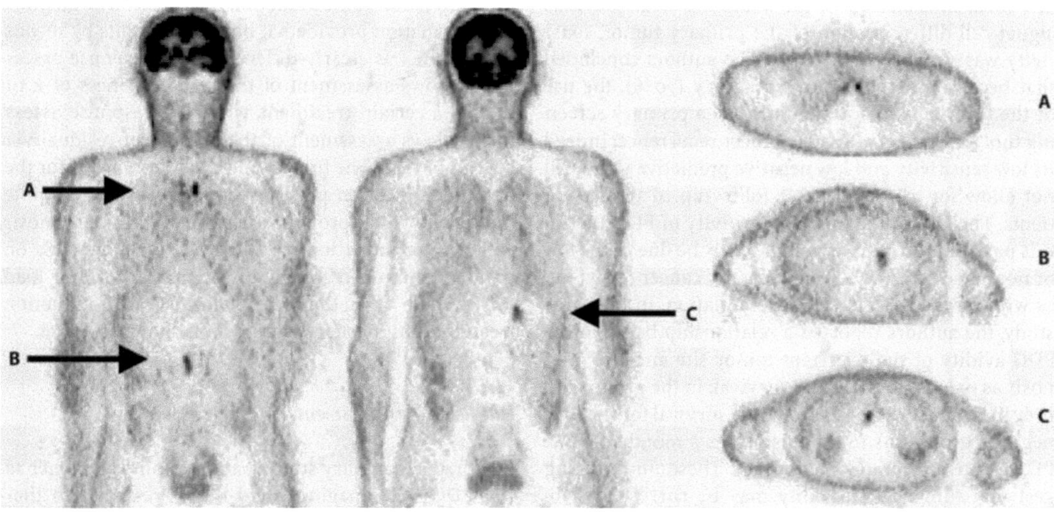

Fig. 6. FDF PET in a symptomatic patient 1 year after resection of an esophageal carcinoma. Endoscopy showed a benign stenosis; CT of chest and abdomen was negative. PET identified multiple true-positive sites of recurrent disease, located peri-anastomotically (**A**), in the retroperitoneal space (**C**), and at the hilus of the spleen (**B**)

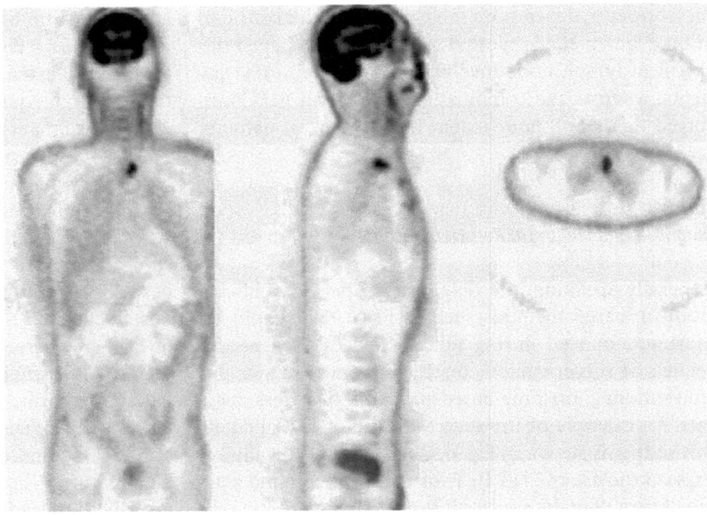

Fig. 7.
False-positive FDF PET finding in a patient with progressive dysphagia after a presumed curative resection of an esophageal carcinoma. The patient underwent a dilatation of the anastomosis some days before the PET scan was performed. Intense FDG accumulation was seen. The patient had a negative follow-up of 1 year

frontation of the PET findings with clinical data, together with close correlation of PET and CT images should neutralize the potential negative impact of these equivocal PET lesions.

De Potter et al. reported a study on the use of FDG PET for recurrent gastric cancer [52]. Thirty-three patients who had surgical treatment for gastric cancer with curative intent and who were suspected for recurrence were studied. The prevalence of recurrent disease was 61%. Sensitivity and specificity of FDG PET for diagnosis of recurrence was 14/20 (70%) and 9/13 (69%). Positive and negative predictive values were 14/18 (78%) and 9/15 (60%). Of the six false-negative cases, four had intra-abdominal lesions (two peritoneal, one liver and one local metastasis). In the subgroup with previous signet cell differentiation of the primary tumor, sensitivity was similarly low (62%). The authors concluded that because of its moderate accuracy (70%), the use of the technique is not warranted as a primary screening tool for suspected gastric cancer recurrence. Indeed, its low sensitivity and low negative predictive value will not allow for a cost-effective follow-up of treated patients. The lack of diagnostic sensitivity of FDG PET in this particular indication might partly be due to the low or non- avidity of FDG seen in gastric cancer recurrences with marked signet cell differentiation. In the same study, the authors reported a relationship between the FDG avidity of the recurrent tumor site and the prognosis as expressed as overall survival: in the group with proven recurrence ($n=20$), median survival for the PET-negative group was 16 months versus 5 months for the PET-positive group ($p=0.05$) [52]. These findings suggest that tumor FDG avidity may be correlated with metabolic aggressiveness and/or patient prognosis. Interestingly, Kawamura et al. recently reported a significantly shorter survival of patients who had gastric tumors that expressed GLUT-1 compared with those with GLUT-1-negative tumors [39]. GLUT-1 negativity reduces the FDG avidity of the lesions. This might explain the correlation between FDG PET positivity of the recurrent tumor sites and the observed reduction of patient survival.

18.2.3 Monitoring of Induction Therapy

The metabolic effects of a non-surgical antitumoral treatment can be assessed at two different time points: early after the start of the treatment (e.g. after 1 week of induction chemotherapy), or late (i.e. some weeks after the completion of the induction treatment). The diagnostic information provided at both time points by means of FDG PET is clearly different: early response assessment allows assessment of the responsiveness of a tumor to a certain treatment, while late response assessment allows assessment of the amount of residual viable tumor load. The first should provide a means for the early identification of non-responding patients, while the second could provide an estimate of the prognosis, which, after induction treatment, strongly depends on the degree of downstaging of the primary tumor load. An example of an early and late FDG PET induction treatment response measurement is shown in Fig. 8.

18.2.3.1 *Late Response Assessment*

The first preliminary study that determined whether serial FDG PET imaging could detect response to therapy in patients with gastro-esophageal tumors was published by Couper et al. [53] Thirteen patients were scanned before and after two or three cycles of 5-fluo-

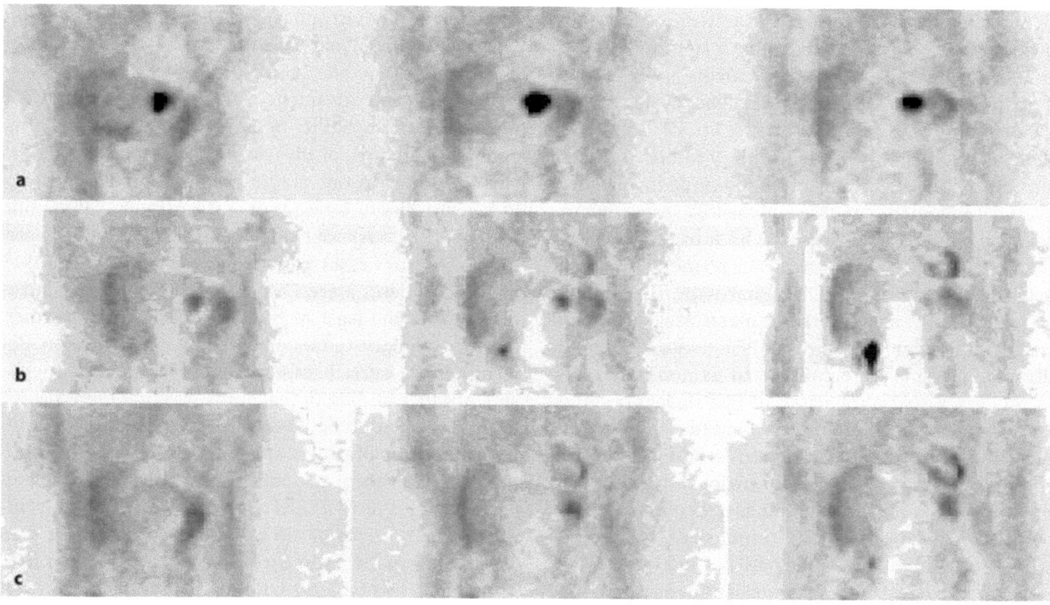

Fig. 8. FDG PET to monitor the effects of induction treatment. A patient with a large tumor of the GEJ underwent an FDG PET scan before (**a**), 1 week after 1 week of chemotherapy alone (**b**), and 4 weeks after a 4-week course of combined chemoradiation (**c**). The early PET indicated a partial response (>50 % reduction of FDG accumulation), the late PET showed a complete normalization of the lesion's FDG uptake. Surgical resection was complete. Pathology revealed a $pT_0N_0M_0$-stage (no residual tumoral activity found)

rouracil and cisplatin-based chemotherapy. Quantification was performed using tumor-to-liver uptake ratios (TLR) and, in seven patients, by calculating the influx constant for FDG (K) using dynamic PET and an image-derived input function. Clinical assessment (dysphagia, weight scores) was used as reference for the response. They found that the FDG accumulation changed in all patients. The median reduction of the TLR was 22 %, ranging from a complete normalization of the FDG uptake to an increase of 15 %. In patients with increased FDG uptake after treatment, CT and the clinical assessment indicated a non-response. The authors also compared the response as measured by using change in TLR with the change of K values in nine lesions in six patients. The correlation between the two methods was strong ($r = 0.87$), justifying the use of a simple TLR change before and after treatment in a clinical setting.

Brücher et al. was the first to report the results of a study evaluating FDG PET for the assessment of the metabolic response to induction CRT in locally advanced squamous cell EC, and related to disease-free and overall survival [54]. Twenty-seven patients underwent neoadjuvant CRT consisting of external-beam radiotherapy and 5-fluorouracil as a continuous infusion. FDG PET was performed before and 3 weeks after the end of the CRT, before surgery. Quantitative measurements of tumor FDG uptake (SUV) were correlated with histopathologic response and patient survival. Histopathologic evaluation revealed less than 10 % viable tumor cells in 13 patients (responder group: consisting of patients with complete or subtotal responses) and more than 10 % viable tumor cells in 11 patients (non-responders: consisting of patients with partial response or stable disease). In responders, FDG uptake decreased by 72 ± 11 %; in non-responders, it decreased by only 42 ± 22 %. A ROC analysis indicated that at a threshold of 52 % decrease of FDG uptake compared with baseline, sensitivity to detect response was 100 %, with a corresponding specificity of 55 %. The positive and negative predictive values were 72 and 100 %. This means that, if in this particular setting the cut-off of about 50 % reduction of SUV is used, about one-quarter of the patients with a larger reduction of FDG uptake will prove to be non-responders, while none of the patients with an FDG reduction of smaller than 50 % will prove to be responders. This indicates that serial FDG PET is particularly well suited for the identification of the non-responding patients. Non-responders to PET scanning had a significantly worse survival after resection than responders: patients with a decrease in the FDG uptake of less than 52 % had a significantly ($p < 0.0001$) shorter median survival time (8.8 ± 2.7 months) compared with patients with an SUV decrease of 52 % or more (22.5 ± 2.5 months).

Flamen et al. confirmed that FDG PET can indeed predict major response to chemoradiation [55]. In that study, major response on histopathology was broadly defined as $pT_{0-2}N_0M_0$ status after treatment ($pT_3N_0M_0$ in selected cases). The protocol included baseline PET,

CRT (cisplatinum, fluorouracil and 40 Gy in 20 fractions) until day 29, follow-up PET 1 month later, followed by surgery in the non-progressive patients 3 weeks thereafter. In contrast to the article by Brücher et al. (in which PET response was defined by using an SUV reduction criterion applied only on the primary tumor, while not considering the PET signs of lymph node involvement after CRT), Flamen et al. assessed the PET response from a clinical point of view. Patients who showed a complete or almost complete normalization of the FDG uptake at the primary tumor site together with the complete normalization of all lymph node metastases seen on the pre-CRT PET were classified as PET major responders. All other patients were considered as non-major PET responders. Visual comparison of PET images obtained before and 1 month after CRT allowed a highly accurate estimate of the CRT response: serial FDG PET had a predictive accuracy of 78% for major response, with a sensitivity of 71% (10/14) and a specificity of 82% (18/22). Misclassifications of CRT-responsiveness based on PET were found in 22% of the patients and were equally based on an overestimation as on an underestimation of the response. The overestimation was due to false-negative PET findings in cases of residual micrometastatic disease. Indeed, PET is prone to false-negativity due to residual micrometastatic cancer foci falling below the detection threshold of the PET device. Consequently, a pathologic complete response cannot be diagnosed accurately by FDG PET. The sensitivity and positive predictive value of a completely normal post-CRT PET for the diagnosis of a pathologic complete response were only 67 and 50%, respectively. The underestimation of CRT response by PET is mainly based on false-positivity at the primary tumor site. The post-therapeutic FDG signal is a result of several intratumoral changes. Death of tumor cells leads to a decreased FDG accumulation. However, inflammatory immune and scavenging reactions may be induced by the therapy, and the influx of leukocytes and macrophages may raise the FDG uptake. These phenomena may cause an underestimation of the effectiveness of a treatment [56].

An important advantage of PET for measuring CRT response is its capability of performing whole-body imaging and, by this, of measuring the response of all lesions together in one single examination. Discordances between the PET response at the primary tumor site with the PET response of the extratumoral sites were found in 8/36 (22%) patients. Importantly, 7/8 (88%) of these patients were CRT non-responders, which indicates that the least responding PET lesion, whether it is the primary tumor or an extratumoral lesion, determines the overall responsiveness (and thus prognosis). Another finding in that study was that there seems to be a correlation between the presence and extent of lymph node involvement as shown by pre-CRT PET and the response rate of patients treated with neo-adjuvant CRT. If only pre-CRT PET was considered as the staging modality, a major CRT response occurred in 9/11 (82%) N_0M_0 patients, in 3/9 (33%) N_1M_0 patients, and in only 2/16 (13%) patients with distant lymphatic spread (M_{1a}). In line with this, pathologic complete responses ($pT_0N_0M_0$) were found in 5/11 (45%) N_0M_0 patients, in only 1/9 (4%) N_1M_0 patients, and in none of the 16 M_{+ly} patients. Most importantly, this correlation between pre-CRT disease extent and response rate was not found using CT or EUS as the staging modality. Thus, PET seems the only imaging modality that can identify those patients who are very likely to attain a major, or even a pathologic complete CRT response. This study also demonstrated a strong relationship between the CRT response as assessed by PET and survival: the median survival according to PET response was 16.3 months vs 6.4 months (log rank test: $p=0.005$). The Kaplan-Meier survival curves are shown in Fig. 9. To prove the added value of assessing PET response in addition to the prognostic information already provided by the pre-CRT

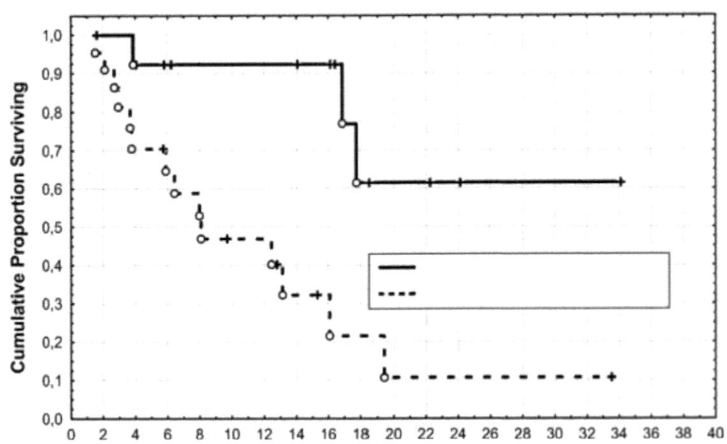

Fig. 9. Kaplan-Meier curves of overall survival after induction chemoradiation therapy in patients with non-metastatic esophageal carcinoma (cT_4) according to the 'late' PET response. PET was performed 4 weeks after completion of a 1-month course of combined chemoradiation therapy

PET, a survival analysis was performed in a more homogeneous subgroup of 25 patients, all showing lymph node involvement on the pre-CRT PET. In this subgroup, six patients had a PET response. Median survival time was 16.7 months in patients with a PET response and 5.9 months in patients without a PET response (log rank testing: $p=0.03$). A Cox regression model confirmed greater predictive power for survival from the reduction in FDG uptake in follow-up scans ($p=0.002$) than from the presence and extent of lymph node involvement in baseline studies ($p=0.087$). The low survival time (5.9 months, starting from the last day of CRT) in the patient subgroup with lymph node metastases seen on the pre-CRT PET, in combination with a poor CRT response observed on PET, clearly indicates very poor prognosis, which raises questions about the value of post-CRT esophagectomy with curative intent in these patients. The finding of a correlation between therapy-induced reduction of the FDG accumulation and prognosis has also been reported in other types of cancer, including non-small-cell lung carcinoma and non-Hodgkin lymphoma [57, 58].

18.2.3.2 *Early Response Assessment*

Generally speaking, about 50 % of patients with EC will not respond to neo-adjuvant CRT. These patients carry the risk for the progression of disease beyond resectability and for the distant spread of therapy-resistant disease. Much futile treatment, with all its toxicity, morbidity and costs, would be avoided if these patients could be identified early after initiating CRT. At the time of writing, only one report is available on the use of serial FDG PET for early therapy monitoring, i.e. after only a few days of treatment [59].

Weber et al. studied 40 consecutive patients with locally advanced adenocarcinomas of the GEJ with FDG PET, performed before and 14 days after initiation of cisplatin-based polychemotherapy. The histopathologic response rate was 24 %. The reduction of tumor FDG uptake after 14 days of therapy was significantly different between responding (-54 ± 17 %) and non-responding tumors (-15 ± 21 %). Using ROC analysis, the optimal differentiation was achieved by a cut-off value of 35 % reduction of initial FDG uptake. Applying this cut-off value as a criterion for a metabolic response predicted clinical response with a sensitivity and specificity of 93 % (14 of 15 patients) and 95 % (21 of 22), respectively. Histopathologically complete or subtotal tumor regression was achieved in 53 % of the patients with a PET metabolic response but only in 5 % of the PET non-responders. Patients without a metabolic response were also characterized by a significantly shorter time to progression/recurrence ($p=0.01$) and shorter overall survival ($p=0.04$): in patients with a PET response, median time to progression or recurrence was 16 months (2-year survival rate, 49 %), whereas it was only 9 months for patients without a PET response (2-year survival rate, 9 %; $p=0.01$). These findings strongly justify further prospective research in this fascinating area. The cut-off of 35 % reduction of FDG signal to differentiate responders from non-responders has been selected based on ROC analysis, and is therefore only applicable to the studied patient population. It is clear that the value of the cut-off depends on the type and dose of therapy given, and the timing of PET after start of therapy. The choice of a cut-off value depends on the therapeutic strategy applied in a particular center: if the oncologist and surgeons aim at a high sensitivity for detecting non-responders, a high cut-off value has to be used (e.g. 50 % reduction); if they aim at a high sensitivity for detecting responders, a lower cut-off value is preferred (e.g. 25 % reduction).

It is clear that we have now entered a new era of metabolism-based imaging for therapy monitoring. Data on response prediction with FDG, [^{18}F]3'-deoxy-3'-fluorothymidine (FLT) and other forms of PET before, during and after treatment should appear in the literature over the next few years. Then, cost-effectiveness studies will be required to convince physicians and public authorities to use this technique [60].

18.3 Indications of PET

According to Medicare Coverage Policy for FDG PET and EC, FDG PET is reimbursed for initial staging and restaging. Coverage for PET is subject to two conditions: (1) the stage of the cancer remains in doubt after completion of a standard diagnostic work-up, including conventional imaging, and (2) clinical management of the patient would differ depending on the stage of the cancer identified. Use of PET would also be considered reasonable and necessary if it could potentially replace one or more conventional imaging studies. Restaging includes both restaging in the setting of recurrence and restaging following completion of a therapeutic regimen or to assess whether a complete response has been achieved. Use of PET to monitor tumor response during the planned course of therapy (i.e. when no change in therapy is being contemplated) is not covered.

18.4 New Tracer Developments

Carbon-11-labeled choline has been proposed as a promising tracer to evaluate mediastinal lymph node metastasis. It has been compared to FDG PET by Kobori et al. in 50 patients with locally advanced EC. The authors found that choline PET was more effective than FDG PET in detecting small lymph node metastases in the mediastinum. An important drawback of this tracer, however, is that it cannot detect metastases in the upper abdomen due to intense physiologic tracer uptake in the liver, spleen and pancreas [61]. The conclusion of that study was that the combination of choline PET and FDG PET was most effective in evaluating the lymph node status of patients with esophageal carcinoma preoperatively. Whether this approach would be cost-effective in the setting of primary staging is very improbable.

There is promise in the FLT ligand, which may become an agent of choice for PET response assessment [62]. FLT is specifically phosphorylated in cells by cytosolic thymidine kinase-1 (TK1). TK1 is a principal enzyme in the DNA-salvage pathway in cells. It is selectively upregulated just before and during the S-phase. Several in-vitro and in-vivo studies have confirmed the relationship between FLT accumulation and the proliferative activity of the tumor cells. This tracer has great promise for therapy monitoring, as it is more specifically related to tumor growth than FDG. Several clinical studies will undoubtedly appear in the near future on the use of this promising new tracer in EC.

18.5 Summary

Based upon the currently available literature data, summarized above, the following general conclusions can be drawn on the present-day use of PET in gastroesophageal cancer.

18.5.1 Initial Preoperative Staging

- FDG PET should be routinely used in patients in whom the standard staging algorithm (i.e. CT scan followed by an EUS) suggests resectable disease. In this patient subset FDG PET improves the detection of metastatic disease (stage IV) and increases the specificity of lymph node staging.
- The diagnostic yield of FDG PET for detection of unsuspected metastatic disease in early-stage EC (Tis and T1) is very low. We do not recommend the routine use of FDG PET in these patients.
- In 10–20% of the adenocarcinomas of the GEJ and proximal stomach the FDG avidity is too low for detection with PET. Almost all of these tumors are poorly differentiated. In case of FDG non-avidity, PET cannot be used for staging nor for further postoperative follow-up.
- The extent of lymph node involvement seen on the initial PET is strongly correlated to prognosis, including the responsiveness to induction CRT.
- The specificity and positive predictive value of FDG PET for lymph node staging are higher than those of conventional modalities. However, false-positivity in inflammatory lesions occurs: correlative imaging of PET and CT, and image-guided biopsies are recommended when a PET finding might affect patient therapeutic management.

18.5.2 Staging Recurrent Disease

- FDG PET allows a highly sensitive diagnosis of recurrent EC.
- False-negative findings have been described in cases of adenocarcinoma with low or absent FDG avidity.
- FDG PET is not accurate for diagnosis of peri-anastomotic recurrence due to frequent false-positive findings based on FDG accumulation in areas of inflammation.

18.5.3 Assessment of Response to Induction Treatment

- Serial PET images allow a highly accurate estimate of the response to induction therapy.
- Simple visual comparison of the PET images allows a clinically based response assessment estimating the degree of downstaging of the tumor load present initially.
- A pathologic complete response cannot be predicted accurately by FDG PET.
- The response assessed by serial FDG PET is strongly correlated with survival.

18.6 Technical Recommendations

18.6.1 Patient Preparation

The incidence of lymph node involvement in the supraclavicular and cervical areas in EC is high. Routine use of myorelaxants (e.g. 5–10 mg diazepam given orally 30 minutes before FDG injection) is therefore strongly recommended to avoid muscular uptake in these areas of interest.

If semiquantitative PET imaging is performed (e.g. for early therapy monitoring), correction for the patient's blood glucose level requires blood sampling.

18.6.2 Attenuation Correction

Attenuation-corrected images are strongly recommended, as these probably enhance the sensitivity of detection of distant lymph node involvement, which, in cases of esophageal and GEJ carcinoma, are often located in the upper abdomen (truncus coeliacus) or neck, two areas in which attenuation correction might increase detection sensitivity.

18.6.3 Pitfalls

Potential false-positive PET findings are a major concern in the use of FDG PET in these patients. It is very important to bear in mind the considerable negative impact of these false-positives on patient comfort, on the referring physician's decision making, and on healthcare costs. Prerequisites for minimizing these PET errors are: (1) experience of the PET reader; (2) complete information available to the PET reader of all clinical (e.g. history; timing, dose and type of chemotherapy) and radiological data; (3) correlative imaging: relating PET information to structural information provided by CT or MRI; (4) good knowledge of the clinical characteristics of the cancer under study (e.g. frequency of the involvement of certain lymph nodes and its impact on patient staging and therapy; (5) multidisciplinary discussion of the integrated PET/CT diagnosis; (6) knowledge of regional incidence of inflammatory (e.g. pneumoconiosis) and infectious disease (e.g. tuberculosis); (7) optimal patient preparation (diazepam, hydration, diuretics, voiding); and (8) histologic or dedicated radiologic confirmation of PET lesions that 'condemn' the patient to a non-curative setting.

There are four major reasons for false-negative PET findings in EC: (1) too small tumor load (e.g. T_1 tumors; peritoneal metastasis); (2) FDG non-avidity; (3) high background activity (e.g. small liver metastasis; omental lymph node involvement; stomach wall); and (4) local, peritumoral lymph nodes, located in the immediate vicinity of the intense uptake of the primary tumor.

References

1. Schrump DS, Altorki NK, Forastiere AA, Minsky BD (2001) Cancer of the esophagus. In: De Vita VT (ed) Cancer. Principles and practice of oncology, vol 33, 6th edn. Lippincott Williams and Wilkins, Philadelphia, pp 1051–1091
2. Lerut T, de Leyn P, Coosemans W et al (1992) Surgical strategies in esophageal carcinoma with emphasis on radical lymphadenectomy. Ann Surg 216:583
3. Beahrs OH, Henson DE, Hutter RVP et al (1998) American Joint Committee on Cancer: manual for staging of cancer, 3rd edn. Lippincott, Philadelphia, pp 63–67
4. Lightdale CJ (1999) Practice guidelines: oesophageal cancer. Am J Gastroenterol 94:20–29
5. Beahrs OH, Henson DE, Hutter RVP et al (1998) American Joint Committee on Cancer: manual for staging of cancer, 3rd edn. Lippincott, Philadelphia, pp 63–67
6. Sobin LH, Wittekind C (1997) TNM classification of malignant tumors, 5th edn. Wiley-Liss, New York
7. Botet JF, Lightdale C (1995) Endoscopic ultrasonography of the gastrointestinal tract. Gastroenterol Clin North Am 24:385–412
8. Siewert JR, Holscher AH, Dittller HJ (1990) Preoperative staging and risk analysis in esophageal carcinoma. Hepatogastroenterology 37:382–387
9. Akiyama H, Masahiko T, Udagawa H, Kihyama Y (1994) Radical lymph node dissection for cancer of the thoracic esophagus. Ann Surg 220:364–373
10. Rice TW, Boyce GA, Sivak MV (1991) Esophageal ultrasound and the preoperative staging of carcinoma of the esophagus. J Thorac Cardiovasc Surg 101:536–544
11. Zuccaro G Jr, Sivak MV, Rice TW (1992) Endoscopic ultrasound and the staging of esophageal and gastric cancer. Gastrointest Endosc Clin North Am 2:625–636
12. Maerz LL, Deveney CW, Lopez RR et al (1993) Role of computed tomographic scans in the staging of esophageal and proximal gastric malignancies. Am J Surg 165:558–560
13. Tio Tl, Coene PP, den Hartog Jager FC et al (1990) Preoperative TNM classification of esophageal carcinoma by endosonography. Hepatogastroenterology 37:376–381
14. Botet JF, Lightdale CJ, Zauber AG et al (1991) Preoperative staging of esophageal cancer: comparison of endoscopic US and dynamic CT. Radiology 181:419–425
15. McLoad TC, Bourgouin PM, Greenberg RW et al (1992) Bronchogenic carcinoma: analysis of staging in the mediastinum with CT by correlative lymph node mapping and sampling. Radiology 182:319–323
16. Sugarbaker DJ, Jalitsch, Liptay MJ (1995) Thoracoscopic staging and surgical therapy for esophageal cancer. Chest 107:218S–223S
17. Bonavina L, Incarbone R, Lattuada E et al (1997) Preoperative laparoscopy in management of patients with carcinoma of the esophagus and of the esophagogastric junction. J Surg Oncol 65:171–174
18. Luketich JD, Schauer P, Landreneau R et al (1997) Minimally invasive surgical staging is superior to endoscopic ultrasound in detecting lymph node metastases in esophageal cancer. J Thorac Cardiovasc Surg 114:817–823
19. Baba M, Aikou T, Yoshinaka H, Natsugoe S, Fukumoto T, Shimazu H et al (1994) Long-term results of subtotal esophagectomy with three-field lymphadenectomy for carcinoma of the thoracic esophagus. Ann Surg 219:310–316
20. Nigro JJ, DeMeester SR, Hagen JA, DeMeester TR, Peters JH, Kiyabu M et al (1999) Node status in transmural esophageal adenocarcinoma and outcome after en bloc esophagectomy. J Thorac Cardiovasc Surg 117:960–968
21. Altorki NK, Girardi L, Skinner DB (1997) En bloc esophagectomy improves survival for stage III esophageal cancer. J Thorac Cardiovasc Surg 114:948–955
22. Van Lanschot JJ, Tilanus HW, Voormolen,MH, van Deelen RA (1994) Recurrence pattern of oesophageal carcinoma after limited resection does not support wide local excision with extensive lymph node dissection. Br J Surg 81:1320–1323
23. Fahn HJ, Wang LS, Huang BS, Huang MH, Chien KY (1994) Tumor recurrence in long-term survivors after treatment of carcinoma of the esophagus. Ann Thorac Surg 57:669–676
24. Mantravardi RV, Lad T, Briele H, Liebner-EJ (1982) Carcinoma of the esophagus: sites of failure. Int J Radiat Oncol Biol Phys 8: 1897–1901
25. Law SYK, Fok M, Wong J (1996) Pattern of recurrence after oesophageal resection for cancer: clinical implications. Br J Surg 83:107–111
26. Raoul JL, Le Prise E, Meunier B, Julienne V, Etienne PL, Gosselin M et al (1995) Combined radiochemotherapy for postoperative recurrence of oesophageal cancer. Gut 37:174–176
27. Carlisle JG, Quint LE, Francis IR, Orringer MB, Smick JF, Gross BH (1993) Recurrent esophageal carcinoma: CT evaluation after esophagectomy. Radiology 189:271–275
28. Barbier PA, Luder PJ, Schupfer G, Becker CD, Wagner HE (1988) Quality of life and patterns of recurrence following transhiatal esophagectomy for cancer: results of a prospective follow-up in 50 patients. World J Surg 12:270–276
29. Katlic MR, Wilkins EW, Grillo HC (1990) Three decades of treatment of esophageal squamous carcinoma at the Massachusetts General Hospital. J Thorac Cardiovasc Surg 99:929–938
30. Bates BA, Detterbeck FC, Bernard SA et al (1996) Concurrent radiation therapy and chemotherapy followed by esophagectomy for localized oesophageal carcinoma. J Clin Oncol 14:156–163
31. Flood WA, Forastiere AA (1998) Oesophageal cancer. In: Al Benson B 3rd (ed) Gastrointestinal oncology. Kluwer Academic, Dortrecht

32. Walsh TN, Noonan N, Hollywood D et al (1996) A comparison of multimodal therapy and surgery for oesophageal adenocarcinoma. N Engl J Med 335:462–467
33. Bosset J-F, Gignoux M, Triboulet J-P et al (1997) Chemoradiotherapy followed by surgery compared with surgery alone in squamous cell cancer of the esophagus. N Eng J Med 33:161–167
34. Van Raemdonck D, van Cutsem E, Menten J et al (1997) Induction therapy for clinical T4 oesophageal carcinoma; a plea for continued surgical exploration. Eur J Cardiothorac Surg 11:828–837
35. Zuccaro G, Rice TW, Goldblum J et al (1999) Endoscopic ultrasound cannot determine suitability for esophagectomy after aggressive chemoradiotherapy for esophageal cancer. Am J Gastroenterol 94:906–912
36. Adelstein DJ, Rice TW, Becker M et al (1996) Concurrent chemotherapy (CCT), accelerated fractionated radiation (AFR) and surgery for esophageal cancer. Proc Am Soc Clin Oncol 15:203
37. Choi CW, Yang WI, Lee JS et al (2000) Dynamic FDG-PET in patients with esophageal cancer. J Nucl Med 5:242P*******
38. Stahl A, Ott K, Weber WA, Fink U, Siewert JR, Schwaiger B (2001) Correlation of FDG uptake in gastric carcinomas with endoscopic and histopathological findings. J Nucl Med 42:78P–79P
39. Kawamura T, Kusakabe T, Sugino T, Watanabe K, Fukuda K, Nashimoto A et al (2001) Expression of glucose transporter-1 in human gastric carcinoma. Association with tumor aggressiveness, metastasis, and patient survival. Cancer 92:634–641
40. Higashi T, Tamaki N, Honda T, Torizuka T, Kimura T, Inokuma T et al (1997) Expression of glucose transporters in human pancreatic tumors compared with increased FDG accumulation in PET study. J Nucl Med 38:1337–1344
41. Flamen P, Lerut A, van Cutsem E et al (2000) Utility of positron emission tomography for the staging of patients with potentially operable esophageal carcinoma. J Clin Oncol 18:3202–3210
42. Fukunaga T, Okazumi S, Koide Y et al (1998) Evaluation of esophageal cancers using fluorine-18-fluorodeoxyglucose PET. J Nucl Med 39:1002–1007
43. Flanagan FL, Dehdashti F, Siegel BA et al (1997) Staging of esophageal cancer with 18F-fluorodeoxyglucose positron emission tomography. AJR 168:417–424
44. Block MI, Patterson GA, Sundaresan RS et al (1997) Improvement in staging of esophageal cancer with the addition of positron emission tomography. Ann Thorac Surg 64:770–777
45. Luketich JD, Friedman DM, Weigel TL et al (1999) Evaluation of distant metastases in esophageal cancer: 100 consecutive positron emission tomography scans. Ann Thorac Surg 68:1133–1137
46. Flamen P, Lerut A, van Cutsem E et al (2000) Utility of positron emission tomography for the staging of patients with potentially operable esophageal carcinoma. J Clin Oncol 18:3202–3210
47. Rice TW, Zuccaro G Jr, Adelstein DJ et al (1998) Esophageal carcinoma: depth of tumor invasion is predictive of regional lymph node status. Ann Thorac Surg 65:787–792
48. Kole AC, Plukker JT, Nieweg OE et al (1998) Positron emission tomography for staging of oesophageal and gastroesophageal malignancy. Br J Cancer 9:1863–1873
49. Kim K, Park SJ, Kim B et al (2001) Evaluation of lymph node metastases in squamous cell carcinoma of the esophagus with positron emission tomography. Ann Thorac Surg 71:290–294
50. Lerut T, Flamen P, Ectors N et al (2000) Histopathologic validation of lymph node staging with FDG-PET scan in cancer of the esophagus and gastroesophageal junction – a prospective study based on primary surgery with extensive lymphadenectomy. Ann Surg 232:743–751
51. Flamen P, Lerut A, van Cutsem E et al (2000) The utility of positron emission tomography (PET) for the diagnosis and staging of recurrent esophageal cancer. J Thorac Cardiovasc Surg 120:1085–1092
52. De Potter T, Flamen P, van Cutsem E et al (2002) Whole-body positron emission tomography (PET) with 18F-fluoro-deoxy-D-glucose (FDG) for diagnosis of recurrent gastric cancer. Eur J Nucl Med 29:525–529
53. Couper GW, McAteer, Wallis F et al (1998) Detection of response to chemotherapy using positron emission tomography in patients with esophageal and gastric cancer. Br J Surg 85:1403–1406
54. Brücher B, Weber W, Bauer M et al (2001) Neoadjuvant therapy of esophageal squamous cell carcinoma: response evaluation by positron emission tomography. Ann Surg 233:300–309
55. Flamen P, van Cutsem E, Lerut A et al (2002) Positron emission tomography for assessment of the response to induction radiochemotherapy in locally advanced oesophageal cancer. Ann Oncol 13:361–368
56. Haberkorn U, Bellemann ME, Altmann A et al (1997) PET 2-fluoro-2-deoxy-D-glucose uptake in rat prostate adenocarcinoma during chemotherapy with Gemcitabine. J Nucl Med 38:1215–1221
57. Vansteenkiste JF, Stroobants SG, de Leyn PR et al (1998) Potential use of FDG-PET scan after induction chemotherapy in surgically staged IIIa-N2 non-small-cell lung cancer: a prospective pilot study. Ann Oncol 9:1193–1198
58. Spaepen K, Stroobants S, Dupont P et al (2001) Prognostic value of positron emission tomography (PET) with fluorine-18 fluorodeoxyglucose ([18F]FDG) after first-line chemotherapy in non-Hodgkin's lymphoma: is [18F]FDG-PET a valid alternative to conventional diagnostic methods? J Clin Oncol 19:414–419
59. Weber WA, Ott K, Becker K et al (2001) Prediction of response to preoperative chemotherapy in adenocarcinomas of the esophagogastric junction by metabolic imaging. J Clin Oncol 19:3058–3065
60. Laking GR, Price PM (2002) FDG-PET for response assessment: answers in search of questions. Ann Oncol 13:345–347
61. Kobori O, Kirihara Y, Kosaka N, Hara T (1999) Positron emission tomography in esophageal cancer using (11)C-choline and (18)F-fluorodeoxyglucose: a novel method of preoperative lymph node staging? Cancer 86:1638
62. Shields AF, Grierson JR, Dohmen BM et al (1998) Imaging proliferation in vivo with [F-18]FLT and positron emission tomography. Nat Med 4:1334–1336

CHAPTER 19

Liver Cancer

J.H. Risse

19.1 Incidence, Etiology and Epidemiology

Liver cancer, or primary hepatobiliary tumors, are among the leading causes of death worldwide. The most important entity, hepatocellular carcinoma (HCC), is the most frequent primary liver cancer (>90%), with an incidence of one million new diagnoses each year; the death rate is about the same (Kew 1998). The incidence of liver cancer varies greatly depending on the geographic region: in endemic regions such as Southeast Asia or equatorial Africa, it is one of the most frequent malignant tumors, with up to 150 cases per 100,000 inhabitants per year, whereas it occurs rarely in developed countries (Fong et al. 2001). In Germany, which is comparable to the USA, only 2.8% (West) and 2.6% (East) of all carcinomas in men are HCC; in women the figures are 1.6 and 2.4%, respectively (Becker and Wahrendorf 1998). The incidence is four new cases per 100,000 inhabitants per year (3,000 men and 1,900 women). The standardized mortality rate in Germany in 1995 was 4.7 (men) and 2.1 (women) per 100,000. Although the incidence of the tumor in Europe and North America is low, that in the developed countries is increasing and the patients are becoming increasingly younger (Becker and Wahrendorf 1998; Okuda et al. 1987; Taylor-Robinson et al. 1997; Deuffic et al. 1998; El-Serag and Mason 1999). In regions with a high incidence, the ratio of men to women is 5:1 and manifestation of the disease is usually before the age of 50 years. In regions with a low incidence, the sex ratio is 2:1 and manifestation of the disease is after 50 years.

Worldwide, risk conditions for the development of HCC are primarily infections with hepatitis B and increasingly hepatitis C, with or without liver cirrhosis. In the western hemisphere, the most important factor is alcoholic liver cirrhosis (Di Bisceglie 1997; Caselmann 1999; Rabe et al. 2001). Other risk factors include hemochromatosis, tyrosinemia, Wilson's disease, primary biliary cirrhosis, aflatoxins, drugs such as oral contraceptives and anabolic steroids, and chemicals such as vinyl chloride, nitrosamines or arsenic. Cirrhosis is an independent risk indicator for the development of liver cancer (Caselmann 1999). Well-known risk conditions for the development of cholangiocellular carcinoma (CCC) are parasitic infection with *Opisthorchis viverrini* (not in the western world), aflatoxins, nitrosamines, liver flukes, and predisposing diseases such as biliary atresia and sclerosing cholangitis (secondary to chronic infectious bowel disease). Prognosis of liver cancer is poor: median survival of untreated patients is 11, 3 and 1 months with 1-year survival rates of 39, 12 and 3% in clinical stage OKUDA I, II and III (see below), respectively.

19.2 Histopathological Classification

For definite diagnosis and grading of suspected liver cancer, biopsy and histological examination are mandatory.

Histologically, primary liver cancer is classified into four groups according to the WHO (1994):

1. Epithelial tumors:
   - Hepatocellular carcinoma (HCC; 91%)
   - Intrahepatic cholangiocellular carcinoma (CCC; 5%)
   - (Cyst-) adenocarcinoma of the bile ducts
   - Combination of HCC and CCC (1%)
   - Hepatoblastoma (childhood; 0.5%)
   - Undifferentiated (anaplastic) carcinoma
2. Not epithelial tumors:
   - Hemangiosarcoma
   - Embryonal (rhabdomyo-) sarcoma
   - Others
3. Other malignant tumors:
   - Teratomas
   - Carcinosarcomas
4. Not classified tumors

The macroscopic appearance of HCC is described as nodular, multicentric, or diffuse infiltrating type.

Histopathological HCC subtypes include the following:

- Trabecular
- Pseudoglandular
- Solid
- Cirrhotic

Fibrolamellar HCC is different because it occurs in younger patients without liver cirrhosis.

Cholangiocellular carcinomas are mostly sclerosing adenocarcinomas, whereas carcinomas of the gall bladder are usually scirrhoid infiltrating adenocarcinomas.

19.3 Conventional Diagnostic Procedures and Treatment Strategies

19.3.1 Diagnostic procedures

Imaging of liver cancer usually begins with ultrasonography, which may be part of a screening program every 6 months in patients with known liver cirrhosis or hepatitis B or C (Caselmann 1999). Any suspicious lesion with or without elevation of the alpha-fetoprotein (AFP; 20 % of HCC are AFP negative) levels has to be clarified. Further conventional imaging procedures for liver cancer include computed tomography (CT) and magnetic resonance imaging (MRI). CT will usually be done as three-phase helical CT:

- Phase 1: the so-called native scan, i.e. before intravenous application of X-ray contrast medium (i.v. contrast); shows tumor tissue (usually hypodense), necroses (hypodense), bleeding (hyperdense), calcifications (very hyperdense)
- Phase 2: arterial phase after i.v. contrast; shows hyperperfused tumor nodules if present
- Phase 3: portal venous phase; shows hypoperfused tumor nodules; recent studies suggest a delayed third phase for even better delineation of the tumor nodules.

Recent developments with multi-slice CT allow imaging of increasingly larger body volumes with better spatial resolution in only one breath-hold cycle. Further information is gathered additionally: regional lymph node enlargement and gross invasion into adjacent organs, vessels (particularly the portal vein) or bile ducts help in classifying the locoregional staging of the patient.

More invasive CT imaging requires a preceding angiography procedure. CT-arteriography (CTA; corresponds to phase 2 after i.v. contrast) is done by injection of contrast medium via a catheter into the hepatic artery and CT-arterio-portography (CTAP; corresponds to phase 3 after i.v. contrast) into the superior mesenteric artery, respectively. Both the invasive methods show enhanced contrast imaging with more and even smaller tumor nodules than the corresponding phases after i.v. contrast. CT after injection of Lipiodol into the hepatic artery is another highly sensitive method for the detection of small HCC (Caselmann 1999; Risse et al. 2001). For treatment strategy planning, [^{131}I]Lipiodol may be given in small diagnostic doses in order to determine scintigraphically whether HCC nodules will accumulate the radiopharmaceutical for therapeutic options (Raoul et al. 1993).

Angiography is another invasive diagnostic method for imaging the pertinent vessels. Because of its invasive nature, angiography will often be combined with or followed by CTA, CTAP or diagnostic Lipiodol administration, if not therapeutic administration of pharmaceuticals in the same session.

Magnetic resonance imaging is done in different sequences (T1, T2, and gradient-echo techniques in multiple variants) before and after intravenous application of gadolinium-DTPA. Improved liver–tumor contrast is achieved by super-paramagnetic iron oxide contrast media (SPIO). SPIO lead to signal loss of liver parenchyma with normal function (hypointense) so that tumor tissue becomes relatively hyperintense. Recent developments have led to the concept of the so-called one-stop shopping, i.e. the combination of the above morphologic information with MR angiography of all pertinent great abdominal vessels (patency of the portal vein, etc.) in one session.

Scintigraphic procedures on the liver (blood pool, colloid and hepatobiliary scintigraphy) are helpful in the differential diagnosis of benign liver lesions but not in liver cancer. Osseous metastases may become positive in bone scintigrams in an advanced stage of the disease. For staging issues, further imaging includes X-ray and/or CT of the thorax.

19.3.2 Staging Classifications

There are two well-recognized staging schemes. Table 1 shows the OKUDA classification for HCC (Okuda et al. 1985) and Table 2 the tumor–node–metastasis (TNM) staging system of the UICC (Union Internationale Contre le Cancer; Sobin and Wittekind 1997) for HCC and intrahepatic CCC.

Table 1. Hepatocellular carcinoma staging according to Okuda (1985)

Stage	Tumor/liver		Ascites		Albumin		Bilirubin	
	>50 % (1)	≤50 % (0)	Yes (1)	No (0)	<3 g/dl (1)	>3 g/dl (0)	>3 mg/dl (1)	≤3 mg/dl (0)
I				0				
II				1 or 2				
III				3 or 4				

Table 2. UICC stages of hepatocellular carcinoma and intrahepatic cholangiocellular carcinoma (Sobin and Wittekind 1997)

Stage I	T1	N0	M0
Stage II	T2	N0	M0
Stage IIIA	T3	N0	M0
Stage IIIB	T1/2/3	N1	M0
Stage IVA	T4	any N	M0
Stage IVB	any T	any N	M1

19.3.3 Treatment Strategies

As shown by the poor prognosis of liver cancer, treatment is not as effective as are diagnostic proceedings. Surgical resection is the only form of treatment with a potential of cure but is feasible only for a minority of patients (Maraj et al. 1988; Brunken et al. 2000): most patients suffer from liver cirrhosis with reduced liver function, so they cannot be operated. Liver transplantation is also feasible only for selected patients. Therefore, the vast majority of patients will be restricted to palliative treatment strategies. Percutaneous radiation has proven ineffective (Robertson et al. 1993), as has systemic chemotherapy (Flickinger et al. 1997). Tamoxifen, an anti-estrogen, which had been the hope for HCC patients in the 1990s, has lost its glamour in recent meta-analyses showing the lack of efficacy (CLIP 1998; Mathurin et al. 1998). Immunotherapy, e.g. interferon alpha, has not proven its efficacy yet, and confirmation of recent good results with somatostatin analogues (octreotide) is pending (Caselmann 1999).

Locoregional treatment strategies for HCC include percutaneous ethanol injection and percutaneous thermal tumor ablation (e.g. radiofrequency thermoablation and laser-induced thermotherapy). These procedures are not indicated in patients with multiple tumor nodules (Bremer et al. 1998; Caselmann 1999; Grasso et al. 2000). Although induction of necroses has been proven with transarterial chemoembolization, it does not ameliorate survival (Bruix et al. 1998; Pelletier et al. 1998), and is not suitable for a significant percentage of patients with portal vein thrombosis because patency of the portal vein is mandatory for the procedure. All these patients are candidates for intra-arterial administration of radiopharmaceuticals such as [^{131}I]Lipiodol (Risse et al. 1999, 2000); unfortunately, this kind of therapy is available in only a few centers.

19.4 PET: Current Status in Liver Cancer

The number of papers dealing with positron emission tomography (PET) in primary liver cancer remains small (recent reviews in Hann et al. 2000; Marienhagen 2000; Stokkel et al. 2001; Gambhir et al. 2001; Kamel and Bluemke 2002). Because HCC has a greater incidence, most papers focus on this form, and there are only a few reports on CCC patients.

Cholangiocellular carcinomas, like hepatic metastases from other primary tumors, usually show increased fluoro-2-deoxy-D-glucose (FDG) uptake with standard uptake value (SUV) tumor/liver ratios greater than 2 and an SUV greater than 3.5 (Lord et al. 1997; Keiding et al. 1998; Delbeke et al. 1998; Shiomi et al. 1999; Iwata et al. 2000; Son et al. 2002). In our own primary liver cancer patient cohort, there are two cases of CCC (one CCC, one combined HCC and CCC), which also both showed up as "hot lesions" (Fig. 1).

In HCC, uptake patterns are more differentiated: soon after the first results in HCC patients with [^{18}F]FDG were published (Paul et al. 1985; Okazumi et al. 1989), it became evident that a significant proportion of HCC do not show an increased FDG uptake and therefore cannot be distinguished from normal liver parenchyma. Some HCC may even show less uptake than the surrounding liver (cold lesion) (Risse et al. 1998a–c, 2000; Grünwald et al. 1998). Table 3 shows the pertinent literature with the relationships of FDG uptake in HCC. Out of 200 HCC in 11 studies, only 107 (53.5 %) were definitely PET positive. There is some evidence that, in patients with moderately or poorly differentiated HCC, tumors >5 cm, or with markedly elevated AFP levels, [^{18}F]FDG PET may contribute to non-invasive staging (Trojan et al. 1999), but others have found no strong correlation between a positive PET finding and the tumor diameter, AFP level or histologic grading of HCC (Risse et al. 2000; Verhoef et al. 2002). Figure 2 shows an example of a positive PET finding in a huge HCC with the corresponding CT image; Figure 3 demonstrates another large HCC, which is PET negative.

The difficulties in imaging HCC in the liver result from the varying relationships of the glucose metabolism in normal liver parenchyma and tumor tissue. The pertinent metabolic patterns in these tissues have been characterized by the metabolic rate constants (k1, k2, k3, k4) using dynamic PET protocols (Enomoto et al. 1991; Okazumi et al. 1992; Torizuka et al. 1995). The normal liver tissue is characterized by low hexokinase activity (phosphorylation; k3) combined with increased glucose-6-phosphatase activity (dephosphorylation; k4). PET images are represented by the ratio k4/k3 (Enomoto et al. 1991), resulting in low-grade diffuse FDG uptake in normal liver tissue (Cook et al. 1999). In malignant liver tumors, this ratio is inverse, with high hexokinase activity and lower glucose-6-phosphatase activity. The pathobiochemical reason for the varying uptake patterns in HCC is their particular k4/k3 ratio. HCC cases without accumulation of FDG had a high ratio of k4/k3, which correlated well with the inverse ratio of FDG-accumulating images on PET so that they could not be

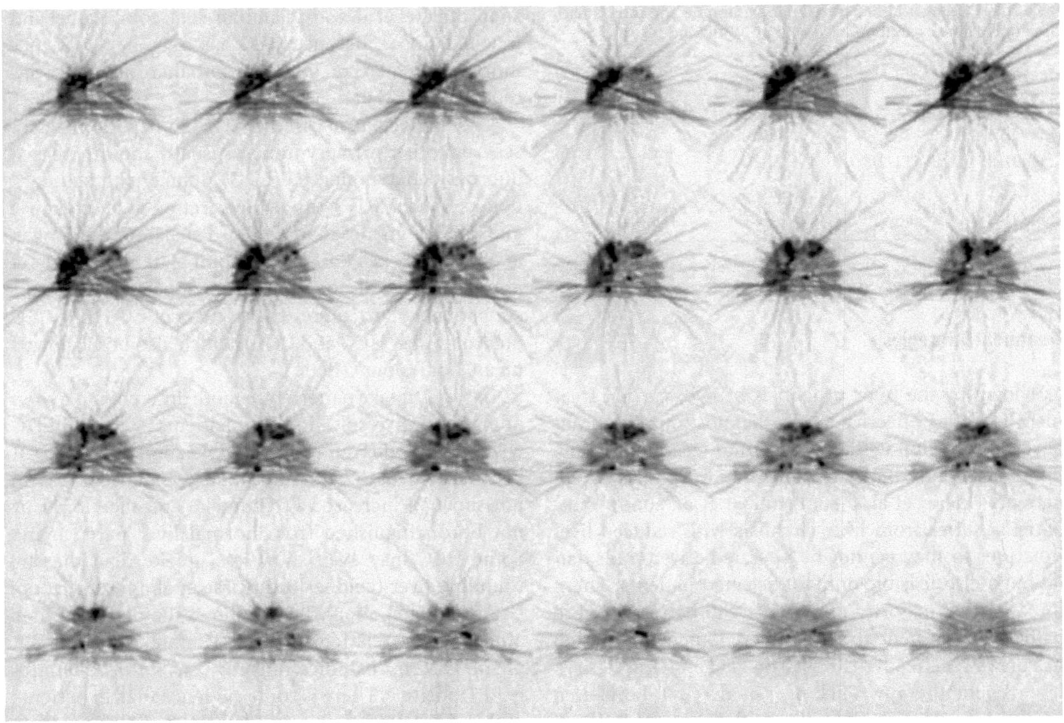

Fig. 1. Diffuse infiltrating cholangiocellular carcinoma. The transmission-corrected axial PET series through the upper abdomen shows multiple diffuse accumulations ("hot spots"; filtered back projection) throughout the liver. No metastases are seen

Table 3.
Relationships of FDG uptake in hepatocellular carcinoma (HCC) as compared to the surrounding liver parenchyma. Not all authors differentiate between similar and lower tumor uptake but give only the number of tumors with increased uptake

Reference	Total number of HCC	Increased tumor uptake	Similar uptake	Lower tumor uptake
Enomoto et al. (1991)	23	12		
Okazumi et al. (1992)	20	11	6	3
Goldberg et al. (1993)	2	0		
Torizuka et al. (1994)	32	19	7	6
Delbeke et al. (1998)	23	16		
Trojan et al. (1999)	14	7	7	
Marienhagen (2000)	11	4	7	
Khan et al. (2000)	20	11		
Risse et al. (2000)	11	5	6	
Verhoef et al. (2002)	10	2		
Son et al. (2002)	34	20		
Total	200	107		

clearly defined from the surrounding non-cancerous hepatic tissue (Enomoto et al. 1991). By determining metabolic rate constants and their ratios, efforts have been made to distinguish benign and malignant liver tumors, to assess the degree of tumor differentiation and histologic grading of HCC, the effectiveness of therapy and tumor viability, and survival rates (Enomoto et al. 1991; Okazumi et al. 1992; Torizuka et al. 1995). However, dynamic PET protocols with calculation of the metabolic rate constants are time consuming and not suitable for a routine setting in clinical practice.

In serial PET studies, delayed scans after intervals of up to 6 hours after injection revealed a better differentiation of malignant versus benign lesions and an advantage of tumor detection in other tumor entities. While normal liver tissue and most benign lesions show sig-

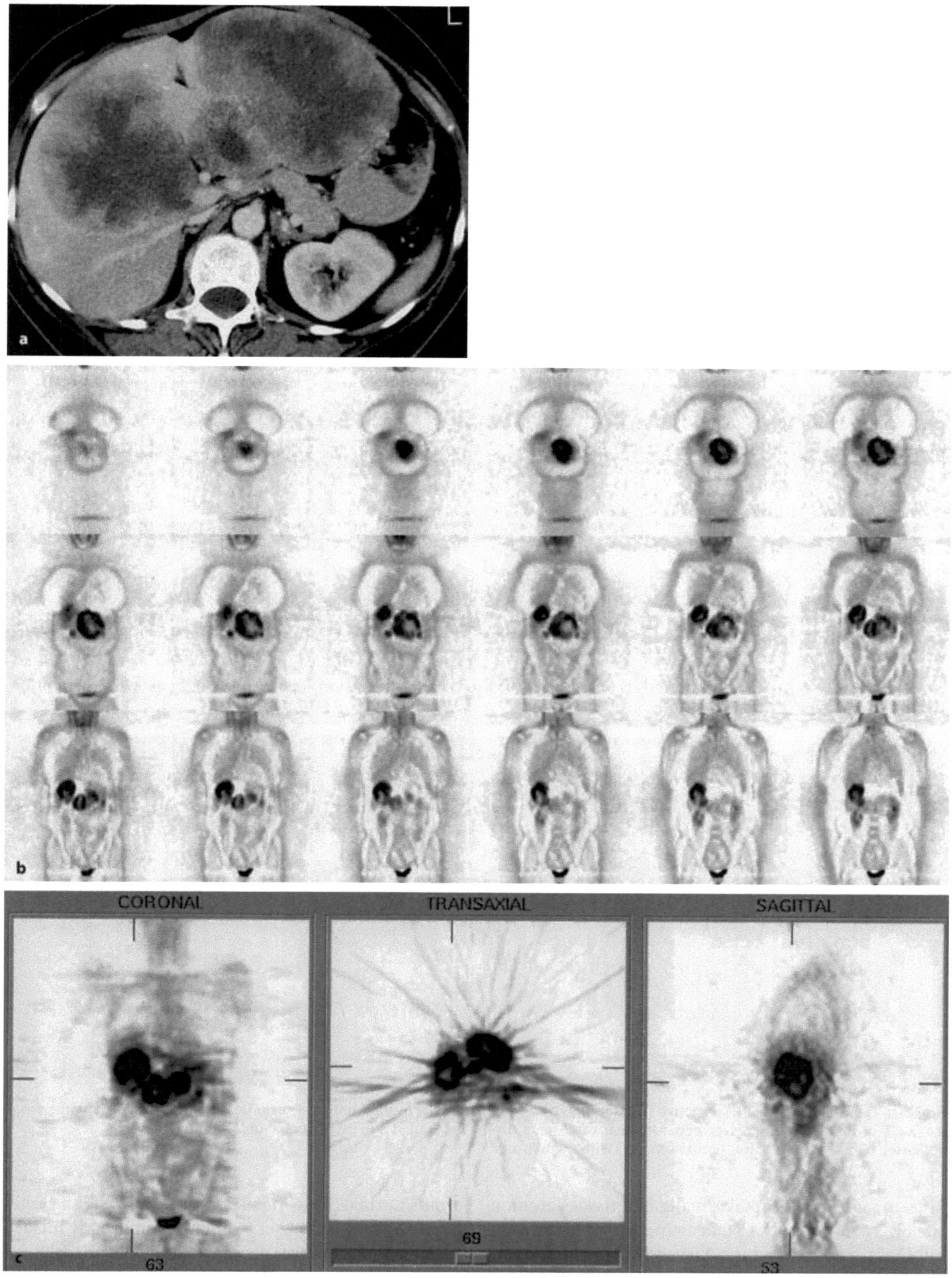

Fig. 2a–c. Typical case of a PET-positive hepatocellular carcinoma. **a** CT of the liver with an oligofocal hepatocellular carcinoma with central necrosis in the tumor nodules. **b** Coronal PET series (emission only) with strong uptake in the outer rim of the tumor nodules but no uptake in the central necroses. **c** Transmission-corrected PET in three planes through the liver ("volume viewer"). No metastases are seen

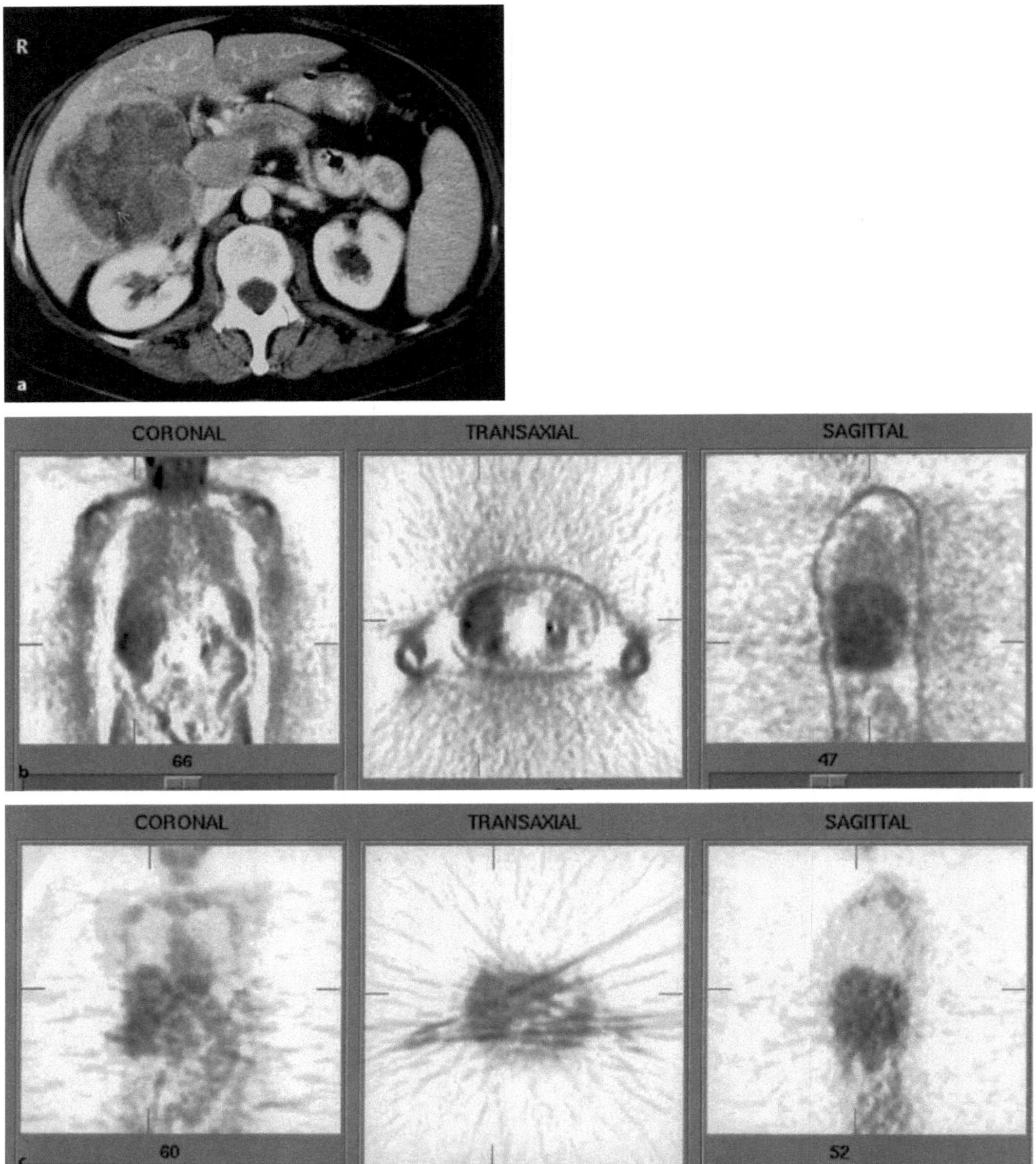

Fig. 3a–c. Typical case of a PET-negative hepatocellular carcinoma. **a** CT of the liver with a large hepatocellular carcinoma (hypodense). **b** PET volume viewer (emission only) with no increased uptake in the tumor. **c** Transmission-corrected PET volume viewer; there is still no increased uptake in the tumor

nificant falls in FDG uptake, malignant tissues accumulate FDG continuously, so that an increasing tumor/non-tumoral tissue contrast is achieved (Kubota et al. 2001). There is only one recent study with this approach in HCC patients so far (Koyama et al. 2002). The authors found that in 11 patients with 18 HCC, visual improvement was observed in 6 of 18 HCC lesions and the tumor/normal liver uptake ratios were significantly higher in delayed images (2 hours) than in early images (50 minutes). However, this means that, by visual analysis, two-thirds of the HCC did not show improved detectability in delayed imaging.

Some authors report follow-up PET studies for the monitoring of HCC after therapy, and it is found that the amount of FDG uptake correlates with response to therapy: a decrease in FDG uptake after therapy indicates a positive response to therapy. However, this conclusion is based on small numbers of patients, whereas the exact response mechanism is still unknown. Moreover, in these case series, the interval between tumor therapy and FDG PET, as well as the method of quantification, SUV or tumor-to-non-tumor ratios, differ between studies. Therefore, it is not possible to draw definite conclusions yet (Risse et al. 2000; Stokkel et al. 2001).

19.5 Judgment of Indications of PET in Liver Cancer

The published data do not yet allow clear statements on PET indications for primary liver cancer. Consequently, this topic is not mentioned in the 3rd German Interdisciplinary Consensus Conference on PET indications in oncology ("Onko-PET III") (Reske and Kotzerke 2001).

However, based on the literature and on our own experience, some distinct indications may be extracted:

- Differential diagnosis of benign versus malignant liver tumors; a positive PET finding is highly suspicious for malignancy (e.g. CCC)
- Staging in case of a positive PET finding in the liver (Fukuda et al. 1994; Khan et al. 2000)
- Therapy monitoring in case of an initial positive PET finding (change in tracer uptake) (Nagata et al. 1990; Vitola et al. 1996; Risse et al. 2000)

As long as there is no validated data base, PET imaging in primary liver cancer should be done in controlled study environments only.

19.6 New Tracer Developments

Besides [^{18}F]FDG, only a few other tracers have been studied in liver cancer. These include [^{13}N]ammonia in HCC (Hayashi et al. 1985; Shibata et al. 1988) and [^{18}F]fluorodeoxygalactose for imaging of bone metastases in a case of HCC (Fukuda et al. 1994). One Japanese study reports on evaluation of oxygen metabolism, blood flow and blood volume of liver cancers using ^{15}O (Okazumi et al. 1991). [^{18}F]5-fluorouracil has been used for monitoring in vivo tumor pharmacokinetics (Blesing and Kerr 1996) and [^{11}C]ethanol for percutaneous intratumoral injection in HCC (Dimitrakopoulou-Strauss et al. 1996,1999). Functional hepatic reserve was evaluated with [^{11}C]methionine ([^{11}C]MET) in major hepatectomy candidates (Enomoto et al. 1994). In its normal distribution, [^{11}C]MET shows high liver activity (Cook et al. 1999) and therefore seems not to be suitable for PET imaging of liver cancer; at least, there is no reported study of [^{11}C]MET in liver cancer yet. In summary, [^{18}F]FDG has proven to be the most efficacious tracer in liver cancer, although there are some limitations, particularly in PET imaging of HCC. Further studies with new tracers are warranted.

19.7 Summary and Outlook

In summary, FDG PET imaging of CCC is highly sensitive and comparable to the ability of demonstrating liver metastases from other primary tumors. However, CCC is a rare tumor entity in the western world, but HCC, being by far the most common primary liver cancer worldwide, is shown by FDG PET in only approximately 50% of cases. Dynamic PET studies revealed the pertinent metabolic patterns, characterized by the metabolic rate constants, which seem to be predictors of histologic grading, the effectiveness of therapy, and survival rates in HCC patients; but dynamic PET is not suitable for a routine setting in clinical practice. Other tracers have been used for imaging of HCC or pharmacokinetic studies but have not gained clinical relevance.

Despite these limitations, indications for PET imaging in suspected liver cancer are differentiation of benign versus malignant liver tumors, and if there is a positive finding, staging and therapy monitoring. In addition, serial PET scans with delayed images might yield better diagnostic results for this tumor entity. Even when the first respective report could demonstrate an improved visual detectability in only one-third of HCC, this method seems to be a possibility to improve HCC detection, which should be investigated further.

19.8 Technical Recommendations

Patient preparation: Fasting period at least 6 hours, blood glucose level <120 mg/dl

Positioning: Supine

Radiopharmaceutical: [^{18}F]FDG, 300–400 MBq intravenously

Data acquisition: Start 60 (at least 45) minutes after injection. Emission scans in at least 4–5 "bed positions" including pelvis, abdomen, chest, cervical region and lower parts of the cerebellum. Optional additional late acquisition after 2–4 hours

Attenuation correction: "Hot transmission" after each emission bed position for accurate reconstruction avoids repositioning artifacts. "Cold transmission" before FDG injection may be better for scheduling many patients but has inherent risks of repositioning artifacts despite skin markers. If a PET CT is available, X-ray CT images are used for transmission

Reconstruction: Iterative reconstruction or filtered back projection (older software)

Dynamic modeling: Calculation of metabolic rate constants in scientific questions/settings

Image evaluation and interpretation: Qualitative/visual analysis: after defining the lesion in CT or MRI, comparison of tumor uptake with the surrounding liver:

- Tumor uptake > liver uptake
- Tumor uptake = liver uptake
- Tumor uptake < liver uptake
- Central necrosis
- Extrahepatic findings

Quantitative analysis: Calculation of normalized tumoral SUV for therapy monitoring (normalization algorithms: Kim and Gupta 1996; Schomburg et al. 1996; Sugawara et al. 1999)

Protocol recommendation: Start acquisition immediately after patient has urinated. The first bed position should include the urinary bladder, which is as empty as possible at that time in order to avoid imaging artifacts in the pelvis due to high urinary bladder activity. In order to diminish these artifacts further, furosemide injection (0.5 mg/kg) prior to FDG application is useful (Diehl et al. 2002). Dual time-point acquisition with a late acquisition after 2–4 hours may help increase the tumor/liver contrast (Koyama et al. 2002).

References

Becker N, Wahrendorf J (1998) Atlas of cancer mortality in the Federal Republic of Germany 1981–1990. Springer, Berlin Heidelberg New York

Blesing CH, Kerr DJ (1996) Intra-hepatic arterial drug delivery. J Drug Target 3:341–347

Bremer C, Allkemper T, Menzel J et al (1998) Preliminary clinical experience with laser-induced interstitial thermotherapy in patients with hepatocellular carcinoma. J Magn Reson Imaging 8:235–239

Bruix J, Llovet JM, Castells A et al (1998) Transarterial embolization versus symptomatic treatment in patients with advanced hepatocellular carcinoma: results of a randomized, controlled trial in a single institution. Hepatology 27:1578–1583

Brunken C, Steiner P, Rogiers X (2000) Perkutane Alkoholinjektion (PEI) und Kryotherapie. Internist 41:205–207

Caselmann W, Blum H, Fleig W, Huppert P, Ramadori G, Schirmacher P, Sauerbruch T (1999) Leitlinien der deutschen Gesellschaft für Verdauungs- und Stoffwechselkrankheiten zur Diagnostik und Therapie des hepatozellulären Karzinoms. Z Gastroenterol 1999; 37:353–365

CLIP group (1998) Tamoxifen in treatment of hepatocellular carcinoma: a randomised controlled trial. Lancet 352:17–20

Cook GJR, Maisey MN, Fogelman I (1999) Normal variants, artefacts and interpretative pitfalls in PET imaging with 18-fluoro-2-deoxyglucose and carbon-11 methionine. Eur J Nucl Med 26:1363–1378

Delbeke D, Martin WH, Sandler MP, Chapman WC, Wright JK Jr, Pinson CW (1998) Evaluation of benign vs malignant hepatic lesions with positron emission tomography. Arch Surg 133: 510–516

Deuffic S, Poynard T, Buffat L, Valleron AJ (1998) Trends in primary liver cancer. Lancet 351:214–215

Di Bisceglie A (1997) Hepatitis C and hepatocellular carcinoma. Hepatology 26 [Suppl 1]:34S–38S

Diehl M, Manolopoulou M, Risse JH, Kranert WT, Menzel C, Grünwald F (2002) FDG excretion with and without application of diuretics. Eur J Nucl Med 29:S262

Dimitrakopoulou-Strauss A, Gutzler F, Strauss LG, Irngartinger G, Oberdorfer F, Doll J, Stremmel W, van Kaick G (1996) PET studies with C-11 ethanol in intratumoral therapy of hepatocellular carcinomas. Radiologe 36:744–749

Dimitrakopoulou-Strauss A, Strauss LG, Gutzler F, Irngartinger G, Kontaxakis G, Kim DK, Oberdorfer F, van Kaick G (1999) Pharmacokinetic imaging of 11C ethanol with PET in eight patients with hepatocellular carcinomas who were scheduled for treatment with percutaneous ethanol injection. Radiology 211:681–686

El-Serag HB, Mason AC (1999) Rising incidence of hepatocellular carcinoma in the United States. N Engl J Med 340:745–750

Enomoto K, Fukunaga T, Okazumi S, Asano T, Kikuchi T, Yamamoto H et al (1991) Can fluorodeoxyglucose-positron emission tomography evaluate the functional differentiation of hepatocellular carcinoma. Kaku Igaku 28:1353–1356

Enomoto K, Matsui Y, Okazumi S, Ioku T, Asano T, Isono K et al (1994) Evaluation of clinical usefulness of 11C-methionine positron emission tomography (11C-MET-PET) as a tool for liver functional imaging. Kaku Igaku 31:271–275

Flickinger JC, Carr BI, Lotze MT (1997) Cancer of the liver. In: DeVita VT Jr, Hellman S, Rosenberg SA (eds) Cancer. Principles and practice of oncology, 5th edn. Lippincott-Raven, Philadelphia, pp 1087–1114

Fong Y, Kemeny N, Lawrence TS (2001) Cancer of the liver and biliary tree. In: De Vita VT Jr, Hellman S, Rosenberg SA (eds) Cancer, principles and practice of oncology, 6th edn. Lippincott Williams and Wilkins, Philadelphia, pp 1162–1203

Fukuda H, Yoshioka S, Takahashi J, Goto R, Tada M, Murata K et al (1994) A case of hepatocellular carcinoma with lumbar bone metastasis with high uptake of 18F-fluorodeoxygalactose in PET. Kaku-Igaku 31:1351–1355

Gambhir SS, Czernin J, Schwimmer J, Silverman DHS, Coleman RE, Phelps ME (2001) A tabulated summary of the FDG PET literature. J Nucl Med 42:1S–93S

Goldberg MA, Lee MJ, Fischman AJ, Mueller PR, Alpert NM, Thrall JH (1993) Fluorodeoxyglucose PET of abdominal and pelvic neoplasms: potential role in oncologic imaging. Radiographics 13:1047–1062

Grasso A, Watkinson AF, Tibballs JM, Burroughs AK (2000) Radiofrequency ablation in the treatment of hepatocellular carcinoma – a clinical viewpoint. J Hepatol 33:667–672

Grünwald F, Risse JH, Menzel C, Bender H, Strunk H, Biersack HJ (1998) 18-FDG-PET and liver CT in intraarterial therapy with I-131-lipiodol in primary liver cancer. J Cancer Res Clin Oncol 124 [Suppl]:R27

Hann LE, Winston CB, Brown KT, Akhurst T (2000) Diagnostic imaging approaches and relationship to hepatobiliary cancer staging and therapy. Semin Surg Oncol 19:94–115

Hayashi N, Tamaki N, Yonekura Y, Senda M, Saji H, Yamamoto K, Konishi J, Torizuka K (1985) Imaging of the hepatocellular carcinoma using dynamic positron emission tomography with nitrogen-13 ammonia. J Nucl Med 26:254–257

Iwata Y, Shiomi S, Sasaki N, Jomura H, Nishiguchi S, Seki S, Kawabe J, Ochi H (2000) Clinical usefulness of positron emission tomography with fluorine-18-fluorodeoxyglucose in the diagnosis of liver tumors. Ann Nucl Med 14:121–126

Kamel IR, Bluemke DA (2000) Imaging evaluation of hepatocellular carcinoma. J Vasc Interv Radiol 13:S173–S184

Keiding S, Hansen SB, Rasmussen HH, Gee A, Kruse A, Roelsgaard K, Tage-Jensen U, Dahlerup JF (1998) Detection of cholangiocarcinoma in primary sclerosing cholangitis by positron emission tomography. Hepatology 28:700–706

Kew MC (1998) Hepatic tumors and cysts. In: Feldman M, Sleisenger MH, Scharschmidt BF (eds) Sleisenger and Fordtran's gastrointestinal and liver disease: pathology/diagnosis/management, 6th edn. Saunders, Philadelphia, pp 1364–1387

Khan MA, Combs CS, Brunt EM, Lowe VJ, Wolverson MK, Solomon H, Collins BT, Di Bisceglie AM (2000) Positron emission tomography scanning in the evaluation of hepatocellular carcinoma. J Hepatol 32:792–797

Kim CK, Gupta NC (1996) Dependency of standardized uptake values of fluorine-18 fluorodeoxyglucose on body size: comparison of body surface area correction and lean body mass correction. Nucl Med Commun 17:890–894

Koyama K, Okamura T, Kawabe J, Ozawa N, Higashiyama S, Ochi H, Yamada R (2002) The usefulness of 18F-FDG PET images obtained 2 hours after intravenous injection in liver tumor. Ann Nucl Med 16:169–176

Kubota K, Itoh M, Ozaki K, Ono S, Tashiro M, Yamaguchi K, Akaizawa T, Yamada K, Fukuda H (2001) Advantage of delayed whole-body FDG-PET imaging for tumour detection. Eur J Nucl Med 28:696–703

Lord DJ, Herrington GD, Stephen MS, Perkins KW, Fulham MJ (1997) FDG-PET in the evaluation of cholangiocarcinoma. J Nucl Med 38:246P

Maraj R, Kew MC, Hyslop RJ (1988) Resectability rate of hepatocellular carcinoma in rural southern Africans. Br J Surg 75: 335–338

Marienhagen J (2000) Hepatobiliary tumors. In: Wieler HJ, Coleman RE (eds) PET in clinical oncology. Springer, Berlin Heidelberg New York, pp 225–233

Mathurin P, Rixe O, Carbonell N et al (1998) Review article: overview of medical treatments in unresectable hepatocellular carcinoma – an impossible meta-analysis? Aliment Pharmacol Ther 12:111–126

Nagata Y, Yamamoto K, Hiraoka M et al (1990) Monitoring liver tumor therapy with 18F-FDG positron emission tomography. J Comput Assist Tomogr 14:370–374

Okazumi S, Enomoto K, Ozaki M, Yamamoto H, Yoshida M, Abe Y et al (1989) Evaluation of the effect of treatment in patients with liver tumors using 18F-fluorodeoxyglucose PET. Kaku Igaku 26:793–797

Okazumi S, Yamamoto H, Enomoto K, Isono K, Ryu M (1991) Evaluation of oxygen metabolism, blood flow and blood volume of liver cancers using 15O and positron emission tomography. Nippon Rinsho 49:1868–1872

Okazumi S, Isono K, Enomoto K, Kikuchi T, Ozaki M, Yamamoto H, et al (1992) Evaluation of liver tumors using fluorine-18-fluorodeoxyglucose PET: characterization of tumor and assessment of effect of treatment. J Nucl Med 33:333–339

Okuda K, Ohtsuki T, Obata H et al (1985) Natural history of hepatocellular carcinoma and prognosis in relation to treatment: study of 850 patients. Cancer 56:918–928

Okuda K, Fujimoto I, Hanai A, Urano Y (1987) Changing incidence of hepatocellular carcinoma in Japan. Cancer Res 47: 4967–4972

Paul R, Ahonen A, Roeda D, Nordman E (1985) Imaging of hepatoma with 18F-fluoro-deoxyglucose. Lancet 1:50–51

Pelletier G, Ducreux M, Gay F et al (1998) Treatment of unresectable hepatocellular carcinoma with lipiodol chemoembolization: a multicenter randomized trial. Group CHC. J Hepatol 29:129–134

Rabe C, Pilz T, Klostermann C, Berna M, Schild HH, Sauerbruch T, Caselmann WH (2001) Clinical characteristics and outcome of a cohort of 101 patients with hepatocellular carcinoma. World J Gastroenterol 7:208–215

Raoul JL, Duvauferrier R, Bretagne JF et al (1993) Usefulness of hepatic artery injection of lipiodol and 131I-lipiodol before therapeutic decision in hepatocellular carcinoma. Scand J Gastroenterol 28:217–223

Reske SN, Kotzerke J (2001) FDG-PET for clinical use: results of the 3rd German Interdisciplinary Consensus Conference, "Onko-PET III", 21 July and 19 Sept 2000. Eur J Nucl Med 28:1707–1723

Risse JH, Grünwald F, Menzel C, Willkomm P, Bender H, Strunk H, Kleinschmidt R, Biersack HJ (1998a) 18-FDG-PET und CT bei intraarterieller J-131-Lipiodol-Therapie bei primären Lebertumoren. Nuklearmedizin 37:A89

Risse JH, Grünwald F, Strunk H, Menzel C, Willkomm P, Bender H, Kleinschmidt R, Biersack HJ (1998b) 3-Phasen-Spiral-CT und 18-FDG-PET zur Verlaufskontrolle bei intraarterieller J-131-Lipiodol-Therapie bei primären Leberkarzinomen. Fortschr Röntgenstr 168 [Suppl 1]:S57–S58

Risse JH, Grünwald F, Strunk H, Bender H, Willkomm P, Menzel C, Biersack HJ (1998c) 18-FDG-PET and 3-phase helical liver CT in intra-arterial therapy with I-131-lipiodol in primary liver cancer. Eur J Nucl Med 25:1032

Risse JH, Grünwald F, Strunk H, Kleinschmidt R, Bender H, Biersack HJ (1999) I-131-Lipiodol therapy in liver neoplasms. Hybridoma 18:83–85

Risse JH, Grünwald F, Kersjes W, Strunk H, Caselmann WH, Palmedo H, Bender H, Biersack HJ (2000) Intraarterial HCC therapy with I-131-lipiodol. Cancer Biother Radio 15:65–70

Risse JH, Caselmann WH, Strunk H, Gallkowski U, Grünwald F, Biersack HJ (2001) Therapy of hepatocellular carcinoma with I-131-lipiodol: a nuclear medicine alternative? Dt Ärztebl 98: A2810–A2815

Robertson JM, Lawrence TS, Dworzanin LM et al (1993) Treatment of primary hepatobiliary cancer with conformal radiation therapy and regional chemotherapy. J Clin Oncol 11:1286–1293

Schomburg A, Bender H, Reichel C, Sommer T, Ruhlmann J, Kozak B, Biersack HJ (1996) Standardized uptake values of fluorine-18 fluorodeoxyglucose: the value of different normalization procedures. Eur J Nucl Med 23:571–574

Shibata T, Yamamoto K, Hayashi N, Yonekura Y, Nagara T, Saji H, Mukai T, Konishi J (1988) Dynamic positron emission tomography with 13N-ammonia in liver tumors. Eur J Nucl Med 14: 607–611

Shiomi S, Sasaki N, Kawashima D, Jomura H, Fukuda T, Kuroki T, Koyama K, Kawabe J, Ochi H (1999) Combined hepatocellular carcinoma and cholangiocarcinoma with high F-18 fluorodeoxyglucose positron emission tomographic uptake. Clin Nucl Med 24:370–371

Sobin LH, Wittekind C (1997) UICC (International Union Against Cancer) TNM classification of malignant tumours. Wiley/Liss, New York

Son HB, Han CJ, Kim BI, Kim J, Jeong SH, Kim YC, Lee JO, Choi CY, Im SM (2002) Evaluation of various hepatic lesions with positron emission tomography. Taehan Kan Hakhoe Chi 8: 472–480

Stokkel MP, Draisma A, Pauwels EK (2001) Positron emission tomography with 2-[18F]-fluoro-2-deoxy-D-glucose in oncology, part IIIb: therapy response monitoring in colorectal and lung tumours, head and neck cancer, hepatocellular carcinoma and sarcoma. J Cancer Res Clin Oncol 127:278–285

Sugawara Y, Zasadny KR, Neuhoff AW, Wahl RL (1999) Reevaluation of the standardized uptake value for FDG: variations with body weight and methods for correction. Radiology 213: 521–525

Taylor-Robinson SD, Foster GR, Arora S, Hargreaves S, Thomas HC (1997) Increase in primary liver cancer in the UK, 1979–1994. Lancet 350:1142–1143

Torizuka T, Tamaki N, Inokuma T, Magata Y, Yonekura Y, Tanaka A et al (1994) Value of fluorine-18-FDG-PET to monitor hepatocellular carcinoma after interventional therapy. J Nucl Med 35: 1965–1969

Torizuka T, Tamaki N, Inokuma T, Magata Y, Sasayama S, Yonekura Y et al (1995) In vivo assessment of glucose metabolism in hepatocellular carcinoma with FDG-PET. J Nucl Med 36:1811–1817

Trojan J, Schroeder O, Raedle J, Baum RP, Herrmann G, Jacobi V, Zeuzem S (1999) Fluorine-18 FDG positron emission tomography for imaging of hepatocellular carcinoma. Am J Gastroenterol 94:3314–3319

Verhoef C, Valkema R, de Man RA, Krenning EP, Yzermans JN (2002) Fluorine-18 FDG imaging in hepatocellular carcinoma using positron coincidence detection and single photon emission computed tomography. Liver 22:51–56

Vitola JV, Delbeke D, Meranze SG, Mazer MJ, Pinson CW (1996) Positron emission tomography with F-18-fluorodeoxyglucose to evaluate the results of hepatic chemoembolization. Cancer 78:2216–2222

CHAPTER 20

Colorectal Cancer

M.T. Kitapci · R.E. Coleman

20.1 Introduction

20.1.1 Definition

The large intestine consists of colon and rectum. The colon is the first 2 meters of the large intestine, and the rectum is the last 25 centimeters. The colon is divided into four parts; the right (ascending), the middle (transverse), the left (descending) and the sigmoid, which continues with the rectum. The rectosigmoid colon is a surgically important region because of the blood supply [1]. Although cancers of the colon and rectum appear to be two distinct entities, pathologic variations of colon and rectal cancer are relatively limited. In this chapter, colorectal cancer, as a general term, will be used to define these two cancers.

20.1.2 Incidence

Colorectal cancer is the third most commonly diagnosed cancer and ranks second among causes of cancer deaths (after lung cancer) in the USA [2–4]. There were an estimated 148,300 new cases and an estimated 56,600 deaths from the disease in the USA in 2002 (Cancer and Facts & Figures 2002). The incidence of colorectal cancer in Europe has increased in the last decade. In 2000, about 52,000 patients were diagnosed with colorectal cancer in Germany, which has a high incidence rate, as does the Czech Republic [2–7].

Although colon cancer is more common in women, rectal cancer is more common in men. The incidence of colorectal cancer is similar among men and women until age 50; then, it becomes higher in men than in women [2, 4, 6]. An individual's lifetime risk of developing colorectal cancer is almost 6%, with more than 90% of cases occurring after age 50 in the USA [3, 4, 6]. There is evidence to support a shift in cancer distribution within the colon during the latter part of the last century. Increasing proportions of cancer are located in the cecum and ascending colon [4–7].

20.1.3 Clinical Presentation

Typically, colon cancers develop slowly. Common clinical presentations of colon cancer are change in bowel habits, abdominal pain, and blood in the stool. In the cecum and ascending colon, the cancer can grow to be large without causing any obstruction or other signs or symptoms. Tumors in the right colon lead to chronic occult blood loss because of ulceration; in the left colon, however, tumors more frequently result in obstruction, which causes abdominal cramping. In the rectosigmoid area, tumors cause tenesmus and changes in stool shape. Subtle symptoms might be the initial evidence of tumor even among patients with an advanced stage of cancer. Symptoms such as fatigue, weakness and weight loss are common in extensive disease [8].

20.1.4 Etiology

The etiology of colorectal cancer is multifactorial. Environmental factors such as diet, occupation, smoking, alcohol intake, physical activity and body weight may play key roles in the etiology of the disease [6, 8].

Although certain relationships with colorectal cancer incidence have not been proven, several important risk factors for colorectal cancer could account for a large proportion of cases. The search for diet, lifestyle, and other factors that can explain an increased risk for colorectal cancer has been driven by two fundamental and powerful observations. First, rates of colorectal cancer differ dramatically among countries, varying by as much as ten-fold, from low-incidence areas in Asia and Africa to much higher incidence areas in northern Europe and the USA. Second, migrants from low-risk areas to western countries experience rapid increases in colorectal cancer risk within the same generation. The incidence of colorectal cancer can also change dramatically over time within countries. Considerable evidence has accumulated that this increased risk may be caused by the presence of carcinogenic heterocyclic amines that are formed during the high-temperature cooking of foods and burning of meat juices [6, 8].

Although smoking has not been shown to be a definite risk factor for colorectal cancer, it is consistently associated with the presence of adenomatous polyps. Cumulative lifetime exposure to smoking might be a risk factor for developing colon cancer. Alcohol is associated with an increased risk of colon cancer. Lifestyle as well as diet might be a predictor of colon cancer development in later life. Physical activity is inversely associated with the risk of colon cancer, whereas increased body weight is associated with an increased mortality rate from cancer, including colon cancer.

Almost 80 % of patients with colorectal cancer have no evidence of genetic disorders; however, the large variation in the incidence of colorectal cancer might be related to genetic predisposition such as familial polyposis, inflammatory bowel disease (ulcerative colitis and Crohn's disease), familial cancer syndromes and, most importantly, adenomatous polyps. For colorectal cancer, mutations in the familial adenomatous polyposis gene are highly penetrant. Familial adenomatous polyposis syndrome has been a focus for screening and pre-emptive surgery before transformation occurs. A person with a family history that is consistent with an autosomal dominant inheritance has an increased risk of colorectal malignancy. A mutation in the familial adenomatous polyposis gene also seems likely to serve as an early event in sporadic colorectal cancer. Other genes that may be involved in colorectal cancer are beta-catenin, Ki-ras, DCC, COX2, and P53 [6, 8].

About one-third of all adenomatous polyps in the colon found in patients over age 60 have dysplastic elements. Most carcinomas are believed to arise from the adenomas; however, only a small percentage of adenomas become carcinomas [8]. The prevalence of adenomas increases with age, and the malignant potential of an adenoma depends on its size, histologic type and degree of atypia. The risk of progression of an adenoma to cancer is less than 10 % over an individual's lifetime [5–8].

20.1.5 Staging

The estimation of prognosis in colorectal cancer is related to pathologic staging that depends on tumor size, histologic type, and tumor grade (Tables 1 and 2). The majority of colorectal cancer is adenocarcinoma. The most common macroscopic type of dysplasia is adenoma. Dysplasia is unequivocal neoplastic epithelial alteration without invasive growth. In contrast to the stomach or the small intestine, a neoplasm in the colon or rectum has metastatic potential only after invasion of at least the submucosa because lymphatic vessels are found only at that level. The life expectancy of a patient with colorectal carcinoma depends on the stage of the tumor. The anatomical extent of colorectal cancer is classified according to the fifth edition of the Union Internationale Contre le Cancer (UICC) TNM classification (primary tumor, nodal involvement, and distant metastases) [5–10]. The TNM classification (Table 1) has replaced the Dukes system described in 1932 and has been modified innumerable times (Table 2).

Staging is based on the natural history of the tumor. For instance, adenocarcinoma of colon spreads sequen-

Table 1. International classification of colorectal cancer

TNM Classification of colorectal cancer	
Primary tumor (T)	
Tx	Primary tumor cannot be assessed
T0	No evidence of tumor in resected specimen (prior polypectomy or fulguration)
Tis	Carcinoma in situ
T1	Invades submucosa
T2	Invades into muscularis propria
T3	Invades through the muscularis propria into the subserosa or into non-peritonealized pericolic or perirectal tissue
T4	Invades directly another organ or structures and/or perforates visceral peritoneum
Regional lymph nodes (N)	
Nx	Nodes cannot be assessed
N0	No regional node metastases
N1	One to three positive nodes
N2	Four or more positive nodes
N3	Central nodes positive
Distant metastases (M)	
Mx	Presence of distant metastases cannot be assessed
M0	No distant metastases
M1	Distant metastases present

Table 2. Staging and comparison of different classifications

Staging comparison of Dukes and Astler-Coller staging with TNM	
Stage	
I	Tis, T1, T2; N0; M0
II	T3, T4; N0; M0
III	Any T; N1; M0
IV	Any T; any N; M1
Dukes	
A	T1, T2; N0; M0
B	T3, T4; N0; M0
C	T1, T2, T3, T4; N1; M0
D	Any T; any N; M1
Astler-Coller	
A	T1; N0; M0
B1	T2; N0; M0
B2	T3; N0; M0
C1	T1, T2; N1
C2	T3, T4; N1
D	Any T; any N; M1

tially from the primary tumor through the bowel wall into pericolonic and perirectal mesentery, into the adjacent lymph nodes, and through lymphatics into the regional and distant organs. In particular, rectal and anal cancers spread to perineal, inguinal and periaortic lymph node basins. Target organs for distant metastases are the liver as well as the lungs. Tumor extent and presence or absence of lymph node involvement is a major determinant for prognosis and risk of recurrence. If the tumor is confined to the submucosa, more than 90 % of cases are cured and the risk for recurrence is 5 %. Recurrence of colorectal carcinoma occurs in 37–45 % of patients within 2 years of curative resection [4–10]. Early detection of resectable tumor recurrence or metastases can improve survival.

The overall 5-year survival rate for colorectal cancer is 61 % (96 % for stage I, 87 % for stage II, 55 % for stage III, and 5 % for stage IV). Survival rates do not vary by anatomic site in the colon and rectum [2–10].

20.1.6 Treatment

Surgical resection is the fundamental treatment for colorectal cancer. The type of surgery depends on preoperative evaluation. The location of the tumor, depth of invasion, and presence or absence of metastasis are important determinant factors that affect the type of surgery [6–8].

Patients with advanced stage disease have a poor prognosis; however, chemotherapy and/or radiotherapy could convert a patient with inoperable stage to the operable category [6, 8]. The benefit of adjuvant radiation therapy and chemotherapy has been observed in several studies. Radiotherapy has several advantages for patients with colorectal cancer, particularly rectal cancer. Radiotherapy results in locoregional tumor control by eliminating microscopic residual disease. Preoperative use of radiation therapy can cause significant tumor regression, so that inoperable lesions may become operable. Third, radiation therapy is used to palliate symptoms in patients with metastatic colorectal cancer. Postoperative radiotherapy has been shown to reduce the number of recurrences. In patients with recurrent tumor, there are several palliative and supportive treatment options, which have an impact on quality of life as well as survival. Compared with untreated controls, systemic chemotherapy has improved the survival and symptoms of patients with recurrent tumor. The chemotherapeutic agent 5-fluorouracil is associated with improved survival and becomes the essential element of treatment of advanced colorectal cancer. New cytotoxic drugs have also been combined with 5-fluorouracil for treatment [8].

20.1.7 Screening

Screening of individuals leads to a reduction in the incidence and mortality of colorectal cancer. Screening of both men and women should be started at age 50. Patients with a family history or predisposing factors should be evaluated at an earlier age [6, 8, 11, 12].

Currently, fecal occult blood test, digital rectal examination, colo-sigmoidoscopy and barium enema are the methods for screening colorectal cancer. The American Cancer Society has recommended screening for colorectal cancer using the fecal occult blood test and flexible sigmoidoscopy every 3–5 years for all persons aged 50 years or older. Double-contrast barium enema is also a standard screening test. Virtual colonoscopy using computed tomography (CT) is being introduced for screening of colorectal cancer. There are several reports that this technique has a significant potential for screening, and studies are underway comparing virtual and actual colonoscopy [11, 12].

Serum carcinoembryonic antigen (CEA) levels cannot localize disease and lack sensitivity for determination of early onset of the disease [6–8].

20.2 Diagnosis

20.2.1 Conventional Imaging Modalities

Barium enema examination and colonoscopy are the common modalities used for the diagnosis of colon cancer. Virtual colonoscopy using CT is being evaluated for its accuracy in detecting colon cancer, but is not routinely used at this time. Ultrasound, CT and magnetic resonance imaging (MRI) do not have a major role in diagnosis of colorectal cancer, but these modalities do have a role in staging the extent of disease.

20.2.2 Nuclear Medicine Techniques

Nuclear medicine techniques are used for the detection and staging of colorectal cancer. A number of promising radiopharmaceuticals and techniques are being evaluated in clinical trials for use in patients with colorectal cancer. Two monoclonal antibodies labeled with gamma emitters have been approved for diagnostic purposes and they are available in kit form. The glucose analog, fluoro-2-deoxy-D-glucose (FDG) is also approved and commercially available. Monoclonal antibody imaging is infrequently used in evaluating patients with colorectal cancer, whereas FDG positron emission tomography (PET) imaging is widely used and its utilization continues to increase [13–15].

20.2.2.1
Immunoscintigraphy

Oncoscint: Satumomab Pendetide

Oncoscint is an IgG murine monoclonal antibody (B72.3) that is directed against the cell surface mucin-like glycoprotein antigen TAG-72, which is commonly found on colorectal cancer as well as ovarian cancer. It is labeled with indium-111 chloride, which has a 67-hour half-life. Planar and single photon emission computed tomography (SPECT) images can be obtained 48 and 96 hours post-injection. Activity is normally seen in the liver, spleen and, to a lesser extent, in bone marrow. Large bowel activity is also seen frequently [16, 17].

Oncoscint has a sensitivity of 70% and a specificity of 75% for primary colorectal cancer. Although these results are similar to those for CT, immunoscintigraphy with Oncoscint and CT are complementary. The combination of Oncoscint and CT increases the patient-based sensitivity. For recurrent colorectal cancer, Oncoscint appears to be more sensitive than CT in the detection of pelvic and/or abdominal recurrence, whereas CT has a higher sensitivity for detection of liver metastases than Oncoscint [16].

Administration of Oncoscint can cause the formation of human anti-murine antibodies (HAMA) in 40% of patients, but HAMA becomes negative in about half of these patients after 4–12 months. The presence of HAMA can alter biodistribution and image interpretation of a subsequent administration of Oncoscint because of increased liver concentration of Oncoscint [17].

20.2.2.2
CEA-Scan: Tc-99m-Arcitumomab

CEA-Scan is a murine monoclonal Fab' fragment generated from IMMU-4 directed against CEA surface antigen. The rapid blood clearance of the fragment provides high target-to-background ratios. Serum CEA levels do not affect the results of imaging [18–21]. CEA-Scan images demonstrate intense renal activity. Bowel and gallbladder activity on early images is not common. Hepatic metastases are typically seen as hot spots on late images, but in early images, a photopenic appearance is common.

Different groups, particularly in Europe, have explored the value of CEA-Scan in patients with colorectal cancer [18–21]. In these studies, CEA-Scan was found to be inferior to conventional modalities in the liver; however, in the evaluation of the extrahepatic abdomen and pelvis, it had higher sensitivity and specificity than the other modalities.

Recently, two different studies with CEA-Scan compared to FDG PET have been published. Willkomm et al. [18] reported that CEA-Scan showed an overall sensitivity, specificity and accuracy of 89, 100 and 96%, respectively, whereas the sensitivity and specificity of FDG PET were 100 and 96%, respectively. On the other hand, Libutti et al. [19] reported a prospective study of FDG PET and CEA-Scan in patients with increased CEA level. They reported low sensitivity (18%) and specificity (30%) for CEA-Scan and a sensitivity of 89% and a specificity of 50% for FDG. It was concluded that CEA-scan is not helpful preoperatively in predicting resectable or unresectable disease.

CEA-Scan produces less immunogenicity than Oncoscint because it is an antibody fragment. HAMA formation has been detected in less than 1% of patients. Minor adverse reactions have been reported.

20.3
FDG PET Imaging for Colorectal Cancer: Current State

20.3.1
Introduction

Increased glucose utilization is one of the important characteristics of cancer cells, and was initially described by Warburg in 1956 [22]. FDG PET relies on the differential uptake of FDG by the high metabolic rate of tumor cells compared to normal cells [23]. Over the past two decades, FDG PET has been shown to provide not only diagnostic information but also prognostic information for several malignancies including colorectal cancers. Thus, FDG PET has gained an important role in the evaluation of patients with colorectal carcinoma [24–29].

Mucinous carcinomas accumulate less FDG than non-mucinous carcinomas. Berger et al. [30] compared the FDG uptake with histopathologic features in 25 patients with mucinous neoplasms and found that FDG PET had an overall sensitivity of 59% for detection of primary and recurrent mucinous carcinoma, a sensitivity that is lower than generally reported for tumors of the gastrointestinal tract and lungs. Thus, mucinous adenocarcinomas are less accurately detected than non-mucinous adenocarcinomas. The reason for the lower sensitivity might be related to the relative cellularity and abundant mucin of the tumor tissue. Higashi et al. observed that low or absent FDG uptake was seen in bronchioloalveolar carcinoma, which often contains abundant amounts of mucin [31].

The presence of extrahepatic metastases is a major determinant of prognosis in patients with suspected recurrence of colorectal cancer. Therefore, highly sensitive whole-body screening modalities are required. A problem with conventional imaging modalities is their limited field-of-view. Consequently, the whole-body capability of FDG PET is helpful for detection of distant metastases. FDG PET has been approved for coverage by Medicare in the USA for diagnosis, staging, and restaging of patients with colorectal cancer. The PET studies in colorectal cancer have been largely performed in patients with recurrent disease. Few studies have been published regarding the use of FDG PET for detection and staging of primary colorectal cancer [22–26].

20.3.2 Diagnosis

Yasuda et al. [32] reported a retrospective study of 119 patients who underwent both FDG PET and colonoscopy for a cancer screening program. The sensitivity of FDG PET increased with increasing adenomatous polyp size. FDG PET detected 24% of adenomas ranging from 5 to 30 mm in size, and 90% of adenomas larger than 13 mm. Drenth et al. [33] evaluated the FDG PET findings of premalignant colonic abnormalities detected with endoscopy. FDG PET had a sensitivity of 74% and a specificity of 84% for the detection of abnormal findings seen by endoscopy [33]. While all patients with colorectal carcinoma in this group were identified by FDG PET, four patients with polyps smaller than 10 mm in size were not detected. The positivity rate for PET images was 61% in patients with polyps >10 mm in size (Fig. 1). In another study, Abdel-Nabi et al. [34] reported that 35 hyperplastic benign polyps that were incidentally discovered during histopathology examination of resected colon specimens were undetectable with FDG PET.

In the same study, Abdel-Nabi et al. compared FDG PET with CT, surgical, and histopathological findings in 48 patients with primary colorectal cancer. FDG PET detected all primary tumors, leading to a sensitivity of 100% compared with 37% for CT; however, the specificity of FDG PET was low (43%) (Fig. 2). Three of four false-positive findings were in patients with acute diverticulitis, and the fourth patient had the FDG PET scan performed soon after polypectomy. Although primary bowel cancers demonstrated high standard uptake values (SUV: 6.32), a significant correlation was not found between the SUV and degree of differentiation or tumor size [34].

20.3.3 Initial Staging

A few studies have been published for initial staging of patients with colorectal cancer. FDG PET has been reported to be superior to CT in the detection of lymph node metastases at the time of initial staging. CT is the major imaging method for detecting lymph node metastases. It relies on the assessment of the size, number and morphology of the nodes; thus lymph node metastases can be difficult to detect on CT. The reported sensitivity of CT ranges from 22 to 73%.

A study by Gupta et al. [35, 36] evaluated 16 patients who were to undergo surgery for colorectal cancer by performing FDG PET and CT imaging. Twenty tumor

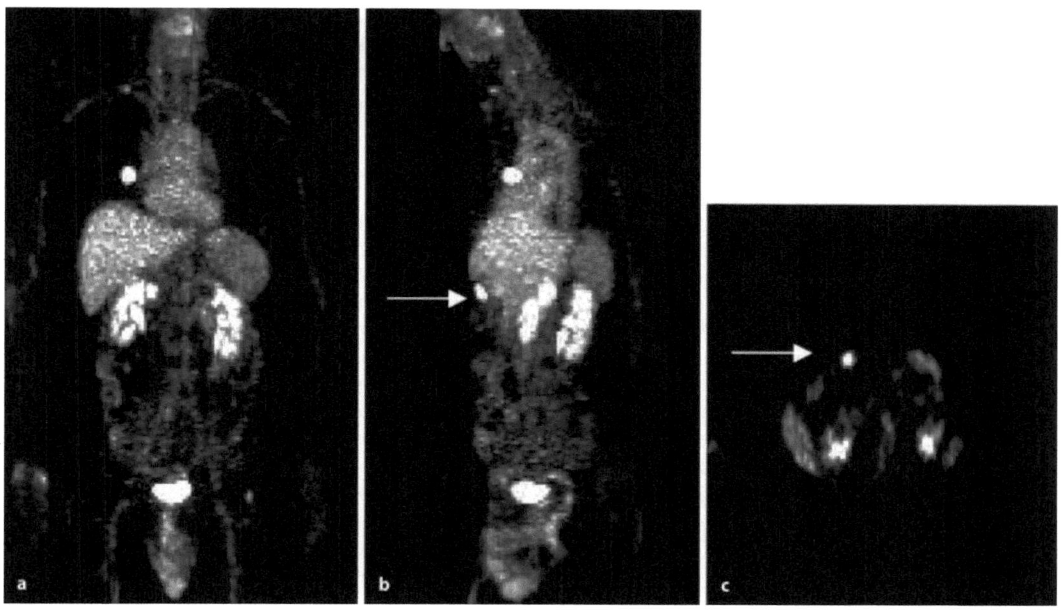

Fig. 1. Anterior (**a**) and 60° (**b**) MIP images and transaxial image (**c**) from 66 year-old male referred for a new diagnosis of a squamous cell carcinoma of the lung. Hypermetabolic right mid-lung nodule corresponds with the known lung malignancy. Additionally, there is a hypermetabolic focus in the right upper abdomen (*arrow*) also worrisome for malignancy that was felt to possibly be a second malignancy. This patient underwent colonoscopy which revealed a 2 cm tubulovillous adenoma in the transverse colon that was completely removed

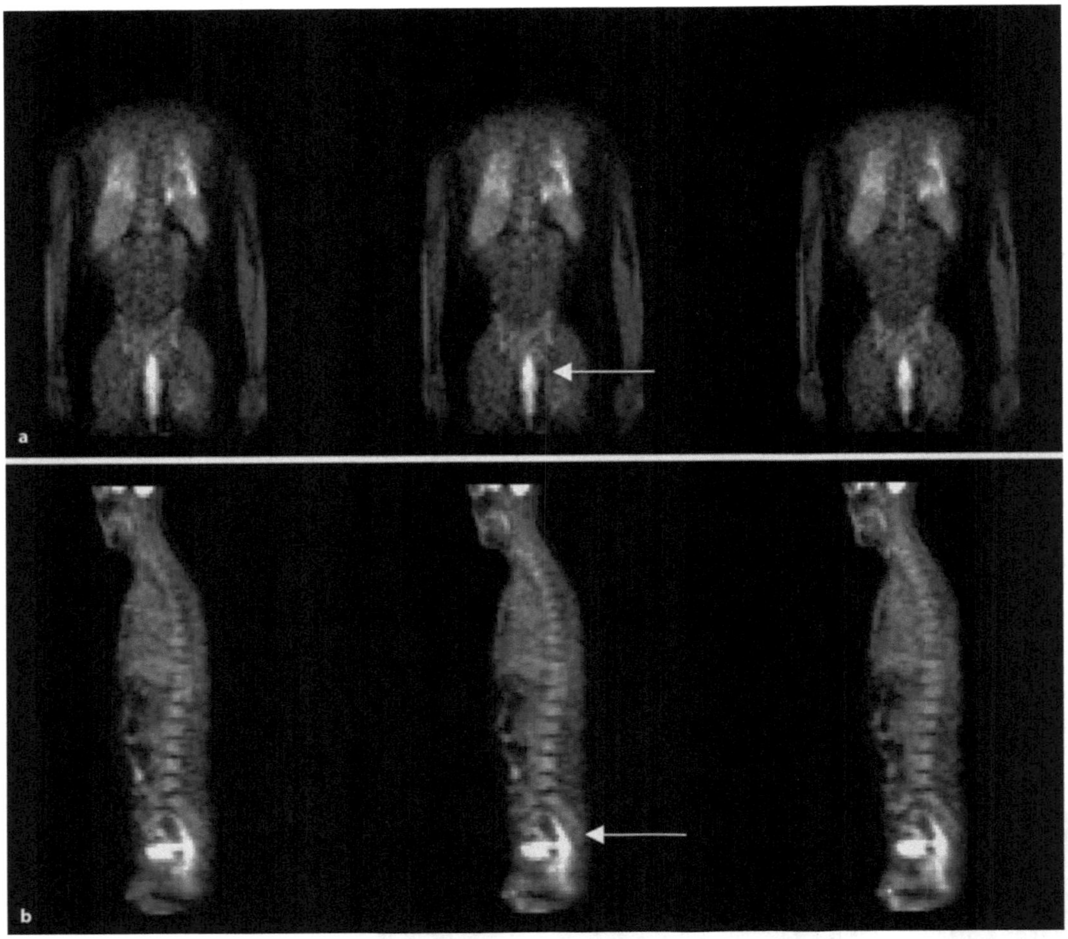

Fig. 2. Coronal (**a**) and sagittal (**b**) images from a 53-year-old male with recent diagnosis of lymphovascular carcinomatosis of the lung of unknown origin. Diffuse hypermetabolism is noted in the lungs. Focal hypermetabolic activity (*arrow*) is seen in the rectal region, and this was biopsied and proven to be adenocarcinoma

sites (five lymph nodes and two liver metastases, and 13 colon and rectum) in 16 patients were found on histology. FDG PET had a 90% sensitivity, 66% specificity and 87% accuracy for detection of tumor sites compared to 60% sensitivity, 100% specificity and 65% of accuracy for CT. They concluded that FDG PET has increased sensitivity for staging colorectal cancer as well as detecting primary as compared to CT scan. On the contrary, Abdel-Nabi et al. [34] reported that FDG PET depicted lymph node metastases in four of the 14 patients for a sensitivity of 29% for detection of regional lymph node involvement. A specificity of 96% was found in 26 patients with negative lymph nodes. FDG PET was false negative for lymph node metastases in patients with either normal or slightly elevated CEA levels, while FDG accumulation was observed in 50% of patients with elevated (7–61 ng/ml) CEA levels. FDG PET had a low sensitivity (29%) and high specificity (96%). Both values are not different from those obtained by CT.

Mukai et al. [37] reported the preoperative FDG PET results in 24 patients with primary colorectal cancer. They found a sensitivity of 22% for the detection of lymph node metastases by FDG PET, while the sensitivity for the detection of the primary tumor was 96%. In both the Abdel-Nabi and Mukai series, FDG PET failed to demonstrate most of the metastases to the regional lymph nodes surrounding the primary lesions. The reason for the low sensitivity was that either most of the lymph nodes were located in close proximity to the primary tumor or they had micrometastatic invasion. The lack of demonstration of lymph node involvement may not cause any changes on treatment because resection of the mesentery along with the primary lesion is part of the standard surgical procedure.

In terms of detecting liver metastases, FDG PET has an important role. Abdel-Nabi reported that FDG PET demonstrated liver metastases in seven of eight patients and was more accurate than CT. The sensitivity and specificity of FDG PET for detecting liver metastases were 88 and 100 %, compared with 38 % for CT.

Even though the use of FDG PET for diagnosis and initial staging of primary colorectal cancer is limited, FDG PET has a high sensitivity for diagnosing primary colon cancer as well as adenomatous polyps that are greater than 13 mm in size and is accurate in the detection of hepatic metastases [34–38].

20.3.4 Staging of Recurrent Colorectal Cancer

Colorectal cancer recurs in 37–44 % of patients, predominantly within 2 years of curative resection. Early detection of tumor recurrence and resectable metastases can lead to improved survival [7, 8, 13]. Colon carcinoma recurrence is more commonly seen in the liver and abdomen, distant from the original site, whereas locoregional recurrence is more commonly seen with rectal carcinoma (Fig. 3).

The presence and location of recurrent disease are crucial factors in the determination of possible curative resection. The likelihood of recurrent tumor following surgery is high; on the other hand, numbers of suitable patients for curative resection are low (12–60 %). After surgery, CT is the primary examination method in the monitoring of patients with colorectal cancer. It has been reported that CT has a sensitivity and specificity in the 65–70 % range. There have been numerous studies showing that FDG PET provides accurate information concerning recurrence and its resectability [13, 39, 40]. Indications for FDG PET in patients with known or suspected recurrent colorectal carcinoma are:

1. A rising CEA level in the absence of known source
2. Equivocal or abnormal lesion on conventional imaging (CT or MRI)
3. Staging prior to curative resection for a known metastasis

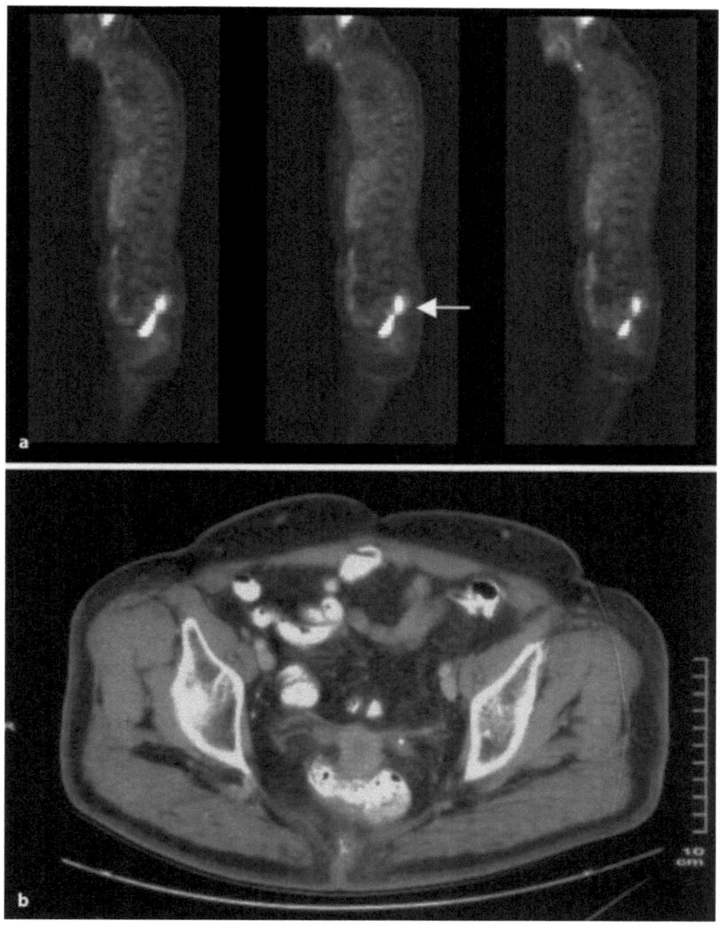

Fig.3. Sagittal images (**a**) from a 66 year-old female with right colon cancer status post right colectomy with rising CEA. Hypermetabolic activity is seen in the presacral region (*arrow*), corresponding to the soft tissue mass on the CT (**b**). This is the finding of recurrent/metastatic disease

4. Distinguishing local recurrence from post-treatment (surgery, radiation, and chemotherapy) changes.

20.3.4.1
Comparison with Rising CEA

Several studies have evaluated the role of FDG PET in patients with elevated CEA levels. Flanagan et al. [41] evaluated the utility of FDG PET in 22 patients with abnormal CEA levels (5.0 ng/ml) and normal conventional imaging studies. Abnormal FDG accumulation was seen in 17 of 22 (77%) patients, with false-positive results in two patients and no true positives. Valk et al. [42] reported a prospective study comparing FDG PET with CT in 155 patients for staging of recurrent colorectal cancer. In a subgroup, FDG PET findings were true positive in 67% of 32 patients with elevated CEA levels and negative CT. They reported that FDG PET had a 90% sensitivity and 92% specificity for this group of patients, while the sensitivity and specificity of FDG PET for the entire group were 95 and 79%, respectively.

In another study, Libutti et al. [19] from the National Cancer Institute compared FDG PET and CEA-scan with second-look laparotomy results for the detection of recurrence in 28 patients with increasing CEA levels. FDG PET had a sensitivity of 89%, and a specificity of 50%, while the CEA-scan had a sensitivity of 18% and a specificity of 33% [16]. FDG PET predicted unresectable disease in 90% of patients who were found to be unresectable at laparotomy. Swanson [43], in his editorial regarding Libutti's article, mentioned the importance of study design and results. He concluded that FDG PET probably will become part of the standard for imaging patients with colorectal cancer and suspected recurrent or metastatic disease.

Flamen et al. [44] evaluated the potential benefit of FDG PET and conventional diagnostic work-up (CDW) in patients with unexplained rising CEA and suspected recurrence. Fifty consecutive patients with elevated CEA levels who had FDG PET and a completely normal or equivocal CDW were retrospectively selected for this study. FDG PET and CDW results were confirmed with tissue or follow-up. The overall sensitivity of FDG PET for the presence of recurrent disease on a patient-basis was 79%. It was concluded that the superior sensitivity of FDG PET would result in a more prominent role in the management of patients with suspected recurrent colorectal cancer, particularly with elevated CEA levels [44]. Willkomm et al. [18] compared the efficacy of FDG PET and CEA-scan in 28 patients with recurrence of colorectal cancer most commonly suspected because of increased CEA level. The CEA-scan had 89% sensitivity and 100% specificity, while FDG PET had 100% sensitivity and 95% specificity. They concluded that both the CEA-scan and FDG PET are suitable for diagnosing local recurrence of colorectal cancer. However, they recommended FDG PET imaging for tumor staging because of its high sensitivity for detecting lymph node and distant metastases.

20.3.4.2
Comparison with Other Conventional Modalities

Flamen et al. [45] studied 103 patients to determine the discrepancies between FDG PET and conventional imaging modalities in lesions that were confirmed by histopathology or follow-up. They concluded that FDG PET had a positive impact on the characterization of lesions that are indeterminate by conventional imaging modalities. In this study, they reported an 81% sensitivity for PET in patients with equivocal CDW findings. In Valk's study [42], 88% of sites that were false negative by CT were true positive by FDG PET. They reported an overall sensitivity of 95% and an overall specificity of 79%, while CT had a 78% sensitivity and 50% specificity. FDG PET was superior to CT in all sites (liver, pelvis, abdomen) for detection of recurrent colorectal cancer.

In a study of 16 patients, Falk et al. [46] reported that FDG PET had a sensitivity of 87%, and a specificity of 67%, whereas CT had a 47% sensitivity and 100% specificity. Although most of the malignant cases were detected by FDG PET, false-negative findings were observed in two patients. One of them had adenocarcinoma with central necrosis and marked fibrosis, and the other one had two lesions, which were next to each other, with the small one being missed by FDG PET.

FDG PET may enable the detection of recurrences before structural changes can be diagnosed by conventional imaging modalities (CT, MRI). Huebner et al. [47] published a meta-analysis of the literature for FDG PET detection of recurrent colorectal cancer. The meta-analysis included 11 studies of 281 patients who underwent whole-body FDG PET. The sensitivity and specificity in the whole-body images of these patients by pooling data were 97 and 76%, respectively. The FDG PET results in local recurrence and in the liver were reported in 366 and 393 patients, respectively. The results in local/pelvic recurrences were 95% sensitivity and 98% specificity, whereas the sensitivity and specificity of recurrences in the liver were 96 and 99%, respectively.

FDG PET has been demonstrated to be more sensitive than CT at all sites except the lung, where both modalities are equivalent. From the results of this literature review, Huebner et al. [47] concluded that FDG PET can effectively direct patients with recurrent colorectal cancer to the most appropriate treatment. Studies regarding sensitivity and specificity of PET and CT for staging recurrent colorectal cancer are shown in Table 3.

Table 3. Comparison of PET and CT results in local/pelvic and distant metastases

Author	No. of patients	PET			CT		
		Sensitivity	Specificity	Accuracy	Sensitivity	Specificity	Accuracy
Ito [52]	15	100	100	100	–	–	–
Gupta [36]	16	90	66	87	60	100	65
Falk [46]	16	87	67	83	47	100	56
Vitola [40]	24	90	100	93	86	58	76
Ruhlmann [29]	59	100	67				
Flanagan [41]	22	89	100				
Valk [42]	155	95	79		78	50	
Whiteford [27]	105	87	68		66	59	
Staib [64]	100	98	90	95	91	72	82
Flamen [45]	50	79–81	89				
Libutti [19]	28	89	50		18	33[a]	
Arulampalam [65]	42	93	58		73	75	
Lonneux[58]	79	97	72		61	36	
Tanaka [56]	23	95		93	83		83

[a] CEA-scan results

20.3.5 Preoperative Staging

The liver is the primary site of hematogenous metastases in colorectal cancer and is a major concern in suspected recurrent colorectal cancer (Fig. 4). Liver resection for hepatic metastases is considered only for patients with one to four lesions confined to one lobe of the liver when no other metastases are present [7, 8, 13].

Superior mesenteric arterial portography is more sensitive than conventional CT for the detection of hepatic metastases, but it has a high rate of false positives. False-positive results from FDG PET in the liver are very rare and occur primarily from hepatic abscesses. In a report by Delbeke et al. [48], FDG PET had a lower sensitivity (91 vs 97%) but higher specificity (95 vs 50%), resulting in a superior overall diagnostic accuracy compared to CT portography.

Ogunbiyi et al. [49] reported high sensitivity (95%) and specificity (100%) of FDG PET for detecting liver metastases. Rohren et al. [50] have published their results for patients being evaluated for potential curative resection of hepatic metastases from colorectal cancer. FDG PET had a sensitivity of 95% and a specificity of 100%. The probability of lesion detection by FDG PET was directly correlated with lesion size. They concluded that FDG PET is accurate for potential curative resection of hepatic masses in patients with colorectal cancer.

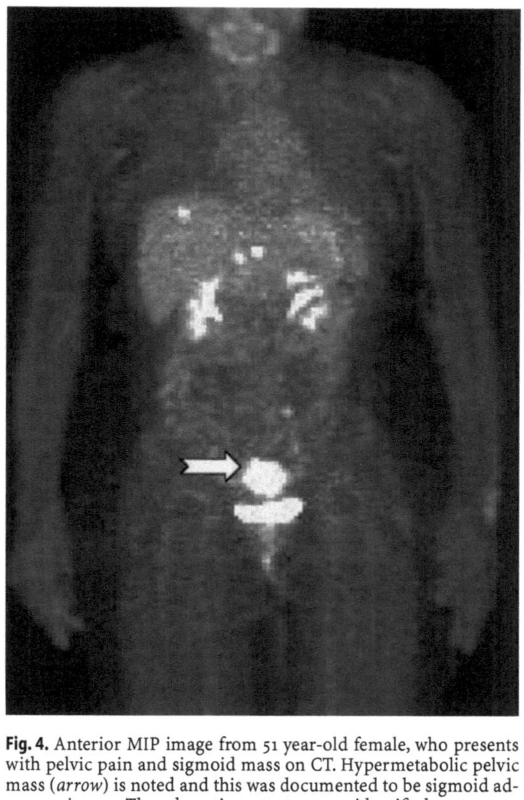

Fig. 4. Anterior MIP image from 51 year-old female, who presents with pelvic pain and sigmoid mass on CT. Hypermetabolic pelvic mass (*arrow*) is noted and this was documented to be sigmoid adenocarcinoma. Three hepatic metastases are identified

Kinkel et al. [51] performed a meta-analysis to compare anatomical diagnostic modalities (ultrasonography, CT, MRI) and FDG PET in the detection of hepatic metastases from colorectal, gastric and esophageal cancer. Among 111 data sets, they found nine PET data sets containing 423 patients, in addition to their own institutional data base of 102 patients. In this study, the prevalence of hepatic metastases was 58% and the number of hepatic metastases per patient was 2.18. The mean

Table 4.
Comparison of PET and CT results in liver metastases

Author	No. of patients	PET			CT		
		Sensitivity	Specificity	Accuracy	Sensitivity	Specificity	Accuracy
Schiepers [55]	76	94	100	98	85	72	93
Ogunbiyi [49]	58	95	100	95	74	85	
Delbeke[48]	52	91	–	92	81	–	78
Staib [64]	100	100	99	99			
Arulampalam [65]	42	100	100		45	100	
Rohren [50]	22	95	100				

Table 5.
Comparison of PET and CT results in local/pelvic recurrence

Author	No. of patients	PET			CT		
		Sensitivity	Specificity	Accuracy	Sensitivity	Specificity	Accuracy
Schiepers [55]	76	93	97	95	60	72	65
Ogunbiyi [49]	58	91	100		52	80	
Willkomm [85]	28	100	95		89	100*	
Staib [64]	45	100	95	96			
Arulampalam [65]	42	100	86		75	100	

weighted sensitivity of the modalities with a specificity higher than 85 % was 55 % for ultrasonography, 72 % for CT, 76 % for MRI, and 90 % for FDG PET. In patients suspected of recurrent hepatic metastases from colorectal cancer, the sensitivity of FDG PET was 88 %, which was lower than reported in the meta-analysis by Huebner [47]. On the basis of their results, they concluded that FDG PET is the most sensitive imaging modality for detecting hepatic metastases from colorectal cancer as well as gastric and esophageal cancer. Other studies also support these findings [52, 53]. The sensitivity and specificity of FDG PET for detection of hepatic metastases in patients with recurrent colorectal cancer are shown in Table 4.

20.3.6 Distinguishing Local Recurrence

The 5-year survival following surgery for local recurrent disease is only about 35 %. Differentiation of recurrence from scar in patients with suspected isolated local recurrence is essential for appropriate patient management. FDG PET has been found to be more sensitive than CT for detection of tumor recurrence [54–57].

In a study reported by Lonneux et al. [58], the results of conventional imaging modalities and FDG PET were compared in 79 patients with known or suspected recurrent colorectal cancer. FDG PET had an overall 97 % sensitivity, and 72 % specificity, which were superior to the conventional imaging modalities for all sites except the liver. FDG PET had a 100 % sensitivity and 98 % specificity for detecting local recurrence, and 97 % sensitivity and 100 % specificity for detecting liver metastases, whereas conventional imaging modalities had a 73 % sensitivity and 95 % specificity for local recurrence and 94 % sensitivity and 96 % specificity for liver metastases [58, 59]. FDG PET demonstrated a sensitivity of 89 % and specificity of 50 % in patients who had second-look laparotomy. The values of sensitivity and specificity of FDG PET and CT for pelvic recurrence are summarized in Table 5.

20.3.7 Assessment of Therapy Response

Infection and inflammation with increased numbers of macrophages can cause abnormal FDG uptake [60]. FDG uptake can occur as a result of radiation therapy. Although there are no systematic studies on the time course of FDG PET accumulation after radiotherapy, Haberkorn et al. [61] reported that most of the inflammatory effects will have disappeared after 6 months. Thus, according to Haberkorn, FDG PET can accurately differentiate recurrent tumor from radiation uptake 6 months after radiation therapy.

Guillem et al. [62] reported a study of 21 patients with primary rectal cancer. Fifteen patients underwent FDG PET imaging for assessment of response to preoperative radiation/chemotherapy. PET identified the primary rectal cancer in all patients, and five parameters were used to assess tumor response: tumor lesion glycolysis, SUV_{max}, SUV_{avg}, PET size and visual response score. It was concluded that the visual response score developed by Larson et al. [63] is the best parameter for evaluating tumor response to therapy; interestingly, all rectal cancers had greatly accelerated glycolysis, after therapy.

20.4
Impact on Patient Management

Several studies have recently documented the impact of FDG PET on managing patients with colorectal cancer. In a report of 100 patients with recurrent colorectal cancer comparing CT, liver ultrasound and CEA levels, Staib et al. [64] evaluated the contribution of FDG PET to surgical decision-making. They found that FDG PET influenced surgical management in 61% of cases. FDG PET had 98% sensitivity, 90% specificity and 95% accuracy, while CT had 91% sensitivity, 72% specificity and 82% accuracy in the detection of recurrent or metastatic colorectal cancer. They reported 100% sensitivity for detection of liver metastases.

Flanagan et al. [34] reported that FDG PET altered clinical management in 40% of the patients with recurrent disease.

Arulampalam et al. [65] evaluated 42 patients previously treated for colorectal cancer with FDG PET and the results were compared with CT in order to assess the impact of FDG on patient management. FDG PET had 93% sensitivity and 58% specificity compared with 73% sensitivity and 75% specificity for CT. FDG PET yielded a correct diagnosis in 83% of patients compared to 74% of patients with CT.

Several consecutive studies have been published regarding the impact of FDG PET on patient management for recurrent colorectal cancer in terms of the referring physician perspective. Meta et al. [66] reported a survey study of 146 patients with colorectal cancer. Changes in clinical stage were reported for 42% of patients, mostly upstaging. In this report, FDG PET resulted in intermodality treatment changes in 37% of patients and intramodality changes in 18% of patients [66–69].

Simo et al. [70] reported the results of a study that evaluated 120 patients with suspected recurrence for assessment of the influence of FDG PET on management of patients. FDG PET detected more lesions than CT and led to a major management change in 48% of patients, particularly those with elevated CEA levels. In another study, Dizendorf et al. [71] reported that FDG PET had a major impact on the management of 27 patients being considered for radiation therapy. The impact of FDG PET imaging on clinical and surgical decision-making is summarized in Table 6.

Table 6. Clinical impact of FDG PET on management of patients with colorectal cancer

	No. of patients	Clinical impact
Vitola [40]	24	25%
Delbeke [48]	61	28%
Ogunbiyi [49]	23	43%
Valk [42]	78	21%
Flamen [44]	103	20%
Simo [70]	120	48%
Lonneux [58]	122	41%
Staib [64]	100	61%
Kalff [67]	102	59%
Arulampalam [65]	42	27%
Meta [66]	57	41%

20.5
Assessment of Prognosis and Cost-Effectiveness

FDG PET predicts which patients are likely to have a good prognosis. Strasberg et al. [72] reported a prospective study of 43 patients with metastatic colorectal carcinoma. In this study, FDG PET identified additional disease not seen on CT in ten patients (25%). They reported that the 3-year survival of patients evaluated by FDG PET before liver resection for metastatic colorectal cancer was 77%, in contrast to the figure of 40% published previously [72].

Decision analysis has been used to determine the cost-effectiveness of FDG in patients with recurrent colorectal cancer [73]. Decision trees based on theoretical models were used to assess the cost-effectiveness of a CT + FDG PET strategy compared with a CT-alone strategy for diagnosis and management of recurrent colorectal cancer. They concluded that despite the relatively high cost of FDG PET compared to other modalities, the use of FDG PET could be more cost-effective because of the increased accuracy of the results. A CT + FDG PET strategy for managing patients can potentially save many patients from unnecessary surgery.

20.6
Limitations

FDG accumulation is frequently seen in the gastrointestinal tract, and the uptake is probably in the mucosa rather than muscle [75, 76]. The linear pattern of uptake in the bowel, which is best seen in coronal images, is easily differentiated from a focal malignant lesion. However, focal intense activity, which is seen with colonic cancers and adenomas, can have other causes, such as inflammation, which occurs with ulcerative colitis [74–77]. Intense colonic FDG uptake has been reported in patients with non-malignant pathology such as acute enterocolitis. Tatlidil et al. [77] reported a study of colonic FDG uptake correlation with colonoscopic and histopathologic findings. They found that a diffuse colonic FDG uptake pattern, regardless of degree, is predictive of a normal finding at colonoscopy, whereas a segmental high uptake pattern implies an inflammatory process. They recommended colonoscopy as a next step for further evaluation of patients who have segmental high uptake [78]. Because excretion of FDG in the bladder may cause difficulties in interpretation of abnormalities in the pelvis, some sites performing FDG PET scans have recommended bladder catheterization when evaluating the pelvis. We have not found it to be necessary.

20.7 Summary

Several studies have shown that FDG PET imaging can detect and stage patients with primary colorectal cancer. False-negative results may be obtained when lesions are small (<1 cm) or necrotic because of a partial volume effect. Mucinous adenocarcinomas are detected less accurately than non-mucinous adenocarcinomas. FDG PET has high sensitivity and specificity in recurrent colorectal cancer. The whole-body capability of FDG PET is useful for detecting tumors that have spread to sites that are not detected by other imaging techniques.

The use of FDG PET has had a considerable impact on patient management. Clinical and correlative imaging improves the specificity of FDG PET [79].

20.8 New Tracers

20.8.1 [^{18}F]Fluorouracil

^{18}Fluorine-labeled fluorouracil ([^{18}F]FU), a cytostatic agent, has been used for therapy monitoring in patients with colorectal carcinoma. Dynamic PET studies with FU demonstrate a relatively low FU uptake in metastases and a large individual variation in uptake [80, 81]. Dual tracer studies using [^{15}O]water and [^{18}F]FU have been performed in patients who were scheduled for intra-arterial chemotherapy. The studies show that the results could be used to select patients who are more likely to benefit from the therapy. [^{18}F]FU can also predict the outcome of therapy. It is possible to predict the tumor response to 5-FU with [^{18}F]FU PET because there is a good correlation between [^{18}F]FU trapping and survival of the patients after chemotherapy.

20.8.2 [^{11}C]Acetate/[11C]Amino Acids

^{11}Carbon acetate has been used for PET imaging in patients with different types of cancer. Yoshimoto et al. [82] evaluated acetate metabolism in human adenocarcinoma cells. They reported higher tumor-to-normal ratios of [^{11}C]acetate in comparison with those of FDG. ^{11}Carbon acetate is potentially a more sensitive tumor imaging tracer than FDG [83].

Wieder et al. [84] reported their results with [^{11}C]methyl-L-methionine (MET) for therapy monitoring in patients with rectal cancer. Although having advantages such as lower radiation dose and less renal clearance, MET PET was not able to assess tumor response in patients with rectal cancer.

20.9 Technical Recommendations

20.9.1 [^{18}F]FDG Whole Body Protocol

20.9.1.1 *Patient Preparation*

Fasting for at least 4–6 hours prior to the study.

Measurement of blood glucose level with finger-stick blood sampling and glucometer.

Patient should remain quiet for a period of 30 minutes.

Patient should be instructed to empty bladder just prior to image acquisition.

20.9.1.2 *Radiopharmaceutical*

Intravenous injection of 140 Ci/kg (minimum 10 mCi, maximum 20 mCi) FDG.

20.9.1.3 *Data Acquisition*

Patient is positioned supine, feet first into the camera.

The laser landmark is set at the external auditory meatus.

- Emission: Four minutes per bed position
  - Six bed positions (for person <64 inches, five bed positions)
- Transmission: 2 minutes 30 seconds per bed position.

20.9.1.4 *Reconstruction*

Iterative reconstruction of transmission and emission scans (OS-EM).

OS-EM, two iterations, 28 subsets, 128 × 128 matrix.

20.9.1.5 *Quantification (Not Routinely Performed)*

Maximum SUV calculation determined using circular region of interest on area of maximum uptake.

20.9.1.6 *Recommendations*

Correlation with anatomical imaging procedures (CT, MRI) is necessary for accurate interpretation. PET/CT facilitates correlative imaging.

References

1. Compton CC (2002) Surgical pathology of colorectal cancer. In: Saltz LB (ed) Colorectal cancer: multimodality management. Humana Press, Totowa NJ, pp 247–265
2. Jemal A, Thomas A, Murray T, Thun M (2002) Cancer statistics, 2002. CA Cancer J Clin 52:23–47
3. Ries LAG, Wingo PA, Miller DS et al (2000) The annual report to the nation on the status of cancer, 1973–1997, with a special section on colorectal cancer. Cancer 88:2398–2424
4. American Cancer Society (2003) Cancer facts and figures. American Cancer Society, Atlanta, Georgia
5. Reske SN, Kotzerke J (2001) FDG PET for clinical use. Results of the 3rd German Interdisciplinary Consensus Conference, "Onko-PET III", 21 July and 19 Sept 2000. Eur J Nucl Med 28: 1707–1723
6. Talbot SM, Newugut AI (2002) Epidemiological trends in colorectal cancer. In: Saltz LB (ed) Colorectal cancer: multimodality management. Humana Press, Totowa NJ, pp 23–46
7. Ed McArdle CS, Kerr DJ, Boyle P (2000) Colorectal cancer. ISIS Medical Media, Oxford
8. Murphy GP, Lawrence W Jr, Lenhard RE Jr (1995) Textbook of clinical oncology, 2nd edn. American Cancer Society, Georgia, USA
9. Greene FL, Page DL, Fleming ID et al (2001) Colon and rectum, part 3. AJCC cancer staging manual, 6th edn. American Joint Committee on Cancer, Chicago
10. Frederick K, Greene FL et al (2002) AJCC cancer staging manual, 6th edn. American Joint Committee on Cancer, Chicago
11. Nakama H, Zhang B, Fukazawa K (2001) Colorectal cancer screening under the age of 50 is less cost-effective. Cancer Invest 20:290–291
12. Frazier AL, Colditz GA, Fuchs CS, Kuntz KM (2000) Cost-effectiveness of screening for colorectal cancer in the general population. JAMA 284:1954–1961
13. Khalkhali I, Maublant JC, Goldsmith SJ (2001) Nuclear oncology: diagnosis and treatment. Lippincott Williams and Wilkins, Philadelphia, PA
14. Goldberg HI, Margulis AR (2000) Gastrointestinal radiology in the United States: an overview of the past 50 years. Radiology 216:1–7
15. Horton K, Abrams RA, Fishman EK (2000) Spiral CT of colon cancer: imaging features and role in management. RadioGraphics 20:419–430
16. Collier BD, Abdel-Nabi H, Doerr RJ et al (1992) Immunoscintigraphy performed with In-111-labeled CYT-103 in the management of colorectal cancer: comparison with CT. Radiology 185:179–186
17. Su WT, Brachman M, O'Connell TX (2001) Use of OncoScint scan to assess resectability of hepatic metastases. Am Surg 67: 1200–1203
18. Willkomm P, Bender H, Bangard M, Decker P, Grunwald F, Biersack HJ (2000) FDG PET and immunoscintigraphy with 99mTc-labeled antibody fragments for detection of the recurrence of colorectal carcinoma. J Nucl Med 41:1657–1663
19. Libutti SK, Alexander RH, Choyke P et al (2001) A prospective study of 2-[f-18] fluoro-2-deoxy-D-glucose/positron emission tomography scan, 99mTc-labeled Arcitumomab (CEA-Scan), and blind second-look laparotomy for detecting colon cancer recurrence in patients with increasing carcinoembryonic antigen levels. Ann Surg Oncol 8:779–786
20. Bridwel R, Thropay J (2003) Economic utility of CEA-scan (arcitumomab) immunoscintigraphy in the evaluation of patients with colorectal cancer. A retrospective financial analysis based on published clinical studies. Alasbimn J 5:1–12
21. Lechner P, Lind P, Goldenberg DM (2000) Can postoperative surveillance with serial CEA immunoscintigraphy detect resectable rectal cancer recurrence and potentially improve tumor-free survival? J Am Coll Surg 191:511–518
22. Warburg O (1956) On the origin of cancer cells. Science 123:309–314
23. Macbeth RAL, Bekesi JG (1962) Oxygen consumption and anaerobic glycolysis of human malignant and normal tissue. Cancer Res 22:244–248
24. Coleman RE (1998) Clinical PET in oncology. Clin Positron Imaging 1:15–30
25. Dobos N, Rubesin SE (2002) Radiologic imaging modalities in the diagnosis and management of colorectal cancer. Hematol Oncol Clin North Am 16:875–895
26. Stokkel MPM, Draisma A, Pauwels EKJ (2001) Positron emission tomography with 2-F-18-fluoro-2-deoxy-D-glucose in oncology, part IIIB. J Cancer Res Clin Oncol 127:278–285
27. Whiteford MH, Whiteford HM, Yee LF et al (2000) Usefulness of FDG PET scans in the assessment of suspected metastatic or recurrent adenocarcinoma of colon and rectum. Dis Colon Rectum 43:759–770
28. Delbeke D, Martin WH (2001) Positron emission tomography in oncology. Radiol Clin North Am 39:883–917
29. Ruhlmann J, Schomburg A, Bender H et al (1997) Fluorodeoxyglucose whole-body positron emission tomography in colorectal cancer patients studied in routine daily practice. Dis Colon Rectum 40:1195–1204
30. Berger KL, Nicholson SA, Dehdashti F, Siegel BA (2000) FDG PET evaluation of mucinous neoplasms: correlation of FDG uptake with histopathologic features. AJR 174:1005–1008
31. Higashi K, Nishikawa T, Seki H et al (1998) Comparison of fluorine-18-FDG PET and thallium-201 SPECT in evaluation of lung cancer. J Nucl Med 39:9–15
32. Yasuda S, Fujii H, Nakahara T et al (2001) 18F-FDG PET detection of colonic adenomas. J Nucl Med 42:989–992
33. Drenth JPH, Nagengast FM, Oyen WJG (2001) Evaluation of (pre) malignant colonic abnormalities: endoscopic validation of FDG PET findings. Eur J Nucl Med 28:1766–1769
34. Abdel-Nabi H, Doerr RJ, Lamonica DM et al (1998) Staging of primary colorectal carcinomas with fluorine-18 fluorodeoxyglucose whole-body PET: correlation with histopathologic and CT findings. Radiology 206:755–760
35. Gupta NC, Bowman BM, Thorson AM et al (1992) F-18 fluorodeoxyglucose (FDG) PET for preoperative staging of colorectal carcinoma (abstract). J Nucl Med 33:975
36. Gupta NC, Falk PM, Frank AL et al. (1993) Pre-operative staging of colorectal carcinoma using positron emission tomography (abstract). Nebr Med J 78:30–35
37. Mukai M, Sadhiro S, Yasuda S et al (2000) Preoperative evaluation by whole-body F18-fluorodeoxyglucose positron emission tomography in patients with primary colorectal cancer (abstract). Oncol Rep 7:85–87
38. Hongming Z, Marc H, Thomas C et al (2002) Incidental detection of colon cancer by FDG positron emission tomography in patients examined for pulmonary nodules. Clin Nucl Med 27: 628–632
39. Strauss LG, Clorius JH, Schlag P (1989) Recurrence of colorectal tumors: PET evaluation. Radiology 170:329–333
40. Vitola JV, Delbeke D, Sandler MP et al (1996) Positron emission tomography to stage metastatic colorectal carcinoma to the liver. Am J Surg 171:21–26
41. Flanagan FL, Dehdashti F, Ogunbiyi OA, Kodner IJ, Siegel BA (1998) Utility of FDG PET for investigating unexplained plasma CEA elevation in patients with colorectal cancer. Ann Surg 227:319–323
42. Valk PE, Abella-Columna E, Haseman A et al (1999) Whole-body PET imaging with F-18Fluoroglucose in management of recurrent colorectal cancer. Arch Surg 134:503–511
43. Swanson RS (2001) Is an FDG PET scan the new imaging standard for colon cancer? Ann Surg Oncol 8:752–753
44. Flamen P, Stroobants S, Custem EV et al (1999) Additional value of whole-body positron emission tomography with fluorine-18-2-deoxy-D-glucose in recurrent colorectal cancer. J Clin Oncol 17:894–901
45. Flamen P, Hoekstra OS, Homans F et al (2001) Unexplained rising carcinoembryonic antigen (CEA) in the postoperative surveillance of colorectal cancer: the utility of positron emission tomography (PET). Eur J Cancer 37:862–869
46. Falk PM, Gupta NC, Thorson AG et al (1994) Positron emission tomography for preoperative staging of colorectal carcinoma. Dis Colon Rectum 37:153–156
47. Huebner RH, Park KC, Shepherd JE et al (2000) A meta-analysis of the literature for whole body FDG PET detection of re-

current colorectal cancer. J Nucl Med 41:1177–1189
48. Delbeke D, Vitola JV, Sandler MP et al (1997) Staging recurrent metastatic colorectal carcinoma with PET. J Nucl Med 38:1196–1201
49. Ogunbiyi OA, Flanagan FL, Dehdashi F et al (1997) Detection of recurrent and metastatic colorectal cancer: comparison of positron emission tomography and computed tomography. Ann Surg Oncol 4:613–620
50. Rohren EM, Paulson EK, Hagge R et al (2002) The role of F-18 FDG positron emission tomography in preoperative assessment of the liver in patients being considered for curative resection of hepatic metastases from colorectal cancer. Clin Nucl Med 27:550–555
51. Kinkel K, Lu Y, Both M, Warren RS, Thoeni RF (2002) Detection of hepatic metastases from cancer of the gastrointestinal tract by using noninvasive imaging methods (US, CT, MRI imaging, PET): a meta-analysis. Radiology 224:748–756
52. Ito K, Kato T, Tadokoro B et al (1992) Recurrent rectal cancer and scar: differentiation with PET and MRI imaging. Radiology 182:549–552
53. Ruers T, Bleichrodt RP (2002) Treatment of liver metastases, an update on the possibilities and results. Eur J Cancer 38:1023–1033
54. Ruers TJM, Langnehoff BS, Neeleeman N, Jager GJ, Strijk S, Wobbes T, Corstens FHM (2002) Value of positron emission tomography with [F-18]fluorodeoxyglucose in patients with colorectal liver metastases: a prospective study. J Clin Oncol 20:388–395
55. Schiepers C, Pennickx F, de Vaddler et al (1995) Contribution of PET in the diagnosis of recurrent colorectal cancer: comparison with conventional imaging. Eur J Surg Oncol 21:517–522
56. Tanaka T, Kawai Y, Kanai M et al (2002) Usefulness of FDG-positron emission tomography in diagnosing peritoneal recurrence of colorectal cancer. Am J Surg 184:433–436
57. Peeyush B, Hongming Z, Marc H, Alavi A (2002) Pelvic kidney mimicking recurrent colon cancer on FDG positron emission tomographic imaging. Clin Nucl Med 27:602–603
58. Lonneux M, Reffad AM, Detry R, Kartheuser A, Gigot JF, Pauwels S (2002) FDG PET improves the staging and selection of patients with recurrent colorectal cancer. Eur J Nucl Med 29: 915–921
59. Ludger S, Schirmeister H, Reske SN, Beger HG (2000) Is 18F-fluorodeoxyglucose positron emission tomography in recurrent colorectal cancer a contribution to surgical decision-making? Am J Surg 180:1–5
60. Kubota R, Kubota K, Yamada S et al (1994) Microautoradiography study for the differentiation of intratumoral macrophages, granulation tissues and cancer cells by the dynamics of fluorine-18-fluorodeoxyglucose uptake. J Nucl Med 35:104–111
61. Haberkorn U, Strauss LG, Dimitrakopoulou A et al (1991) PET studies of fluorodeoxyglucose metabolism in patients with recurrent colorectal tumors receiving radiotherapy. J Nucl Med 32:1485–1490
62. Guillem JG, Calle JP Jr, Akhurst T et al (2000) Prospective assessment of primary rectal cancer response to preoperative radiation and chemotherapy using 18-fluorodeoxyglucose positron emission tomography. Dis Colon Rectum 43:18–24
63. Larson SM, Erdi Y, Akhurst T et al (1999) Tumor treatment response based on visual and quantitative changes in global tumor glycolysis using PET-FDG imaging. Clin Positron Imaging 2:159–171
64. Staib L, Schirrmeister H, Reske SN, Beger HG (2000) Is F-18-fluorodeoxyglucose positron emission tomography in recurrent colorectal cancer a contribution to surgical decision-making? Am J Surg 180:1–5
65. Arulampalam T, Costa D, Visvikis D, Boulos P, Taylor I, Ell P (2001) The impact of FDG PET on the management algorithm for recurrent colorectal cancer. Eur J Nucl Med 28:1758–1765
66. Meta J, Seltzer M, Schiepers C et al (2001) Impact of 18F-FDG PET on managing patients with colorectal cancer: the referring physician's perspective. J Nucl Med 42:586–590
67. Kalff V, Hicks RJ, Ware RE, Hogg A, Binns D, McKenzie AF (2002) The clinical impact of 18F-FDG PET in patients with suspected or confirmed recurrence of colorectal cancer: a prospective study. J Nucl Med 43:492–499
68. Tucker R, Coel M, Ko J, Morris P, Druger G, McGuigan P (2001) Impact of fluorine-18 fluorodeoxyglucose positron emission tomography on patient management: first year's experience in a clinical center. J Clin Oncol 19:2504–2508
69. Bombardieri E, Crippa F (2002) The increasing impact of PET in the diagnostic work-up of cancer patients. In: Freeman LM (ed) Nuclear medicine annual. LWW, PA, USA
70. Simo M, Lumen F, Setoain AJ et al (2002) FDG PET improves the management of patients with suspected recurrence of colorectal cancer. Nucl Med Commun 23:975–982
71. Dizendorf EV, Baumert BG, von Schulthess GK (2003) Impact of whole-body F18-FDG PET on staging and managing patients for radiation therapy. J Nucl Med 44:24–29
72. Strasberg SM, Dehdashti F, Siegel BA, Drebin JA, Linehan D (2001) Survival of patients evaluated by FDG PET before hepatic resection for metastatic colorectal carcinoma: a retrospective database study. Ann Surg 233:293–299
73. Park K, Schwimmer J, Shepherd J et al (2001) Decision analysis for the cost-effective management of recurrent colorectal cancer. Ann Surg 233:310–319
74. Yasuda S, Takahashi W, Takagi S, Ide M, Shohtsu B (1998) Primary colorectal cancers detected with PET. Jpn J Clin Oncol 28: 638–643
75. Jadvar H, Schambye RB, Segall GM (1999) Physiologic source of intestinal FDG uptake: effect of atropine and Sincalide. Clin Positron Imaging 2:318 (abstract)
76. Kim S, Chung JK, Kim BT et al (1999) Relationship between gastrointestinal F-18-fluorodeoxyglucose accumulation and gastrointestinal symptoms in whole-body PET. Clin Positron Imaging 2:273–280
77. Tatlidil R, Jadvar H, Bading JR, Conti PS (2002) Incidental colonic fluorodeoxyglucose uptake: correlation with colonoscopic and histopathologic findings. Radiology 224:783–787
78. Seok-ki K, June-Key C, Byung TK et al (1998) Relationship between gastrointestinal F-18-fluorodeoxyglucose accumulation and gastrointestinal symptoms in whole-body PET. Clin Pos Imag 2:273–280
79. Hany TF, Steinert HC, Goerres GW, Buck A, von Schulthess GK. (2002) PET diagnostic accuracy: improvement with in-line PET-CT system: initial results. Radiology 225:575–581
80. Moehler M, Strauss AD, Gutzler F et al (1998) F-18-labeled fluorouracil positron emission tomography and the prognosis of colorectal carcinoma patients with metastases to the liver treated with 5-fluorouracil. Cancer 83:245–253
81. Aboagye EO, Saleem A, Cunningham VJ, Osman S, Price PM. (2001) Extraction of 5-fluorouracil by tumor and liver: a noninvasive positron emission tomography study of patients with gastrointestinal cancer. Cancer Research 61:4937–4941
82. Yoshimoto M, Waki A, Yonekura Y et al (2001) Characterization of acetate metabolism in tumor cells in relation to cell proliferation: acetate metabolism in tumor cells. Nucl Med Biol 28:117–122
83. Liu RS (2000) Clinical application of C-11 acetate in oncology. Clin Positron Imaging 3:185 (abstract)
84. Wieder H, Ott K, Zimmermann F et al (2002) PET imaging with [11C]methyl-L-methionine for therapy monitoring in patients with rectal cancer. Eur J Nucl Med 29:789–796
85. Willkomm (2001)

CHAPTER 21

Ovarian Cancer

M. Zimny

21.1 Incidence, Etiology, Epidemiology

Ovarian cancer accounts for approximately 4% of cancer related deaths worldwide with an estimated number of 131000 patients dying from this disease in 2000 (World Health Report 2002). There is a high incidence in Northern Europe and in the United States, and a low incidence in Japan [18]. Major risk factors include nulliparity, family history of ovarian cancer in first-degree relatives, late age at menopause, low intake of green vegetables, and a high fat score [15, 37, 48]. The risk is significantly reduced in patients with a history of use of oral contraceptives, hysterectomy, or unilateral oophorectomy [2, 15, 18, 37, 48]. About 5–10% of ovarian cancers are familial. In the majority of cases with hereditary forms of ovarian cancer mutations of the tumor suppressor genes BRCA1 and BRCA2 are found [18, 28, 34]. The hereditary forms can be separated into three syndromes; the breast-ovarian cancer syndrome, the site-specific ovarian cancer syndrome and a syndrome which also includes colon cancer [30, 35]. According to Nahhas the risk to develop ovarian cancer by an age of 70 years is 44% in women with a mutation of BRCA1 compared to a risk of 1.4% for the general population [35]. The overall twenty-year survival rate of patients with ovarian cancer is about 50% [3]. With aggressive treatment the stage-related five-year survival is 93% in Stage I, 70% in Stage II, 37% in Stage III, and 25% in patients with Stage IV [18]. Recent data from the Saarland cancer registry indicate that in the last decades the survival rates have increased for younger patients, whereas the prognosis of older patients is still poor [4].

21.2 Histological Classification

A variety of malignant tumors arises from the ovaries. Epithelial ovarian cancer accounts for more than 90% of primary malignancies of the ovaries. Less frequent malignancies are stromal tumors, mixed tumors, or germ cell tumors. Epithelial carcinoma can be further subdivided in the most common serous cystadenocarcinoma and the less frequent mucinous cystadenocarcinoma, endometrioid adenocarcinoma, and clear cell cystadenocarcinoma. In addition, benign differentiations and tumors of low malignant potential exist for all subgroups. Ovarian carcinoma arises from the surface epithelium and infiltrates adjacent structures such as the fallopian tube, the uterus and the contralateral ovary. The pelvic wall, bladder, rectum, and the cul-de-sac can be involved by both infiltration and peritoneal metastases. If the tumor extends beyond the capsule of the ovary shedding of tumor cells into the peritoneal cavity causes peritoneal carcinomatosis, which predominately affects the cul-de-sac, the paracolic gutters, the infradiaphragmatic surface, and the omentum. Via lymph vessels of the diaphragm pleural effusions may occur. Depending on the tumor stage lymph node metastases of the pelvic and para-aortic nodes are found in as many 75% of the patients [6].

Staging of ovarian cancer is based on the TNM and FIGO classification [22]. T1 or FIGO I describes tumors limited to the ovaries, T2 or FIGO II tumors of one or both ovaries limited to the pelvis, T3 or FIGO III describes peritoneal metastases beyond the pelvis and/or lymph node metastases. Metastases of the capsule of the liver are also staged as T3 or FIGO III, whereas metastases of the liver parenchyma or any other distant metastases are classified as T4 or FIGO IV. Subclassifications take into account the presence of tumor cells in the peritoneal lavage or the size of peritoneal metastases. Staging of ovarian cancer is usually performed with a thorough staging laparotomy, including bilateral salpingo-oophorectomy, hysterectomy, peritoneal washings, pelvic and para-aortic lymph node sampling, infradiaphragmatic smears, and biopsies [11].

21.3 Diagnosis and Treatment of Ovarian Cancer

21.3.1 Screening

Bimanual rectovaginal examination, transvaginal sonography, and the tumor marker CA-125 are diagnostic tools for screening of ovarian cancer. The effectiveness of mass screening for ovarian cancer is discussed controversially [10, 43]. However, screening may be effective in women with a high risk to develop ovarian cancer [11, 35].

21.3.2 Diagnosis

Because of the late onset of often unspecific symptoms related to the extension of the disease outside the pelvis, ovarian cancer is rarely detected in patients with limited disease [7]. In about 80% of patients with advanced ovarian cancer the antigen CA-125 is elevated. However, this tumor marker is not specific for ovarian cancer. Elevated levels may be found in lung, breast, or gastrointestinal cancer or in benign conditions such as cysts or endometriosis [1, 7, 35]. Moreover, the sensitivity of CA-125 is limited in early stage disease [52]. Transvaginal sonography is a sensitive tool to detect ovarian masses. However, the specificity to differentiate benign and malignant lesions of the ovaries is limited, even with the use of Doppler sonography [16, 49]. Magnetic resonance imaging can accurately depict some benign ovarian tumors such as dermoid cysts and endometrial cysts, however, all other cases require surgical exploration [39]. Computed tomography is of limited value for the differential diagnosis of ovarian cystic masses [17]. CT may be helpful to assess tumor spread and resectability, however small peritoneal metastases can be missed with CT [25]. Thus, the exploratory laparotomy is often necessary to diagnose and stage ovarian cancer [5, 7].

21.3.3 Treatment

Surgery alone may be the appropriate therapeutic approach for Stage Ia (disease limited to one ovary), especially if preservation of fertility is intended [7]. Standard therapy of advanced ovarian cancer is extensive cytoreductive surgery followed by chemotherapy. Aim of the surgical approach is to remove all visible tumor tissue [5]. Cytoreductive surgery includes bilateral salpingo-oophorectomy, hysterectomy, resection of the omentum, and resection of all gross tumor deposits [11, 19]. In patients with bulky disease neoadjuvant chemotherapy can improve the rate of optimal surgical debulking [26]. Chemotherapy of advanced ovarian cancer usually consists of a combination of cisplatin or carboplatin and paclitaxel [11, 32].

21.3.4 Recurrent Disease

Despite the fact that ovarian cancer is very sensitive to platinum-based chemotherapy with response rates up to 80%, the majority of patients will ultimately relapse [7]. Secondary cytoreductive surgery can be appropriate for localized recurrence or macronodular disease in patients with a good performance status [9]. Second-line platinum-based chemotherapy is effective in patients with platinum-sensitive disease [42]. The development of recurrent disease is often indicated by a progressive rise of the tumor marker CA-125. However, CA-125 cannot differentiate between localized and diffuse tumor recurrence and the diagnosis has frequently to be completed by imaging modalities [11]. The most common imaging modality in this situation is computed tomography. In contrast to good results for the detection of pelvic recurrences the value of computed tomography to detect small nodule-disease is discussed controversially [13, 14, 25, 31, 33, 51]. Furthermore, positive findings of computed tomography may be considerably preceded by a rise of CA-125 [47].

21.4 Positron Emission Tomography

21.4.1 Primary Diagnosis of Ovarian Cancer

A typical example of primary ovarian cancer is shown in Fig. 1. The tumor presents as a large pelvic mass with high FDG uptake in the periphery of the lesion and virtually no uptake in the center corresponding to solid and cystic parts of the tumor. Figure 2 shows a benign fibroma with low and homogenous FDG uptake of the solid mass.

The initial study by Hubner et al. which comprised fifty-one patients with suspected primary or metastatic ovarian cancer revealed encouraging results for FDG PET [20]. The sensitivity of PET (83%) was similar to CT (82%), while the specificity was higher for PET (80% vs. 53%). These results were later on confirmed by Schröder et al. with only three false negative cases (two borderline tumors and one well-differentiated adenocarcinoma FIGO Ia) and one false positive result (abscess of the ovary) in a series of twenty-eight patients [44]. However, there is evidence that the specificity of FDG PET is closely related to the prevalence of benign lesions in the patients cohort. Recently, Fenchel et al. reported the results of FDG PET in a large number of patients with asymptomatic adnexal tumors [12]. FDG PET correctly excluded ovarian cancer in 66 of 87 patients with benign lesions (specificity 76%). A number of false positive findings were related to misinterpretation of unspecific bowel activity and correctly classified after re-evaluation together with magnetic resonance imaging. In agreement with the observations by Schröder et al. already cited above [44], Fenchel showed that FDG PET fails to detect tumors of low malignant potential or early stage adenocarcinoma.

So far, only one group used a dual head coincidence gamma camera for FDG PET of ovarian cancer. Al-

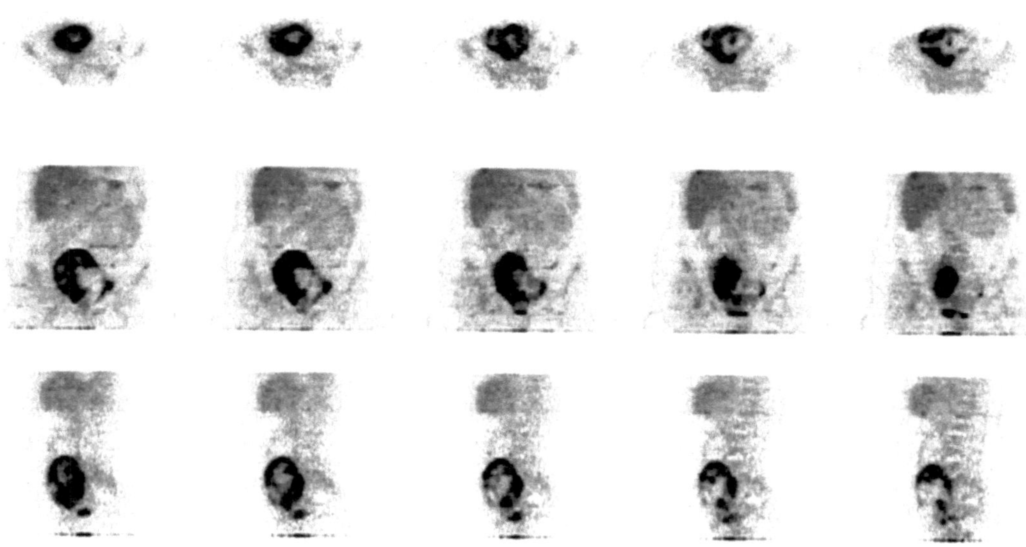

Fig. 1. Transverse (*top row*), frontal (*middle row*), and sagittal slices (*bottom row*) showing serous adenocarcinoma without peritoneal carcinomatosis or lymph node metastases (FIGO IIIa)

Fig. 2. Transverse slices of a large pelvic mass with only moderate FDG uptake (SUV 1.5). Histology revealed benign fibroma

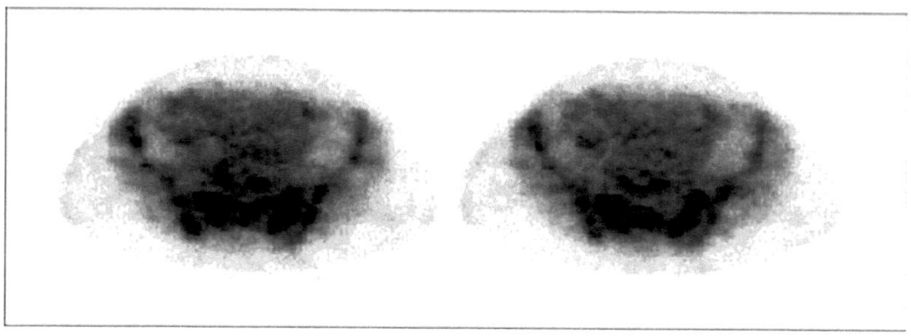

though the study comprised only a small number of patients, the results for gamma camera PET were comparable to the data presented for dedicated PET [29]. Table 1 gives a summary of the PET results for the primary diagnosis of ovarian cancer. The broad range for sensitivity and specificity of FDG PET can be explained by the limited number of patients in some of the studies and the patient selection criteria of each study with a different prevalence of borderline or early stage tumors and inflammatory lesions.

21.4.2 Staging of Ovarian Cancer

The detection of extra-pelvic disease was addressed by Liebermann et al. [29] using gamma camera PET and Schröder et al. [44] using dedicated PET. With gamma camera PET extra-pelvic disease was correctly identified in 8/8 and excluded in 1/3 patients. Schröder et al. reported a sensitivity and specificity of 73% and 92% for the diagnosis of lymph node metastases and 71% and 100% for the diagnosis of peritoneal carcinomatosis. False negative findings are most frequently related to microscopic or micronodular disease.

21.4.3 Diagnosis of Recurrent Disease

Figure 3 shows an example of extra-pelvic recurrent disease before and after second-line chemotherapy. One of the first studies on FDG PET in ovarian cancer published by Karlan et al. addressed the diagnostic accuracy in patients who were scheduled for second-look laparotomy [24]. The authors observed that FDG PET accurately localized the tumor recurrence in patients with suspected recurrent disease, whereas PET failed to de-

Table 1.
Results of FDG PET for the primary diagnosis of ovarian carcinoma

Author	Year	N	TP Sens.	TN Spec.	PPV	NPV	Comments
Hubner [20]	1993	32	14/15 93%	14/17 82%	 82%	 93%	1/2 LMP* tumors FN Stage information not provided
Römer [40]	1997	19	5/6 83%	7/13 54%	 46%	 88%	1/1 LMP tumors FN 1/1 FIGO Ia adenocarcinoma TP 4/6 FP findings due to inflammatory lesions
Schröder [44]	1999	24	11/14 79%	9/10 90%	 92%	 75%	2/2 LMP tumors FN 1/1 FIGO Ia adenocarcinoma FN 1/1 tubo-ovarian abscess FP
Kubik-Huch [27]	2000	7	4/4	2/3			1/1 FP finding due to tuberculosis 4/4 FIGO ? IIIc
Liebermann [29]	2001	17	9/10 90%	5/7 71%	 82%	 83%	1/1 LMP* tumor FN Stage information not provided Coincidence gamma camera was used for PET imaging
Fenchel [12]	2002	99	7/12 58%	66/87 76%	 25%	 93%	2/3 FIGO Ia FN 3/4 LMP tumors FN only asymptomatic tumors FP findings frequently caused by misinterpretation of bowel activity

* Tumors of low malignant potential, TP = true positive, TN = true negative, PPV = positive predictive value, NPV = negative predictive value

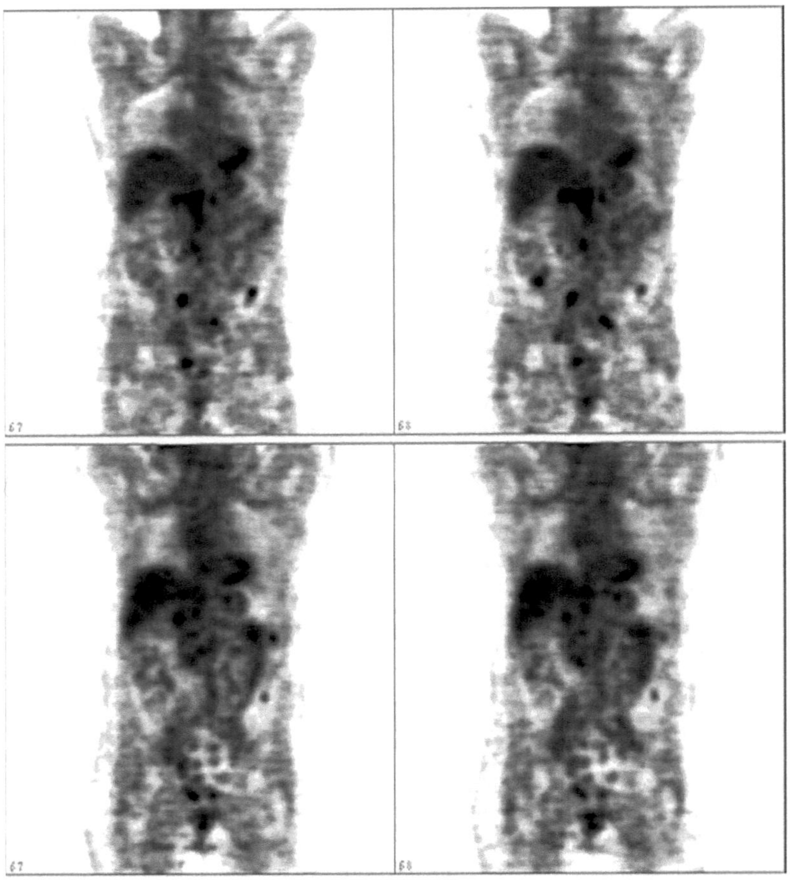

Fig. 3.
Frontal slices showing recurrent ovarian cancer 15 months after cytoreductive surgery and chemotherapy (*top*). One month after second-line chemotherapy FDG PET demonstrates partial remission with decreasing metabolic activity of the peritoneal implants (*bottom*)

Table 2. Results of FDG PET for the diagnosis of recurrent ovarian cancer in patients with suspected recurrence and in clinically disease-free patients

Author	Year	N	TP	TN	Comments
Karlan [24]	1993	12	6/6		suspected recurrence
			1/5	1/1	clinically free of disease (FN findings in microscopic disease)
Casey [8]	1994	9	5/5		suspected recurrence
			1/1	3/3	clinically free of disease
Yuan [54]	1999	5	5/5		suspected recurrence
Kubik-Huch [27]	2000	10	8/8	2/2	suspected recurrence
Jiminez-Bonilla [23]	2000	14	12/12	1/2	suspected recurrence
Rose [41]	2001	22	1/11	5/11	clinically free of disease (FN findings in micronodular disease)
Nakamoto [36]	2001	24	8/10	1/2	suspected recurrence
			2/3	8/9	clinically free of disease
Zimny[a)] [56]	2001	106	51/54	3/4	suspected recurrence
			22/36	10/12	clinically free of disease
Makhija[b)] [31]	2002	6	1/2		suspected recurrence
			2/4		clinically free of disease
Torizuka [50]	2002	25	16/20	5/5	suspected recurrence
Σ		257[c)]	122/133	24/28	suspected recurrence
			29/60	27/36	clinically free of disease
Sens.	Spec.	NPV	PPV	Acc.	
92%	86%	67%	97%	91%	suspected recurrence
48%	75%	47%	76%	58%	clinically free of disease

a) 106 scans in 48 patients
b) combined PET/CT scanner
c) total number of PET scans

tect recurrent disease in all patients presenting with microscopic tumor deposits at second-look laparotomy. The latter observation was recently confirmed by Rose et al. [41]. The authors prospectively investigated the role of FDG PET to replace second-look laparotomy in patients with complete clinical and radiological remission and normal CA-125 levels after completion of chemotherapy. In a series of twenty-two patients only 1/9 patients with macroscopic disease and none of four patients with microscopic disease were correctly diagnosed with PET. A retrospective study that re-evaluated 48 scans in patients with complete clinical remission revealed a sensitivity of 63%, a specificity of 86%, a negative predictive value of 50%, and a positive predictive value of 92% [56]. The low negative predictive value indicates that a negative PET scan cannot rule out later relapse. However, a positive scan is a very reliable indicator of an overt tumor relapse in the further course of the disease. In fact, a positive PET scan preceded the conventional diagnosis or clinical symptoms of recurrent disease by a median of 6 months. In contrast to this, the median relapse-free interval after a negative PET scan was 20 months. Thus, a PET scan in clinically disease-free patients followed up after chemotherapy and cytoreductive surgery is not an alternative to second-look laparotomy – itself an invasive procedure of doubtful clinical relevance [45] – however, it may provide relevant prognostic information.

As expected the sensitivity of FDG PET to detect recurrent disease in patient with clinical symptoms, elevated CA-125 levels and/or abnormal results of imaging studies is far better compared to the results obtained in clinically disease-free patients (Table 2). A compilation of data retrieved from studies published between 1993 and 2002 revealed a sensitivity of 92% and a specificity of 86% in patients with suspected recurrent disease compared to 48% and 75% in patients without suspected recurrence. Perhaps of more clinical relevance is the detection of recurrent disease in patients with elevated CA-125 levels as the only sign of tumor relapse. This issue was recently addressed by three publications [23, 50, 56]. The sensitivity was in the range of 87%–100 %.

21.4.4 Assessment of Treatment Response

Recommendations for the assessment of metabolic therapy response based on the standardized uptake value SUV have been published by the EORTC Functional Imaging Group in 1999 [53]. As yet, monitoring of chemotherapy with FDG PET in ovarian cancer has not been investigated systematically. However, a report of six cases by Zimny et al. showed that the SUV of peritoneal tumor deposits or lymph node metastases determined before and three weeks after completion of chemotherapy paralleled the course of the tumor marker CA-125 [55].

21.4.5
Indications of FDG PET in Ovarian Cancer

In the United States FDG is approved for ovarian cancer by the Food and Drug Administration, whereas in Germany FDG still awaits approval for the majority of malignancies including ovarian cancer. As yet, there are no generally accepted (and reimbursed) clinical indications for the routine use of FDG PET in ovarian cancer. Based on the available data it is doubtful that FDG PET will gain clinical relevance for the primary diagnosis of ovarian cancer. However, encouraging results for the early detection of recurrent disease justify the use FDG PET as the first-line imaging modality in patients with suspected recurrence based on CA-125 levels or clinical symptoms. Accordingly, the 3rd German Interdisciplinary Consensus Conference classified FDG PET for the detection of recurrent disease as useful in individual cases [38]. If assessment of treatment response with FDG PET is superior to conventional parameters such as the CA-125 level has, as yet, not been investigated systematically.

21.5
Summary

FDG PET allows the early detection of recurrent ovarian cancer in patients with elevated CA-125 levels and thus, should be considered as the first-line imaging modality in this setting. Although it cannot rule out microscopic or micronodular disease in clinically disease-free patients, a negative PET scan in these patients predicts a longer time interval until an overt tumor relapse occurs than a positive PET scan. However, as long as the intent of second-line treatment is palliative, the clinical relevance of early detection of tumor relapse with FDG PET in asymptomatic patients is unclear. While FDG PET enables comprehensive diagnosis and staging of advanced primary ovarian cancer, low FDG uptake of early stage tumors or tumors of low malignant potential and high FDG uptake of a number of benign lesions limit the clinical relevance of FDG PET for the differential diagnosis of unclear adnexal tumors.

21.6
Technical Recommendations

The only radiopharmaceutical for PET that gained widespread use in ovarian cancer is FDG. Thus, the following sections will focus on FDG PET. Considering the patterns of tumor spread in patients with ovarian cancer a PET scan should at least encompass the trunk of the body. To obtain semiquantitative parameters of glucose metabolism non-uniform attenuation correction is necessary. Furthermore, attenuation correction improves diagnostic accuracy and anatomic orientation in the abdomen [21]. Alternating acquisition of transmission and emissions using singles transmission and/or segmented attenuation maps reduces imaging time and avoids repositioning errors. The minimal FDG dose that ensures good image quality depends on the scanner, the acquisition protocol, the body-weight and the time between FDG administration and imaging. The following protocol using an ECAT EXACT 922/47 tomograph (Siemens/CTI) proofed to be adequate: 2D Mode, 8 min emission scanning and 4 min transmission scanning for each bed position, an uptake period of 60 min after 200 to 300 MBq FDG (depending on the body-weight), and iterative reconstruction (OSEM).

21.6.1 Patient Preparation

A fasting period of at least four hours is mandatory. Hyperglycemia should be excluded before the administration of FDG. Regular insulin can be used to achieve normal blood glucose concentrations in patients with diabetes. However, insulin increases the muscular uptake of glucose via the glucose transport protein GLUT IV. Thus, FDG administration after insulin should be delayed until the glucose levels are stable, which can take 30 to 60 min. Supervision of the patient and serial controls of the blood glucose levels are mandatory after intravenous administration of insulin. An isotonic saline infusion of 500 ml combined with 10–20 mg furosemide reduces the radioactivity concentration in the kidneys and the bladder and thus improves the image quality of the abdomen and the pelvis. Bladder catheters for the time of the scan are advisable to facilitate evaluation of the pelvis. Some authors also recommend the use of scopolamine to reduce unspecific bowel activity [46].

21.6.2
Image Analysis

21.6.2.1
Visual Analysis

It is recommended to use both, attenuation corrected and non-attenuation corrected data sets for image analysis. Modern processing software allows parallel viewing of orthogonal slices as well as maximum intensity projections in cine mode. Especially the latter is helpful for anatomical orientation and the differentiation of, for example, peritoneal carcinomatosis and unspecific bowel activity. Most frequently benign lesions such as cystadenomas or serous cysts demonstrate a low FDG uptake of the solid parts [12]. However, there are a number of benign lesions that can show an increased FDG uptake and can therefore mimic malignant tumors. A survey of reported benign lesions misinterpreted as ovarian cancer is shown in Table 3.

Peritoneal carcinomatosis commonly presents as multiple, focal lesions with intense FDG uptake, predom-

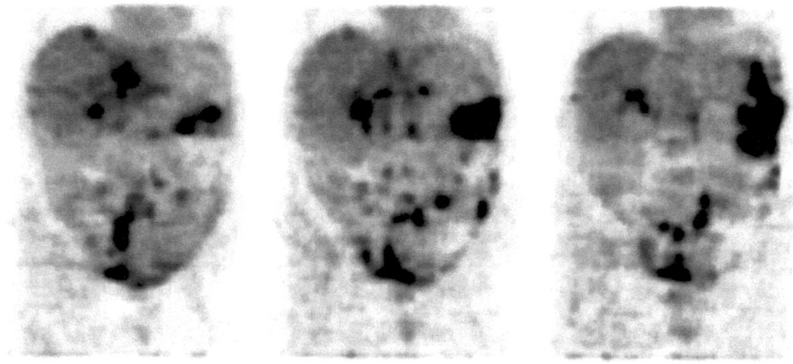

Fig. 4.
Frontal slices demonstrating extensive peritoneal carcinomatosis with tumor deposits at the liver capsule, the paracolic gutters, the omentum, and the cul-de-sac

Table 3. Survey of benign lesions/conditions that can mimic ovarian cancer

Inflammation	Tubo-ovarian abscess Salpingitis Tuberculosis of the ovaries
Benign germ cell tumors	Benign teratoma
Benign epithelial tumors	Mucinous cystadenoma Serous cystadenoma
Retention cysts	Corpus luteum cyst Hemorrhagic follicle cyst
Others	Endometrioma Schwannoma

Compiled from [12, 20, 27, 29, 40, 55]

inately located in the cul-de-sac, the pelvic walls, the omentum and the paracolic gutters. Especially in the latter location unspecific FDG uptake in the intestine has to be excluded, which is a common phenomenon in patients with primary ovarian cancer. Peritoneal carcinomatosis is unlikely if long segments of the bowels with rather homogenous FDG uptake are visible. Figure 4 shows an example of extensive peritoneal carcinomatosis.

21.6.2.2
Quantitative Analysis

The quantitative analysis of FDG uptake of ovarian tumors is predominately based on the semiquantitative "Standardized uptake value; SUV". Römer et al. showed that the SUV of ovarian tumors correlates with the transport rate of FDG determined by Patlaks's graphical analysis [40]. Hubner et al. [20] and Zimny et al. [55] reported significantly higher SUVs of ovarian cancer compared to benign lesions. Unfortunately, there is evidence that the SUV cannot reliably differentiate benign inflammatory lesions and ovarian cancer or benign non-inflammatory lesions and tumors of low malignant potential [20, 40, 55]. However, quantitative analysis is useful to differentiate unspecific FDG uptake in the intestine from peritoneal carcinomatosis with significantly higher uptake values for the latter (4.9±1.5 vs. 10.8±6.5) [55].

References

1. Bast RCJ, Xu FJ, Yu YH, Barnhill S, Zhang Z, Mills GB (1998) CA 125: the past and the future. Int J Biol Markers 13:179–187
2. Beard CM, Hartmann LC, Atkinson EJ, O'Brien PC, Malkasian GD, Keeney GL, Melton LJ 3rd (2000) The epidemiology of ovarian cancer: a population-based study in Olmsted County, Minnesota, 1935–1991. Ann Epidemiol 10:14–23
3. Brenner H (2002) Long-term survival rates of cancer patients achieved by the end of the 20th century: a period analysis. Lancet 360:1131–1135
4. Brenner H, Stegmaier C, Ziegler H (1999) Trends in survival of patients with ovarian cancer in Saarland, Germany, 1976–1995. J Cancer Res Clin Oncol 125:109–113
5. Bristow RE (2000) Surgical standards in the management of ovarian cancer. Curr Opin Oncol 12:474–480
6. Burghardt E, Girardi F, Lahousen M, Tamussino K, Stettner H (1991) Patterns of pelvic and paraaortic lymph node involvement in ovarian cancer. Gynecol Oncol 40:103–106
7. Cannistra, SA (1993) Cancer of the ovary. N Engl J Med 329: 1550–1559
8. Casey MJ, Gupta NC, Muths CK (1994) Experience with positron emission tomography (PET) scans in patients with ovarian cancer. Gynecol Oncol 53:331–338
9. Chen LM, Karlan BY (2000) Recurrent ovarian carcinoma: is there a place for surgery? Semin Surg Oncol 19:62–68
10. Crayford TJ, Campbell S, Bourne TH, Rawson HJ, Collins WP (2000) Benign ovarian cysts and ovarian cancer: a cohort study with implications for screening. Lancet 355:1060–1063
11. Deutsche Krebsgesellschaft (2002) Kurzgefasste Interdisziplinäre Leitlinien, 3rd edn.
12. Fenchel S, Grab D, Nuessle K, Kotzerke J, Rieber A, Kreienberg R, Brambs HJ, Reske SN (2002) Asymptomatic adnexal masses: correlation of FDG PET and histopathologic findings. Radiology 223:780–788
13. Ferrozzi F, Bova D, de Chiara F, Garlaschi G, Draghi F, Cocconi G, Bassi P (1998) Thin-section CT follow-up of metastatic ovarian carcinoma correlation with levels of CA-125 marker and clinical history. Clin Imaging 22:364–370
14. Giunta S, Venturo I, Mottolese M, Salzano M, Diotallevi F, Squillaci S, Bigotti A, Curcio CG, Atlante G, Natali PG (1994) Noninvasive monitoring of ovarian cancer: improved results using CT with intraperitoneal contrast combined with immunocytology. Gynecol Oncol 53:103–108
15. Gonzalez-Diego P, Lopez-Abente G, Pollan M, Ruiz M (2000) Time trends in ovarian cancer mortality in Europe (1955–1993): effect of age, birth cohort and period of death. Eur J Cancer 36:1816–1824

16. Grab D, Flock F, Stohr I, Nussle K, Rieber A, Fenchel S, Brambs HJ, Reske SN, Kreienberg R (2000) Classification of asymptomatic adnexal masses by ultrasound, magnetic resonance imaging, and positron emission tomography. Gynecol Oncol 77:454–459
17. Guerriero S, Mallarini G, Ajossa S, Risalvato A, Satta R, Mais V, Angiolucci M, Melis GB (1997) Transvaginal ultrasound and computed tomography combined with clinical parameters and CA-125 determinations in the differential diagnosis of persistent ovarian cysts in premenopausal women. Ultrasound Obstet Gynecol 9:339–343
18. Holschneider CH, Berek JS (2000) Ovarian cancer: epidemiology, biology, and prognostic factors. Semin Surg Oncol 19:3–10
19. Hoskins WJ (1993) Surgical staging and cytoreductive surgery of epithelial ovarian cancer. Cancer 71:1534–1541
20. Hubner KF, McDonald TW, Niethammer JG, Smith GT, Gould HR, Buonocore E (1993) Assessment of primary and metastatic ovarian cancer by positron emission tomography (PET) using 2-[18F]deoxyglucose (2-[18F]FDG). Gynecol Oncol 51:197–204
21. Hustinx R, Dolin RJ, Benard F, Bhatnagar A, Chakraborty D, Smith RJ, Jang S, Alavi A (2000) Impact of attenuation correction on the accuracy of FDG-PET in patients with abdominal tumors: a free-response ROC analysis. Eur J Nucl Med 27:1365–1371
22. International Union Against Cancer (UICC) (1997) TNM classification of malignant tumours, 5th edn. Wiley-Liss, New York, pp 87–90
23. Jimenez-Bonilla J, Maldonado A, Morales S, Salud A, Zomeno M, Roman J, Belon J, Moya F (2000) Clinical impact of 18F-FDG-PET in the suspicion of recurrent ovarian carcinoma based on elevated tumor marker serum levels. Clin Positron Imaging 3: 231–236
24. Karlan BY, Hawkins R, Hoh C, Lee M, Tse N, Cane P, Glaspy J (1993) Whole-body positron emission tomography with 2-[18F]-fluoro-2-deoxy-D-glucose can detect recurrent ovarian carcinoma. Gynecol Oncol 51:175–181
25. Kawamoto S, Urban BA, Fishman EK (1999) CT of epithelial ovarian tumors. Radiographics 19:S85–S102
26. Kayikcioglu F, Kose MF, Boran N, Caliskan E, Tulunay G (2001) Neoadjuvant chemotherapy or primary surgery in advanced epithelial ovarian carcinoma. Int J Gynecol Cancer 11:466–470
27. Kubik-Huch RA, Dorffler W, von Schulthess GK, Marincek B, Kochli OR, Seifert B, Haller U, Steinert HC (2000) Value of (18F)-FDG positron emission tomography, computed tomography, and magnetic resonance imaging in diagnosing primary and recurrent ovarian carcinoma. Eur Radiol 10:761–767
28. Kuschel B, Lux MP, Goecke TO, Beckmann MW (2000) Prevention and therapy for BRCA1/2 mutation carriers and women at high risk for breast and ovarian cancer. Eur J Cancer Prev 9:139–150
29. Lieberman G, MacLean AB, Buscombe JR, Hilson AJ, Adamson K, Reid WM, Green A, Begent RH (2001) The clinical application of a dual head gamma camera with coincidence detection in 20 women with suspected ovarian cancer. BJOG 108:1229–1236
30. Lynch HT, Watson P, Lynch JF, Conway TA, Fili M (1993) Hereditary ovarian cancer. Heterogeneity in age at onset. Cancer 71: 573–581
31. Makhija S, Howden N, Edwards R, Kelley J, Townsend DW, Meltzer CC (2002) Positron emission tomography/computed tomography imaging for the detection of recurrent ovarian and fallopian tube carcinoma: a retrospective review. Gynecol Oncol 85:53–58
32. Markman M (2000) The genetics, screening, and treatment of epithelial ovarian cancer: an update. Cleve Clin J Med 67:294–298
33. Method MW, Serafini AN, Averette HE, Rodriguez M, Penalver MA, Sevin BU (1996) The role of radioimmunoscintigraphy and computed tomography scan prior to reassessment laparotomy of patients with ovarian carcinoma. A preliminary report. Cancer 77:2286–2293
34. Moslehi R, Chu W, Karlan B, Fishman D, Risch H, Fields A, Smotkin D, Ben David Y, Rosenblatt J, Russo D, Schwartz P, Tung N, Warner E, Rosen B, Friedman J, Brunet JS, Narod SA (2000) BRCA1 and BRCA2 mutation analysis of 208 Ashkenazi Jewish women with ovarian cancer. Am J Hum Genet 66: 1259–1272
35. Nahhas WA (1997) Ovarian cancer. Current outlook on this deadly disease. Postgrad Med 102:112–120
36. Nakamoto Y, Saga T, Ishimori T, Mamede M, Togashi K, Higuchi T, Mandai M, Fujii S, Sakahara H, Konishi J (2001) Clinical value of positron emission tomography with FDG for recurrent ovarian cancer. AJR Am J Roentgenol 176:1449–1454
37. Parazzini F, Chatenoud L, Chiantera V, Benzi G, Surace M, La Vecchia C (2000) Population attributable risk for ovarian cancer. Eur J Cancer 36:520–524
38. Reske SN, Kotzerke J (2001) FDG-PET for clinical use. Results of the 3rd German Interdisciplinary Consensus Conference, «Onko-PET III», 21 July and 19 Sept 2000. Eur J Nucl Med 28: 1707–1723
39. Rieber A, Nussle K, Stohr I, Grab D, Fenchel S, Kreienberg R, Reske SN, Brambs HJ (2001) Preoperative diagnosis of ovarian tumors with MR imaging: comparison with transvaginal sonography, positron emission tomography, and histologic findings. AJR Am J Roentgenol 177:123–129
40. Römer W, Avril N, Dose J, Ziegler S, Kuhn W, Herz M, Janicke F, Schwaiger M (1997) Metabolic characterization of ovarian tumors with positron-emission tomography and F-18 fluorodeoxyglucose. Rofo Fortschr Geb Rontgenstr Neuen Bildgeb Verfahr 166:62–68
41. Rose PG, Faulhaber P, Miraldi F, Abdul-Karim FW (2001) Positive emission tomography for evaluating a complete clinical response in patients with ovarian or peritoneal carcinoma: correlation with second-look laparotomy. Gynecol Oncol 82:17–21
42. Rose PG, Fusco N, Fluellen L, Rodriguez M (1998) Second-line therapy with paclitaxel and carboplatin for recurrent disease following first-line therapy with paclitaxel and platinum in ovarian or peritoneal carcinoma. J Clin Oncol 16:1494–1497
43. Sato S, Yokoyama Y, Sakamoto T, Futagami M, Saito Y (2000) Usefulness of mass screening for ovarian carcinoma using transvaginal ultrasonography. Cancer 89:582–588
44. Schröder W, Zimny M, Rudlowski C, Büll U, Rath W (1999) The role of 18-F-fluoro-deoxyglucose positron emission tomography (18-F-FDG PET) in diagnosis of ovarian cancer. Int J Gynecol Cancer 9:117–122
45. Sijmons EA, Heintz AP (2000) Second-look and second surgery: second chance or second best? Semin Surg Oncol 19:54–61
46. Stahl A, Weber WA, Avril N, Schwaiger M (2000) Effect of N-butylscopolamine on intestinal uptake of fluorine-18-fluorodeoxyglucose in PET imaging of the abdomen. Nuklearmedizin 39: 241–245
47. Sugiyama T, Nishida T, Komai K, Nishimura H, Yakushiji M (1996) Comparison of CA 125 assays with abdominopelvic computed tomography and transvaginal ultrasound in monitoring of ovarian cancer. Int J Gynaecol Obstet 54:251–256
48. Sutcliffe S, Pharoah PD, Easton DF, Ponder BA (2000) Ovarian and breast cancer risks to women in families with two or more cases of ovarian cancer. Int J Cancer 87:110–117
49. Tekay A, Joupila P (1996) Controversies in assessment of ovarian tumors with transvaginal color Doppler ultrasound. Acta Obstet Gynecol Scand 75:316–329
50. Torizuka T, Nobezawa S, Kanno T, Futatsubashi M, Yoshikawa E, Okada H, Takekuma M, Maeda M, Ouchi Y (2002) Ovarian cancer recurrence: role of whole-body positron emission tomography using 2-[fluorine-18]-fluoro-2-deoxy- D-glucose. Eur J Nucl Med Mol Imaging 29:797–803
51. Uysal U, Kostakoglu L, Elahi N, Aydingoz U, Firat D, Bekdik CF (1997) Can bone scintigraphy detect additional metastatic sites unrevealed by CT in patients with recurrent ovarian carcinoma? Radiat Med 15:55–58
52. Verheijen RH, von Mensdorff-Pouilly S, van Kamp GJ, Kenemans P (1999) CA 125: fundamental and clinical aspects. Semin Cancer Biol 9:117–124
53. Young H, Baum R, Cremerius U, Herholz K, Hoekstra O, Lammertsma AA, Pruim J, Price P (1999) Measurement of clinical and subclinical tumour response using [18F]-fluorodeoxyglucose and positron emission tomography: review and 1999

EORTC recommendations. European Organization for Research and Treatment of Cancer (EORTC) PET Study Group. Eur J Cancer 35:1773–1782
54. Yuan CC, Liu RS, Wang PH, Ng HT, Yeh SH (1999) Whole-body PET with (fluorine-18)-2-deoxyglucose for detecting recurrent ovarian carcinoma. Initial report. J Reprod Med 44:775–778
55. Zimny M, Schröder W, Wolters S, Cremerius U, Rath W, Büll U (1997) 18F-fluorodeoxyglucose PET in ovarian carcinoma: methodology and preliminary results. Nuklearmedizin 36:228–233
56. Zimny M, Siggelkow W, Schröder W, Nowak B, Biemann S, Rath W, Buell U (2001) 2-[Fluorine-18]-fluoro-2-deoxy-d-glucose positron emission tomography in the diagnosis of recurrent ovarian cancer. Gynecol Oncol 83:310–315

CHAPTER 22

Cancer of the Uterus

M.-J. Reinhardt

22.1 Preface

The uterus is divided anatomically in two parts, the cervix and the corpus uteri. Currently there are no sufficient data justifying the use of ^{18}F-FDG PET in carcinoma of the corpus uteri. Thus, the following chapter focuses on the invasive carcinoma of the cervix uteri.

22.2 Epidemiology

Cancer of the cervix is the second most common cancer among women world-wide [1]. The American Cancer Society estimated that there were approximately 15.000 new cases of invasive cervical cancer diagnosed in the United States in 1999 [2]. The incidence of cervical cancer is 9 per 100.000 and the mortality is 3 per 100.000 [1]. The peak age at diagnosis of invasive cervical cancer is between 45 and 50 years [1]. The age-adjusted mortality of cervical cancer has declined nearly 70% in the last half-century, which is at least in part due to the adoption of routine screening programs with pelvic examinations and cervical cytology [3]. However, cancer of the cervix continues to be the leading cause of cancer deaths for women in many second and third world countries [3].

22.3 Pattern of Spread and Histology

Most cervical cancer arise from the junction between the primary columnar epithelium of the endocervix and squamous epithelium of the ectocervix [3]. Once the tumour has broken through the basement membrane, it may penetrate the cervical stroma. Tumour may extend superiorly to the lower uterine segment, inferiorly to the vagina, or into the para-cervical spaces via the broad or uterosacral ligaments. The cervix has a rich supply of lymphatics, which drain to the obturator nodes, the inferior and superior gluteal, common iliac, presacral, and sub-aortic nodes. Thus, the incidence of lymph-node metastases in cervical cancer is high except for the micro-invasive cancer FIGO stage IA, which is associated with a risk of pelvic lymph node metastases of less than 1% [4, 5]. Pelvic node involvement in patients who underwent lymphadenectomy is reported to be 16% in FIGO stage IB, 25 % in FIGO stage IIA, 32% in FIGO stage IIB and 41% in FIGO stage III cervical cancer [3]. Para-aortic nodes are rarely involved in patients with negative pelvic nodes, but about one third of patients with positive pelvic nodes present with additional para-aortic lymph node metastases. Para-aortic node involvement is observed in 6% of patients with FIGO stage IB, 16% in FIGO stage II, 28% in FIGO stage III and 33% in FIGO stage IV [6]. Distant metastases were rarely observed in the early stages. The most frequent sides of distant recurrence are lung, extra-pelvic nodes, liver, and bone [7].

Between 80% and 90% of all cervical carcinomas are squamous and the remainders are adenocarcinoma or adenosquamous carcinoma [1]. Most authors reported similar survival rates and pelvic control rates for both squamous and adenocarcinoma. However, the incidence of distant metastases is significantly higher in patients with adenocarcinomas. While the prognostic significance of histologic grade has been a matter of debate for squamous carcinomas, adenocarcinomas show a clear correlation between degree of differentiation and clinical course [3].

22.4 Diagnosis, Staging and Prognostic Factors

The International Federation of Gynecology and Obstetrics (FIGO), has defined the most widely accepted staging system for patients with cervical cancer [8]. This is a clinical staging system which based on careful clinical examination, abdominal and/or endovaginal ultrasound, chest radiography and intravenous urography as well as cystoscopy and proctoscopy in bulky disease. TNM pathologic staging system is sometimes applied to surgically treated patients but has not been widely accepted because it can hardly be applied to patients who are treated with primary radio- and/or chemotherapy [3].

In FIGO stage I, the tumour is confined to the cervix and extends beyond the cervix in stage II but not onto the pelvic wall, which is allotted as stage III. In stage IV, the tumour has invaded the mucosa of bladder or rectum. FIGO suggests to assign the clinical stage of a particular case before definitive treatment is performed and should not be changed due to subsequent findings. In cases of doubt, FIGO recommends to chose the earlier stage. Treatment of the earlier stages of cervical cancer can be surgery, radiation therapy or a combined radio-chemotherapy with similar results [9]. More advanced stages are favourably treated with a combination of radio- and chemotherapy. The 5-year survival rate decreases progressively from FIGO stage I through stage IV: 80%–100% in stage IB, 60%–75% in stage II, 30%–60% in stage III, and 10%–20% in stage IVA [9]. Although the survival and pelvic disease control rates of patients with cervical cancer correlate with FIGO stage, the prognosis of disease is also influenced by a number of tumour characteristics that are not included in the staging system. Beside the tumour diameter the extent of lymphatic spread is the most important predictor of prognosis. Survival rates of patients with FIGO stage IB cervical cancer treated with radical hysterectomy and pelvic lymphadenectomy decrease from 85%–95% for patients with negative nodes to 45%–55% for those with lymph node metastases [10]. Even in stage II cervical cancer, the survival rate is correlated with the number of pelvic lymph-nodes involved [11, 12]. Survival rates for patients with positive para-aortic nodes treated with extended-field radiation therapy vary between 10% and 50% depending on the extent of pelvic disease and para-aortic lymph node involvement [3].

Lymphangiography (LAG), computed tomography (CT) and magnetic resonance (MR)-imaging are frequently performed to evaluate regional nodes, but the accuracy of these studies is compromised by their failure to depict small metastases, and because patients with bulky necrotic tumours often have enlarged reactive nodes [3]. In a meta-analysis of 38 studies fulfilling stringent inclusion criteria, sensitivity of CT and MR-imaging ranged from 0.38 to 0.89 and specificity ranged from 0.78 to 0.99 [13]. FIGO states that findings by LAG, CT and MR-imaging are of value for therapy planning but should not be used to change the clinical stage. Thus, the non-invasive detection of nodal disease remains a difficult task. Identification of a sensitive and specific imaging modality would be a useful adjunct to the clinical evaluation of cervical cancer, as it might improve the individual therapy planning.

22.5 Evidence for the Use of ^{18}F-FDG PET in the Management of Cervical Cancer

Since 1999, 11 studies including 379 patients have been published to evaluate the feasibility of ^{18}F-FDG PET imaging in cervical cancer [14–24]. A total of 10 papers with 310 patients focussed on the detection of lymph-node metastases [14–19, 21–24], and 4 papers with 31 patients focussed on the detection of recurrence [14, 16, 19, 20]. 1 paper dealt with the use of ^{18}F-FDG PET for therapy control in 38 patients [24]. Furthermore, the prognostic value of pre-treatment ^{18}F-FDG PET was addressed in 1 paper including 101 patients [18].

Sugawara and co-workers [14] compared ^{18}F-FDG PET and CT for detection of lymph node metastases in 17 newly diagnosed and 4 recurrent cervical cancer patients of stages FIGO IB to IVA. From 7 patients with confirmed lymph node metastases, ^{18}F-FDG PET detected 6 (86%) and CT detected 4 (57%). No false positive findings on either ^{18}F-FDG PET and CT were reported.

Rose and co-workers [15] studied 32 patients with cervical cancer of stages FIGO IIB to IVA with ^{18}F-FDG PET prior to staging lymphadenectomy. All 10 of 17 patients with lymph-node metastases were identified by ^{18}F-FDG PET, while CT identified only 5 of them. The authors observed a higher sensitivity of ^{18}F-FDG PET for pelvic (1.00) than for para-aortic (0.75) nodes. The positive predictive value was 0.75 for ^{18}F-FDG PET. Only 2 cases with para-aortic micro-metastases were missed on ^{18}F-FDG PET images.

Umesaki and co-workers [16] studied 9 patients with newly diagnosed and 4 patients with recurrent cervical cancer. Local recurrence could be reliably detected, as well as metastatic spread when compared with MR-imaging.

Reinhardt and co-workers [17] compared ^{18}F-FDG PET and MR-imaging results with histologic findings of 35 patients with cervical cancer stage FIGO IB and II prior to radical hysterectomy and pelvic and para-aortic lymphadenectomy. On a patient basis, sensitivity and specificity of ^{18}F-FDG PET was 0.91 and 1.00 and of MR-imaging it was 0.73 and 0.83, respectively. The positive predictive value was 1.00 for ^{18}F-FDG PET and 0.67 for MR-imaging. An example is shown in Fig. 1. This was a 42-year old patient with stage FIGO II cervical cancer. MR-imaging showed lymph-nodes of less than 1 cm in the left external and common iliac lymph node chain, which were not suspicious for malignancy. PET-imaging displayed slightly increased FDG-uptake in these areas. Histology confirmed small lymph-node metastases. Similar to the study from Rose and co-workers, only few micro-metastases were missed on ^{18}F-FDG PET images.

Grigsby and co-workers [18] compared ^{18}F-FDG PET and CT for lymph-node staging in 101 patients of stages FIGO IA to IVB prior to standard irradiation and chemotherapy. CT identified enlarged pelvic lymph nodes in 20%, and enlarged para-aortic nodes in 7% of the patients, while ^{18}F-FDG PET showed focally increased uptake in pelvic nodes in 67%, in para-aortic nodes in 21%, and in supra-clavicular nodes in 8% of all patients. Based on the pelvic lymph node status, the 2-year pro-

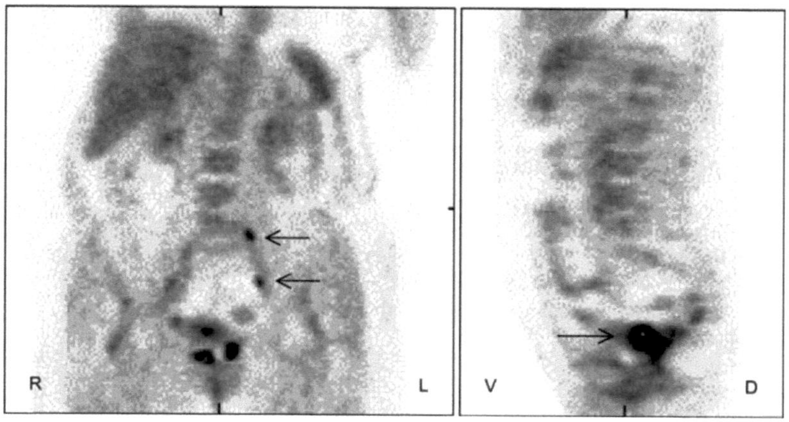

Fig. 1.
Coronal (*left*) and sagittal (*right*) ^{18}F-FDG PET images of a 42-year old patient with cervical cancer FIGO stage II. ^{18}F-FDG shows high uptake at the primary tumour site (*arrow, right image*) and two lymph-node metastases at the left external iliac and common iliac vessels (*arrows, left image*). The urinary bladder was continuously irrigated during emission scan

gression free survival rate was significantly higher for ^{18}F-FDG PET and CT negative patients than for CT negative and ^{18}F-FDG PET positive or CT and ^{18}F-FDG PET positive patients (0.73 versus 0.49 and 0.39, $p < 0.001$). This difference became even more obvious when the para-aortic lymph node status was evaluated. The 2-year progression free survival was 64% for CT and ^{18}F-FDG PET negative patients but dropped to 18% or 14%, if ^{18}F-FDG PET was positive and CT was either negative or positive ($p < 0.0001$). In a multivariate analysis of patient age, tumour stage, tumour histology, lymph node status by CT in the pelvis and para-aortic region, and lymph node status by ^{18}F-FDG PET in the pelvis and para-aortic region, the para-aortic lymph node metastases as determined by ^{18}F-FDG PET were identified as the most significant independent prognostic factor for progression free survival.

Kerr and co-workers [19] studied 10 patients with newly diagnosed and 3 patients with recurrent cervical cancer with ^{18}F-FDG PET. ^{18}F-FDG PET identified 3 tumour sites not detected by other imaging techniques including CT.

Sun and co-workers [20] studied 20 patients with recurrent cervical cancer with ^{18}F-FDG PET. ^{18}F-FDG PET identified 12 of 14 patients with local recurrence, all 16 patients with pelvic lymph node metastases and all 14 patients with para-aortic lymph node metastases and 4 patients with distant metastases as confirmed by histology or clinical follow-up for longer than 1 year. There were 2 false positive findings (1 patient without local recurrence and 1 patient without pelvic lymph-node metastasis). Sensitivity and specificity of ^{18}F-FDG PET for differentiation of local recurrence was 0.86 and 0.92, for detection of pelvic lymph node metastases it was 1.00 and 0.94, and for para-aortic metastases it was 1.00 and 1.00, same as for distant metastases.

Narayan and co-workers [21] compared ^{18}F-FDG PET and MR-imaging for pre-surgical staging of 27 patients with locally advanced cervical cancer. Sensitivity and specificity of ^{18}F-FDG PET in 24 patients evaluable for pelvic lymph node status were 0.83 and 0.92, and the positive predictive value was 0.91. MR-imaging identified only 50% of patients with pelvic lymph node metastases, all of which were seen by ^{18}F-FDG PET. However, para-aortic involvement was identified by ^{18}F-FDG PET in only 4 of 7 patients (57%). All histologically confirmed metastatic sites not visualised on ^{18}F-FDG PET images were less than 1 cm in diameter.

Kühnel and co-workers [22] analysed the feasibility of ^{18}F-FDG PET for pre-surgical evaluation of the extent of lymphatic spread in 15 cervical cancer patients. The accuracy of ^{18}F-FDG PET for assessment of pelvic lymph node metastases was 0.73 and 0.86 for para-aortic metastases. Only 2 cases with micro-metastases were missed on ^{18}F-FDG PET images.

Yeh and co-workers [23] evaluated the feasibility of ^{18}F-FDG PET for pre-surgical detection of para-aortic lymph node metastases in 42 patients with locally advanced cervical cancer and negative abdominal MR-imaging results. ^{18}F-FDG PET was true positive in 10 of 12 patients with histologically confirmed para-aortic lymph node metastases and false positive in 1 case. Thus, sensitivity and specificity of ^{18}F-FDG PET for para-aortic lymph node staging in cervical cancer patients was 0.83 and 0.97, respectively.

Belhocine and co-workers [24] compared the contribution of ^{18}F-FDG PET and MR-imaging to the management of cervical cancer in 22 patients for pre-surgical staging and in 38 patients for therapy control. ^{18}F-FDG PET identified 9 unsuspected extra-pelvic lymph node sites but missed 8 micro-metastases in the pelvis. In 18% of the patients, ^{18}F-FDG PET significantly influenced the therapeutic procedure. In the follow-up, ^{18}F-FDG PET detected 13 cases of recurrent disease while morphological imaging methods were false negative.

In summary, sensitivity of ^{18}F-FDG PET for pre-treatment lymph-node staging in cervical cancer patients ranged from 0.75 to 1.00, and specificity ranged from 0.92 to 1.00, which is significantly better than that reported for CT and MR-imaging with sensitivity between 0.38 and 0.89 and specificity between 0.78 and 0.99 [13]. On the basis of the presented literature, ^{18}F-FDG PET should be applied to lymph node staging in cervical cancer patients. Despite several positive estimates, the database is just to small to recommend the use of ^{18}F-FDG PET for therapy control, detection of recurrent disease and of distant metastases.

As a consequence, ^{18}F-FDG PET has been included in the guideline cervical cancer from the German Cancer Society as useful imaging modality if other imaging studies are negative [25].

22.6 Technical Recommendations

Several methodological procedures have been proposed to improve the detectability of the primary tumour and its metastases in the pelvis due to the small distance between cervix uteri, urinary bladder on the one side and rectum on the other side. This includes post-void scans [14], intravenously administered hydration and diuretic administration [18] as well as bladder catheterization and continuous bladder irrigation during emission scan [17]. From our experience continuous bladder irrigation is a very effective and simply approach to minimize artefacts from urinary excretion of ^{18}F-FDG PET in the pelvis. The accuracy of anatomical localization of hypermetabolic foci in projection to the pelvic and para-aortic lymph nodes sites might further benefit from fusion of ^{18}F-FDG PET with CT or MR images.

22.7 Conclusion

^{18}F-FDG PET appears feasible to improve the pre-treatment evaluation of lymphatic spread in cervical cancer patients compared to morphologic imaging methods. Thus, ^{18}F-FDG PET might significantly influence patient management as the assessment of the extent of lymph-node metastasis is essential for either surgical and radiation therapy planning. Even detection of recurrence might be improved by ^{18}F-FDG PET. Finally, pre-treatment ^{18}F-FDG PET imaging results are strongly associated with prognosis of cervical cancer patients.

References

1. Hempling RE (1996) Cervical cancer. In: Piver MS (ed) Handbook of gynecologic oncology, 2nd edn. Little Brown, Boston, pp 103–130
2. Wingo PA, Tong T, Bolden S (1999) Cancer statistics 1999. CA: Cancer J Clin 49:8–31
3. Eifel PJ, Berek JS, Thigpen JT (1997) Cancer of the cervix, vagina and vulva. In: De Vita VT, Hellman S, Rosenberg SA (eds) Cancer. Principles and practice of oncology, 5th edn. Lippincott-Raven, Philadelphia, pp 1433–1478
4. Boyce J, Fruchter RG, Nicastri AD, Ambiavagar PC, Reinis MS, Nelson JH Jr (1981) Prognostic factors in stage I Carcinoma of the cervix. Gynecol Oncol 12:154–165
5. Kolstad P (1989) Follow-up study of 232 patients with stage Ia1 and 411 patients with stage Ia2 squamous cell carcinoma of the cervix (microinvasive carcinoma). Gynecol Oncol 33:265–272
6. Piver MS (1987) Current management of lymph-node metastasis in early and locally advanced cervical cancer. In: Rutledge FN, Freedman RS, Gershenson DM (eds) Diagnosis and treatment strategies for gynecologic cancer. University of Texas Press, Houston, pp 251–264
7. Fagundes H, Perez CA, Grigsby PW, Lockett MA (1992) Distant metastases after irradiation alone in carcinoma of the uterine cervix. Int J Radiat Oncol Biol Phys 24:197–204
8. International Federation of Gynecology and Obstetrics (1995) FIGO staging of gynecologic cancers: cervical and vulva. Int J Gynecol Cancer 5:319–324
9. Beck L, Smit BJ, Roth SL (1999) Gynäkologische Tumoren. Zervixkarzinom. In: Schmitt G (ed) Onkologie systematisch. UNI-MED Verlag, Bremen, pp 121–125
10. Delgado G, Bundy B, Zaino R, Sevin BU, Creasman WT, Major F (1990) Prospective surgical-pathological study of disease-free interval in patients with stage IB squamous cell carcinoma of the cervix: a Gynecologic Oncology Group study. Gynecol Oncol 38:352–357
11. Kamura T, Tsukamoto N, Tsuruchi N, Saito T, Matsuyama T, Akazawa K, Nakano H (1992) Multivariate analysis of the histopathologic prognostic factors of cervical cancer in patients undergoing radical hysterectomy. Cancer 69:181–186
12. Inoue T, Morita K (1990) The prognostic significance of number of positive nodes in cervical carcinoma stages IB, IIA, and IIB. Cancer 65:1923–1927
13. Scheidler J, Hricak H, Yu KK, Subak L, Segal MR (1997) Radiological evaluation of lymph node metastases in patients with cervical cancer. A meta-analysis. JAMA 278:1096–1101
14. Sugawara Y, Eisbruch A, Kosuda S, Recker BE, Kison PV, Wahl RL (1999) Evaluation of FDG-PET in patients with cervical cancer. J Nucl Med 40:1125–1131
15. Rose PG, Adler LP, Rodriguez M, Faulhaber PF, Abdul-Karim FW, Miraldi F (1999) Positron emission tomography for evaluating para-aortic nodal metastasis in locally advanced cervical cancer before surgical staging: a surgicopathologic study. J Clin Oncol 17:41–45
16. Umesaki N, Tanaka T, Miyama M, Kawabe J, Okamura T, Koyama K et al (2000) The role of 18F-fluoro-2-deoxy-D-glucose positron emission tomography (18F-FDG-PET) in the diagnosis of recurrence and lymph node metastasis of cervical cancer. Oncol Rep 7:1261–1264
17. Reinhardt MJ, Ehritt-Braun C, Vogelgesang D, Ihling C, Högerle S, Mix M, Moser E, Krause TM (2001) Metastatic lymph nodes in patients with cervical cancer: detection with MR imaging and FDG PET. Radiology 218:776–782
18. Grigsby PW, Siegel BA, Dehdashti F (2001) Lymph node staging by positron emission tomography in patients with carcinoma of the cervix. J Clin Oncol 17:3745–3749
19. Kerr IG, Manji MF, Powe J, Bakheet S, Al Suhaibani H, Subhi J (2001) Positron emission tomography for the evaluation of metastases in patients with carcinoma of the cervix: a retrospective review. Gynecol Oncol 81:477–480
20. Sun SS, Chen TC, Yen RF, Shen YY, Changlai SP, Kao A (2001) Value of whole body 18F-fluoro-2-deoxyglucose positron emission tomography in the evaluation of recurrent cervical cancer. Anticancer Res 21:2957–2961
21. Narayan K, Hicks RJ, Jobling T, Bernshaw D, McKenzie AF (2001) A comparison of MRI and PET scanning in surgically staged loco-regionally advanced cervical cancer: potential impact on treatment. Int J Gynecol Can 11:263–271
22. Kühnel G, Horn LC, Fischer U, Hesse S, Seese A, Georgi P, Kluge R (2001) 18F-FDG positron-emission-tomography in cervical carcinoma: preliminary findings. Zentralbl Gynäkol 123:229–235
23. Yeh LS, Hung YC, Shen YY, Kao CH, Lin CC, Lee CC (2002) Detecting para-aortic nodal metastasis by positron emission tomography of 18F-fluorodeoxyglucose in advanced cervical

cancer with negative magnetic resonance imaging findings. Oncol Rep 9:1289–1292
24. Belhocine T, Thille A, Fridman V, Albert A, Seidel L, Nickers P, Kridelka F, Rigo P (2002) Contribution of whole-body 18FDG PET imaging in the management of cervical cancer. Gynecol Oncol 87:90–97
25. Deutsche Krebsgesellschaft eV (ed) (2002) Qualitätssicherung in der Onkologie. Kurzgefasste Interdisziplinäre Leitlinien 2002. Informationszentrum für Standards in der Onkologie (ISTO). Zuckschwerdt, Munich, pp 260–272

CHAPTER 23

PET in Bladder, Renal, and Prostate Cancer

M. Seltzer · O. Shvarts

23.1 Introduction

The general application of FDG-PET to malignancies of the bladder, kidney, and prostate has been limited compared to other cancers primarily because the primary tumor and regional lymph node site for each cancer type is often masked or difficult to visualize against a background of excreted FDG in the urinary tract. Complicating matters further is the observation that primary and metastatic prostate cancers typically have lower rates of glucose metabolism, and renal cell cancers have a more variable biologic behavior than most other common cancers. With these considerations in mind, the following review summarizes the strengths and limitations of PET in these three malignancies.

23.2 Bladder Cancer

Carcinoma of the bladder is the second most common cancer of the genitourinary tract affecting men more commonly then women (2.7:1) with an average age at diagnosis of sixty five years [1]. Risk factors include smoking (implicated in 50% and 31% of cases in men and women, respectively) as well as occupational exposure to chemicals (benzidine, beta-naphthylamine, and 4-aminobiphenyl) found in the dye, rubber, and petroleum industries [2, 3]. These chemicals likely serve as initiators in the multifactorial process of neoplastic transformation of urothelial cells through alteration in the DNA of normal cells. This alteration in DNA is thought to involve the activation of oncogenes and the inactivation of tumor suppressor genes [4]. The most common type of bladder cancer is transitional cell carcinoma (90% of cases) while adenocarcinoma (2%) and squamous cell carcinoma (5–10%) occur at a lower frequency in select patient populations [1].

The majority of patients with bladder cancer present with either microscopic or gross hematuria but some patients present with only irritative symptoms such as frequency, urgency, or dysuria. The primary diagnosis is typically made by cystoscopy with biopsy. Localized, low stage tumors usually appear as exophytic, papillary lesions while more invasive tumors are often sessile or ulcerated. Imaging with intravenous pyelograms, CT scanning, and ultrasonography can sometimes demonstrate large primary lesions but they are not as accurate as pathological staging. Approximately 15% of patients present with local extension outside the bladder and/or metastasis to regional lymph nodes or distant organs [1]. Patients with histologically proven invasive disease are often clinically understaged, underscoring the need for more reliable imaging.

CT and MRI are commonly used for preoperative staging of invasive bladder cancer but both modalities have significant limitations. CT is the most commonly used test for this purpose and has been reported to detect gross tumor extension beyond the bladder wall with an overall accuracy ranging from 64%–92% [5]. The accuracy of CT for detecting lymph node metastasis ranges from 70 to 90% with false negative rates as high as 40% [6]. MRI has not been proven superior to CT, with accuracies ranging from 60–75% [7]. Both CT and MRI have the propensity for overstaging because their findings are based on anatomical changes that may represent an inflammatory response to the tumor or recent biopsies and may not correlate with malignancy [5, 8].

FDG-PET has been used with limited success to identify both local and distant spread of bladder cancer (Fig. 1). Kosuda et al. employed PET to assess 12 patients with histologically proven recurrent or residual bladder cancer [9]. This study demonstrated a sensitivity of only 67% for detecting primary tumors (33% false negative rate) in spite of performing continuous bladder irrigation and Foley catheter drainage. PET correctly identified two of three patients with spread to regional lymph nodes and was particularly successful in its ability to identify 100% (17/17) of distant metastatic sites (lung, bone, and remote lymph node stations) [9]. Other small series have reported a similar accuracy for detecting metastatic disease [10, 11].

In the study by Kosuda et al. [9], the average SUV in the primary tumors was 4.5±2.2 (range 2.2 to 8.9) compared to 3.1±1.2 (range 1.5 to 4.8) in organ metastases which included an average SUV of 3.6 in lymph node metastases. By comparison, the SUV of urine in the bladder and ureters was 6.3±1.6 (range 2.8 to 8.9), high-

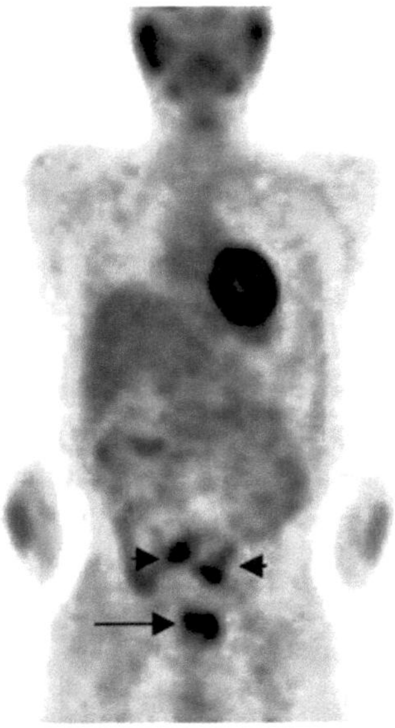

Fig. 1. FDG-PET images of a 65-year-old man with invasive bladder cancer (*large arrow*) in the native urinary bladder and a remote history of urinary bladder diversion. Excreted urine activity pooling in an intestinal neobladder is seen in the upper central pelvis (*arrowheads*). The absence of excreted urine within the native bladder allows complete visualization of the primary tumor activity

lighting the importance of minimizing bladder and ureteral activity when performing FDG-PET. Other studies have attempted to improve the sensitivity of PET for detecting the primary tumor by using tracers that do not undergo primary renal excretion. Ahlstrom et al., for example, compared the use of FDG with 11-C-Methionine and found the latter to be superior [12]. However, the primary tumor was still only identified with a sensitivity of 78%(18/23) using this method. This study also found that tracer uptake was proportional to tumor stage. Carbon-11 choline was recently demonstrated to have a higher sensitivity than FDG-PET in staging bladder tumors [13].

In summary, FDG-PET appears to be a useful modality in conjunction with conventional imaging studies for identifying distant sites of metastases. The detection of the primary tumor, local tumor recurrence, and regional pelvic lymph node metastases is limited due to the presence of excreted FDG in the urinary tract. With the advent of new tracers that are not renally excreted, PET may play a greater role in the diagnosis and locoregional staging of bladder cancer.

23.3 Renal Cancer

Renal cell carcinoma (RCC) comprises approximately 3% of all adult malignancies, with approximately 30,000 new cases diagnosed and 12,000 resultant deaths each year [14]. RCC afflicts twice as many men as women, most commonly in the fifth and sixth decades. The etiology of RCC is unknown although several theories have attributed the malignancy to environmental and occupational exposures as well as chromosomal abnormalities. RCC occurs in both sporadic and inherited forms. Inherited forms include hereditary papillary RCC [15], Von Hippel-Lindau disease [16], and chromosome 8-chromosome 3 translocation [17]. Cigarette smoking has been consistently linked to RCC [18]. In addition, hemodialysis patients with acquired cystic disease have a 30 times greater risk of RCC than the general population [19].

RCC originates from the proximal tubule epithelium [20]. The histological subtypes include clear cell, granular cell, sarcomatoid, and mixed cell type. The classic triad of presenting symptoms – flank pain, hematuria, and flank mass – occurs in approximately 10–15% of patients [1]. Approximately one third of patients present with metastatic disease to such sites as lung, liver, bone, and adrenal gland [21]. The increasing use of CT and ultrasound to help diagnosis a variety of medical conditions has led to the incidental diagnosis of RCC in a higher proportion of patients [22].

FDG-PET has a limited role in the initial diagnosis of renal tumors. In one study of 29 patients with solid renal masses, FDG PET demonstrated a sensitivity of (77%) (20/26) in histologically confirmed cases of RCC, with 3 false positives [23]. Ramdave et al. [24] compared CT and PET in evaluating 17 patients presenting with a primary renal mass and then verified the imaging diagnoses through histological examination or clinical follow up. PET and CT were found to have equivalent accuracies of 94%. PET confirmed 15/16 true positives with one true negative, while CT demonstrated 16/16 true positives and one false positive. In addition, PET demonstrated an added advantage of identifying pulmonary metastases in 2 patients [24].

PET has been used successfully to monitor the progression of RCC in the form of local recurrence or metastasis. Hoh et al. [25] followed 21 patients obtaining PET scans every three to six months during their evaluation for interleukin 2 based therapy. PET was able to identify progression in 10/10 cases versus 7/10 cases by CT, and PET accurately demonstrated absence of disease in 5/5 patients. Ramdave et al. [24] similarly demonstrated the superior value of PET over CT in his evaluation of 8 patients with suspected recurrent RCC. PET was 100% accurate in demonstrating local tumor recurrence and metastases as opposed to 88% for CT. PET was able to better differentiate between recurrent malignancy in the renal fossa and radiation necrosis when compared to CT.

A recent study by Safei et al. [26] employed FDG-PET for restaging 36 patients with advanced renal cell cancer.

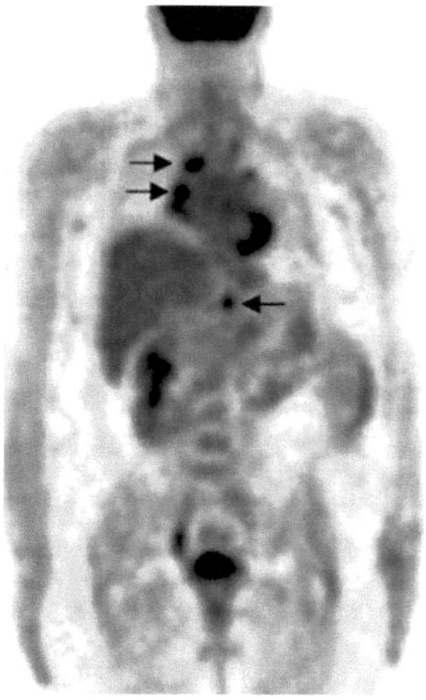

Fig. 2. FDG-PET imaging in a 56-year-old woman with history of left renal cell carcinoma status post left radical nephrectomy. The scan shows lymph node metastases in the right paratracheal, right hilar, and celiac axis nodal regions (*arrows*). Subsequent mediastinal biopsy confirmed metastatic RCC

PET classified the clinical stage correctly in 32/36 patients (89%) and was incorrect in 4/36 (11%) for a sensitivity and specificity of 87% and 100%, respectively [26]. Safei also investigated the accuracy of PET in classifying lesions that were later biopsied and found that PET correctly classified 21/25 (84%) of the biopsied lesions (sensitivity and specificity: 88% and 75%) [26]. Other studies have also demonstrated the utility of PET in detecting metastatic spread of RCC as compared with other imaging modalities [27, 28]. Because PET is routinely performed as a whole body survey, it may identify metastases in areas that would not otherwise be suspected by conventional region specific staging exams (Fig. 2). One study, for example, demonstrated the use of PET in identifying an RCC metastasis to the intramedullary spinal cord [29]. Another study confirmed the superiority of FDG-PET over bone scan in detecting active osseous metastasis [30].

In summary, FDG-PET appears to have its greatest role in staging RCC when used as an adjunct to conventional imaging for identifying local tumor recurrence, distant sites of metastases, and for monitoring response to therapy.

23.4 Prostate Cancer

Prostate Cancer is the most commonly diagnosed cancer and the second most common cause of cancer related death in American men [1]. The prevalence of prostate cancer increases with age [31]. Other risk factors include African American race, family history, and high dietary fat [32–34]. Early stage prostate cancer is usually asymptomatic and is diagnosed by digital rectal exam and serum Prostate Specific Antigen (PSA) testing. The routine use of PSA as a screening tool in men over the age of 50 has revolutionized the detection of prostate cancer, leading to the diagnosis of a greater number of low stage, impalpable tumors [1]. Once prostate cancer is suspected, the diagnosis is confirmed through an ultrasound guided prostate needle biopsy. Ninety five percent of pathologically identified prostate cancers are adenocarcinoma [1]. Rare forms include transitional cell carcinoma, neuroendocrine carcinomas, and sarcomas. Prostate Cancer is pathologically graded according to a Gleason Score (scale of 2–10) which is the sum of the two most commonly observed cancer grades (scale of 1–5) within the specimen [35].

The treatment of prostate cancer depends on the stage of the disease at the time of diagnosis. If the tumor has not spread beyond the capsule of the prostate – also referred to as organ confined disease – the likelihood of cure with specific local treatments such as surgery or radiation therapy is very high [37]. Unfortunately, a high percentage of patients who present with newly diagnosed prostate cancer have disease that is not organ confined and is therefore unlikely to be cured with local therapies [38].

Current staging after initial diagnosis is based on a variety of parameters: digital rectal examination, serum PSA, tumor histology (Gleason score), transrectal ultrasound findings, and the results of systematic random biopsies of the prostate. Nomograms that incorporate all of these parameters are available and can be used to determine the patient's likelihood of having metastatic disease [39, 40]. In spite of improvements in staging techniques, a high percentage (20–50%) of patients following primary local treatment for presumed «organ confined» disease develop local tumor recurrence and/or distant metastases. Imaging performed prior to definitive treatment is primarily limited to transrectal ultrasound or endorectal MRI to evaluate the extent of local disease, pelvic CT to assess the presence of regional lymph node metastases and bone scintigraphy to assess the presence of bone metastases [41, 42]. Imaging performed when patients develop a rising serum PSA following local therapy includes transrectal ultrasound with anastomotic biopsy, pelvic CT, and bone scintigraphy [41].

The most common sites of early metastatic disease are the axial skeleton and the pelvic and abdominal retroperitoneal lymph nodes [35] Current recommended imaging modalities used for evaluating the presence of metastatic disease include bone scintigraphy for determining the presence of osseous metastases, and computed tomography (CT) of the pelvis to determine the presence of regional lymph node metastases [41]. While bone scintigraphy is a highly sensitive test for detecting bone metastases, it is often nonspecific; positive findings may be related to degenerative joint disease or to benign bone disease such as skeletal trauma or Paget's disease. For the assessment of regional pelvic lymph node metastases, cross-sectional imaging with CT or MRI is not routinely performed due to its generally low sensitivity, averaging approximately 35%, [43]. CT and MRI identification of nodal metastases is based on a size criteria that requires a lymph node to measure at least 1.0 to 1.5 cm in diameter before it is considered positive for metastasis [44]. By definition, therefore, CT will miss small less than 1 cm metastatic lymph nodes. In addition, the anatomic criteria of CT does not allow one to differentiate reactive from neoplastic nodal involvement.

Primary Diagnosis: FDG-PET has not proven to be a useful test for evaluating primary prostate malignancies. In one study of 48 patients, the degree of FDG uptake by primary tumors of low, intermediate, and high grade histology was similar to the degree of FDG uptake in benign prostate tissue [45]. There was no correlation between the amount of FDG accumulation and the tumor grade or stage. The average SUV (body weight method) was 4.5 ± 1.4 for prostate cancer compared to 4.1 ± 1.0 for benign tissue. In another study of 24 patients with biopsy proven and clinically organ confined tumors, FDG-PET identified only 1 of 24 primary tumors [46]. Both previously mentioned studies employed a method to minimize urinary activity in the bladder either with continuous bladder irrigation [45] or with a pre-scan diuretic administration [46].

Other investigational PET tracers used to study primary prostate cancer include C-11 and F-18 labeled choline derivatives and C-11 acetate. Both acetate and choline are key components of the lipid synthesis pathways. As a major advantage over FDG, C-11 choline and C-11 acetate have negligible renal excretion of tracer allowing for improved visualization of the prostate bed and regional pelvic lymph nodes. Early investigations of these tracers suggested that they have an improved ability over FDG to detect locally advanced primary tumors [47–49]. One recent study suggested that C-11 acetate PET was a highly sensitive test for diagnosing primary prostate cancer but this study could not evaluate the test's specificity [50]. A more recent investigation of C-11 acetate PET demonstrated that there is significant overlap between the degree of C-11 accumulation in benign and malignant prostate tissue [51]. The mean SUV of prostate cancer was 1.9 ± 0.6 which was not significantly different from benign prostatic hyperplasia (mean SUV of 2.1 ± 0.6). This result, which has also been replicated in our own laboratory, indicates that C-11 acetate PET is not a reliable tracer for making the diagnosis of primary prostate cancer [51]. The radiolabeled choline derivatives have yet to be rigorously studied for this purpose.

Staging/Restaging: FDG-PET has met with limited success for the purpose of initial staging of patients with newly diagnosed prostate cancer. FDG-PET has a reported lower sensitivity than bone scintigraphy for the detection of osseous metastases in newly diagnosed untreated prostate cancer patients. In one study of 22 untreated prostate cancer patients with 202 osseous metastases detected by bone scintigraphy, the sensitivity of FDG-PET was only 65% [52]. The positive predictive value of FDG-PET in this study was 98%. For restaging patients following systemic therapy, FDG-PET holds great promise to help distinguish between active and quiescent bone metastases (See Fig. 3) [53].

The evaluation of patients with a rising PSA after radical prostatectomy or radiation therapy is a diagnostic challenge that could have a major impact on subsequent clinical management. At our own institution, we investigated the ability of FDG-PET to detect lymph node metastases in 45 patients with a rising PSA after primary local therapy [54]. The detection rate of metastases by FDG-PET was highly dependent on the level of the serum PSA and on the rate of change of the serum PSA level over time (PSA velocity). FDG-PET detected evidence of lymph node metastases in 50% of patients with a PSA greater than 4 ng/ml or a PSA velocity greater than 0.2 ng/ml/month. In contrast, FDG-PET was positive for distant disease in only 4% of patients with a PSA level less than 4 ng/ml or a PSA velocity less than 0.2 ng/ml/month. The low detection rate of metastases by FDG-PET in patients with a low PSA or low PSA velocity may indicate that the incidence of metastasis is low in this group of patients. Alternatively, it may mean that there exists a small tumor burden which is below the spatial resolution of PET or that the tumor has a low glycolytic rate which is below the metabolic resolution of FDG-PET. In the same study, we compared the imaging results of FDG-PET to conventional imaging with helical computed tomography of the abdomen and pelvis and to the monoclonal antibody scan, ProstaScint. In this comparison the detection rate of metastases was similar for PET and helical CT – 50% of patients with a high PSA or PSA velocity had a positive PET and CT scan – but our data suggested that CT and PET were superior to ProstaScint for the detection of lymph node metastases. Of those patients that had biopsy proven lymph node metastases, FDG-PET was true positive in 6 of 9 patients while ProstaScint was true positive in only 1 of 6 patients.

Finally, C-11 acetate and C-11 or F-18 choline derivatives are being actively investigated for the purpose of staging and restaging prostate cancer. Preliminary findings from our laboratory and others indicate that PET imaging with these new tracers can provide important

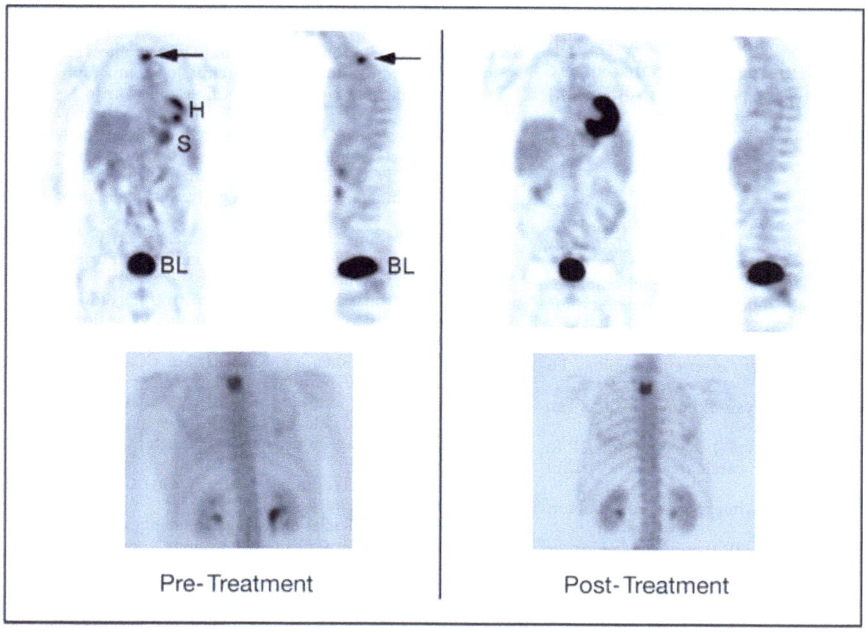

Fig. 3. A 78-year-old man with hormone refractory prostate cancer and a solitary osseous metastasis in the T3 vertebral body (*arrow*) confirmed on bone scan and MRI. Following 6 months of second-line hormonal therapy, PSA decreased from 10 to 1.3 ng/ml. Top row: complete metabolic response measured by FDG-PET. Bottom row: Persistent abnormality on bone scintigraphy. H=heart, S=stomach, BL=bladder

Fig. 4. Comparison of C-11 acetate and FDG-PET scans in a 55-year-old man with metastatic prostate cancer. The C-11 acetate PET scan (**a**) demonstrates multiple sites of osseous metastases in the right scapula, thoracolumbar spine, and pelvis (*small arrows*) and local tumor recurrence in the prostate bed (*large arrow*). The corresponding FDG-PET scan (**b**) markedly underestimates the extent of active disease in the axial skeleton and in the prostate bed. Renally excreted activity in the ureters and bladder (open arrowheads) is noted only on the FDG-PET study

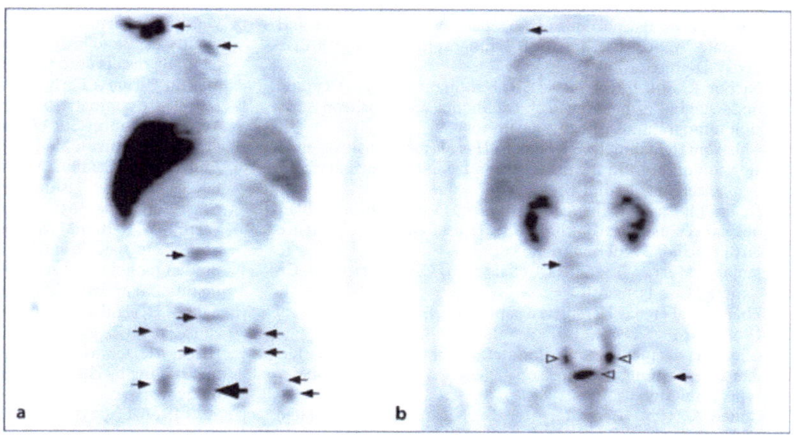

complementary staging information to anatomic imaging and FDG-PET (see Fig. 4) [55–57].

23.5 Summary

Positron Emission Tomography using the tracer FDG has a limited role in the evaluation of bladder, renal, and prostate malignancies for two basic reasons. Firstly, the tracer FDG is primarily excreted via the kidneys and the presence of urine activity in the renal collecting system and urinary bladder can mask the presence of a metabolically active primary malignancy or regional lymph nodes. Secondly, many of these cancers, particularly those of the prostate and kidney, may have low rates of glucose utilization at the time the cancer is first detected or has begun to metastasize to other sites in the body. In spite of these limitations, FDG-PET has been demonstrated to be a useful imaging modality when applied to specific indications in selected patients that have a high pre-test likelihood of harboring metabolically active disease. The availability of new metabolic tracers with more favorable properties with regard to no urinary excretion and higher tumor tracer concentration should improve our ability to image these cancer types.

References

1. Tanagho E et al (2000) Urothelial carcinoma: cancers of the bladder, ureter and renal pelvis in Smith's General Urology, 15th edn. McGraw-Hill, New York
2. Thompson I, Fair W (1990) Occupational and environmental factors in bladder cancer. In: Chisolm G, Fair W (eds) Scientific foundations of urology, 2nd edn. Heinemann Medical Books, London
3. Matonoski G, Elliott E (1981) Bladder cancer epidemiology. Epidemiol Rev 3:203
4. Olumi A et al (1990) Molecular analysis of human bladder cancer. Semin Urol 4:270
5. Nurmi M, Katevuo K, Puntala P (1988) Reliability of CT in preoperative evaluation of bladder carcinoma. Scand J Urol Nephrol 22:125
6. Lantz E, Hattery R (1984) Diagnostic imaging of urothelial cancer. Urol Clin North Am 11:567
7. Buy J, Moss A, Guinet C et al (1988) MR staging of bladder carcinoma: correlation with pathologic findings. Radiology 169: 695
8. Kim B, Semelka R, Aschner S et al (1994) Bladder tumor staging: comparison of contrast-enhanced CT, T1 and T2 weighted MR imaging, dynamic gadolinium-enhanced imaging, and gadolinium-enhanced imaging. Radiology 193:239
9. Kosuda S, Kison P, Greenough R et al (1997) Preliminary assessment of fluorine-18 fluorodeoxyglucose positron emission tomography in patients with bladder cancer. Eur J Nucl Med 24: 615
10. Heicappell R, Muller-Mattheis V, Reinhardt M et al (1999) Staging of pelvic lymph nodes in neoplasms of the bladder and prostate by positron emission tomography with 2-[(18)F]-2-deoxy-D-glucose. Eur Urol 36:582
11. Bachor R, Kotzerke J, Reske SN, Hautmann R (1999) Lymph node staging of bladder neck carcinoma with positron emission tomography. Urologe A 38:46–50
12. Ahlstrom H, Malmstrom P, Letocha H et al (1996) Positron emission tomography in the diagnosis and staging of urinary bladder cancer. Acta Radiol 37:180
13. De Jong I, Pruim J, Elsinga P et al (2002) Visualisation of bladder cancer using (11)C-choline PET: first clinical experience. Eur J Nucl Med Mol Imag 29:1283
14. Jemal A, Murray T, Samuels A et al (2003) Cancer statistics. CA Cancer J Clin 53:5–26
15. Zbar B et al (1994) Hereditary papillary renal cell carcinoma. J Urol 151:561
16. Chen F et al (1995) Germline mutations in the von-Hippel-Lindau disease tumor suppressor gene: correlation with phenotype. Hum Mutat 5:66
17. Cohen A (1979) Hereditary renal-cell carcinoma associated with chromosomal translocation. N Engl J Med 301:592
18. La Vecchia C et al (1990) Smoking and renal cell carcinoma. Cancer Res 50:5231
19. Brennan J et al (1991) Acquired renal cystic disease: implications for the urologist. Br J Urol 67:342
20. Makay B et al (1987) The ultrastructure and immunocytochemistry of renal cell carcinoma. Ultrastruct Pathol 11:483
21. Middleton R (1967) Surgery for metastatic renal cell carcinoma. J Urol 97:973
22. Tsui K et al (2000) Renal cell carcinoma: prognostic significance of incidentally detected tumors. J Urol 163:426
23. Bachor R, Kotzerke J, Gottfried H (1996) Positron emission tomography in diagnosis of renal cell carcinoma. Urology 35:146
24. Ramdave S, Thomas G, Berlangieri S (2001) Clinical role of F-18 fluorodeoxyglucose positron emission tomography for detection and management of renal cell carcinoma. J Urol 166:825
25. Hoh C, Figlin R, Belldegrun A (1996) Evaluation of renal cell carcinoma with whole body FDG PET. J Nucl Med 37:141P
26. Safaei A, Figlin R, Hoh CK et al (2002) The usefulness of F-18 deoxyglucose whole-body positron emission tomography(PET) for re-staging of renal cell cancer. Clin Nephrol 57:56
27. Brouwers AH, Dorr U, Lang O, Boerman OC, Oyen WJ, Steffens MG, Oosterwijk E, Mergenthaler HG, Bihl H, Corstens FH (2002) 131 I-cG250 monoclonal antibody immunoscintigraphy versus [18 F]FDG-PET imaging in patients with metastatic renal cell carcinoma: a comparative study. Nucl Med Commun 23: 229–236
28. Kocher F, Grimmel S, Hautmann R et al (1994) Preoperative lymph node staging in patients with kidney and urinary bladder neoplasm. J Nucl Med Suppl 35:233P
29. Poggi M, Patronas N, Buttman J (2001) Intramedullary spinal cord metastasis from renal cell carcinoma: detection by positron emission tomography. Clin Nucl Med 26:837
30. Wu HC, Yen RF, Shen YY, Kao CH, Lin CC, Lee CC (2002) Comparing whole body 18F-2-deoxyglucose positron emission tomography and technetium-99m methylene diphosphate bone scan to detect bone metastases in patients with renal cell carcinomas – a preliminary report. J Cancer Res Clin Oncol 128:503–506
31. Jemal A, Murray T, Samuels A et al (2003) Cancer statistics. Cancer statistics. Cancer J Clin 53:5–26
32. Morton R (1994) Racial differences in adenocarcinoma of the prostate in North American men. Urology 44:637
33. Carter H et al (1993) Hereditary prostate cancer: epidemiologic and clinical features. J Urol 150:797
34. Whittemore A et al (1995) Prostate cancer in relation to diet, physical activity and body size in blacks, whites, and Asians in the United States and Canada. J Natl Cancer Inst 87:652
35. Gleason D et al (1974) Prediction of prognosis for prostatic adenocarcinoma by combined histologic grading and clinical staging. J Urol 111:58
36. Saitoh H, Hida M, Shimbo T et al (1984) Metastatic patterns of prostatic cancer. Correlation between sites and number of organs involved. Cancer 54:3078–3084
37. Walsh PC, Partin AW, Epstein JI (1994) Cancer control and quality of life following anatomical radical retropubic prostatectomy: results at 10 years. J Urol 152:1831–1836
38. Mettlin C (1993) Early detection of prostate cancer following repeated examinations by multiple modalities: results of the American Cancer Society National Prostate Cancer Detection Project. Clin Invest Med 16:440–447
39. Andriole GL, Catalona WJ (1993) Using PSA to screen for prostate cancer: the Washington University experience. Urol Clin North Am 20:647–651
40. Partin AW, Kattan MW, Subong ENP et al (1997) Combination of prostate-specific antigen, clinical stage, and gleason score to predict pathological stage of localized prostate cancer, a multi-instutional update. JAMA 277:1445–1451
41. Baker LH, Hanks G, Gershenson D et al (1996) NCCN prostate cancer practice guidelines. Oncology 10:265–288
42. Hricak H, Dooms GC, Jeffrey RB et al (1987) Prostatic carcinoma: staging by clinical assessment, CT, and MR imaging. Radiology 162:331
43. Wolf JS et al (1995) The use and accuracy of cross-sectional imaging and fine needle aspiration cytology for detection of pelvic lymph node metastases before radical prostatectomy. J Urol 153:993
44. Hricak H, Dooms GC, Jeffrey RB et al (1987) Prostatic carcinoma: staging by clinical assessment, CT, and MR imaging. Radiology 162:331
45. Effert PJ, Bares R, Handt S, Wolff JM, Bull U, Jakse G (1996) Metabolic imaging of untreated prostate cancer by positron emission tomography with 18F-fluorine-labeled deoxyglucose. J Urol 155:994
46. Liu I, Zafar M, Lai Y, Segall G, Terris M (2001) Fluorodeoxyglucose positron emission tomography studies in diagnosis and staging of clinically organ-confined prostate cancer. Urology 57:108
47. Kotzerke J, Prang J, Neumaier B, Volkmer B, Guhlmann A, Kleinschmidt K, Hautmann R, Reske SN (2000) Experience with car-

bon-11 choline positron emission tomography in prostate carcinoma. Eur J Nucl Med 27:1415–1419
48. Hara T, Kosaka N, Kishi H (1998) PET imaging of prostate cancer using carbon-11-choline. J Nucl Med 39:990–995
49. DeGrado TR, Coleman RE, Wang S, Baldwin SW, Orr MD, Robertson CN, Polascik TJ, Price DT (2001) Synthesis and evaluation of 18F-labeled choline as an oncologic tracer for positron emission tomography: initial findings in prostate cancer. Cancer Res 61:110–117
50. Oyama N, Akino H, Kanamaru H, Suzuki Y, Muramoto S, Yonekura Y, Sadato N, Yamamoto K, Okada K (2002) Accumulation of [(11)C]acetate in normal prostate and benign prostatic hyperplasia: comparison with prostate cancer. J Nucl Med 43: 181–186
51. Kato T, Tsukamoto E, Kuge Y, Takei T, Shiga T, Shinohara N, Katoh C, Nakada K, Tamaki N (2002) Accumulation of [(11)C]acetate in normal prostate and benign prostatic hyperplasia: comparison with prostate cancer Eur J Nucl Med Mol Imag 29:1492–1495
52. Shreve PD, Grossman HB, Gros MD, Wahl RL (1996) Metastatic prostatic cancer: initial findings of PET with 2-deoxy-2-[F-18]fluoro-D-glucose. Radiology 199:751–756
53. Morris MJ, Akhurst T, Osman I, Nunez R, Macapinlac H, Siedlecki K, Verbel D, Schwartz L, Larson SM, Scher HI (2002) Fluorinated deoxyglucose positron emission tomography imaging in progressive metastatic prostate cancer. Urology 59: 913–918
54. Seltzer MA, Barbaric Z, Belldegrun A, Naitoh J, Dorey F, Phelps ME, Gambhir SS, Hoh CK (1999) Comparison of helical computerized tomography, positron emission tomography and monoclonal antibody scans for evaluation of lymph node metastases in patients with prostate specific antigen relapse after treatment for localized prostate cancer. J Urol 162:1322–1328
55. Price DT, Coleman RE, Liao RP, Robertson CN, Polascik TJ, DeGrado TR (2002) Comparison of [18 F]fluorocholine and [18 F]fluorodeoxyglucose for positron emission tomography of androgen dependent and androgen independent prostate cancer. J Urol 168:273–280
56. De Jong IJ, Pruim J, Elsinga PH, Vaalburg W, Mensink HJ. 2002Visualization of prostate cancer with 11C-choline positron emission tomography. Eur Urol 42:18–23
57. Fricke E, Machtens S, Hofmann M, van den Hoff J, Bergh S, Brunkhorst T, Meyer GJ, Karstens JH, Knapp WH, Boerner AR (2003) Positron emission tomography with (11)C-acetate and (18)F-FDG in prostate cancer patients. Eur J Nucl Med Mol Imag 30:607–611

CHAPTER 24

Testicular Tumors

P. Albers

24.1 Incidence, Epidemiology and Clinical Diagnosis

The incidence of testicular cancer has increased threefold over the past 40 years, with the highest incidence being in Northern European countries. The overall survival in Germany is 94%, but this varies according to region and can be as low as 75%. This can stem from variation in treatment and standardization is necessary. The increasing incidence of the disease could be as a result of genetic predisposition or exogenic effects, such as prenatal influences, which have also resulted in a shift in the age of diagnosis. In the 1940s, the disease occurred primarily in men aged 20–40 years, whereas at present, this has shifted to even younger men.

24.1.1 Risk Factors

The most important risk factor for testicular cancer is a tumor in the contralateral testis, with a 5% risk of developing a second tumor. In the general population, a maldescended testis is an important risk factor for the disease and is associated with a ten-fold increase in risk. Another risk factor is having a relation with the disease, particularly a sibling rather than a father. Estrogen consumption by the mother during pregnancy has been shown in the past to have an influence on the disease, although this practice has now been discontinued.

24.1.2 Clinical Diagnosis of Testicular Cancer

The diagnosis of testicular cancer is usually made by self-examination. The palpable mass can then be confirmed as a tumor using ultrasound examination or in cases such as cystic lesions, by magnetic resonance imaging (MRI). In the presence of microlithiasis on ultrasound the patient should be informed that a biopsy may be indicated, as up to 30% of such patients will be found to have testicular intraepithelial neoplasia (TIN). The risk for TIN without microlithiasis in case of a contralateral testicular tumor is about 5% and TIN can also be excluded with a biopsy. In patients with low volume testes (<12 ml) and of young age (<34 years), the risk for TIN is much higher (about 15%), thus, contralateral biopsy is recommended. Frozen section histology before orchidectomy is used in cases where a benign lesion is suspected and where testes-sparing surgery can be conducted.

Tumor markers are beneficial in differentiating germ cell tumors from each other and from other malignancies. Initial assessment should include the following markers: alpha-fetoprotein (AFP), the beta chain of choriogonadotrophin (HCG), lactate dehydrogenase (LDH) and placental alkaline phosphatase (PLAP). Markers are also of importance in staging of tumors after removal of the primary tumor (see below). The combined elevation of markers or excessive elevation (>1000 ng/ml AFP; >5000 IU/l HCG) is an indication to commence treatment without histological findings in the case of an extragonadal tumor. Biopsy of the testes should be conducted in these cases, as around 30% of extragonadal tumors derive from burned-out testicular tumors.

Nodal assessment is conducted through abdominal and chest computerized tomography (CT) in a primary testes cancer patient. Pelvis CT is indicated for scrotal violation as it is a highly sensitive means of detecting metastases. PET scan in low stage disease is not more sensitive in detecting metastasis with accurately performed CT scan. Generally, PET scan is of very high specificity and is useful for further investigation of CT identified tumors, but it cannot detect nodal invasion below 10 mm in diameter [1, 3, 7, 9].

24.2 Pathological Diagnosis and Classification

Tumor-bearing testes should be assessed histopathologically and classified according to the 1997 WHO recommendation (Table 1). Patients with advanced disease should additionally be classified according to the International Germ Cell Cancer Collaborative Group (IGCCCG) classification (Table 2). Immunostaining using CD31 is used for identification of vascular invasion; PLAP for testicular intraepithelial neoplasia (TIN); and CK20 to identify epithelial cells. The staging system used for testicular cancer is shown in Table 3.

Table 1. The 1997 TNM staging system for testicular cancer

pT	Primary tumor
pTx	Primary tumor cannot be assessed (if no radical orchidectomy has been performed Tx is used)
pTo	No evidence of primary tumor (e.g. histological scar in testis)
pTis	Intratubular germ cell neoplasia (carcinoma in situ)
pT1	Tumor limited to testis and epididymis without vascular/lymphatic invasion; tumor may invade tunica albuginea, but not tunica vaginalis
pT2	Tumor limited to testis and epididymis with vascular/lymphatic invasion, or tumor extending through tunica albuginea with involvement of tunica vaginalis
pT3	Tumor invades spermatic cord with or without vascular/lymphatic invasion
pT4	Tumor invades scrotum with or without vascular/lymphatic invasion
pN	Regional lymph nodes
pNx	Regional lymph nodes cannot be assessed
pN0	No regional lymph node metastasis
pN1	Metastasis with a lymph node mass 2 cm or less in greatest dimension and five or fewer positive nodes, none more than 2 cm in greatest dimension
pN2	Metastasis with a lymph node mass more than 2 cm but not more than 5 cm in greatest dimension, or more than five nodes positive, none more than 5 cm, or evidence of extranodal extension of tumor
pN3	Metastasis with a lymph node mass more than 5 cm in greatest dimension
pM	Distant metastasis
The pM category corresponds to the M category	
S	Serum tumor markers
Sx	Serum marker studies not available or not performed
So	Serum marker study levels within normal limits
LDH	β-hCG (mIU/ml) AFP (ng/ml)
S1	<1.5×N[a] and <5000 and <1000
S2	1.5–10×N or 5000–50,000 or 1000–10,000
S3	>10×N or >50,000 or >10,000

LDH, lactate dehydrogenase; β-hCG, beta-human chorionic gonadotrophin; AFP, alpha-fetoprotein.
[a] Indicates the upper limit of normal for the LDH assay.

Table 2. A prognostic-based staging system for metastatic germ-cell (International Germ Cell Cancer Collaborative Group)

Non-seminoma	Seminoma
Good prognosis group	
56 % of cases	90 % of cases
5-year PFS: 89 %	5-year PFS: 82 %
5-year survival: 92 %	5-year survival: 86 %
All of the following:	*All of the following:*
Testis/retroperitoneal primary	Any primary site
No non-pulmonary visceral metastases	No non-pulmonary visceral metastases
AFP <1000 ng/ml	Normal AFP
β-hCG <5000 mIU/l (1000 ng/ml)	Any β-hCG
LDH <1.5×ULN	Any LDH
Intermediate prognosis group	
28 % of cases	10 % of cases
5-year PFS: 75 %	5-year PFS: 67 %
5-year survival: 80 %	5-year survival: 72 %
All of the following:	*Any of the following:*
Testis/retroperitoneal primary	Any primary site
No non-pulmonary visceral metastases	Non-pulmonary visceral metastases
AFP >1,000 and <10,000 ng/ml or	Normal AFP
β-hCG >5,000 and <50,000 mIU/l or	Any β-hCG
LDH >1.5 and <10 ULN	Any LDH
Poor prognosis group	
16 % of cases	No patients classified as poor prognosis
5-year PFS: 41 %	
5-year survival: 48 %	
Any of the following:	
Mediastinal primary	
Non-pulmonary visceral metastases	
AFP >10,000 ng/ml or	
β-hCG >50,000 mIU/l (10,000 ng/ml) or	
LDH >10×ULN	

AFP, alpha-fetoprotein; β-hCG, beta-human chorionic gonadotrophin; LDH, lactate dehydrogenase; PFS, progression-free survival.

Table 3. Staging of testicular cancer

I	No evidence of metastases
IM	Rising markers
IIA	Abdominal nodes <2 cm diameter
IIB	Abdominal nodes 2–5 cm diameter
IIC	Abdominal nodes >5 cm diameter
III	Supradiaphragmatic lymphadenopathy
IV	Extra-lymphatic disease (L+, lung metastases; H+, liver metastases; Br+, brain metastases; Bo+, bone metastases)

24.3 PET in Diagnosis and Treatment

Verification of testicular tumor by ultrasound is an indication for ablation of the testis. A high inguinal incision is used with removal of the spermatic cord up to the inguinal ring, with separation of the ductus deferens and gonadal vessels. Based on the German experience, organ sparing surgery is only recommended in solitary testis with normal preoperative testosterone levels. This is done in conjunction with post-operative irradiation and should be restricted to specialized centers.

24.3.1 Stage I Seminoma

24.3.1.1 *Clinical Stage I Seminoma*

There is a 20% risk of occult metastases in stage I disease; however, the cure rate is nearly 100%. This can be achieved through two strategies: adjuvant radiotherapy reducing the risk for recurrence to 3%–4%, or 'surveillance' with definite therapy for recurrence only (radiotherapy or chemotherapy). Recurrence rates are currently 20% with surveillance and it occurs almost exclusively in the retroperitoneal area. Salvage radiotherapy/chemotherapy for recurrence involves intensive treatment and this is associated with more toxicity.

The target volume of adjuvant radiotherapy includes the infradiaphragmal paraaortal/paracaval lymph nodes. The overall dose is 26 Gy, applied in individual doses of 2.0 Gy each. Latest data from a randomized Medical Research Council Trial suggest the reduction of the overall dose to 20 Gy as equivalent to 30 Gy. Radiation should be applied using linear accelerators. An extension of the radiation field to ipsilateral iliacal, inguinal or scrotal areas is not indicated. At present, adjuvant carboplatinum therapy has not been proven to produce similar results to radiotherapy and the optimum number of cycles still remains unclear. Consequently, carboplatin treatment should only be given within a current clinical trial.

24.3.1.2 *Role of PET in Clinical Stage I Seminoma*

As in non-seminomatous germ cell tumors, the clinical staging error is due to micrometastases mostly in the retroperitoneal region that are overlooked by conventional CT. In most cases, these micrometastases consist of small tumor cell conglomerates that are invisible to imaging modalities. In clinical stage I seminoma, the clinical staging error is about 20%. In all series of FDG-PET in the primary clinical staging, PET was not superior to the CT scan to detect these micrometastases. As long as there is no visible enlargement of lymph nodes in the retroperitoneal area, PET is not able to reliably detect metastases. The sensitivity of PET is not better than the CT sensitivity (75%–80%) [1].

Therefore, with the currently used tracer FDG, PET is not recommended over CT in the primary staging of seminoma patients.

24.3.2 Stage II Seminoma

24.3.2.1 *Treatment of Clinical Stage II A/B Seminoma*

The standard treatment of clinical stage II seminoma is radiotherapy, with the target volume including the paraaortal and ipsilateral iliacal lymph nodes. In stage IIA, 30 Gy are administered homogeneously, while in IIB, 36 Gy are applied. The 4-year recurrence-free survival rate is 92.5% for both IIA/B. Owing to recurrence rates of 5% for stage IIA and 11% for stage IIB, chemotherapy is being investigated as an alternative to radiotherapy in some countries.

24.3.2.2 *Role of PET in Clinical Stage II Seminoma*

In contrast to non-seminomatous germ cell tumors, metastases from testicular seminoma without AFP elevation are homogeneous tumors that do not harbor teratoma elements. Clinical stage IIA describes a metastatic seminoma with a solitary lymph node metastases in the paraaortal region of less than 2 cm in transverse diameter. This lesion is easy to detect with CT scan and in these circumstances PET may be useful to exclude a benign enlargement.

Seminoma as a homogeneous tumor will be visible with PET and, therefore, clinical staging may potentially improve. There are no consecutive data providing enough evidence to recommend PET as a routine staging in clinical stage II seminomas; however, from the experience of the published series so far, PET will be able to better classify stage IIA versus stage IIB and larger masses [4–6]. Most importantly, PET will be able to exclude non-tumorous enlargement and, therefore, may avoid over-treatment in patients with benign lesions. In contrast to non-seminomas, with a correct histopathological diagnosis, there is no chance for teratoma elements in seminomatous tumors that have proven to be negative in PET scan.

24.3.3
Stage I Non-seminoma

24.3.3.1
Treatment of Clinical Stage I NSGCT

The cure rate for clinical stage I non-seminomatous germ cell testicular cancer (NSGCT) is 99% and this can be achieved through two therapeutic strategies: retroperitoneal lymph node dissection (RPLND) or a risk-adapted therapy involving surveillance for low-risk patients and adjuvant chemotherapy for high-risk groups. On correctly performed clinical staging, 20%–25% of these patients have occult retroperitoneal metastases, while 8% will develop pulmonary metastases. Vascular invasion is the only risk factor for occult metastases identified so far in prospective clinical trials; 48% of these patients (high-risk group) will develop recurrent disease: 61% in the retroperitoneum and 25% in the lungs. For patients without any evidence of vascular invasion (low-risk group), recurrence occurs in 14%–22%.

RPLND is the classical treatment option for this disease stage. Advantages include correct pathological staging, low short-term morbidity (10%) and exclusively pulmonary recurrence rates of 8%. In terms of risk-adapted strategy, salvage therapy for patients following surveillance consists of three cycles of cisplatin, etoposide and bleomycin (PEB). Two cycles of cisplatin-based chemotherapy are the standard therapy for high-risk patients; recurrence rates are of the order of 3% [2].

24.3.3.2
Role of PET in Clinical Stage I Non-seminoma

In numerous retrospective trials [1, 3, 10], PET was tested to improve the clinical staging of non-seminoma patients in clinical stage I. The staging error with conventional clinical staging is about 30%, and hence, it would be useful to improve on this using PET.

However, none of the trials was able to show a benefit for PET regarding the sensitivity. Lesions below 10 mm usually are not visible in PET. In addition, most of the cases that have been reported with positive findings during RPLND or surveillance with an initially negative PET scan histologically were teratomatous tumors. However, there are no data of a prospective series so far that is able to report on a statistically valid number of patients with clinical stage I non-seminoma comparing PET with CT staging. From the experience with the CT scan it may be possible to carefully check patients using PET with traditionally negative CT scans but with lymph node enlargement in the range of 3–5 mm. In most of these cases, the number of visible lymph nodes has also increased and using the combination of PET and CT it may be possible to detect signals below 10 mm in projection of these borderline lymph nodes. Currently, there is a German multicenter trial ongoing to investigate the role of PET in low-stage non-seminoma. Until this trial is finished, PET cannot be recommended in clinical stage I disease.

24.3.4
Stage II Non-seminoma

24.3.4.1
Treatment of Non-seminoma Clinical Stage II A/B

There are two treatment options for non-seminoma stage IIA/B: RPLND and chemotherapy. A risk-adapted treatment is not possible because of the lack of prospectively evaluated risk factors. Cure rates achieved are of the order of 98%.

The advantage of RPLND is that it provides information on clinical overstaging, which is important as 13% of patients will not have stage II disease and might be treated unnecessarily. Chemotherapy can be conducted as an adjuvant to surgery or as the primary therapy. Toxicity resulting from chemotherapy usually starts from the third cycle onwards. The pros and cons of each treatment option should be discussed with the patient, particularly with regard to fertility issues, acute and long-term toxicity and quality of life. There are no properly randomized trials available to favor any particular treatment option. Limited data are available that suggest that quality of life following treatment was greatest in patients undergoing RPLND plus chemotherapy rather than either therapy alone.

24.3.4.2
Role of PET in Clinical Stage II Non-seminoma

As opposed to clinical stage I non-seminoma, patients with enlarged lymph nodes may benefit from an additional PET scan. In up to 13% of these patients, the enlarged lymph nodes do not harbor germ cell cancer and this may be detected by PET [9]. However, PET is not able to rule out teratoma with the currently used tracers and the patients that initially benefit from a negative PET have to undergo close surveillance and surgery if the mass grows. As in seminomas, PET will improve the clinical staging of stage IIA versus IIB and larger and in cases with positive PET scan the technique may be used for monitoring during chemotherapy as in advanced cases. Taken together, PET may be useful for stage II lesions for following reasons: (1) to rule out benign disease and, therefore, to avoid treatment; (2) to improve the differential staging between IIA and IIB and, therefore, to avoid surgery in cases with advanced disease.

24.3.5 Advanced Stages

24.3.5.1 *Advanced Disease*

Treatment options for advanced disease are chemotherapy in the first instance followed by residual tumor resection if the tumor is still present. For patients with a 'good prognosis,' according to IGCCCG the standard treatment consists of three cycles of PEB or for cases of contraindication against bleomycin, four cycles of PE.

Patients with 'intermediate risk' are treated with four cycles of PEB. Due to the generally less favorable prognosis of this patient group, in comparison to patients with 'good prognosis,' they should principally be treated in prospective studies.

For patients with 'poor prognosis,' the standard therapy consists of four cycles of PEB; four cycles of PEI are of the same efficacy, but more toxic. A 5-year progression-free survival in this group is 45% – 50% and it has not yet been proven that high-dose chemotherapy increases the survival rate.

24.3.5.2 *Role of PET in Advanced Stages*

There are numerous trials that suggest the use of PET for the monitoring of patients with chemotherapy of advanced germ cell tumors.

For *advanced seminoma*, a large prospective multicenter trial has been published that nicely showed the usefulness of PET after chemotherapy [5]. PET after chemotherapy of advanced seminoma was able to predict necrosis at a negative predictive value level of 97% in 33 patients. Even more important, PET in this clinical setting was able to detect all patients with residual active tumor after chemotherapy. With this trial of DeSantis et al., PET has gained an important role in the clinical management of advanced seminoma. From previous trials of RPLND after chemotherapy of seminoma it has been suggested to avoid surgery in these patients because more than 95% of patients will show necrotic tissue only after chemotherapy and, thus, surgery after chemotherapy would have staging reasons only. Now it is possible to identify these patients using PET and, therefore, avoid surgery at a much higher level of confidence. Detection and localization of a vital tumor by PET-CT is shown as an example in Fig. 1 in a patient with stage Lugano IIIA advanced seminoma (IGCCCG good prognosis) and restaging after three courses of BEP chemotherapy, with PET-positive signals in retroperitoneal lymph nodes as a sign of residual vital tumor.

As opposed to advanced seminoma, the use of PET in *advanced non-seminoma* is much more critical. If non-teratoma elements are present after chemotherapy, PET may be useful to detect these aggressive cancer residuals and, therefore, further treatment (salvage chemotherapy) may be based on this finding. However, this has not been proven in a prospective fashion. In advanced non-seminoma, there is a high chance of relapse and consecutive death of tumor, if potentially aggressive tumor residuals after chemotherapy have not been completely resected. If resection is delayed, the tumor might progress

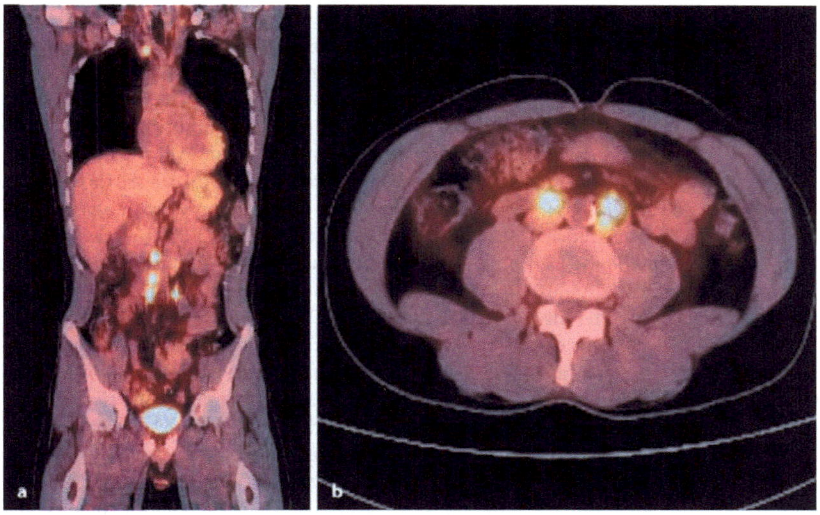

Fig. 1. PET-CT imaging of a residual vital tumor after chemotherapy of seminoma with retroperitoneal metastasis. Clinical data: 40-year-old patient with stage Lugano IIIA advanced seminoma (IGCCCG good prognosis). Restaging after three courses of BEP chemotherapy, with PET positive signals in retroperitoneal lymph nodes as a sign of residual vital tumor. Technical data: Injection of 404 MBq F-18-FDG; CT without contrast 40 mAs/130 kV. Start of measurements 90 min p.i. acquisition 5 min/position. **a** Coronal image PET-CT. **b** Transversal Image PET-CT

as chemorefractory disease. In about 5 % of patients after chemotherapy for non-seminoma without residual tumor resection the tumor may occur as a late relapse and these patients cannot be cured in about 30 %–50 % of cases. Therefore, the decision to avoid residual tumor resection after chemotherapy is difficult and PET has not yet proven to be as safe as surgery to diagnose completely necrotic tissue. If properly performed, PET is currently able to detect vital non-teratoma residual disease. However, the negative predictive value of PET is low (60 %) since teratoma and small vital residuals are overlooked [8, 11, 12]. Even in positive PET scans after chemotherapy, the consecutive management should not be based on the PET finding, since some of the patients have false-positive signals. The reason for this is a too short time period after the end of chemotherapy, inflammatory reactions or benign sarcoid differentiation of tumors [11].

24.3.6 Salvage Therapy

Salvage therapy for seminoma includes cisplatinum and this can result in long-term remission in up to 50 % of patients. It is debated whether a high-dose regimen provides an advantage and consequently treatment of these patients within centers or clinical trials is of utmost importance.

Standard salvage therapy for non-seminoma includes cisplatin, etoposide and ifosfamide (PEI)/vinblastine, ifosfamide and cisplatin (VIP) or Velban, ifosfamide and cisplatin (VEIP). Conventional dosing can result in long-term remission in 15 % – 40 % of patients, depending on the risk factors.

24.3.7 Relapse

24.3.7.1 *Late Relapse*

Increasing data are becoming available on late relapse patients. Late relapse is defined as tumor recurrence >2 years after complete remission. Overall, 3 % – 3.5 % of patients will experience late relapse and it should be noted that these tumors have a completely different cell biology. Patients usually show up with symptoms or with slowly elevating AFP. Histologically, in most cases carcinoma or undifferentiated teratoma is found. In more than two thirds of patients with late relapse the disease occurs in the retroperitoneum ("in-field"). This suggests that improper RPLND or postchemotherapy RPLND may be one reason for late relapse. Most of the patients (>50 %) will die of this relapse and in the currently published series only patients with complete resection of the late relapse tumors have survived. Thus, surgery is the mainstay of treatment in these patients.

24.3.7.2 *Role of PET in the Management of Relapsing Tumors*

Again, there is no standard application of PET in this setting. However, in the case of late relapse, more than half of patients recur with vital cancer (no teratoma). Therefore, PET is able to visualize relapse even in cases of marker-negative relapsing tumors. However, in this clinical setting it is again true that PET will detect tumor masses only if they are large enough. With slowly rising markers, PET usually will only be positive if the marker level increases to several hundred units. Taken together, PET is of value in detecting relapsing tumors if they surmount a certain level of tumor mass and if they consist of non-teratoma elements.

24.4 Summary and Future Directions

In the management of testicular tumors, PET has gained importance in diagnosis as well as in monitoring during chemotherapy. The precise indication of PET will be clarified after analysis of the currently ongoing German multicenter trial in low-stage non-seminomatous and advanced testicular tumors.

In the primary staging, PET yields a very high specificity as long as enlarged lymph nodes are visible on CT scan. However, the sensitivity compared to the initial staging CT is not higher and, therefore, PET may not contribute to the initial clinical staging of stage I tumors (seminoma and non-seminoma). This is mainly due to the lower limit of detection (about 5–10 mm lesions). In stage II tumors (lymph nodes >2 cm), PET is able to visualize aggressive tumor components like embryonal carcinoma, yolk sac tumor, or choriocarcinoma. However, with the currently available tracers, PET is not able to exclude teratoma. Therefore, its use in the management of non-seminomatous tumors currently is limited. In advanced seminoma, however, PET clearly visualizes vital seminoma (in clinical stage II as well as residual disease after chemotherapy) with a very high sensitivity and specificity. Hence, PET is already a valuable tool in the management of metastatic seminoma, and PET-CT improves the specific localization (Fig. 1).

In order to use PET in the initial clinical staging, the lower limit of detection must be below 5 mm and a correlation to CT scans is necessary (PET-CT). With these features it might be realistic to improve the clinical staging of seminomas as well as non-seminomas at a very early stage. In advanced tumors, it is crucial to exclude slowly progressing teratoma elements within residual tumors. New tracers and dynamic analysis of PET signals might help to solve this problem.

References

1. Albers P, Bender H, Yilmaz H, Schoeneich G, Biersack HJ, Müller SC (1999) Positron emission tomography in the clinical staging of patients with stage I and II testicular germ cell tumors, Urology 53:808–811
2. Albers P, Siener R, Kliesch S, Weissbach L, Krege S, Sparwasser C, Schulze H, Heidenreich A, De Riese W, Loy V, Bierhoff E, Wittekind C, Fimmers R, Hartmann M for the GTCSG and the German Association of Urologic Oncology (Trial # AH 01/94) (2003) Risk factors for relapse in clinical stage I non-seminomatous testicular germ cell tumors (NSGCT) - results of the German Testicular Cancer Study Group (GTCSG) trial. J Clin Oncol 21:1505–1512
3. Cremerius U, Effert PJ, Adam G, Sabri O, Zimmy M, Wagenknecht G, Jakse G, Buell U (1998) FDG PET for detection and therapy control of metastatic germ cell tumor. J Nucl Med 39: 815–822
4. Cremerius U, Wildberger JE, Borchers H, Zimny M, Jakse G, Gunther RW, Buell U (1999) Does positron emission tomography using 18-fluoro-2-deoxyglucose improve clinical staging of testicular cancer? Results of a study in 50 patients. Urology 54: 900–904
5. De Santis M, Bokemeyer C, Becherer A, Stoiber F, Oechsle K, Kletter K, Dohmen BM, Dittrich C, Pont J (2001) Predictive impact of 2-18fluoro-2-deoxy-D-glucose positron emission tomography for residual postchemotherapy masses in patients with bulky seminoma. J Clin Oncol 19:3740–3744
6. Ganjoo KN, Chan RJ, Sharma M, Einhorn LH (1999) Positron emission tomography scans in the evaluation of postchemotherapy residual masses in patients with seminoma. J Clin Oncol 17:3457–3460
7. Hain SF, O´Doherty MJ, Timothy AR, Leslie MD, Partridge SE, Huddart RA (2000) Fluorodeoxyglucose PET in the initial staging of germ cell tumours. Eur J Nucl Med 27:590–594
8. Hain SF, O'Doherty MJ, Timothy AR, Leslie MD, Harper PG, Huddart RA (2000) Fluorodeoxyglucose positron emission tomography in the evaluation of germ cell tumors at relapse. Br J Cancer 83:863–869
9. Krege S, Suchon R, Schmoll HJ (2001) Interdisciplinary consensus on diagnosis and treatment of testicular germ cell tumors: result of an update conference on evidence-based medicine (EBM). Eur Urol 40:372–391
10. Muller-Mattheis V, Reinhardt M, Gerharz CD, Furst G, Vosberg H, Muller-Gartner HW, Ackermann R (1998) Positron emission tomography with [18 F]-2-fluoro-2-deoxy-D-glucose (18FDG-PET) in diagnosis of retroperitoneal lymph node metastases of testicular tumors. Urologe A 37:609–620
11. Muggia FM, Conti PS (1998) Seminoma and sarcoidosis: a cause for false positive mediastinal uptake in PET? Ann Oncol 9:924
12. Nuutinen JM, Leskinen S, Elomaa I, Minn H, Varpula M, Solin O, Soderstrom KO, Joensuu H, Salminen E (1997) Detection of residual tumors in postchemotherapy testicular cancer by FDG-PET. Eur J Cancer 33:1234–1341

CHAPTER 25

Malignant Melanoma

P. Paquet · R. Hustinx · P. Rigo · G.E. Piérard

25.1 Introduction

The incidence of cutaneous melanoma is increasing at a rate greater than that of any other malignancy [1]. UK data indicate an incidence of 10/100,000/year, with a lifetime risk of one in 200 [2]. The prognosis is linked to the neoplastic progression stage at diagnosis. Hence, accurate staging is essential to implement appropriate management and improve the prognosis. Substantial progress has been made in identifying the most significant clinical and histological criteria that predict melanoma metastasis and survival.

The American Joint Committee on Cancer (AJCC) staging system for cutaneous melanoma is the current authoritative guideline [1, 3]. The most powerful prognostic parameters include the primary stage of tumour (melanoma thickness, ulceration), nodal staging (number of involved lymph nodes, micrometastases vs macrometastases, satellites and in transit metastases) and metastasis staging (site of metastases, and elevated serum lactate dehydrogenase (LDH) (Table 1). Brought together, these TNM data led to a four-stage classification of cutaneous melanoma (Table 2). Clinical staging should be performed after complete excision of the primary melanoma (including microstaging) with clinical

Table 1. Melanoma TNM classification

T classification	Thickness	Ulceration status
T1	≤ 1.0 mm	a: without ulceration and level II/III b: with ulceration or level IV/V
T2	1.01 – 2.0 mm	a: without ulceration b: with ulceration
T3	2.01 – 4.0 mm	a: w/o ulceration b: with ulceration
T4	>4.0 mm	a: w/o ulceration b: with ulceration
N classification	**No of metastatic nodes**	**Nodal metastatic mass**
N1	1 node	a: micrometastasis* b: macrometastasis†
N2	2–3 nodes	a: micrometastasis* b: macrometastasis† c: in transit met(s)/satellite(s) without metastatic nodes
N3	or more 4 metastatic nodes, or matted nodes, or in-transit metastases/ satellite(s) with metastatic node(s)	
M classification	**Site**	**Serum LDH**
M1a	Distant skin, SQ or nodal mets. Lung metastases	Normal Normal
M1b	All other visceral metastases	Normal
M1c	Any distant metastasis	Elevated

* Micrometastases are diagnosed after sentinel or elective lymphadenectomy.
† Macrometastases are defined as clinically detectable nodal metastases confirmed by therapeutic lymphadenectomy or when nodal metastasis exhibits gross extracapsular extension.
Reprinted with permission from Balch et al. [3]

Table 2.
Proposed stage groupings for cutaneous melanoma

Clinical staging*				Pathologic staging†			
0	Tis	N0	M0	0	Tis	N0	M0
IA	T1a	N0	M0	IA	T1a	N0	M0
IB	T1b	N0	M0	IB	T1b	N0	M0
	T2a	N0	M0		T2a	N0	M0
IIA	T2b	N0	M0	IIA	T2b	N0	M0
	T3a	N0	M0		T3a	N0	M0
IIB	T3b	N0	M0	IIB	T3b	N0	M0
	T4a	N0	M0		T4a	N0	M0
IIC	T4b	N0	M0	IIC	T4b	N0	M0
III	Any T	N1	M0	IIIA	T1–4a	N1a	M0
		N2			T1–4a	N2a	M0
		N3		IIIB	T1–4b	N1a	M0
					T1–4b	N2a	M0
					T1–4a	N1b	M0
					T1–4a	N2b	M0
					T1–4a/b	N2c	M0
				IIIC	T1–4b	N1b	M0
					T1–4b	N2b	M0
					Any T	N3	M0
IV	Any T	Any N	Any M1	IV	Any T	Any N	Any M1

* Clinical staging includes microstaging of the primary melanoma and clinical/radiologic evaluation for metastases. By convention, it should be used after complete excision of the primary melanoma with clinical assessment for regional and distant metastases.
† Pathologic staging includes microstaging of the primary melanoma and pathologic information about the regional lymph nodes after partial or complete lymphadenectomy. Pathologic stage 0 or stage IA patients are the exception: they do not require pathologic evaluation of their lymph nodes.
Reprinted with permission from Balch et al. [3]

assessment of regional lymph nodes. Pathologic staging uses information gained from microstaging the primary tumour and from microscopic evaluation of lymph nodes after selective sentinel or complete lymphadenectomy.

Patients with primary melanoma without evidence for regional or distant metastases are divided into two stages. Stage I refers to early-stage patients at „low risk" for metastases and melanoma-specific mortality. Stage II applies to those patients with „intermediate risk" for metastases and melanoma specific mortality. Patients with regional metastases (regional lymph nodes, cutaneous satellites and in-transit metastases) belong to stage III melanoma. Patients with metastases to distant skin, subcutaneous tissue, lymph nodes or viscera belong to stage IV melanoma.

The survival rates for these stages are presented in Table 3.

25.2 Rationale for Using 18-FDG as a Radiotracer in Melanoma

The most commonly used PET radiotracer for melanoma imaging is the glucose analogue 2-[F-18] fluoro-2-deoxy-D-glucose (FDG) [4]. FDG uptake in cancer tissue is based on the aerobic glycolysis (degradation of glucose to lactic acid in the presence of oxygen) that is increased in malignancy compared with most normal tissues [5]. This phenomenon is linked to the increase both in the glucose membrane transporters and in the activity of the principal enzymes controlling the glycolytic pathways [5]. Melanoma is one of the tumours with the highest glycolytic metabolism, FDG uptake and tumour: blood ratio [6].

Table 3. Survival rates for melanoma TNM and staging categories (reprinted with permission from [3])

Pathologic stage	TNM	Thickness (mm)	Ulceration	No + nodes	Nodal size	Distant Metastasis	No of patients	Survival±SE			
								1-year	2-year	5-year	10-year
IA	T1a	1	No	0	–	–	4,510	99.7±0.1	99.0±0.2	95.3±0.4	87.9±1.0
IB	T1b	1	Yes or level IV,V	0	–	–	1,380	99.8±0.1	98.7±0.3	90.9±1.0	83.1±1.5
	T2a	1.01–2.0	No	0	–	–	3,285	99.5±0.1	97.3±0.3	89.0±0.7	79.2±1.1
IIA	T2b	1.01–2.0	Yes	0	–	–	958	98.2±0.5	92.9±0.9	77.4±1.7	64.4±2.2
	T3a	2.01–4.0	No	0	–	–	1,717	98.7±0.3	94.3±0.6	78.7±1.2	63.8±1.7
IIB	T3b	2.01–4.0	Yes	0	–	–	1,523	95.1±0.6	84.8±1.0	63.0±1.5	50.8±1.7
	T4a	>4.0	No	0	–	–	563	94.8±1.0	88.6±1.5	67.4±2.4	53.9±3.3
IIC	T4b	>4.0	Yes	0	–	–	978	89.9±1.0	70.7±1.6	45.1±1.9	32.3±2.1
IIIA	N1a	Any	No	1	Micro	–	252	95.9±1.3	88.0±2.3	69.5±3.7	63.0±4.4
	N2a	Any	No	2–3	Micro	–	130	93.0±2.4	82.7±3.8	63.3±5.6	56.9±6.8
IIIB	N1a	Any	Yes	1	Micro	–	217	93.3±1.8	75.0±3.2	52.8±4.1	37.8±4.8
	N2a	Any	Yes	2–3	Micro	–	111	92.0±2.7	81.0±4.1	49.6±5.7	35.9±7.2
	N1b	Any	No	1	Macro	–	122	88.5±2.9	78.5±3.7	59.0±4.8	47.7±5.8
	N2b	Any	No	2–3	Macro	–	93	76.8±4.4	65.6±5.0	46.3±5.5	39.2±5.8
IIIC	N1b	Any	Yes	1	Macro	–	98	77.9±4.3	54.2±5.2	29.0±5.1	24.4±5.3
	N2b	Any	Yes	2–3	Macro	–	109	74.3±4.3	44.1±4.9	24.0±4.4	15.0±3.9
	N3	Any	Any	4	Micro/ macro	–	396	71.0±2.4	49.8±2.7	26.7±2.5	18.4±2.5
IV	M1a	Any	Any	Any	Any	Skin, SQ	179	59.3±3.7	36.7±3.6	18.8±3.0	15.7±2.9
	M1b	Any	Any	Any	Any	Lung	186	57.0±3.7	23.1±3.2	6.7±2.0	2.5±1.5
	M1c	Any	Any	Any	Any	Other visceral	793	40.6±1.8	23.6±1.5	9.5±1.1	6.0±0.9
Total							17,600				

25.3 Sensitivity and Specificity of 18-FDG-PET in Cutaneous Melanoma

25.3.1 Overall Sensitivity and Specificity

The major benefit for using FDG-PET in melanoma is the detection of metastatic disease. We will therefore use this clinical situation to define the overall sensitivity and specificity of FDG-PET. We will later analyse the sensitivity at the various stages of the disease. According to the currently published studies, FDG-PET has an overall sensitivity of 74–100% and a specificity of 67–100% in the detection of melanoma metastases [2]. A meta-analysis of eleven clinical studies regarding FDG-PET and cutaneous melanoma showed that the mean sensitivity and specificity for FDG-PET in the detection of melanoma metastases were 79% (95% CI: 0.66 – 0.93) and 86% (95% CI: 0.78–0.95), respectively [7]. The pooled diagnostic odds ratio was 33.1 (95% CI: 21.9–54) suggesting high diagnostic accuracy for PET [7].

Another meta-analysis about FDG-PET in the detection of recurrent melanoma determined an overall sensitivity of 92% (95% CI: 88.4–95.8) and an overall specificity of 90% (95% CI: 83.2–96) [8]. Furthermore, data available for change-in-management suggested a 22% overall FDG-PET directed change in management [8].

Thus, meta-analyses indicate the potential benefits of using FDG PET as a diagnostic and management tool in melanoma [7, 8].

25.3.2 Sensitivity with Respect to Clinical Stages of Melanoma

25.3.2.1 *Stages I and II Disease*

FDG-PET has a low sensitivity in clinical melanoma stages I or II. When sentinel lymph node microstaging using conventional microscopy and immunohistochemistry was performed in these stages, detection of subclinical nodal metastases reached 86–94% in sensitivity whereas FDG-PET detected only 14–17% of these metastases [9, 10].

As FDG-PET sensitivity in melanoma lymph node metastases depends on the tumour volume [11], the low detection rate of FDG-PET is probably due to the small size of nodal metastases in stages I and II. Indeed, FDG-PET detects only 23% of lymph nodes metastases up to 5 mm in diameter [12]. PET inability to disclose microscopic disease suggests that FDG-PET is not a sensitive indicator of occult melanoma metastases in regional lymph nodes and is of limited value for evaluating patients with early stage disease [9, 13].

As a practical consequence, metabolic imaging is not recommended for staging regional lymph nodes in patients with melanoma stages I and II. Sentinel node lymphoscintigraphy remains the procedure of choice for detecting subclinical lymph node involvement from primary cutaneous melanoma [10].

25.3.2.2
Stage III Disease

Contribution of FDG-PET to regional staging is gained in clinical stage III melanoma compared to clinical stages I and II. Indeed, the larger tumour burden in stage III disease is more likely to be detected with PET [9]. FDG-PET has a sensitivity of 85% in stage III melanoma [13]. Metastatic foci smaller than 1 cm are generally a cause of misdiagnosis [13]. In fact, FDG-PET detects almost all metastases larger than 10 mm, 83% of metastases in the range 6–10 mm and 13% of metastases smaller than 5 mm [12]. Moreover, only those metastases with more than 50% lymph node involvement or with capsular infiltration were detected with a high sensitivity (above 93%) [12].

25.3.2.3
Stage IV Disease

FDG-PET appears to be more accurate for the detection of distant metastases (diagnostic odds ratio: 36.4) than for the detection of regional lymph node metastases (diagnostic odds ratio: 19.5) [7]. It demonstrates an overall sensitivity of 80–100% for detecting visceral melanoma metastases [14–18]. However, great regional differences in sensitivity have been pointed out. FDG-PET is especially valuable in melanoma patients with suspected intra-abdominal involvement with a nearly 100% sensitivity in detecting these metastases [14, 16, 19, 20]. However, some treated liver metastases show a liver-equivalent uptake and cannot be differentiated from the normal liver parenchyma [21]. FDG-PET yielded only a 70% sensitivity in detecting lung metastases [14, 22]. Such a low figure was attributed to blurring caused by respiratory movement and to limited spatial resolution [2]. It has thus been argued that once metastases have been identified by CT-scan, the complementary use of FDG-PET may not be of value for diagnosing lung and liver metastases [23].

25.4
FDG-PET Versus Conventional Imaging in Melanoma

Overall, FDG-PET imaging appears to be superior to conventional imaging in the detection of regional and distant melanoma metastases (Table 4). FDG-PET is likely to have a substantial effect on the clinical management of a large number of patients [20], although to date, its actual impact has not been appropriately studied. In addition, the comparative effectiveness depends on the different metastatic sites.

FDG-PET is reported to be more sensitive and specific than CT-scan for detecting melanoma metastases in bones, small-bowel and lymph nodes [14–16, 18–20, 24]. However, FDG-PET was found to be inferior to CT scan in diagnosing lung metastases (sensitivity 70 vs 87%) [14, 23, 25]. The ability of FDG-PET to detect liver metastases from melanoma as accurately as CT-scan remains controversial [15, 23, 25]. Larger series including different tumour types clearly show however that, at equivalent specificity, PET is more sensitive than US, CT and MRI for diagnosing liver metastatic involvement [26].

The comparison of FDG-PET and ultrasonography in the detection of regional lymph nodes indicates that both imaging modalities have similar sensitivities and specificities, reaching 74% and 93%, respectively, for FDG-PET and 76% and 96%, respectively, for ultrasonography [27]. Conversely, a recent study comparing FDG-PET with high-dose gallium-67 imaging encompassing whole-body scanning and comprehensive single-photon emission tomography (SPET) shows that FDG-PET provides incremental and clinically important information missed by SPET in about 10% of the patients [28].

In fact, FDG-PET and conventional imaging should be regarded as complementary rather than competing imaging modalities, each of them displaying specific advantages and drawbacks. FDG-PET has greater overall sensitivity and specificity than CT-scan in melanoma. Whole-body FDG-PET can also disclose neoplastic masses inside multiple organ systems and lymph nodes in a single imaging session. However, FDG-PET provides less accurate anatomical localization of metastatic disease. Hence, it typically requires complementary conventional imaging. CT-scan shows a low sensitivity particularly for neoplastic infiltrations in normal-sized lymph nodes and for small metastases in the abdomen. In fact, structural imaging methods are limited in that the criteria for malignancy are solely based on the size of the lymph nodes. Furthermore, not all the body is simultaneously accessible. Lesions may also be overlooked due to unexpected lymphatic drainage pat-

Table 4. Comparison of FDG-PET and CT-scan sensitivity and specificity in malignant melanoma metastases

Reference	Number of patients	Sensitivity (%)		Specificity (%)	
		PET	CT	PET	CT
18	104	84	58	97	70
16	38	97	62	56	22
15	76	94	55	83	84
14	100	100	85	95	68

terns, particularly for melanoma of the head and trunk. Although whole-body FDG-PET is expensive, it remains less costly than whole-body MRI [4]. FDG-PET is also cost effective in melanoma stages II and III with a saving cost ratio 2:1 when used as an additional procedure and 4:1 when CT scan of the chest and abdomen can be discarded [29].

25.5 Pitfalls of FDG-PET in Melanoma

False-negative FDG-PET results may occur when the lesion is close to or within a structure that naturally takes FDG up, such as the brain. Since the spatial resolution of the technique remains limited (4–6 mm FWHM), PET is more affected by partial volume effect than CT or MRI. Lesions smaller than 0.5–1 cm are thus more frequently missed than larger lesions. In addition, FDG-PET obviously cannot detect discrete microscopic neoplastic infiltrations [30].

Factors other than tumour size may contribute to PET false-negative results in melanoma. Indeed, the glucose metabolic rate and the density in glucose transporter proteins may vary according to oncogene expressions [31].

FDG is not a tumour-specific probe which may result in a high rate of false positive results [32]. It accumulates in various physiologic and non-neoplastic pathologic conditions including infectious and granulomatous diseases. Uptake can also be enhanced by inflammatory processes such as post-operative healing and post-radiotherapy change [30]. The specificity of the test may however be improved when reading the studies with knowledge of the patients' clinical history [13].

Even if whole-body FDG-PET scan is a useful tool in searching for metastatic melanoma, the histological assessment and long term clinical follow-up remain of paramount importance [30].

Representative examples are showed in Figs. 1 and 2.

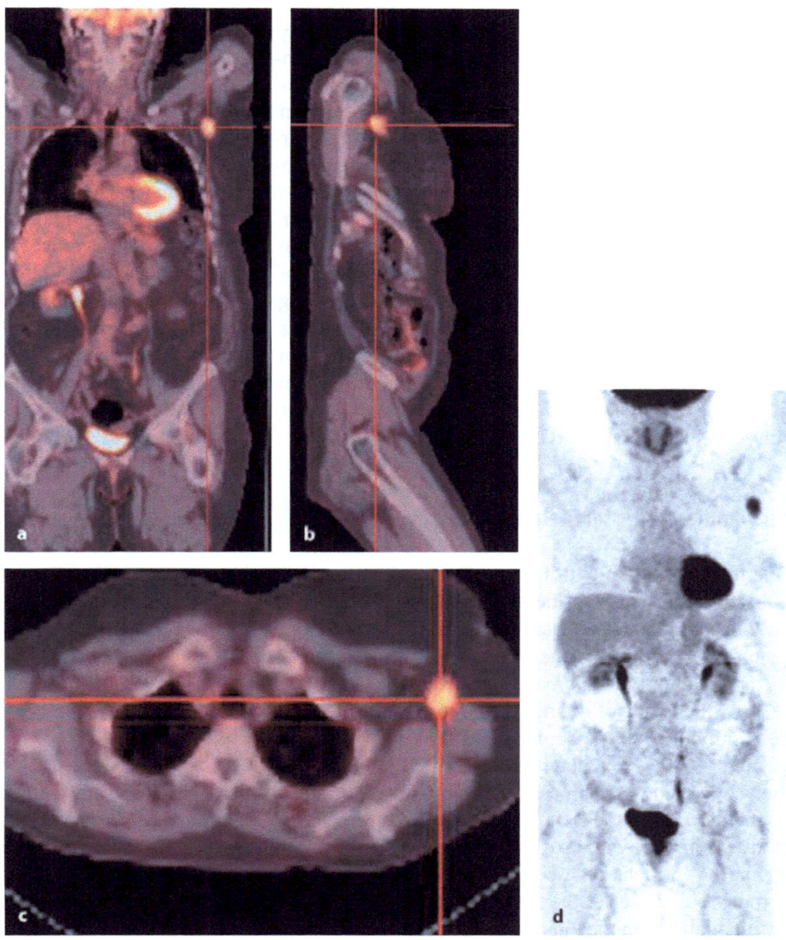

Fig. 1. Left axillary lymph node from a melanoma. Fused PET/CT images are showed in **a** (coronal section), **b** (sagittal section) **c** (transverse section). 3D projection PET images are shown in **d**

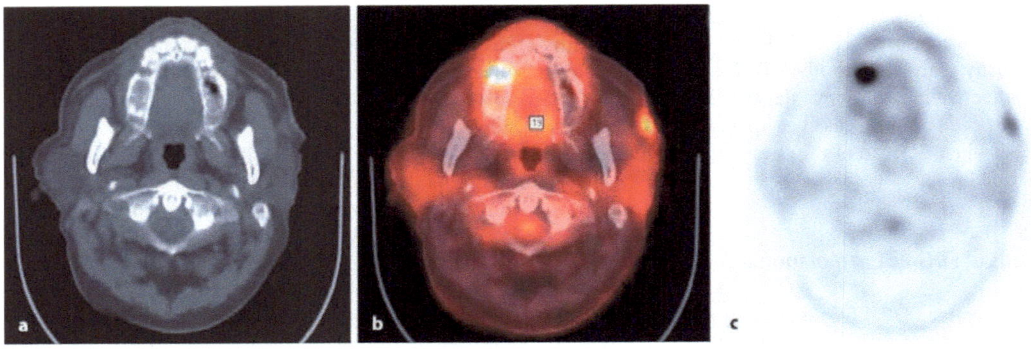

Fig. 2. Small cutaneous melanoma lesion on the left cheek. There is also a focus of increased activity in the right jaw, corresponding in fact to an abscess. This illustrates the high sensitivity of PET for tumour lesions but also the non specific uptake by inflammatory or infectious processes. CT transverse section (**a**), fused PET/CT (**b**) and PET images (**c**) are shown

25.6 FDG-PET in Ocular Melanoma

PET appears to be of limited value for the diagnosis of primary ocular melanoma. It exhibits low sensitivity (25–50%) in uveal melanoma [33–35]. This low sensitivity could be due to the size of the tumour or to biochemical differences. Ocular tumour with a diameter less than 7.5 mm are generally not detected by FDG PET [34]. Furthermore, it seems likely that the rate of glucose metabolism in some ocular melanomas is not high enough to correspond to an activity level suitable for imaging purposes [35]. The extent in increased glucose metabolism by malignant cells is correlated with the growth rate of the tumour. Uveal melanoma is often a slow-growing neoplasm in which few mitotic figures can be seen. This slow melanoma growth may be due to a low expression of some proto-oncogenes which manage the expression of glucose transport and the glucose metabolic rates involved in FDG uptake and metabolism [35].

25.7. New Radiotracers for Melanoma

One major problem with FDG-PET is the low specificity in the neoplasm identification. FDG accumulates not only in malignant neoplasm but also in inflammatory lesions. New radio-pharmaceuticals providing more information about melanoma lesions would be welcome.

Tyrosine is one of the main components of melanin. The amino acid is transported into the cells and transformed to dihydroxyphenylalanine (DOPA). DOPA is then converted to melanin after several metabolic steps. F-labelled-L-DOPA (FDOPA), labelled in the 6-position of the aromatic ring, provides primarily transport information in melanoma cells because ^{18}F label is likely to be removed after the first metabolic steps [36]. Experimental data in the mouse showed a high uptake and a preferential accumulation of FDOPA in cells engaged in the S-phase [37].

In human pretreated melanoma, the overall sensitivity of FDOPA reached 64% versus 86% to 18-FDG [36]. The uptake of FDOPA was indeed low, the label was lost early in the metabolic sequences, the metabolism was slow compared with the period of imaging and no metabolic trapping occurred [36]. FDG led to higher uptake concentrations in tumour cells. FDG uptake was 1.5 fold higher than FDOPA uptake in 18 of 22 melanoma metastases whereas FDOPA uptake was 1,5 fold higher than FDG uptake in 2 patients with liver metastases [37]. Moreover as FDOPA is lost early in the metabolic sequence, its uptake is then simply an indicator of large neutral amino acid transport [38]. Hence, although FDOPA is unlikely to be a specific imaging agent for melanoma [38], it may prove to be of value for oncological imaging, as protein metabolism is less affected in inflammatory tissues than in tumour lesions. At this time, FDOPA should not be used as the primary tracer in PET, but it might be considered in combination with FDG.

Detection of melanoma metastases was indeed enhanced when both tracers were used in combination (sensitivity 95%) [36]. Multitracer studies are potentially powerful because different parameters can be used to improve the accuracy of parameter estimates or can be combined to create new parameters [38].

25.8 Conclusion

FDG-PET generally contributes to additional important diagnostic information that often have significant effect on the clinical treatment of patients with cutaneous melanoma. The sensitivity and specificity of FDG-PET vary according to the clinical stage and the localization of the melanoma lesions. Conventional radiological imaging remains valuable in some circumstances in bringing information not provided by FDG-PET. Hence, these two methods are synergistic rather than redundant in managing melanoma.

Other tracers should be identified in order to probe alternative metabolic pathways and reduce the false-positive findings that remain a problem with FDG imaging.

References

1. Thompson JA (2002) The revised American Joint Committee on Cancer staging system for melanoma. Semin Oncol 29:361–369
2. Prichard RS, Hill ADK, Skehan SJ, O'Higgins NJ (2002) Positron emission tomography for staging and management of malignant melanoma. Br J Surg 89:389–396
3. Balch CM, Buzaid AC, Soong SJ, Atkins MB, Cascinelli N et al (2001) Final version of the American Joint Committee on Cancer staging system for cutaneous melanoma. J Clin Oncol 19: 3635–3648
4. Hoh CK, Schiepers C, Seltzer MA, Gambhir SS, Silverman DHS et al (1997) PET in oncology: will it replace the other modalities? Semin Nucl Med 27:94–106
5. Waki A (1998) Recent advances in the analyses of the characteristics of tumors on FDG uptake. Nucl Med Biol 25:589–592
6. Wahl RL, Hutchins GD, Buchsbaum DJ (1991) Fluorine-18-2-deoxy-2-fluoro-D-glucose (FDG) uptake into human tumor xenografts: feasibility studies for cancer imaging with PET. Cancer 67:1544–1549
7. Mijnhout GS, Hoekstra OS, van Tulder MW, Teule JJ, Deville WLJM (2001) Systematic review of the diagnostic accuracy of 18F-fluorodexyglucose positron emission tomography in melanoma patients. Cancer 91:1530–1542
8. Schwimmer J, Essner R, Patel A, Jahan SA, Shepherd JE et al (2000) A review of the literature for whole-body FDG PET in the management of patients with melanoma. Q J Nucl Med 4: 153–167
9. Wagner JD, Schauwecker D, Davidson D, Coleman JJ, Saxman S et al (1999) Prospective study of fluorodeoxyglucose-positron emission tomography imaging of lymph node basins in melanoma patients undergoing sentinel node biopsy. J Clin Oncol 19:1508–1515
10. Belhocine T, Piérard G, de la Brassinne M, Lahaye T, Rigo P (2002) Staging of regional node in AJCC stage I and II melanoma: 18 FDG PET imaging versus sentinel node detection. Oncologist 7:271–278
11. Wagner JD, Schauwecker DS, Davidson D, Wenck S, Jung SH et al (2001) FDG-PET sensitivity for melanoma lymph node metastases is dependent on tumor volume. J Surg Oncol [Suppl] 77:237–242
12. Crippa F, Leutner M, Belli F, Gallino F, Greco M et al (2000) Which kinds of lymph node metastases can FDG PET detect? A clinical study in melanoma. J Nucl Med 41:1491–1494
13. Tyler DS, Onaitis M, Kherani A, Hata A, Nicholson E et al (2000) Positron emission tomogrpahy scanning in malignant melanoma. Clinical utility in patients with stage III disease. Cancer 89: 1019–1025
14. Rinne D, Baum RP, Hör G, Kaufmann R (1998) Primary staging and follow-up of high risk melanoma patients with whole-body 18F-fluorodeoxyglucose positron emission tomography. Results of a prospective study of 100 patients. Cancer 82:1164–1171
15. Holder WD, White RL, Zuger JH, Easton EJ, Greene FL (1998) Effectiveness of positron emission tomography for the detection of melanoma metatases. Ann Surg 227:764–769
16. Eigtved A, Andersson AP, Dahlstrom K, Rabol A, Jensen M et al (2000) Use of fluorine-18 fluorodeoxyglucose positron emission tomography in the detection of silent metastases from malignant melanoma. Eur J Nucl Med 27:70–75
17. Paquet P, Henry F, Belhocine T, Hustinx R, Najjar F et al (2000) An appraisal of 18-fluorodeoxyglucose positron emission tomography for melanoma staging. Dermatology 200:167–169
18. Swetter SM Caroll LA, Johnson DL, Segall GM (2002) Positron emission tomography is superior to computed tomography for metastatic detection in melanoma patients. Ann Surg Oncol 9: 646–653
19. Tatlidil R, Mandelkern M (2001) FDG-PET in the detection of gastrointestinal metastases in melanoma. Melanoma Res 11: 297–301
20. Jadvar H, Johnson DL, Segall GM (2000) The effect of fluorine-18 fluorodeoxyglucose positron emission tomography on the management of cutaneous malignant melanoma. Clin Nucl Med 25:48–51
21. Mantaka P, Dimitrakopoulou-Strauss A, Strauss LG (1999) Detection of treated liver metastases using fluorine-18-fluorodeoxyglucose (FDG) and positron emission tomography (PET). Anticancer Res 19:4443–4450
22. Gritters LS, Francis IR, Zasaduy KR, Wahl RL (1993) Initial assessment of positron emission tomography using 2-fluorine-18-fluoro-2-deoxy-D-glucose in the imaging of malignant melanoma. J Nucl Med 34:1420–1428
23. Krug B, Dietlein M, Groth W, Stutzer H, Psaras E et al (2000) Fluor-18-fluorodeoxyglucose positron emission tomography (FDG-PET) in malignant melanoma. Acta Radiol 41:446–452
24. Kuvskinoff BW, Kurtz C, Coit DG (1997) Computed tomography in evaluation of patients with stage III melanoma. Ann Surg Oncol 4:252
25. Dietlein M, Krug B, Groth W, Smolarz K, Scheidhauer K et al (1999) Positron emission tomography using 1F-fluorodeoxyglucose in advanced stage of malignant melanoma: a comparison of ultrasonographic and radiological methods of diagnosis. Nucl Med Comm 20:255–261
26. Kinkel K, Lu Y, Both M, Warren RS, Thoeni RF (2002) Detection of hepatic metastases from cancers of the gastrointestinal tract by using noninvasive imaging methods (US, CT, MR imaging, PET): a meta-analysis. Radiology 224:748–756
27. Blessing C, Feine U, Geiger L (1995) Positron emission tomography and ultrasonography. Arch Dermatol 131:1394–1398
28. Kalff VH, Hicks RJ, Ware RE, Greer B, Binns DS et al (2002) Evaluation of high-risk melanoma: comparison of 18F-FDG-PET and high dose 67 Ga SPET. Eur J Nucl Med Mol Imag 29:506–515
29. Valk PE, Pounds TR, Tesar RD, Hogkins DM, Haeman MK (1996) Cost effectiveness of PET imaging in clinical oncology. Nucl Med Biol 23:737–743
30. Paquet P, Hustinx R, Rigo P, Piérard GE (1998) Malignant melanoma staging using whole-body positron emission tomography. Melanoma Res 8:59–62
31. Flier J, Mueckler MM, Usher P, Lodish HF (1987) Elevated levels of glucose transport and transporter messenger RNA are induced by ras or src oncogenes. Science 235:1492–1495
32. Acland KM, Healy C, Calonje E et al (2001) Comparison of positron emission tomography scanning and sentinel node biopsy in the detection of micrometastases of primary cutaneous malignant melanoma. J Clin Oncol 19:2674–2678
33. Lucignani G, Paganelli G, Modorati G, Pieralli S, Rizzo G et al (1992) MRI, antibody-guided scintigraphy and glucose metabolism in uveal melanoma. J Comput Assist Tomogr 16:77–83
34. Modorati G, Lucignani G, Landoni C, Freschi M, Trabucchi G et al (1996) Glucose metabolism and pathological findings in uveal melanoma: preliminary results. Nucl Med Commun 17:1052–1056
35. Spraul CW, Long GE, Lang GK (2001) Value of positron emission tomography in the diagnosis of malignant ocular tumors. Ophtalmologica 215:163–168
36. Dimitrakopoulou-Strauss A, Strauss LG, Burger C (2001) Quantitative PET studies in pretreated melanoma: comparison of 6-(18F) fluoro-L-Dopa with 18F-FDG and 15O-water using compartment and noncompartment analysis. J Nucl Med 42:248–256
37. Ishiwata K, Kubota K, Kubota R, Iwata R, Takahashi T et al (1991) Selective 2-(18F) fluorodopa uptake for melanogenesis in murine metastatic melanomas. J Nucl Med 32:95–101
38. Graham MM (2001) Combined 18F-FDG-FDOPA tumor imaging for assessing response to therapy. J Nucl Med 42:257–258

CHAPTER 26

Malignant Lymphomas

C. Menzel

26.1 Hodgkin's Disease

26.1.1 Incidence, Etiology and Epidemiology

In general, Hodgkin's disease (HD) is a rare cause of tumor-related death in the population. However, within the group of patients under 30 years of age, it is – after leukemias and the Non-Hodgkin's lymphomas (NHL) – a major cause for tumor-related death [51]. Annually there are approximately 40,000 new cases of HD and 16,000 HD-related deaths. HD thus represents less than 1% of all malignancies, and there is a three-fold increased chance of dying from HD in less well-developed countries. The incidence is higher in the white population and HD affects more male than female patients [54].

Since its first description by Thomas Hodgkin in 1828, an infectious association was discussed [15] and epidemiological data point towards an association with HD and previous viral infections, especially the Epstein-Barr virus (EBV) [12, 45]. EBV, however, is no prerogative for HD which is documented by the number of EBV-negative HD patients and vice versa by the high number of EBV-positive but HD-negative persons in the population.

26.1.2 Histopathologic Classification

In contrast to any other solid tumor, HD shows the unique phenomenon that only a minor part of the tumor volume accounts for truly malignant cells, such as the Reed-Sternberg and Hodgkin cells. In contrast, the majority of the tumor volume consists of a benign mass of inflammatory lymphocytic cells. HD can be traced back to clonal populations of transformed B- and, less frequently, T-lymphocytes.

Histopathologic HD-subtypes are based on the historical classifications according to Rye and REAL, which were recently revised in the current WHO classification [19]. Here, the classic morphological criteria, like nodularity and Hodgkin cells or Reed-Sternberg cells, are complemented by the immunophenotype (CD20+, CD15–, CD30–, J-Kett+, EBV–) (Table 1 and 2).

The most frequent subtype is the nodular sclerosing HD which accounts for roughly two thirds of all cases. In about 25% of all cases a mixed type is diagnosed and the "classic" HD with dominance of lymphocytes is a rather rare type accounting for about 3% of all HD lymphomas. Lymphocyte depleted HD is even less common. All other cases are represented by an HD of lymphocyte predominance, typically associated with an EBV-negative status [2].

Table 1. WHO classification of HD

Subtypes	Entities
Nodular lymphocyte predominant Hodgkin's disease (NLPHD)	Nodular lymphocyte predominant Hodgkin's disease (NLPHD)
Classic, lymphocyte-rich HD Nodular sclerosis Mixed cellularity Lymphocyte depleted	Classic HD

26.1.3 Conventional Diagnostics and Current Therapy

HD is treated according to its stage which is defined by an increasingly less aggressive algorithm. This consists initially of a clinical evaluation and laboratory tests (e.g. BSR, LDH, AP). This approach is complemented by di-

Table 2. Immunophenotype of the classic HD and the NLPHD

	Classic HD	NLPHD
CD 15	(+)	–
CD 20	(–)	+
CD 30	+	–
EMA	(–)	+
J-chain	–	+
Vimentin	+	–
EBV association	Mixed type 75% Nodular sclerosis 25%	– –
Background TIA1/CD57	≠	Ø

Table 3. Stages of HD according to the Ann Arbor classification

Stage I	affection of a single lymph node (LN) region or a lymphoid structure (e.g. thymus or spleen or tonsils)
Stage I E	affection of a single LN region and growth into adjacent tissue or a single tumor manifestation in an extralymphatic organ (not liver)
Stage II	affection of 2 or more KN region on one side of the diaphragm
Stage II E	localized affection of one extralymphatic organ and one or more affected LN region on the same side of the diaphragm
Stage III	affected LN on both sides of the diaphragm with or without additional splenic involvement (III S)
Stage III E	affected LN on both sides of the diaphragm with or without splenic involvement plus a localized affection of extranodal tissue
Stage IV	non-localized, diffuse or disseminated affection of one or more extralymphatic organs with or without additional affection of the lymphatic system

Further categories according to the presence or absence of clinical signs or symptoms as A or B, with A indicating no symptoms and B indicating the presence of unexplained weight loss of more than 10% in the past 6 months, fever of unknown origin, drenching night sweats; letter X will indicate a bulky disease

agnostic imaging that more or less routinely includes a chest X-ray, an abdominal sonography and a X-ray computed tomography (CT) of the thoracic organs and the abdomen/pelvis. Furthermore, bone scintigraphy, bone marrow biopsy and sometimes liver biopsy are included in the staging algorithm.

This staging algorithm has changed significantly in recent years, partly driven by new therapeutic strategies towards a less invasive approach. Invasive diagnostic procedures, e.g. a staging laparotomy, or more aggressive therapies, e.g. an extended field radiotherapy, today do not play a major role in the routine management of HD. These changes have been made possible due to advances of CT, allowing a sufficient whole-body staging, and the development of further chemotherapy concepts that allow a primarily systemic approach with moderate side effects. Nevertheless, the exact staging remains important for both a sufficiently planned therapy regimen and an estimate of prognosis.

Regarding prognosis, there are known, easily accessible factors associated with its establishment, such as the presence of large mediastinal tumor, whether extranodal structures are affected, a massively increased BSR (>50 mm in A- and >30 mm in B-stages) or the involvement of three or more lymph node sites. The definition of the HD stages can be found in Table 3.

Based on this algorithm, the early stages (I–II) are treated with a favorable prognosis by polychemotherapy, if there are no additional risk factors. This therapy may or may not include an involved-field (IF) radiotherapy. Chemotherapy follows a scheme mainly according to the ACVB-protocol (Doxorubicin, Bleomycin, Vinblastine and Dacarbazine). Regarding the number of necessary cycles or the need for an additional IF-radiotherapy, many questions remain unanswered to date. Patients in early stages with unfavorable prognosis do undergo IF-radiotherapy after completion of the chemotherapy which results in up to 80% long-term survival. More advanced stages (II–IV) may undergo escalated chemotherapy (e.g. BEACOPP using Cyclophosphamide, Adriamycin, Etoposide, Procarbazine, Prednisone, Vincristine and Bleomycin). Here, both the number of cycles and the doses of the pharmaceuticals are increased, e.g. eight cycles of escalated BEACOPP plus four cycles of baseline BEACOPP optionally including radiotherapy of bulk or residual lymphoma. A detailed review of the protocols of the current HD-10 to -12 therapy studies can be found in Wolf et al. [53].

26.1.4 Positron Emission Tomography

There are different aspects and views that allow an integration of PET into the investigation of HD. The main criteria, however, include the initial staging and restaging following completion of therapy. These aspects will be discussed in more detail, but the emphasis will be put on dedicated PET using FDG only, because this is currently the most effective technique and also because tumor scintigraphy with Gallium-68 is far less sensitive than PET [37, 40, 49].

26.1.5 Staging

The use of PET for the initial staging of newly diagnosed HD was recently summarized in a paper by Reske and Kotzerke [36] which included all studies up to the year 2000. In 11 studies and 514 patients with lymphomas, PET showed a 10% increased sensitivity and a specificity of 85%–90% compared to conventional imaging like CT. Since then, similar results were found in approximately 200 patients with the main focus on HD staging [18, 22, 27, 33, 41, 46, 50]. The available data, therefore, suggest a superior sensitivity of PET for the detection of nodal HD of approximately 90%, and slightly better results were found for cervical and mediastinal LN compared to abdominal LN. Overall, the results of PET for nodal and extranodal staging of HD were clearly superior to conventional radiological imaging. Hueltenschmidt et al. [18] found an accuracy of PET of 96% versus 56% for the conventional CT-based staging. In 30%–50% of all cases the results of PET indicated a change of stage of the disease. Although these data clearly favor PET, a number of questions remain since the therapy concept is primarily systemic and also because the histopathologic gold standard is missing in most lesions found by PET. For example, there were false-negative LN in the PET scan in patients who otherwise showed

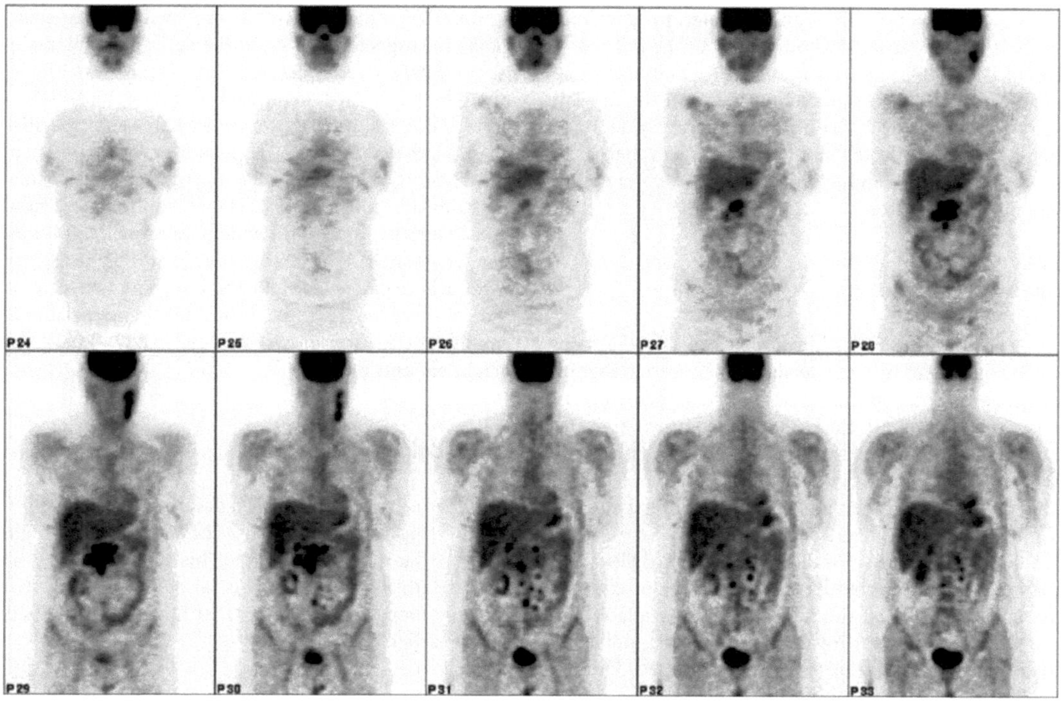

Fig. 1. Coronal sequence of slices including the typical field-of-view for a routine PET scan in oncology. This patients suffers from a known NHL affecting the left cervical lymph nodes. The further staging showed no additional tumor sites. The abdominal CT scan described some accentuated abdominal lymph nodes of sub-critical size. The FDG-PET clearly depicts the cervical chain of affected lymph nodes and leaves no doubt about the abdominal tumor growth. Accordingly, the patient was upstaged from I to III

clearly increased FDG uptake in other tumor sites. The LN were considered as false-negative PET findings because these LN were enlarged on CT and showed a regression of size to normal after chemotherapy [40, 50]. These findings should not be overestimated as enlarged LN on a CT scan do lack the missing gold standard even more than lesions described to be hypermetabolic in a PET. Thus, the CT results of LN may also have been false-positive, but this matter is not completely settled.

In 58 histopathologically controlled extranodal lesions, PET had a sensitivity of 100% and a specificity of 97%, also clearly superior to that of CT (sensitivity 63%, specificity 93%) [29].

Regarding histopathologic subtypes of HD, a recent study conducted by Döbert et al. [10] showed no major differences of FDG uptake. In a total of 44 cases of HD, all subtypes had mean SUV above or equal to 2.5.

FDG-PET may be false negative in up to 5% of cases with known bone marrow infiltration [7, 31], which was related in most cases to a tumor cell fraction of less than 10% of the total cellularity. On the other hand there is a rate of up to 10% false-negative bone marrow biopsies due to the fact that the HD manifestation was located elsewhere and thus missed.

26.1.6 Restaging/Therapy Control

In comparison to its primary staging the data pool for the restaging of HD is more elaborate. This holds especially true for the detection of tumor viability after chemotherapy if there are remnants seen on CT. For this indication the sensitivity of PET lies within a range of 71%–88% and the specificity is 83%–86%. This corresponds to an X-ray CT sensitivity/specificity of 88% and 31%, respectively [36]. These data are further underlined by current studies that do propose the routine use of PET with FDG for the follow-up of HD after therapy [9, 21, 55]. Maintained FDG utilization correlates with the incidence of recurrence. In a mixed collective of HD and NHL, Cremerius et al. were able to show that there was early recurrence in 16/19 cases with tumor remnants according to PET, but in only 3/22 with a normal/negative PET scan. In these patients the mean follow-up was 21 months [8]. Progression-free survival was above 90% in PET-negative patients, while no patients remained in remission who had a PET scan indicating viable tumor remnants [42]. Thus, the general inclusion of PET in the restaging algorithm of HD, even if no tumor rest is seen of the CT, is required [25]. The correct time for the PET scan after therapy is currently about 4 weeks after the completion of the fist 4–8 cycles of chemotherapy. In demanding cases it may be applied earlier after the completion of the treatment. The use of PET for early identification of responders and non-responders to the therapy is – although there is little doubt that this can be achieved with PET – currently still under evaluation.

26.1.7 Summary and Outlook

HD is one of the most striking indications for PET using FDG. This relates not only to staging but also to therapy control and work-up in a situation of a suspected recurrence. The method is clearly superior to the combined information gained by the conventional algorithm, and in particular superior to CT, as well as bone scan. This holds true for both the nodal and extranodal staging/restaging of HD and PET should therefore be routinely used in these patients. For this group of primarily young patients, and supported by the availability of effective therapies, the method should generally be available.

PET remains a non-invasive imaging technique and its limitations should not be underestimated. There is still some controversy about the potential of false-negative results and there are still a number of factors that might influence FDG uptake by tumors or result in nonspecific uptake, some of them being known and some not. False-positive findings in the cervical and paravertebral structures compared to other tumors occur more frequently in HD/NHL. This so-called lobster-sign may influence the specificity of PET for the detection of HD remnants. A PET scan today cannot and should not be used as a substitute for CT-based staging until larger studies are available that define the extent to which either parts of the conventional test battery or the additional PET may be unnecessary. A bone marrow biopsy should be performed after PET has been conducted.

26.1.8 Technical Recommendations – Tips and Tricks

A routine protocol including a transmission correction and a scan area between the base of the skull and the proximal femora is strongly recommended. The patients preparation, dose application, latency/voiding and imaging itself, as well as the reconstruction and evaluation of the tomograms, should follow a routine course, thus allowing reproducible imaging conditions. Depending on the clinical question, an additional scan of the neurocranium may be included. Also, a routine application of intravenous furosemide is recommended in all relevant cases in order to allow optimal evaluation of the abdomen and pelvis. At least some tumor manifestations should be routinely quantified using the SUV technique. In all cases where nonspecific uptake is suspected and/or in the setting of unclassifiable lesions a second, delayed PET scan of this region should be performed. Malignant lesions should show a stable or increasing SUV over time whereas nonspecific/inflammatory uptake may decrease over time. This approach may be used in uncertain situations also associated with the "lobster-sign". The reason for these nonspecific uptake sites is still widely unknown and it has been postulated to resemble muscular uptake [4, 11]. More recent studies using PET/CT suggest that at least some of these foci resemble brown fat tissue [14], but it remains unclear why this shows such a high uptake in certain patients only.

26.2 Non-Hodgkin's Lymphoma

A number of considerations as described for HD apply in the setting of NHL also. This is especially true of high-grade NHL in younger patients. This chapter focuses in more detail, therefore, on clinical specialties of NHL and only makes reference to what has been described for HD earlier.

26.2.1 Incidence, Etiology and Epidemiology

In 2000 there were approximately 14,000 new cases of NHL in Western Europe [51]. More than 6500 cancer-related deaths were related to NHL. In contrast to HD, NHL thus represents a far more frequent cause of cancer and of cancer-related morbidity. During the past decades a continuous increase of newly diagnosed NHL was noticed [35]. Like HD, NHL have a higher incidence in the white population and affect more males than females. Some subtypes show a regional predominance. In adults, B-cell lymphomas represent 85% of all NHL, consisting mainly of follicular and diffuse large-cell B-cell NHL. In contrast, T-cell NHL represent about two thirds of all NHL in childhood. There are a number of immunodeficiencies and viral infections, as well as radiogenic and toxic causes, known to be associated with a higher incidence of NHL.

26.2.2 Histopathologic Classification

The tumor clone dominates the histopathology of the NHL proportionally to its volume. Clinically, biologically and histopathologically, NHL are a very heterogeneous group of diseases which – in contrast to HD – cannot be all and unrestrictedly be recommended as a potential indication for PET scanning.

Their common characteristic is a clonal malignancy of lymphatic cells, and pathologic manifestations com-

Table 4. Ann Arbor classification of non-Hodgkin's lymphoma

Stage I	Involvement of a single lymph node region (LN) (I) or a single extralymphatic structure (I E)
Stage II	Involvement of 2 or more LN on the same side of the diaphragm (II) or a localized affection of a single extralymphatic organ (II E)
Stage III	Involvement of LN both sides of the diaphragm (III) or localized involvement of extralymphatic structures (III E), of the spleen (III S) or both (III ES)
Stage IV	Diffuse or disseminated involvement of extralymphatic organs with or without additional lymph node involvement

Further categories in analogy to HD, see Table 3

prise the spectrum of primary nodal involvement (typical lymphomas), leukemia's and plasmocytomas. They are complexly classified according to the recent WHO classification which has finally adopted an international consensus [20]. Even though from the viewpoint of oncology this must be seen as a major step forward, for the use of FDG-PET it currently remains a less complex approach to evaluate the method according to the working classification of the NHL, namely the definition of low-grade, intermediate and high-grade NHL. Approximately 40% of cases are low-grade NHL which – apart from a few cases – can currently not be treated with curative intention. Another 40% are intermediate NHL, which are in their early stages in about one third of all cases at the time of diagnosis. The remaining 20% account for high-grade NHL which will show rapid progression and lethal course unless adequately treated.

26.2.3 Conventional Diagnostics and Current Therapy

Current therapy of high- and intermediate-grade NHL relies almost exclusively on chemotherapy and is based on the histopathologic subtype. While lymphoblastic and Burkitt NHL directly undergo an ALL protocol which is adapted to age and type, the therapy of other NHL also considers risk factors (such as age, LDH, stage II/IV, nodal or extranodal involvement, etc.) first (Table 4). Together with an exact staging, the cornerstones of therapy are defined (see also IPI-score [47]). Conventional staging includes radiological (CT, sonography) and nuclear medicine methods and it may in relation to the availability of PET be judges for its specific advantages and disadvantages alike the HD. For chemotherapy, the current strategies mainly rely on a CHOPP-protocol (Cyclophosphamide, Doxorubicin, Vincristine and Prednisone), that may be followed by radiotherapy in the case of bulky disease or extranodal manifestations. Using such concepts, less than half of the patients with high-grade NHL may finally be cured [26]. New promising therapies like immuno- or radioimmunotherapy and stem cell transplantation are currently under evaluation.

26.2.4 Positron Emission Tomography

The potential clinical indications for PET using FDG in the NHL reflect the same as already described in the context of HD. However, the heterogenous nature and growth pattern of NHL require a more profound dealing with the clinical and especially histopathological background of the individual patient.

26.2.5 Staging

With regard to the initial staging of high-grade and intermediate-grade NHL, the same arguments which have already been mentioned in the context of HD apply. The studies published to date often represent a combination of HD and NHL patients and thus the results found for sensitivity and specificity are quite similar. In general, it can be said that FDG-PET quite reliably outperforms the conventional staging. The use of FDG-PET may result in a change of stage in up to 44% of patients, and a modification of the therapeutic strategy was noticed in up to 62% of all cases [3, 17, 30, 40]. PET results obtained during childhood and adolescence are similarly good [47].

Compared to these figures, the use of PET for imaging in low-grade NHL is by far less well evaluated and the available data in the literature suggest a much more restrained employment of PET in these malignancies. Regarding plasmocytomas there are some observations reported that PET may be useful to detect occult [32] or extranodal disease [23]. In MALT lymphoma the data are even more contradictory with some positive but mainly disappointing results [1, 16, 38]. Thus, while it remains to be shown that FDG-PET is useful in these indications, considerable doubt remains.

26.2.6 Restaging/Therapy Control

Regarding the restaging and therapy control, the available body of data in the literature relating to NHL is – again similar to HD – much larger. The results of mixed patient populations of HD/NHL – a sensitivity in the range of 71%–88% and a specificity of 83%–86% have been mentioned already [36, 55]. Although large prospective studies of well-defined collectives are still few, those data available indicate that the superiority of functional imaging using FDG-PET over conventional radiological imaging that has been shown for HD also holds true for the restaging of the more aggressive NHL also.

A recently published study of Montravers et al. [28] was able to show FDG-PET to be of major relevance not only in the staging and restaging of adults suffering from HD/NHL, but also in children and adolescents. In 50%

of all cases, the staging had to be corrected on the basis of the PET results. Two cases of false-positive results in PET related to FDG uptake in thymus remnants, a well known "pitfall", and one which needs to be given particular consideration in young patients. Since this pitfall generally has a typical location and formation, it should nowadays be interpreted correctly in most cases [5, 13].

Another important indication for FDG-PET is the early control of therapy and its effectiveness. Since there is a wider spectrum of therapeutic choices available, an early assessment of therapy response and a consequent adjustment of therapy is essential. This, again, is an approach which cannot be sufficiently solved by morphologically oriented, conventional imaging. FDG-PET is able to make an early differentiation between fibrotic tissue remnants and viable tumor rests [34].

Also, responders to chemotherapy can be differentiated early [44]. This could be demonstrated in 93 patients with a high-grade NHL. An inconspicuous PET scan after a first line chemotherapy was related with a significantly better prognosis. In contrast, patients with pathologic FDG uptake all had suffered recurrence within 3 months. According to this investigation, the PET may be used as early as after the first three to four cycles of therapy, thus still in the middle of the first treatment block. Other studies even suggest that this prognostic information may be obtained as early as after the first cycle of chemotherapy, but this has not been sufficiently evaluated to date [24, 39]. Spaepen et al. [43] confirmed earlier results in 70 patients with histopathologically known aggressive NHL. The patients were treated with an average of eight cycles according to standard- or intensified CHOP protocol and a control of therapy efficiency was done using PET after the third or fourth cycle. In 68/70 patients there was also a PET scan available that had been carried out prior to the initiation of chemotherapy. In 31/37 cases with normal PET results, a complete remission could be obtained and this related to a follow-up of almost 3 years. Minimal residual disease could thus not be ruled out definitively in some patients. On the other hand, of 33 patients with an abnormal PET scan after three to four cycles of CHOP, none (0/33) reached a permanent remission.

26.2.7
Summary and Outlook

PET is a well established method for the staging and re-staging of intermediate and high-grade NHL. Due to the interindividual differences in response to chemotherapy, PET most probably will become the most suitable method to obtain an early estimate about therapy effectiveness. Whenever possible, this should be compared to an initial PET scan being obtained prior to the initiation of therapy. FDG-PET and new radiopharmaceuticals hold promise to enable oncologists to embark on a new approach to a more individual therapy for their patients. The lymphomas in general serve as a good example of this. They often occur in young patients and a number of very efficient therapies are available. Using standardized approaches to such patients, a number of patients are certainly being overtreated and may experience the sometimes significant side-effects of, e.g. chemotherapy. Others may be insufficiently treated and with PET this is most likely detectable at an early stage, prior to the clinically evident recurrence.

References

1. Aigner RM, Schwarz T, Wurzinger G, Karpf E (2000) Detection of unsuspected gastric MALT-lymphoma with F-18-FDG-PET. Nuklearmedizin 39:N107
2. Anagnostopoulos I, Hanmann ML, Franssila K, Harris M, Harris NL, Jaffe ES, van Krieken HJM, Poppema S, Marafioti T, Franklin J, Sextro M, Diehl V, Stein H (2000) European Task Force on Lymphoma Project on Lymphocyte Predominance Hodgkin's Disease: histological and immunohistological analysis of submitted cases reveals two types of Hodgkin's disease with a nodular pattern growth and abundant lymphocytes. Blood 96:1889–1899
3. Bangerter M, Moog F, Buchmann I et al (1998) Whole body 2-[18F]-fluoro-2-deoxy-D-glucose positron emission tomography (FDG PET) for accurate staging of Hodgkin's disease. Ann Oncol 89:1117–1122
4. Barrington SF, Maisey MN (1996) Skeletal muscle uptake of fluorine-18-FDG: effect of oral diazepam. J Nucl Med 37:1127–1129
5. Bomanji JB, Syed R, Brock C, Janowska P, Dogan A, Costa DC, Ell PJ, Lee SM (2002) Challenging cases and diagnostic dilemmas: case 2. Pitfalls of positron emission tomography for assessing residual mediastinal mass after chemotherapy for Hodgkin's disease. J Clin Oncol 20:3347–3349
6. Canellos GP (1988) Residual mass in lymphoma may not be residual disease. J Clin Oncol 6:931–933
7. Carr R, Barrington SF, Madan B, O'Doherty MJ, Saunders CA, van der Walt J, Timothy R (1998) Detection of lymphoma in bone marrow by whole-body positron emission tomography. Blood 91:3340–3346
8. Cremerius U, Fabry U, Neuerburg J, Zimny M, Bares R, Osieka R, Büll U (2001) Prognostic significance of positron emission tomography using fluorine-18-fluorodeoxyglucose in patients treated for malignant lymphoma. Nuklearmedizin 40:23–30
9. De Wit M, Bumann D, Beyer W et al (1997) Whole-body positron emission tomography (PET) for diagnosis of residual mass in patients with lymphoma. Ann Oncol 8 [Suppl 1]:S57–S60
10. Döbert N, Menzel C, Berner U, Hamscho N, Diehl M, Wördehoff N, Mitrou P, Grünwald F Positron emission tomography in patients with Hodgkin's disease – correlation to histopathologic subtypes.
11. Engel H, Steinert H, Buck A, Berthold T, Huch Boni RA, von Schulthess GK (1996) Whole- body PET: physiological and artifactual fluorodeoxyglucose accumulations. J Nucl Med 37:441–446
12. Garcia JF, Camacho FI, Morente M, Fraga M, Montalban C, Alavaro T, Bellas C, Castano A, Diez A, Flores T, Martin C, Martinez MA, Mazorra F, Menarguez J, Mestre MJ, Mollejo M, Saez AI, Sanchez L, Piris MA (2003) Hodgkin's and Reed-Sternberg cells harbor alterations in the major tumor suppressor pathways and cell-cycle checkpoints: analyses using tissue-microarrays. Blood 101:601–609
13. Glatz S, Kotzerke J, Moog F et al (1996) Vortäuschung eines, mediastinalen Non-Hodgkin Lymphomrezidivs durch diffuse Thymushyperplasie. RöFo 165:309–310
14. Hany TF, Gharehpapagh E, Kamel EM, Buck A, Himms-Hagen J, von Schulthess GK (2002) Brown adipose tissue: a factor to consider in symmetrical tracer uptake in the neck and upper chest region. Eur J Nucl Med 29:1393–1398

15. Hodgkin T (1832) On some morbid appearances of the absobent glands and splen. Med Chir Trans 17:68
16. Hoffmann M, Kletter K, Diemling M, Becherer A, Pfeffel F, Petkov V, Chott A, Raderer M (1999) Positron emission tomography with fluorine-18-2-fluoro-2-deoxy-D-glucose (F18-FDG) does not visualize extranodal B-cell lymphoma of the mucosa-associated lymphoid tissue (MALT)-type. Ann Oncol 10:1185–1189
17. Hoh CK, Glaspy J, Rosen P et al (1997) Whoöe body FDG PET imaging for staging of Hodgkin's disease and lymphoma. J Nucl Med 38:343–348
18. Hueltenschmidt B, Sautter-Bihl ML, Lang O, Maul FD, Fischer J, Mergenthaler HG, Bihl H (2001) Whole body positron emission tomography in the treatment of Hodgkin disease. Cancer 91:302–310
19. Jaffe ES, Harris NL, Diebold J, Müller-Hermelink HK (1999) World Health Organization classification of neoplastic diseases of the hematopoietic and lymphoid tissues. Am J Clin Pathol 111:S8–S12
20. Jaffe ES, Harris NL, Stein H, Vardiman JW (2001) World Health Organization classification of tumours. Pathology and genetics of tumours of haematopoietic and lymphoid tissues. IARC Press, Lyon
21. Jerusalem G, Beguin Y, Fassotte MF et al (1999) Whole-body positron emission tomography using fluorine-18-fluorodeoxyglucose for post-treatment evaluation in Hodgkin's disease and non-Hodgkin's lymphoma has a higher diagnostic and prognostic value than classical computed tomography scan imaging. Blood 94:429–433
22. Jerusalem G, Beguin Y, Fassotte MF, Najjar F, Paulus P, Rigo P, Fillet G (2001) Whole-body positron emission tomography using 18F-fluorodeoxyglucose compared to standard procedures for staging patients with Hodgkin's disease. Haematologica 86: 266–273
23. Kato T, Tsukamoto E, Nishioka T, Yamazaki A, Shirato H, Kobayashi S, Asaka M, Imamura M, Tamaki N (2000) Early detection of bone marrow involvement in extramedullary plasmacytoma by whole-body F-18 FDG positron emission tomography. Clin Nucl Med 25:870–873
24. Kostakoglu L, Coleman M, Leonard JP, Kuji I, Zoe H, Goldsmith SJ (2002) PET predicts prognosis after 1 cycle of chemotherapy in aggressive lymphoma and Hodgkin's disease. J Nucl Med 43: 1018–1027
25. Lang O, Bihl H, Hultenschmidt B, Sautter-Bihl ML (2001) Clinical relevance of positron emission tomography (PET) in treatment control and relapse of Hodgkin's disease. Strahlenther Onkol 177:138–144
26. Lymphoma 2000 (2001) The first international symposium on biology and treatment of aggressive lymphomas. The stagnation seems to be over. Ann Hematol 80:B1–B2
27. Menzel C, Döbert N, Mitrou P, Mose S, Diehl M, Berner U, Grünwald F (2002) Positron emission tomography for the staging of Hodgkin's lymphoma. Acta Oncol 41:430–436
28. Montravers F, McNamara D, Landman-Parker J, Grahek D, Kerrou K, Younsi N, Wioland M, Leverger G, Talbot JN (2002) [18F] FDG in childhood lymphoma: clinical utility and impact on management. Eur J Nucl Med 29:1155–1165
29. Moog F, Bangerter M, Diederichs CG, Guhlmann A, Merkle E, Frickhofen N, Reske SN (1998) Extranodal malignant lymphoma: detection with FDG PET versus CT. Radiology 206:475–481
30. Moog F, Bangerter M, Diederichs C et al (1998) Extranodal malignant lymphoma: detection with FDG PET versus CT. Radiology 206:475–481
31. Moog F, Bangerter M, Kotzerke J, Guhlmann A, Frickhofen N, Reske SN (1998) 18-F-fluorodeoxyglucose-positron emission tomography as a new approach to detect lymphomatous bone marrow. J Clin Oncol 16:603–609
32. Orchard K, Barrington S, Buscombe J, Hilson A, Prentice HG, Mehta A (2002) Fluorodeoxy-glucose positron emission tomography imaging for the detection of occult disease in multiple myeloma. Br J Haematol 117:133–135
33. Partridge S, Timothy A, O'Doherty MJ, Hain SF, Rankin S, Mikhaeel G (2000) 2-Fluorine-18-fluoro-2-deoxy-D glucose positron emission tomography in the pretreatment staging of Hodgkin's disease: influence on patient management in a single institution. Ann Oncol 11:1273–1279
34. Paul R (1987) Comparison of fluorine-18-2-fluorodeoxyglucose and gallium-67 citrate imaging for the detection of lymphoma. J Nucl Med 28:288–292
35. Rabkin C, Devesa S, Zahm SH, Gail MH (1993) Increasing incidence of non-Hodgkin's lymphoma. Semin Hematol 30:286
36. Reske SN, Kotzerke J (2001) FDG-PET for clinical use. Eur J Nucl Med 28:1707–1723
37. Rini JN, Manalili EY, Hofmann MA, Karayalcin G, Mehrotra B, Tomas MB, Palestro CJ (2002) F-18 FDG versus Ga-67 for detecting splenic involvement in Hodgkin's disease. Clin Nucl Med 27:572–577
38. Rodriguez M, Ahlstrom H, Sundin A, Rehn S, Sundstrom C, Hagberg H, Glimelius B (1997) [18F] FDG PET in gastric non-Hodgkin's lymphoma. Acta Oncol 36:577–584
39. Romer W, Hanauske A, Ziegler S, Todtman R, Weber W, Fuchs C et al (1998) Positron emission tomography in non-Hodgkin's lymphoma: assessment of chemotherapy with fluorodeoxyglucose. Blood 91:4464–4471
40. Sasaki M, Kuwabara Y, Koga H, Nakagawa M, Chen T, Kaneko K, Hyashi K, Nakamura K, Masuda K (2002) Clinical impact of whole body FDG-PET on the staging and therapeutic decision making for malignant lymphoma. Ann Nucl Med 16:337–345
41. Schöder H, Meta J, Yap C, Ariannejad M, Rao J, Phelps ME, Valk PE, Sayre J, Czernin J (2001) Effect of whole-body (18)F-FDG PET imaging on clinical staging and management of patients with malignant lymphoma. J Nucl Med 42:1139–1143
42. Spaepen K, Stroobants S, Dupont P, Thomas J, Vandenberghe P, Balzarini J, de Wolf-Peeters C, Mortelmans L, Verhoef G (2001) Can positron emission tomography with [(18)F]-fluorodeoxyglucose after first-line treatment distinguish Hodgkin's disease patients who need additional therapy from others in whom additional therapy would mean avoidable toxicity? Br J Haematol 115:272–278
43. Spaepen K, Stroobants S, Dupont P, Vandenberghe P, Thomas J, de Groot T, Balzarini J, De Wolf-Peeters C, Mortelmans L, Verhoef G (2002) Early restaging positron emission tomography with 18F-fluorodeoxglucose predicts outcome in patients with aggressive non-Hodgkin's lymphoma. Ann Oncol 13:1356–1363
44. Spaepen K, Stroobants S, Dupont P et al (2001) Prognostic value of positron emission tomography with fluorine-18 fluorodeoxyglucose after first line chemotherapy in non-Hodgkin's lymphoma: is [18F]FDG-PET a valid alternative to conventional diagnostic methods? J Clin Oncol 19:414–419
45. Stark GL, Wood KM, Jack F, Angus B, Proctor SJ, Taylor PR (2002) Hodgkin's disease in the elderly: a population-based study. Br J Haematol 119:432–440
46. Stumpe KDM, Urbinelli M, Steinert HC, Glanzmann C, Buck A, von Schulthess GK (1998) Whole-body positron emission tomography using fluorodeoxyglucose for staging of lymphoma: effectiveness and comparison with computed tomography. Eur J Nucl Med 25:721–728
47. The international Non-Hodgkin's Lmyphoma Prognostic Factors Project (1993) A predictive model for aggressive non-Hodgkin's lymphoma. N Engl J Med 329:987–994
48. Thomas F, Cosset JM, Cherel P et al (1988) Thoracis CT: scanning follow-up of residual masses after treatment of Hodgkin's disease. Radiother Oncol 11:119–122
49. Van den Bossche B, Lambert B, De Winter F, Kolindou A, Dierckx RA, Noens L, van de Wiele C (2002) 18FDG PET versus high-dose 68 Ga scintigraphy for restaging and treatment follow-up of lymphoma patients. Nucl Med Commun 23:1079–1083
50. Weihrauch MR, Re D, Bischoff S, Dietlein M, Scheidhauer K, Krug B, Textoris F, Ansen S, Franklin J, Bohlen H, Wolf J, Schicha H, Diehl V, Tesch H (2002) Whole-body positron emission tomography using 18F-fluorodeoxyglucose for initial staging of patients with Hodgkin's disease. Ann Hematol 81:20–25
51. WHO/IARC cancer mortality statistics, database 2000
52. Wiedmann E, Baican B, Hertel A, Baum RP, Chow KU, Knupp B, Adams S, Hor G, Hoelzer D, Mitrou PS (1999) Positron emission tomography (PET) for staging and evaluation of response to treatment in patients with Hodgkin's disease. Leuk Lymphoma 34:545–551

53. Wolf J, Franklin J, Diehl V (2000) Primärtherapie des Morbus Hodgkin. Onkologe 6:1169–1177
54. Wun LM (1992) Hodgkin'disease. In: Miller BA, Ries LAG, Hankey BF (eds) Cancer statistics review 1973–1989. NIH Publ no 92–2789
55. Zinzani PL, Chierichetti F, Zompatori M, Tani M, Stefoni V, Garraffa G, Albertini P, Alinari L, Ferlin G, Baccarani M, Tura S (2002) Advantages of positron emission tomography (PET) with respect to computed tomography in the follow-up of lymphoma patients with abdominal presentation. Leuk Lymphoma 43:1239–1243

CHAPTER 27

Musculoskeletal Tumors

A.K. Buck · H. Schirrmeister · S.N. Reske

The majority of bone tumors correspond to bone metastases from extraskeletal malignancies. In contrast primary malignant bone or soft tissue tumors are rare events. A high prevalence of bone manifestations is further on present in plasma cell neoplasms. This chapter gives an overview of the clinical data of FDG-PET for diagnosis and management of these tumors.

27.1 Incidence, Etiology, Epidemiology

27.1.1 Primary Musculoskeletal Tumors

Primary tumors originating from soft tissue or bone comprise various tumor entities with different grades of malignancy, biological behavior and therapeutic options. The incidence of malignant soft tissue tumors is 2–3 per 100.000 and 1 per 100.000 for primary malignant bone tumors. Approximately 7800 new cases with soft tissue sarcoma and 2600 primary bone tumors are diagnosed per year in the USA [1]. Compared to epithelial derived solid cancers these tumors are less frequently observed and account for 0.6% of all malignant tumors.

Soft tissue sarcomas can appear in the entire body with a majority arising from muscles of the extremities, retroperitoneum, chest wall or mediastinum. Some tumor entities demonstrate a typical age distribution (Table 1). Neuroblastoma, for example, occurs exclusively in childhood, whereas malignant fibrous histiocytoma or liposarcoma commonly appear predominantly in the 5th and 6th decade. Characteristic age distributions and preferential localization sites were also described for malignant bone tumors (Table 2). Osteosarcoma and Ewing's sarcoma are most frequently found in children and young adults whereas the majority of chondrosarcomas occur after the 4th decade.

Most musculoskeletal tumors have no clearly defined etiology but some predisposing factors have been identified. Alterations in the retinoblastoma gene (RB) and the tumor suppressor gene p53 are frequently observed

Table 1. Classification of soft tissue sarcomas

Histologic subtype	Relative frequency	Preferential age	Primary manifestation site
Fibrosarcoma	10%	30–50	Extremities, trunk
Malignant fibrous histiocytoma (MFH)	20–30%	50–70	Proximal extremities, retroperitoneum
Liposarcoma	15–18%	40–60	70% lower extremities, retroperitoneum
Leiomyosarcoma	7%	50–60	Retroperitoneum, cutis, subcutis of lower extremities
Rhabdomyosarcoma			
Embryonal	14%	7–11	Head and neck, urogenital
Alveolar	4%	15–25	Extremities, head and neck
Pleomorphic	1%	40–60	Extremities, urogenital
Angiosarcoma	<1%	50–70	Cutis and subcutis of the head, lower extremities
Synovial sarcoma	8–10%	20–35	Joints of lower extremities, preferentially extraarticular
Malignant schwannoma (MPNST)	5–10%	25–50	Trunk, proximal extremities
Neuroblastoma	10–12%	1–2	40% adrenal gland, retroperitoneum, sympathetic ganglia
Primitive neuroectodermal tumor (PNET)	1%	15–35	Trunk, lower extremities
Extraskeletal Ewing's Sarcoma	rare	10–30	30% preferentially lower extremities, 30% paravertebral, 15% chest wall

Table 2. Classification of malignant bone tumors

Histologic subtype	Relative frequency	Preferential age	Primary manifestation site
Osteosarcoma			
Central	24%	10–20	80% long bones, 45% knee, 10% humerus
Periosteal	0.2%	10–20	diaphysis of tibia/femur
Parosteal	1%	15–40	metaphysis of lower extremities, 65% femur
Chondrosarcoma			
Classic	13%	30–60	Trunk, pelvis, prox. extremities, facial bones
Dedifferentiated	1%	50–80	Similar to classic variant
Clear-cell	rare	30–40	Epiphysis of long bones
Mesenchymal	rare	20–40	Entire skeleton
Malignant giant cell tumor	0.5%	20–40	Epiphysis of long bones (knee region)
Fibrosarcoma	3.3%	15–60	Entire skeleton
Malignant fibrous histio-cytoma (MFH)	1.6%	10–70	Long bones
Ewing's sarcoma	6.6%	10–20	Entire skeleton, preferentially diaphyses of long bones
Malignant lymphoma of bone	6.6%	20–70	Entire skeleton, preferentially lower extremities and trunk
Plasmacytoma, multiple myeloma	40%	40–70	Skull, spine, pelvis, prox. extremities; extramedullary in 5%

in sarcomas [2, 3]. Unlike malignant epithelial tumors, those entities do not arise from in situ changes or benign tumors. Patients with a history of external beam irradiation have an increased risk for developing bone or soft tissue sarcoma. In a retrospective study, various sarcomas such as malignant fibrous histiocytoma, angiosarcoma and osteosarcoma were described in patients following radiation therapy [4]. For certain entities viral factors (e.g. Kaposi sarcoma) are discussed.

27.1.2 Multiple Myeloma and Plasmacytoma

Multiple myeloma accounts for approximately 10% of hematological malignancies with a peak incidence in the 7th decade [1]. Commonly, the bone marrow is infiltrated with clonal, proliferating plasma cells. The release of paracrine factors like IL-6 by myeloma cells activates osteoclasts and leads to an increasing bone demineralization and hypercalcaemia. Approximately 10% of the patients have a solitary manifestation of myeloma which can appear either as extramedullary plasmacytoma or solitary plasmacytoma of bone.

27.1.3 Secondary Bone Tumors

Bone metastases are more frequently observed than primary bone tumors. The majority of bone metastases are related to breast, thyroid, lung, renal and prostate cancer. In autopsy studies, the incidence of bone metastases was 33–85% in prostate cancer, 30–55% in bronchogenic and 47–85% in breast cancer [5].

27.2 Histopathological Classification

Soft tissue sarcomas are malignant tumors evolving from connective tissue, muscle or peripheral nerves. An abbreviated list of the most relevant tumor entities is shown in Table 1.

Bone tumors are classified on the basis of respective cell type and the product of proliferating cells. 20% of malignant primary tumors are chondrogenic (chondrosarcoma), 40% hematopoietic (myeloma), 18% osteogenic (osteosarcoma) and 4% fibrogenic (fibrosarcoma). For Ewing's sarcoma the histologic origin is unknown. Vascular derived malignomas like hemangiopericytoma and hemangioendothelioma account for only 1.6% of soft tissue sarcomas (Table 2).

Grading of the primary tumor is an important prerequisite for choice of therapy and estimation of prognosis. Four grades of differentiation are defined for musculoskeletal tumors: grade 1 (well differentiated), grade 2 (intermediate), grade 3 (poor), and grade 4 (undifferentiated). Ewing's sarcoma and primary lymphoma of bone are generally classified as grade 4. Malignant bone and soft tissue tumors metastasize hematogenously to the lungs and skeleton. Intraosseous metastases of osteosarcoma, so called 'skip lesions', are a typical but less frequently observed event.

Plasma cell neoplasms comprise several tumor entities characterized by clonal proliferation. They share common features as plasma cell morphology, production of immunoglobulins and immune dysfunction. Dysfunctional plasma cells can secrete either the immunoglobulin IgA, IgG, IgE, IgD or IgM. The excessive production of free light chain molecules leads to their urinary excretion (Bence-Jones proteinuria).

Based on their appearance on radiographs bone metastases can be differentiated in osteoblastic, osteolytic and mixed type. Predominantly osteolytic metastases are observed in patients with thyroid, bronchogenic or renal cancer. Osteoblastic metastases are typical in prostate cancer. Bone metastases are most frequently localized in the vertebral column, thorax, pelvis, proximal femur or humerus. In contrast to other cancers, bone metastases from thyroid cancer occur frequently solitary in the flat bones such as the skull, pelvis or ribs.

27.3 Conventional Diagnostic Procedures and Treatment Strategies

27.3.1 Musculoskeletal Tumors

Multimodal treatment protocols including chemotherapy, radiotherapy and surgery are used for high grade sarcomas whereas surgery is the therapy of choice for low-grade tumors. Pretherapeutic imaging is performed to evaluate the exact extent of the local tumor, to assess the dignity of the process and to screen for distant metastases. Contrast enhanced spiral CT and MRI are standard techniques for the evaluation of the extent of the primary tumor, vascularisation, invasiveness and integrity of surrounding tissue. CT of the thorax is generally recommended since pulmonary metastases were often missed on planar radiographs.

Bone scintigraphy is the standard imaging modality for estimation of the local extent of the primary tumor and for exclusion of bone metastases. Prior to biopsy and operative resection performance of angiography provides detailed information about the vascularization of the tumor. Alkaline phosphatase is commonly elevated in malignant bone tumors. However, laboratory tests are often unspecific.

Incisional biopsy is mandatory to obtain the histopathological diagnosis. For exact information, vascularized tumor tissue with a size of $1 \times 2 \times 2$ cm has to be excised. In certain tumors such as Ewing's sarcoma or Non-Hodgkin's lymphoma bone marrow biopsy is recommended for the exclusion of bone marrow infiltration.

27.3.2 Plasmacytoma

True solitary plasmacytoma can be cured with local radiotherapy. Indolent myeloma patients are typically not treated with chemotherapy until they become symptomatic. Palliative chemotherapy is performed when progression to symptomatic myeloma occurs including lytic bone lesions and high serum myeloma protein levels. Because of their osteolytic appearance with low osteosclerotic bone reaction technetium bone scans are regarded as less sensitive in detecting myeloma associated bone lesions [6]. Commonly radiographs of the skull, thorax, spine, pelvis and long bones are performed for staging of the skeleton. However, the superior sensitivity of MRI over planar radiographs for detection of vertebral myeloma lesions has been proven recently by Lecouvet and coworkers [7]. Moulopoulos [8] reported that additional foci are revealed by MRI at the vertebral column in one third of patients considered to have solitary plasmacytoma. In the series reported by Lecouvet and coworkers MRI of the vertebral column and pelvis showed a higher extent of disease in 34% of patients with stage III multiple myeloma [7]. Disadvantages of MRI making this technique impracticable for routine whole-body surveys are motion artifacts at the ribs and the long imaging time. Substitution of planar radiographs by an MRI imaging survey limited to the spine and pelvis would have caused understaging in 10% of patients in Lecouvet's series [7].

27.3.3 Bone Metastases

Multiple therapeutic options are available for the management of metastatic bone disease. Besides local radiation therapy and surgery, systemic therapies can be performed including chemotherapy, bone marrow transplantation, hormone therapy, immunotherapy and medication with bisphosphonates. Bone scanning using ^{99m}Tc-labeled polyphosphonates has been demonstrated to reveal bone lesions several months before they become apparent on conventional radiographs but is considered less sensitive in osteolytic compared to osteosclerotic metastases. For detection of osteolytic metastases, bone marrow scintigraphy, CT and MRI were shown to be clearly more sensitive [9, 10]. MRI was shown to be more precise than CT in detecting bone metastases [9]. Recently it was reported that bone scans provide a sufficient sensitivity in detecting bone lesions in the peripheral skeleton but are significantly less sensitive in detecting vertebral lesions [11]. Hence, substitution of conventional bone scans with SPECT improved the sensitivity in detecting bone metastases significantly [12]. In a study by Kosuda et al. [13] routine SPECT was as sensitive as MRI for detection of vertebral metastases. Both MRI and CT are impracticable for whole-body imaging [9]. At present MRI is used to clarify indeterminate lesions detected with bone scintigraphy. Planar X-ray and CT are not useful for the screening of metastatic bone disease but are adequate for estimating fracture risk and for confirmation of metastases detected with bone scintigraphy.

27.4
Positron Emission Tomography

27.4.1
Staging of Primary Bone and Soft Tissue Tumors

First results for differential diagnosis and staging of bone tumors with PET were published 1988 by Kern and coworkers [14]. Several studies confirmed the opportunity to differentiate benign from malignant bone tumors with PET (15–21, Figs. 1, 2). Accurate differentiation of high grade from low grade and benign tumors and a close correlation between the FDG-uptake and tumor grading was reported in the vast majority of studies [14–21]. Additionally, FDG-PET can improve selection of the optimal site for tumor biopsy by determination of the most aggressive region. However, FDG-PET is inadequate to discriminate between low grade malignant lesions and benign tumors. Furthermore, false positive PET-findings were reported in aggressive benign tumors and in inflammatory lesions. Therefore, histopathological tissue analysis cannot be replaced by PET. In a study from Schulte et al. [22] bone tumors with a tumor to background ratio >3.0 were defined as malignant and <1.5 as benign. This definition resulted in a sensitivity of 93% and a specificity of 67% for detecting malignant bone tumors. For soft tissue tumors similar sensitivity and specificity values of 97% and 66% were reported [21].

The accuracy of PET in detecting distant metastases was evaluated in 71 patients with primary bone tumors [23]. The sensitivity in detecting lung metastases was as low as 50% (specificity 98%) with PET and 75% (specificity 100%) with spiral CT. However, FDG-PET was superior to bone scintigraphy in detecting bone metastases (sensitivity 100%, specificity 96%, for bone scintigraphy 68% and 87%) [24].

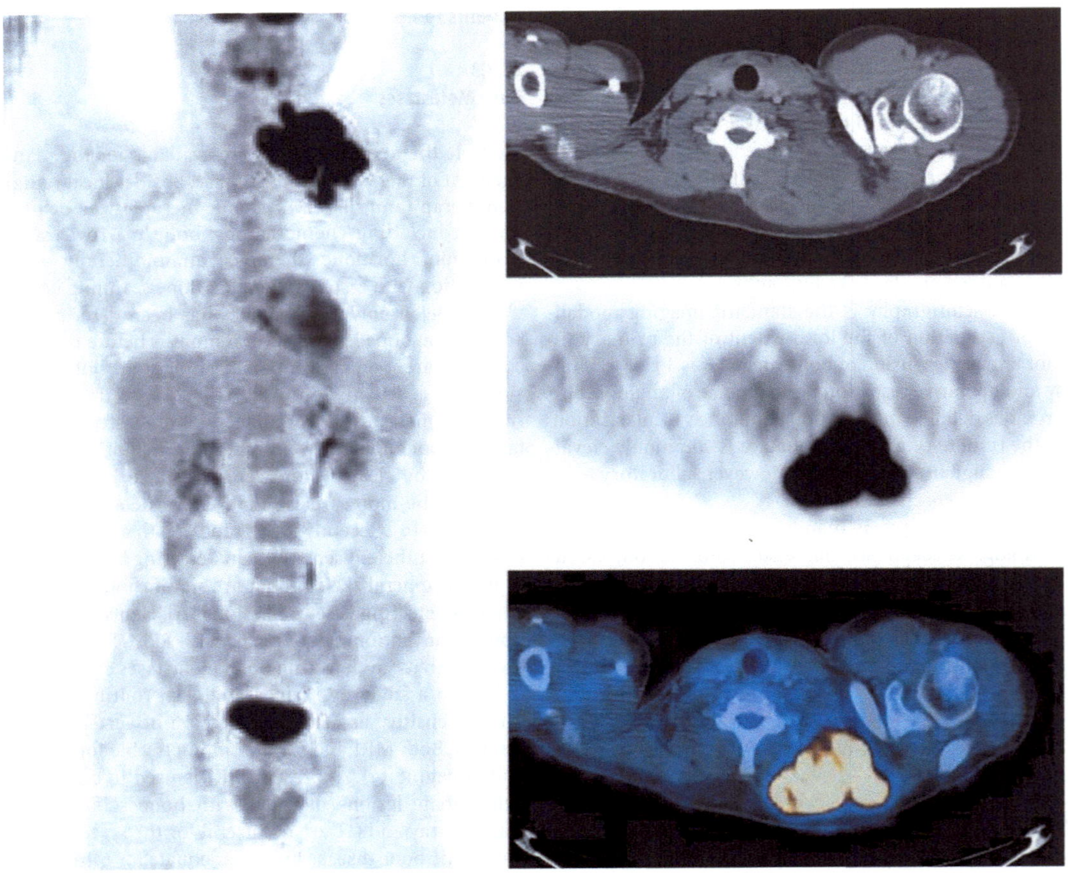

Fig. 1. Spiral CT shows a hypodense tumor in the left neck of a 25-year-old patient. FDG-PET demonstrates increased tracer accumulation of the entire lesion. Histopathology revealed rhabdomyosarcoma grade 3 (*left*: maximum intensity projection of FDG-PET, *upper right*: spiral CT, transaxial section; *middle right*: FDG-PET, transaxial section; *lower right*: image fusion)

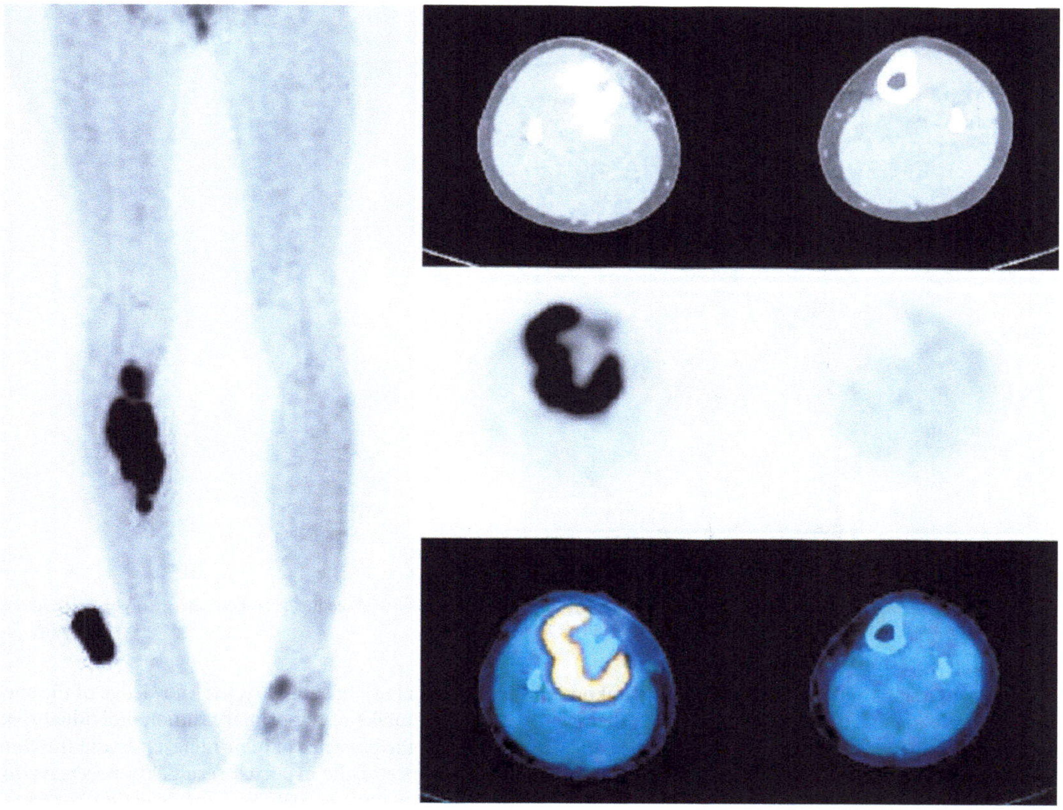

Fig. 2. A 23-year-old female patient reported new onset of bone pain and soft tissue swelling at the right tibia. Histopathology revealed osteosarcoma grade 3. Intense tumoral FDG-uptake as demonstrated by image fusion (*left*: maximum intensity projection of FDG-PET, *upper right*: spiral CT, transaxial section; middle right: FDG-PET, transaxial section; *lower right*: image fusion)

27.4.2
Therapy Control

Assessment of therapy response after neoadjuvant chemotherapy is a major factor for determination of the therapeutic strategy and estimation of prognosis in malignant bone or soft tissue tumors. Several preliminary studies (9–30 patients per study) reported decreased FDG-uptake in musculoskeletal tumors responsive to chemotherapy [16, 25–28]. Consecutively, they suggested that early discrimination between responders and non-responders with PET could be useful to adjust the therapeutic regimen in non-responders. However, large prospective clinical trials have to be performed before a definite conclusion concerning the use of PET for therapy control can be drawn.

27.4.3
Recurrent Disease

For soft tissue sarcoma several authors reported possible detection of recurrent disease with FDG-PET [29–32]. Garcia and coworkers reported a sensitivity of 98% and a specificity of 90% for detection of recurrent disease in 48 patients with bone or soft tissue sarcomas [33]. In another study recurrent osseous sarcoma was detected with a sensitivity of 96% and a specificity of 81% [34]. In the latter study PET was as sensitive as the combination of MRT, spiral CT and whole-body bone scintigraphy.

27.4.4
Plasmacytoma and Multiple Myeloma

To date, only two groups evaluated glucose utilization in plasma cell neoplasms with FDG-PET [35,36]. In our own series FDG-PET was true positive in 91,2% of radiographically detected osteolytic lesions and indicated a higher extent of disease compared to planar radiographs in 11 out of 23 patients (47,8%) with osteolytic bone lesions (Fig. 3). The potential of detecting medullary and extramedullary lesions in one single examination is an important advantage over x-ray, CT or MRI. In extramedullary multiple myeloma FDG-PET was true positive in all out of

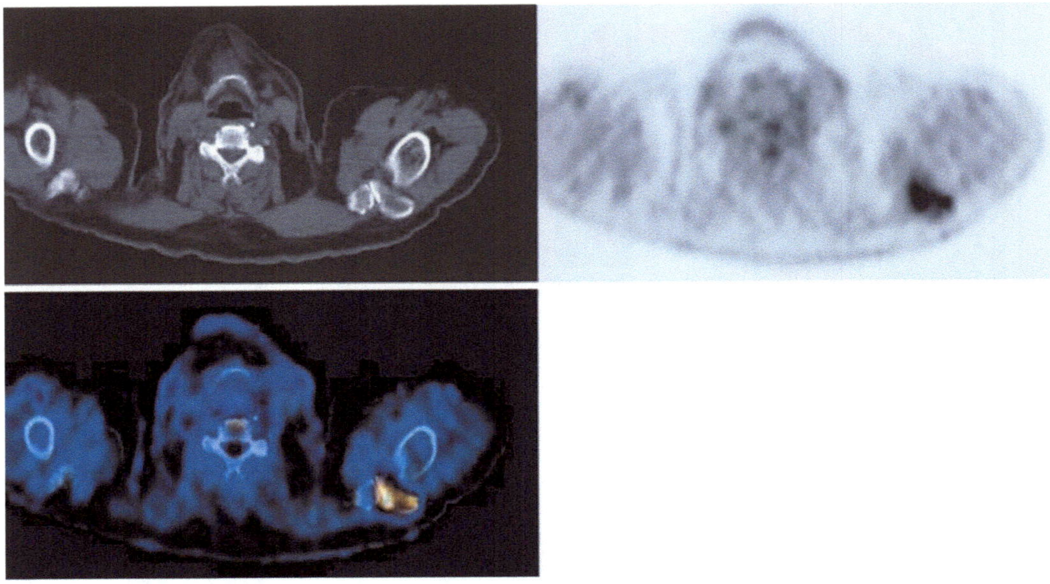

Fig. 3. A 53-year-old patient with newly diagnosed multiple myeloma. Spiral CT (transaxial section, *left*) shows an osteolytic lesion in the left acromion; *middle*: intense FDG-uptake within the lesion; *right*: image fusion

5 pre-known lesions and revealed 5 previously unknown lesions in 2 patients. As a result of FDG-PET, therapeutic management was influenced in 5 (14%) of the patients and was potentially influenced in further 2 patients.

27.4.5 Secondary Bone Tumors

For detection of bone metastases from breast cancer Cook [37] reported an intense uptake of FDG in osteolytic metastases whereas osteoblastic metastases presented with significantly lower FDG-uptake. In an own series of 117 patients [38] with newly diagnosed breast cancer, bone metastases were correctly detected with bone scintigraphy and FDG-PET (Fig. 4). In this study the incidence of bone metastases was as low as 2%. Due to the low incidence at initial diagnosis the different sensitivity in detecting osteolytic or osteoblastic bone metastases, as described by Cook et al. [37], seems not relevant at primary staging.

In 34 patients with bone metastases from prostate cancer only 131 from 202 metastases were correctly detected (sensitivity 65%) with PET [39]. The limited sensitivity was suggested to be related to the generally lower FDG-uptake in osteoblastic metastases and to the limited glucose utilization of the primary tumor.

Different glucose metabolism of bone metastases were also reported in primary bone tumors. In a series of 70 patients the sensitivity of PET for detection of bone metastases from Ewing's sarcoma was significantly higher than for detection of bone metastases from osteosarcoma [24]. In summary, the knowledge of the specific FDG-uptake of the primary tumor, individual risk factors for the presence of bone metastases and the clinical relevance of the expected results are necessary to determine the use of FDG-PET for detecting bone metastases.

27.5 Judgment of Indications for FDG-PET

Estimation of the clinical value of FDG-PET for the assessment of musculoskeletal tumors is difficult due to the heterogeneity of tumor entities. In 2000, the 3rd German interdisciplinary consensus conference considered five publications which examined a total of 301 patients [40]. For differentiation of benign from malignant tumors and determination of the biological aggressiveness PET was judged to have a probable clinical use (classified as 1b). For T-Staging, morphologically based imaging techniques such as spiral CT and MRI provide detailed information about tumor size, invasiveness and integrity of proximate normal tissues and are therefore more suitable for T-Staging than PET. Encouraging results implicate the ability of FDG-PET for the accurate determination of tumor viability after chemotherapy but yet there are only limited data which do not justify a definite judgment of the usefulness of FDG-PET. Also, in a tabulated summary of the PET literature the authors conclude that the number of data is yet too small to describe the evidence of FDG-PET for disease management [41]. Therefore clinical studies with large

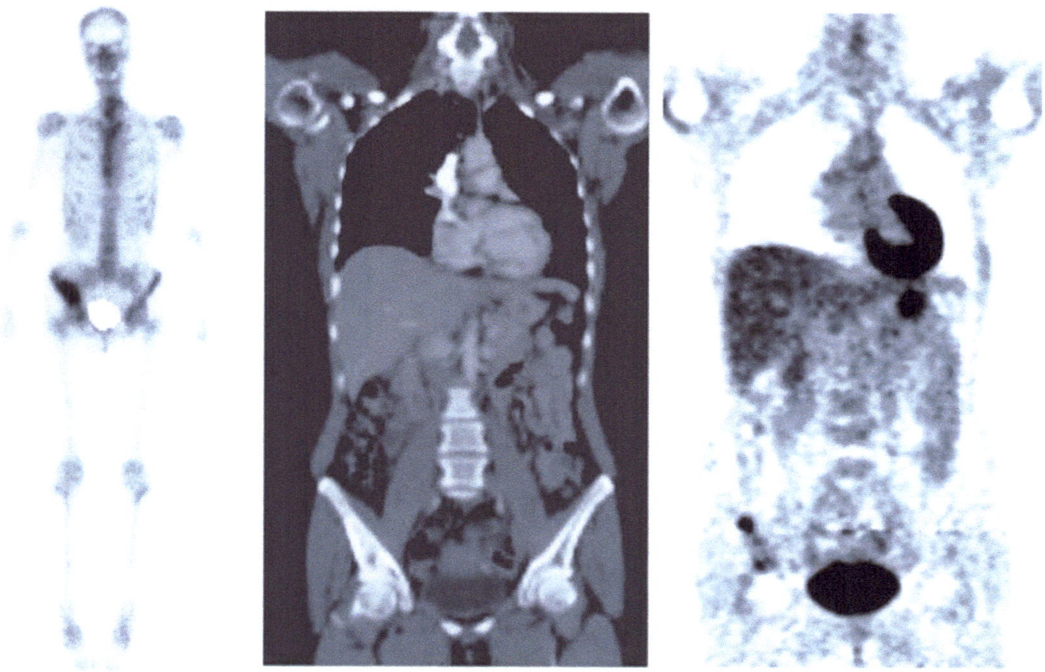

Fig. 4. Bone scan (*left*) of a 42-year-old female patient with a history of breast cancer shows focal tracer uptake in the right iliac bone. Spiral CT (coronal section) displays an osteolytic lesion (*middle*). Intense FDG-accumulation at the margin of the lesion (coronal section, *right*). Biopsy revealed a solitary bone metastasis

patient numbers are needed to further clarify the potential benefits of FDG-PET in these indications.

27.6 New Tracer Developments

FDG-PET proved efficient for visualization of malignant bone and soft tissue tumors but may also visualize benign lesions. Therefore, efforts had been made to develop innovative tracers which are more specific for malignant tumors. ^{11}C labeled thymidine analogs were introduced in the early 1990's for specific imaging of proliferative activity. However, due to the short half life of ^{11}C and decreased in-vivo stability this tracer was estimated to be of less utility for clinical routine studies. Recently, an ^{18}F labeled thymidine analog, ^{18}F-FLT was introduced to clinical medicine [42]. To date, there are no data available to estimate the diagnostic accuracy of FLT-PET for assessment of musculoskeletal tumors. In a first clinical trial soft tissue and bone tumors could be visualized with FLT (unpublished data, Fig. 5). However, preferential assessment of proliferative activity with FLT remains to be determined.

Another approach is the use of radiolabeled amino acids [43] such as tyrosine (^{18}F-FMT). In 75 cases with musculoskeletal tumors, Watanabe [44] reported that FMT is equally efficient for imaging sarcoma and exhibited a better specificity compared to FDG (85 vs 66%, respectively). In contrast to FDG-PET, there was no correlation between FMT-uptake and tumor grading.

Recently, high accuracy values for detection of bone metastases were reported for ^{18}F fluoride PET which are discussed in chapter 28.

27.7 Summary and Outlook

Due to the low incidence of primary musculoskeletal tumors and the heterogeneity of this group only limited data are available to estimate the clinical use of FDG-PET. Judgment of useful clinical applications is further complicated by the multitude of tumor entities. However, FDG-PET proved accurate for differentiation of low grade from high grade sarcomas. Therefore, preoperative analysis of glucose metabolism can help to choose the appropriate therapeutic regimen. Additionally, accuracy of incisional biopsy can be enhanced by detection of tumor areas with the highest metabolic activity.

The high sensitivity of FDG-PET for detecting primary tumors implicates a similar relevance for the detection of skip lesions, lymph node and distant metastases. For detection of primary bone tumors, FDG-PET

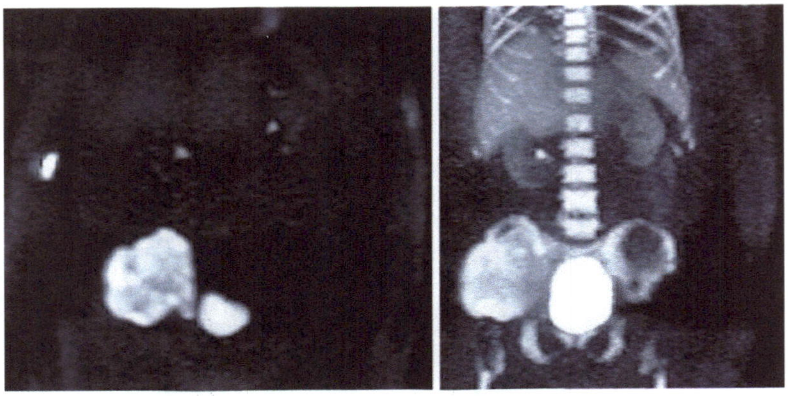

Fig. 5. Osteosarcoma of the right iliac bone in a 28-year-old patient. Intense tumoral FDG-uptake (maximum intensity projection, *left*). The *right* image shows a maximum intensity projection of F-18 FLT-PET with additional visualization of the proliferating bone marrow in the vertebral column, pelvis and thorax

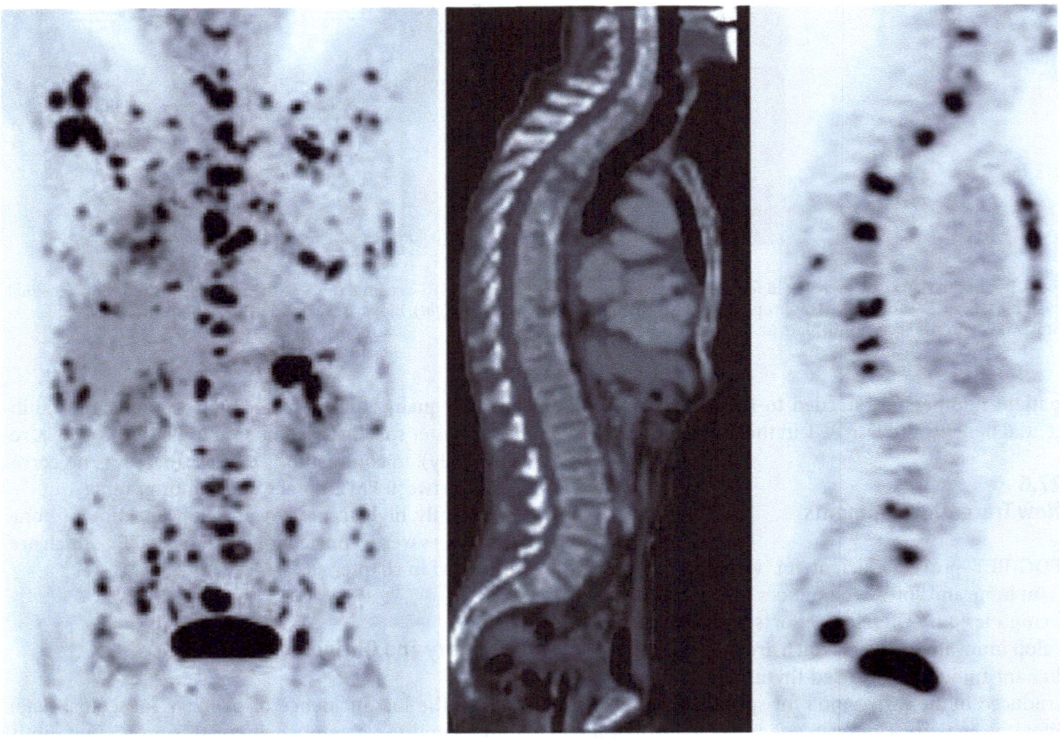

Fig. 6. A 49-year-old patient with non-small cell lung cancer in the right upper lobe. FDG-PET shows disseminated osseous metastases (*left*: maximum intensity projection; *middle right*: spiral CT, sagittal section; *right*: FDG-PET, sagittal section)

was superior compared to bone scintigraphy. However, large clinical trials are needed to prove the diagnostic accuracy of FDG-PET compared to the standard staging modalities.

Imaging glucose utilization is a unique tool to discriminate between scar tissue and vital tumor tissue. In several studies, PET was useful for early detection of local recurrence in soft tissue sarcoma. Additionally, PET can be used for evaluation of therapy response after chemo- or radiotherapy. Consequently the therapeutic regimen can be modified or started at an earlier stage of the disease. This possibility is especially useful in patients with Ewing's sarcoma or osteosarcoma since only patients responsive to neoadjuvant therapy benefit from a limb salvage procedure. Hence, FDG-PET might play an increasing role for therapy control of musculoskeletal tumors [45]. Another advantage of PET over standard tomographic imaging modalities is that follow-up examinations are not compromised by artifacts caused by metal implants and other osteosynthetic materials. A promising role of FDG-PET can be expected in staging multiple myeloma and plasmacytoma. Furthermore, FDG-PET proved to be highly sensitive in detecting distant metastases from various malignancies (Fig. 6).

However, limitations are the differentiation of low grade malignant from benign tumors and a probably lower sensitivity in detecting osteosclerotic bone metastases from extraskeletal malignancies with FDG. The accuracy of PET may be increased by using more selective biomarkers such as ^{18}F fluoride, ^{18}F-FMT and ^{18}F-FLT.

27.8 Technical Recommendations

27.8.1 Patient Preparation

Patients should be fasted for at least 8 hours. Blood glucose level should be lower than 130 mg/dl. To prevent unspecific tracer uptake in the muscle, patients should rest during the waiting period. In the case of tumor localization in the upper extremity, tracer has to be injected at the opposite arm. The needle should be removed after tracer administration.

27.8.2 Positioning

For assessment of the lower extremities, legs should rest in a straight position to exclude movement related artifacts. For thoracic imaging, arms should be placed in an elevated position. If the primary tumor is localized in the upper extremity, the arms should be positioned straight next to the body.

27.8.3 Radiopharmaceutical

Standard radiopharmaceutical is the glucose analog 2-[18F]-2-deoxy-D-glucose (FDG). A single dose of 370 MBq is sufficient for whole body imaging.

27.8.4 Data Acquisition

60 min after injection of FDG, static acquisition of upper or lower extremities is recommended. In primary bone tumors, both adjacent joints have to be included for exclusion of skip lesions. Additionally, PET imaging of the thorax is necessary to exclude pulmonary metastases in primary bone or soft tissue tumors. The PET scan should cover the skull, trunk and the upper legs in patients with multiple myeloma or with skeletal metastases.

27.8.5 Attenuation Correction/Image Reconstruction

An iterative reconstruction algorithm is recommended. Transmission scanning should be performed to allow quantitative analysis of the FDG-uptake within the lesion.

27.8.6 Image Evaluation and Interpretation (Qualitative and Quantitative Analysis)

When available, the PET scans should be interpreted in combination with all available morphological imaging modalities (CT, MRI, X-ray and ultrasound). For qualitative analysis, the intensity and shape of the lesion has to be interpreted and its localization defined as soft tissue, bone or bone marrow (medullary cavity). Semiquantitative analysis of the glucose uptake of the primary tumor using standardized uptake values or tumor to background ratios are helpful for therapy monitoring.

27.8.7 Pitfalls

Moderate FDG-uptake can be observed in the epiphyseal growth plates in children and must not be misinterpreted as malignant. In diabetic patients tumoral FDG-uptake may be reduced. Patients using crutches before the examination may present with intense FDG-uptake in muscles of the shoulder region.

References

1. Landis SH, Murray T, Bolden S, Wingo PA (1999) Cancer statistics, 1999. CA Cancer J Clin 49:8–31
2. Cance WG, Brennan MF, Dudas ME, Huang CM, Cordon-Cardo C (1990) Altered expression of the retinoblastoma gene product in human sarcomas. N Engl J Med 323:1457–1462
3. Latres E, Drobnjak M, Pollack D, Oliva MR, Ramos M, Karpeh M, Woodruff JM, Cordon-Cardo C (1994) Chromosome 17 abnormalities and TP53 mutations in adult soft tissue sarcomas. Am J Pathol 145:345–355
4. Brady MS, Gaynor JJ, Brennan MF (1992) Radiation-associated sarcoma of bone and soft tissue. Arch Surg 127:1379–1385
5. Rubens RD, Fogelman I (1991) Bone metastases. Springer, Berlin Heidelberg New York
6. Watanabe N, Shimizu M, Kageyama M, Tanimura K, Kinuya S, Shuke N, Yokoyama K, Tonami N, Watanabe A, Seto H, Goodwin DA (1999) Multiple myeloma evaluated with 201Tl scintigraphy compared with bone scintigraphy. J Nucl Med 40:1138–1142
7. Lecouvet FE, Malghem J, Michaux L, Maldague B, Ferrant A (1999) Skeletal survey in advanced multiple myeloma: radiographic versus MR imaging survey. Br J Haemtol 106:35–39
8. Moulopoulos LA, Varma DG, Dimopoulos MA, Leeds NE, Kim EE, Johnston DA, Alexanian R, Libshitz HI (1992) Multiple myeloma: spinal MR imaging in patients with untreated newly diagnosed disease. Radiology 185:833–840
9. Frank JA, Ling A, Patronas NJ, Carrasquillo JA, Horvath K, Hickey AM, Dwyer AJ (1990) Detection of malignant bone tumors: MR imaging vs scintigraphy. AJR Am J Roentgenol 155: 1043–1048

10. Venz S, Hosten N, Friedrichs R, Neumann K, Cordes M, Nagel R, Felix R (1994) Osteoplastic bone metastases in prostatic carcinoma: magnetic resonance tomography and bone marrow scintigraphy (in German). Röfo – Fortschr Rontgenstr 161:64–69
11. Schirrmeister H, Glatting G, Hetzel J, Nussle K, Arslandemir C, Buck AK, Dziuk K, Gabelmann A, Reske SN, Hetzel M (2001) Prospective evaluation of the clinical value of planar bone scans, SPECT, and (18)F-labeled NaF PET in newly diagnosed lung cancer. J Nucl Med 42:1800–1804
12. Sedonja I, Budihna NV (1999) The benefit of SPECT when added to planar scintigraphy in patients with bone metastases in the spine. Clin Nucl Med 24:407–413
13. Kosuda S, Kaji T, Yokoyama H, Yokokawa T, Katayama M, Iriye T, Uematsu M, Kusano S (1996) Does bone SPECT actually have lower sensitivity for detecting vertebral metastasis than MRI? J Nucl Med 37:975–978
14. Kern KA, Brunetti A, Norton JA, Chang AE, Malawer M, Lack E, Finn RD, Rosenberg SA, Larson SM (1988) Metabolic imaging of human extremity musculoskeletal tumors by PET. J Nucl Med 29:181–186
15. Adler LP, Blair HF, Markley JT, Wiliams RP, Joyce MJ, Leisure G, al-Kaisi N, Miraldi F (1991) Noninvasive Grading of musculoskeletal tumors using PET. J Nucl Med 32:1508–1512
16. Kole AC, Plaat BE, Hoekstra HJ, Vaalburg W, Molenaar WM (1999) FDG and L-[1-11C]-tyrosine imaging of soft-tissue tumors before and after therapy. J Nucl Med 40:381–386
17. Eary JF, Conrad EU, Bruckner JD, Folpe A, Hunt KJ, Mankoff DA, Howlett AT (1998) Quantitative [F-18]fluorodeoxyglucose positron emission tomography in pretreatment and grading of sarcoma. Clin Cancer Res 4:1215–1220
18. Lodge MA, Lucas JD, Marsden PK, Cronin BF, O'Doherty MJ, Smith MA (1999) A PET study of 18FDG uptake in soft tissue masses. Eur J Nucl Med 26:22–30
19. Lucas JD, O'Doherty MJ, Cronin BF, Marsden PK, Lodge MA, McKee PH, Smith MA (1999) Prospective evaluation of soft tissue masses and sarcomas using fluorodeoxyglucose positron emission tomography. Br J Surg 86:550–556
20. Nieweg OE, Pruim J, van Ginkel RJ, Hoekstra HJ, Paans AM, Molenaar WM, Koops HS, Vaalburg W (1996) Fluorine-18-fluorodeoxyglucose PET imaging of soft-tissue sarcoma. J Nucl Med 37:257–261
21. Schulte M, Brecht-Krauss D, Heymer B, Guhlmann A, Hartwig E, Sarkar MR, Diederichs CG, Schultheiss M, Kotzerke J, Reske SN (1999) Fluorodeoxyglucose positron emission tomography of soft tissue tumours: is a non-invasive determination of biological activity possible? Eur J Nucl Med 26:599–605
22. Schulte M, Brecht-Kraus D, Heymer B, Guhlmann A, Hartwig E, Sarkar MR, Diederichs CG, von Baer A, Kotzerke J, Reske SN (2000) Grading of tumors and tumorlike of bone: evaluation by FDG-PET. J Nucl Med 41:1695–1701
23. Franzius C, Daldrup-Link HE, Sciuk J, Rummeny EJ, Bielack S, Jurgens H, Schober O (2001) FDG-PET for detection of pulmonary metastases from malignant primary bone tumors: comparison with spiral CT. Ann Oncol 12:479–486
24. Franzius C, Sciuk J, Daldrup-Link HE, Jurgens H, Schober O (2000) FDG-PET for detection of osseous metastases from malignant primary bone tumours: comparison with bone scintigraphy. Eur J Nucl Med 27:1305–1311
25. Van Ginkel RJ, Hoekstra HJ, Pruim J, Nieweg OE, Molenaar WM, Paans AM, Willemsen AT, Vaalburg W, Koops HS (1996) FDG-PET to evaluate response to hyperthermic isolated limb perfusion for locally advanced soft-tissue sarcoma. J Nucl Med 37: 984–990
26. Schulte M, Brecht-Krauss D, Werner M, Hartwig E, Sarkar MR, Keppler P, Kotzerke J, Guhlmann A, Delling G, Reske SN (1999) Evaluation of neoadjuvant therapy response of osteogenic sarcoma using FDG PET. J Nucl Med 40:1637–1643
27. Franzius C, Sciuk J, Brinkschmidt C, Jurgens H, Schober O (2000) Evaluation of chemotherapy response in primary bone tumors with F-18 FDG positron emission tomography compared with histologically assessed tumor necrosis. Clin Nucl Med 25:874–881
28. Jones DN, McCowage GB, Sostman HD, Brizel DM, Layfield L, Charles HC, Dewhirst MW, Prescott DM, Friedman HS, Harrelson JM, Scully SP, Coleman RE (1996) Monitoring of neoadjuvant therapy response of soft-tissue and musculoskeletal sarcoma using fluorine-18-FDG PET. J Nucl Med 37:1438–1444
29. Kole AC, Nieweg OE, van Ginkel RJ, Pruim J, Hoekstra HJ, Paans AM, Vaalburg W, Koops HS (1997) Detection of local recurrence of soft-tissue sarcoma with positron emission tomography using [18F]fluorodeoxyglucose. Ann Surg Oncol 4:57–63
30. Lucas JD, O'Doherty MJ, Wong JC, Bingham JB, McKee PH, Fletcher CD, Smith MA (1998) Evaluation of fluorodeoxyglucose positron emission tomography in the management of soft-tissue sarcomas. J Bone Joint Surg Br 80:441–447
31. Schwarzbach M, Willeke F, Dimitrakopoulou-Strauss A, Strauss LG, Zhang YM, Mechtersheimer G, Hinz U, Lehnert T, Herfarth C (1999) Functional imaging and detection of local recurrence in soft tissue sarcomas by positron emission tomography. Anticancer Res 19:1343–1349
32. Hain SF, O'Doherty MJ, Lucas JD, Smith MA (1999) Fluorodeoxyglucose PET in the evaluation of amputations for soft tissue sarcoma. Nucl Med Commun 20:845–848
33. Garcia R, Kim EE, Wong FC, Korkmaz M, Wong WH, Yang DJ, Podoloff DA (1996) Comparison of fluorine-18-FDG PET and technetium-99m-MIBI SPECT in evaluation of musculoskeletal sarcomas. J Nucl Med 37:1476–1479
34. Franzius C, Daldrup-Link HE, Wagner-Bohn A, Sciuk J, Heindel WL, Jurgens H, Schober O (2002) FDG-PET for detection of recurrences from malignant primary bone tumors: comparison with conventional imaging. Ann Oncol 13:157–160
35. Durie BG, Waxman AD, D'Agnolo A, Williams CM (2002) Whole-body (18)F-FDG PET identifies high-risk myeloma. J Nucl Med 43:1457–1463
36. Schirrmeister H, Bommer M, Buck AK, Muller S, Messer P, Bunjes D, Dohner H, Bergmann L, Reske SN (2002) Initial results in the assessment of multiple myeloma using 18F-FDG PET. Eur J Nucl Med Mol Imaging 29:361–366
37. Cook GJ, Houston S, Rubens R, Maisey MN, Fogelman I (1998) Detection of bone metastases in breast cancer by 18FDG PET: differing metabolic activity in osteoblastic and osteolytic lesions. J Clin Oncol 16:3375–3379
38. Schirrmeister H, Kuhn T, Guhlmann A, Santjohanser C, Horster T, Nussle K, Koretz K, Glatting G, Rieber A, Kreienberg R, Buck AC, Reske SN (2001) Fluorine-18 2-deoxy-2-fluoro-D-glucose PET in the preoperative staging of breast cancer: comparison with the standard staging procedures. Eur J Nucl Med 28: 351–358
39. Shreve PD, Grossman HB, Gross MD, Wahl RL (1996) Metastatic prostate cancer: initial findings of PET with 2-deoxy-2-[F-18]fluoro-D-glucose. Radiology 199:751–756
40. Reske SN, Kotzerke J (2001) FDG-PET for clinical use. Results of the 3rd German Interdisciplinary Consensus Conference, "Onko-PET III", 21 July and 19 September 2000. Eur J Nucl Med 28:1707–1723
41. Gambhir SS, Czernin J, Schwimmer J, Silverman DH, Coleman RE, Phelps ME (2001) A tabulated summary of the FDG PET literature. J Nucl Med 42 [Suppl 5]:1S–93S
42. Shields AF, Grierson JR, Dohmen BM, Machulla HJ, Stayanoff JC, Lawhorn-Crews JM, Obradovich JE, Muzik O, Mangner TJ (1998) Imaging proliferation in vivo with [F-18]FLT and positron emission tomography. Nat Med 4:1334–1336
43. Plaat B, Kole A, Mastik M, Hoekstra H, Molenaar W, Vaalburg W (1999) Protein synthesis rate measured with L-[1-11C]tyrosine positron emission tomography correlates with mitotic activity and MIB-1 antibody-detected proliferation in human soft tissue sarcomas. Eur J Nucl Med 26:328–332
44. Watanabe H, Inoue T, Shinozaki T, Yanagawa T, Ahmed AR, Tomiyoshi K, Oriuchi N, Tokunaga M, Aoki J, Endo K, Takagishi K (2000) PET imaging of musculoskeletal tumours with fluorine-18 alpha-methyltyrosine: comparison with fluorine-18 fluorodeoxyglucose PET. Eur J Nucl Med 27:1509–1517
45. Hawkins DS, Rajendran JG, Conrad EU 3rd, Bruckner JD, Eary JF (2002) Evaluation of chemotherapy response in pediatric bone sarcomas by [F-18]-fluorodeoxy-D-glucose positron emission tomography. Cancer 94:3277–3284

CHAPTER 28

Skeletal Imaging with F-18

H. Palmedo

28.1 Background

28.1.1 Lung Cancer

Lung cancer is the most common malignant tumor in male patients [1]. In Germany, 29,000 men died due to lung cancer in 1995. The mortality rate has decreased slightly within the last decades to a level of 45 cases per 100,000 inhabitants. For women, lung cancer represents the third most common malignant tumor increasing steadily over recent decades. Therefore, the standardized mortality rate reached a level of 9.6 cases per 100,000 inhabitants per year for the year 1995 [1].

Due to their different biological properties, lung cancer is classified as belonging to the group of non-small-cell lung cancer (NSCLC) with a frequency of about 76%, or to the group of small-cell lung cancer (SCLC) being diagnosed in about 21% of the cases [2, 3]. An exact staging of any lung cancer following the TNM classification is essential to be able to establish a stage-relevant therapy plan [4]. Besides the histopathological diagnosis of the primary tumor, imaging modalities for the staging of the mediastinum, liver, skeleton and adrenal glands are indispensable. For small-cell lung cancer, patients with limited disease (stage I–IIIb) have to be distinguished from patients with extensive disease (presence of distant metastases) [5].

The probability of having distant metastases is correlated with the T- and the N-stage of the tumor. Distant metastases will be found in 20%–40% of patients with the early stage I–II (T1–2 cancer with N0 or with N1 = ipsilateral-hilus lymph node). However, this patient group only accounts for about 25% of all lung cancers [6–10]. For all lung cancers, frequent locations of distant metastases are the liver, bones, bone marrow, lymph nodes, brain and adrenal glands [11, 12]. In patients with SCLC, distant metastases and therefore extensive disease is present in 45%–60% of cases at the time of primary diagnosis [13]. In patients with a higher stage of disease, bone marrow disease is found three to four times as often for SCLC compared to NSCLC [14]. Consequently, lung cancer has the tendency to metastasize to the bones at a very early stage, demonstrating the need for diagnostic work-up at this time point.

Although different staging modalities like bone scintigraphy are performed, it must be supposed that also patients showing no evidence of metastases at the time of imaging frequently present an advanced stage of disease. For lung cancer, an imaging modality detecting as early as possible and with high diagnostic accuracy osseous metastases is required for to the following reasons:

- Clearly bone metastases have a high prognostic relevance for all types of lung cancer [16–18]. The broad range of the 5-year-survival in stage I (50%–80%) and stage II (35%–60%) may be the result of a very early developing osseous metastasizing. Moreover, early detection of bone metastases could be helpful for the planning and evaluation of therapy studies by enabling the clinician to build special subgroups of patients.
- Mainly for NSCLC (rarely in SCLC patients), curative therapy by performing surgery is only indicated if bone metastases have been excluded [15]. If bone metastases were detected at an early stage, a high-risk operation could be avoided for the concerned patients. Additionally, early detection would mean better patient selection what would result in an improvement of the survival rate after curative therapy.
- Neoadjuvant chemotherapy of lung cancer for stage III (mainly IIIa) patients could be a curative approach if followed by surgical tumor elimination. Also in this patient group, exclusion of metastatic bone disease is extremely important [19].
- It is necessary to determine the exact extent of bone disease to localize regions having a high fracture risk and being appropriate for external beam radiotherapy.
- In patients with SCLC, the evidence of osseous metastases will modify the chemotherapeutic regimen. In patients in who bone disease has been excluded, aggressive chemotherapy has shown some advantage in survival [20, 21].

28.1.2
Prostate Cancer

Prostate cancer is the second leading cause of cancer-related mortality in men [22]. In 1994, mortality had a level of 30 cases per 100,000 male inhabitants, and the incidence has steadily increased in recent years [23]. The mean age at diagnosis is about 70 years.

Depending on the stage prostate cancer generally metastasizes in the locoregional lymph nodes of the pelvis. Subsequently, tumor extension follows the lymphatic vessels to the retroperitoneal and paraaortal region or will disseminate into bones, lung and liver [24, 25]. Typically, prostate cancer generates osteoblastic bone metastases that are mainly located in the vertebral column (lumbar region), in the pelvis and the ribs [24].

The exact TNM staging of prostate cancer which is a precondition for adequate therapy planning is a particular problem. About 50%–60% of the tumors preoperatively staged as T1 and T2 and subsequently operated on in curative intention are identified as in fact advanced T3 cancers, therefore, have been understaged [26, 27].

To determine the T-stage of the tumor a digital rectal examination (DRE), the transrectal sonography (TRS) and the measurement of PSA are performed. The understaging rate for DRE and TRS was found to lie at a level of 60% and 38%, respectively [28, 29]. The measurement of PSA has been integrated as a valuable parameter in the diagnostic work-up and the follow-up of prostate cancer patients [30]. There is a positive correlation between clinical and pathological stage and the extent of the tumor disease [31]. However, a significant overlap with regard to PSA measurements exists between malignant and benign tumors of the prostate because also benign prostate tumors produce PSA [32]. Therefore, when evaluating the PSA value one has to take into account different factors like the volume of the prostate gland. PSA has not been reliable for differentiating T2 from T3 tumors [33]. Consequently, prostatovesiculectomy is still the gold standard to determine the T-stage.

A similar situation can be found for lymph node staging. In spite of PSA measurements and modern imaging modalities like sonography, computer tomography, MRI and PET pelvic lymphadenectomy is the only exact staging method for the lymph nodes [34]. There is still is some controversy about in which patients pelvic lymphadenectomy is necessary [35, 36].

If local tumor growth is present (maximal T2) curative therapy by radical prostatectomy or external beam radiation is possible [37–40]. About 50%–60% of patients account for the T1–2 stage. If advanced local tumor (pT3) or lymph node or bone metastases are present the disease is considered as a systemic cancer disease necessitating a palliative therapy regimen [41]. The incidences of distant metastases at T1–2 and stage T3 are 20% and 40%, respectively [42]. Since a strong correlation between the PSA value and the frequency of bone metastases has been proven, bone scintigraphy is recommended only for prostate cancer patients with PSA values over 10 ng/ml [43].

Early detection of metastatic bone diseases in prostate cancer is extremely important at the time of primary diagnosis because it has to be decided if a palliative or a curative (radical prostatectomy or external beam radiation) treatment is appropriate for the patient. In this context it is important to recall that in spite of systematic biopsies of the prostate gland 30%–50% of pT3 tumors are operated on because they had been staged as T2 tumor before surgery [44, 45]. The number of operated T3 patients could be reduced if early detection of bone metastases was possible preoperatively. Moreover, it is helpful if the exact extent of bone disease can be defined to plan potential external beam radiotherapy.

28.1.3
Breast Cancer

Carcinoma of the breast represents the most common malignant tumor in women [46–48]. Every ninth woman in the modern countries of the western world will develop breast cancer during her lifetime. The incidence in West and North Europe is approximately 70–100 cases per 100,000 women and mortality lies at 29 per 100,000. Disease will appear mainly in women between 45 and 65 years of age. For women in the 35 to 45 year age group, breast cancer is the leading cause for death overall [49].

Dynamics of tumor growth differ from breast tumor to breast tumor and the time for the doubling of tumor volume lies between 23 and 209 days [50]. It has been observed that 75% of tumors first metastasize via the lymphatic vessels and subsequently develop distant metastases via the blood vessels [51]. However, in about 25% of patients it must be supposed that tumor cells spread out primarily via the blood vessels because patients demonstrate distant metastases without having lymphatic disease. The preferred locations for breast cancer metastases are the lungs, the liver and the bones [52]. The size of the primary tumor correlates strongly with the probability of having lymph node and distant metastases [53, 54]. Due to the aforementioned biological behavior of early hematological spread of some of the breast cancers, even small tumors with a size of 1–2 cm can generate distant metastases in 25% of cases during the course of disease [54]. In contrast to this observation, in 10% of the big breast cancers over 8 cm or more distant metastases are absent and, in 25% of patients with axillary lymph node metastases at the time of primary diagnosis, no distant metastases will appear [53]. This makes it clear that the predictive value of the tumor size alone is of limited value.

Most patients discover breast cancer on their own during self-examination of the breasts detecting tumors with a mean diameter of 2 cm [55, 56]. Mammography screening is able to detect occult breast carcinoma and has led to an increase in the detection rate and the surgical treatment of such early cancers [57–59]. Still, having a patient with a solid breast cancer, a clinically detectable distant metastasis must be assumed in about 30 % of patients at the time of primary diagnosis [60]. One of the first locations often concerned is the skeleton [61]. Bone marrow involvement (proof of cancer cells) in T1/T2 tumors and in T3/T4 tumors can be found in 22 % and 40 % of cases, respectively [62]. At the time of primary diagnosis, bone scintigraphy demonstrates metastatic disease in approximately 2 %–3 % of patients, whereas this rate increases up to 30 % in patients with recurrent disease [63, 64]. Frequently, osseous metastases are observed in patients with well-differentiated estrogen-positive tumors [65].

The early detection of bone metastases in breast cancer at the time of primary staging is important because the result will influence the further therapeutic management of the patient. Consequently, the surgeon will confine the graft to a pure palliative treatment like tumorectomy or mastectomy if osseous disease is present. Moreover, in patients who only have distant metastases confined to the bone, often hormonal treatment is preferred to chemotherapy [66]. In combination with chemotherapy, the administration of bisphosphonates inhibits activity of osteoclasts and results in a delay of progression and extension of bone metastases [67–69]. In patients with newly diagnosed local recurrence, it is important to exclude osseous metastases since a curative approach is possible in this patient group [70, 71]. For the palliative treatment strategy, it is valuable to determine the exact extent of bone disease to be able to monitor therapy success and to apply external beam radiotherapy. This question is also of significance in patients with a singular sternal metastases in whom surgical resection is considered [72]. It is not clear if early detection of bone metastases can prolong survival in patients in whom no further organs are affected.

28.2 Conventional Screening for Bone Metastases

The method of choice for screening of bone metastases in lung, prostate and breast cancer is bone scintigraphy. This imaging modality has the advantage that the whole body is examined within a relatively short time interval [73]. Bone scintigraphy including SPECT imaging has a high sensitivity for detecting metastatic bone disease. Moreover, the administration of technetium labeled phosphonates does not have any side effects except for a low radiation burden. One disadvantage of bone scintigraphy is its limited specificity that regularly necessitates further modalities like X-ray imaging. It has been shown that MRI detects more osteolytic metastatic lesions in the vertebra column than planar scintigraphy. However, in these studies, no systematic SPECT imaging was performed. This seems to be important because there is evidence that SPECT increases sensitivity for detecting bone metastases in the vertebra column and the pelvis. With regard to the ribs, the sternum and the skull, bone scintigraphy revealed highest sensitivity of all imaging modalities.

28.3 PET With F-18 Sodium Fluoride for Metastatic Bone Disease

F-18 sodium fluoride (NaF-18) represents a new PET tracer that is actually under investigation for imaging of metastatic bone disease. Similar to the use of technetium-99m labeled phosphonates, NaF-18 is able to visualize bone metabolism. However, in comparison to whole-body scintigraphy, PET with NaF-18 delivers high resolution cross-sectional imaging of the whole body (Fig. 1).

F-18 sodium fluoride has been used earlier for conventional bone scintigraphy [75, 79–81]. When new technetium-99m labeled radiopharmaceuticals were introduced into clinical routine NaF-18 scintigraphy was dropped due to worse physical characteristics for the gamma camera. Since positron emission tomography has been introduced as a clinical routine procedure NaF-18 has gained new interest. One underlying reason for this is the high spatial resolution of PET [74]. The spatial resolution of PET is about 5 mm whereas that of single-photon-emission computer tomography (SPECT)

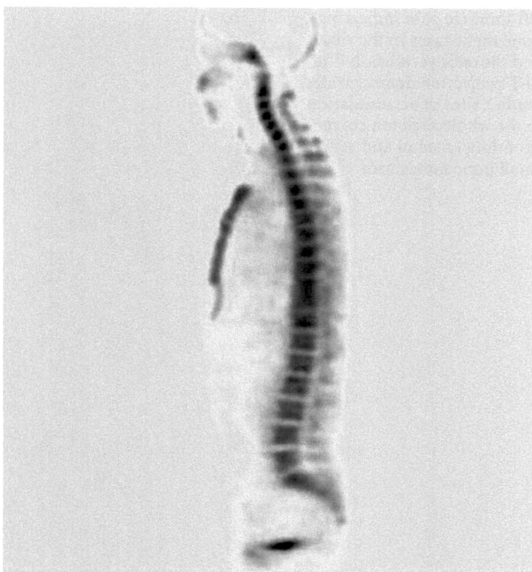

Fig. 1. Sagittal slice of a F-18 PET showing the high resolution and good anatomical correlation of images. The scan depicts no metastatic disease

lies between 1cm and 1.5cm [76]. A further advantage of NaF-18 is that its bone uptake in regions of pathologically elevated bone metabolism is clearly higher compared to that of technetium-99m labeled phosphonates [77]. Moreover, it has been shown that the absolute tracer uptake in normal bone of NaF-18 is twice as high as that of the phosphonates [78]. These properties of NaF-18 result in an enhanced image contrast of metastasis to normal bone and, consequently, lead to the better visualization and detection rate of PET. Additionally, tracer elimination from the vascular compartment is more rapid for NaF-18 than for the polyphosphonates [77]. Therefore, the time interval between injection of the agent and start of acquisition can be shortened when using NaF-18.

Initial results with NaF-18 PET are very encouraging [73, 82–85]. Schirrmeister et al. conducted a study in breast cancer patients comparing the diagnostic accuracy for detecting osseous metastases between F-18 PET and planar whole body scintigraphy [73]. In this study, MRI was used as a gold standard reference method. The authors found that the extent of metastatic bone disease was underestimated in 11 of 17 patients by bone scintigraphy, but correctly identified in all patients by F-18 PET. Furthermore, F-18 PET could reveal bone metastases in three patients with negative scintigraphy. The authors concluded that F-18 PET had an impact on clinical patient management in 18% of the cases. Also, for prostate, lung and thyroid cancer patients, F-18 PET seems to deliver superior results in comparison to conventional bone scintigraphy [83–85]. In our study including lung, breast and prostate cancer patients, we found that F-18 PET revealed metastatic bone disease even though bone scintigraphy was negative or indeterminate in 32% of patients with bone metastases (Fig. 2) [85]. Furthermore, in 13 of 17 patients with scintigraphically positive bone metastases, F-18 PET detected additional sites of bone disease. It has been demonstrated that SPECT can increase the sensitivity of planar bone scintigraphy. However, it seems that SPECT cannot reach the same diagnostic accuracy as F-18 PET [84, 85]. Furthermore, whole body SPECT (at least of the whole vertebra column to be comparable to PET) would require an unacceptable long examination time not being feasible for clinical routine. Compared to bone scintigraphy, also specificity of bone screening can be increased by NaF-18 PET due to better anatomical visualization of the skeleton [82, 85].

In conclusion, early data show that F-18 PET is able to detect earlier and more accurately with regard to the extent of metastatic osseous disease in different cancer patients (breast, lung, prostate cancer). Further studies are needed to clarify which patient groups will have the highest benefit from NaF-18 PET.

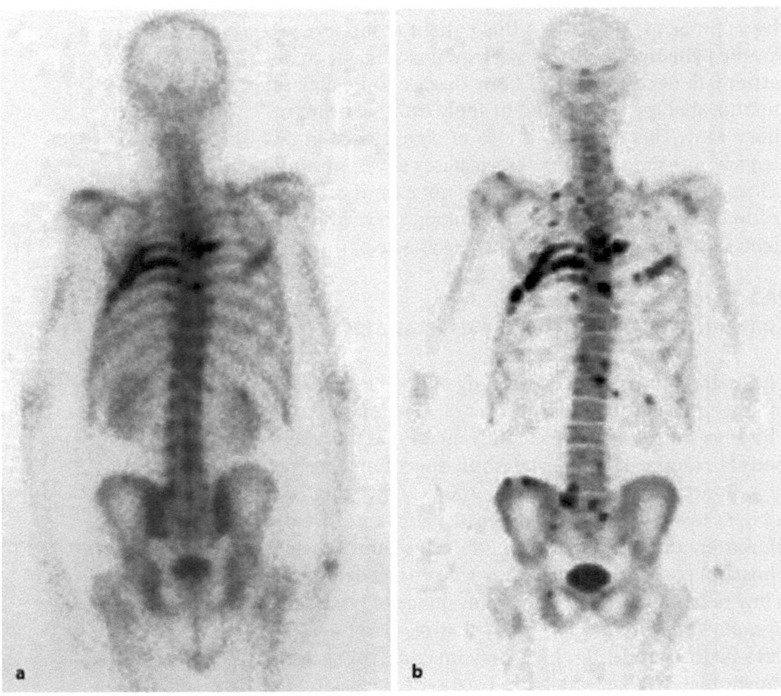

Fig. 2.
a Bone scintigraphy of a patient with lung cancer and left thoracic pain indicating bone metastases in the ribs and thoracic vertebra. **b** F-18 PET projection demonstrates further sites of accumulation in the whole skeleton corresponding to small and very small bone metastases

28.4 Technical Recommendations

- Patient Preparation:
  Patients require no special preparation for this procedure.
- Radiopharmaceuticals:
  370 MBq (ca. 10 mCi) sodium fluoride-18 i.v.
- Data acquisition:
  Beginning 60–90 min after injection, hydration with 1 l of water, voiding of the bladder. Emission scan of 8–10 min, optionally transmission scan 3–5 min or CT-corrected attenuation.
- Reconstruction:
  Iterative reconstruction.
- Image evaluation:
  Visual analysis (focally increased activity), quantification of regional tracer uptake (e.g. standard uptake value).
- Pitfalls:
  Tracer uptake in benign bone lesions and degenerative disease of bone and joints, additionally pitfalls known for bone scintigraphy.

References

1. Becker N, Wahrendorf J (1998) Krebsatlas der Bundesrepublik Deutschland 1981–1990. Springer, Berlin Heidelberg New York
2. Schalhorn A (1985) Bronchialkarzinom: Möglichkeiten und Grenzen der Chemotherapie. Fortschr Med 103:309–311
3. Schalhorn A (1985) Bronchialkarzinom: Möglichkeiten und Grenzen der Chemotherapie. Fortschr Med 103:453–456
4. Sobin LH, Wittekind C (1997) TNM classification of malignant tumors, 5th edn. Wiley-Liss, New York
5. Stahel RA, Ginsberg R, Havemann K, et al (1989) Staging and prognostic factors in small cell lung cancer: a consensus report. Lung Cancer 5:119–126
6. Stuschke M, Heilmann HP (1996) Lunge und Mediastinum. In: Scherer E, Sack H (eds) Strahlentherapie. Springer, Berlin Heidelberg New York
7. Holmes EC (1989) Surgical adjuvant therapy of NSCLC. J Surg Oncol 42 [Suppl 1]:26–33
8. Dosoretz D, Galmarini D, Rubenstein JH et al (1993) Local control in medically inoperable lung cancer: analysis of its importance in outcome and factors determining the probability of tumor eradication. Int J Radiat Oncol Biol Phys 27:507–516
9. Noordijk EM, van der Poest, Hermans J, Wever AMJ, Leer JWH (1988) Radiotherapy as an alternative to surgery in elderly patients with resectable lung cancer. Radiother Oncol 13:83–89
10. Sandler HM, Curran WJ, Turrisi AT (1990) The influence of tumor size and pre-treatment staging on outcome following radiation therapy alone for stage I NSCLC. Int J Radiat Oncol Biol Phys 10:9–13
11. Bülzebruck H, Danzer B, Hilkemeier G et al (1998)Metastasierung und Prognose des kleinzelligen Bronchialkarzinoms. Onkologe 4:1039–1047
12. Line D, Deeley TJ (1971) The necropsy findings in carcinoma of the bronchus. Br J Dis Chest 65:238
13. Wolf M (1998) Kleinzelliges Bronchialkarzinom: klinische Präsentation, Diagnostik und prognostische Faktoren. Onkologe 4:1005–1018
14. Hansen HH, Muggia FM (1972) Staging of inoperable patients with bronchogenic carcinoma with special reference to bone marrow and peritoneoscopy. Cancer 30:1395–1401
15. Schalhorn A, Sunder-Plassmann L (2000) Maligne Tumoren der Thorakal- und Mediastinalorgane. In: Wilmanns W, Huhn D, Wilms K (eds) Internistische Onkologie. Thieme, Stuttgart
16. Bonomi PD, Finkelstein DM, Ruckdeschel JC et al (1989) Combination chemotherapy vs. single agents followed by combinations chemotherapy in stage IV NSCLC: a study of the eastern cooperative oncology group. J Clin Oncol 7:1602–1613
17. Drings P, Becker H, Bülzebruck H, Manke HG, Tessen HW (1990) Chemotherapie des fortgeschrittenen nichtkleinzelligen Bronchialkarzinoms mit Ifosfamid und Etoposid. Tumordiagn Ther 11:79–84
18. Spiegelman D, Maurer H, Ware JH (1989) Prognostic factors in SCLC: an analysis of 1521 patients. J Clin Oncol 7:344–354
19. Rosell R, Lopez-Cabrerizo MP, Astudillo J (1997) Preoperative chemotherapy for stage IIIA NSCLC. Curr Opin Oncol 9:149–155
20. Albain KS, Crowley JJ, Leblanc M, Livingston RB (1990) Determinants of improved outcome in SCLC: an analysis of the 2580-patients southwest oncology group data base. J Clin Oncol 8: 1563–1574
21. ManegoldC, Bülzebruck H, Drings P, Vogt-Moykopf I (1989) Prognostische Faktoren beim kleinzelligen Bronchialkarzinom. Onkologe 12:240–245
22. Golz R, Störkel S (1999) Anatomie und Pathologie des Prostatakarzinom. In: Hinkelbein W, Miller K, Wiegel T (eds) Prostatakarzinom. Springer, Berlin Heidelberg New York
23. Statistisches Bundesamt (1994) Gesundtheitswesen. Fachserie 12, Reihe 4: Todesursachen in Deutschland, Wiesbaden
24. Saitoh H, Hida M, Shimbo T et al (1984) Metastatic patterns of prostatic cancer. Cancer 54:3078–3084
25. De la Monte SM, Moore GW, Hutchins GM (1986) Metastatic behaviour of prostate cancer. Cancer 58:985–993
26. Ravery V, Schmid HP, Toublanc M, Boccon-Gibod L (1996) Is the percentage of cancer in biopsy cores predictive of extracapsular disease in T1-T2 prostate cancer? Cancer 78:1079–1084
27. Badalament RA, Miller MC, Peller PA et al (1996) An algorithm for predicting nonorgan confined prostate cancer using the results obtained from sexant core biopsies with prostate specific antigen level. J Urol 156:1375–1380
28. Breul J et al (1991) Fehler bei der präoperativen Bestimmung des lokalen Tumorstadiums bei der radikalen Prostatektomie . In: Hartung, Kropp (eds) Urologische Beckenchirurgie. Springer, Berlin Heidelberg New York
29. Rorvik J, Halvorsen OJ, Servoll E, Haukaas S (1994) Transrectal ultrasonography to assess local extent of prostatic cancer before radical prostatectomy. Br J Urol 73(1):65–9
30. Partin A et al (1990) PSA in the staging of localized prostate cancer: influence of tumor differentiation tumor volume and benigne hyperplasia. J Urol 143:747
31. Kleer E, Oesterlin JE (1993) PSA and staging of localized prostate cancer. Urol Clin North Am 20:695–705
32. Catalona WJ, Smith DS, Ratliff TL, Basler JW et al (1991) Measurement of PSA in serum as a screening test for prostate cancer. N Engl J Med 324:1156–1161
33. Wirth MP, Frohmüller HGW (1992) PSA and prostate acid phosphatase in the detection of early prostate cancer and the prediction of regional lymph node metastases. Eur Urol 22:27–32
34. Shreve PD, Grossman HB, Gross MD, Wahl RL (1996) Metastatic prostate cancer: initial findings of PET with F-18 fluoro-D-glucose. Radiology 199:751–756
35. Partin AW, Kattan MW, Subong EN et al (1997) Combination of PSA, clinical stage, and Gleason Score to predict pathological stage of localized prostate cancer. JAMA 277:1445–1451
36. Klän R, Meier T, Knispel HH, Wegner HE, Miller K (1995) Laparoscopic pelvic lymphadenectomy in prostatic cancer. Urol Int 55:78–83
37. Catalona WJ, Smith DJ (1994) 5-year tumor recurrence rates after anatomical radical retropubic prostatectomy for prostate cancer. J Urol 152:1837–1842
38. Ohori M, Goag JR, Wheeler TM et al (1994) Can radical prostatectomy alter the progression of poorly differentiated prostate cancer? J Urol 152:1843–1849
39. Hanks GE, LeeWR, Haulon MS et al (1996) Conformal technique dose escalation for prostate cancer. Int J RadiatOncol Biol Phys 35:861–868

40. Zietman AL, Shipley WU (1993) Randomized trials in locoregionally confined prostate cancer: past present and future. Semin Radiat Oncol 3:210–220
41. Epstein J et al (1993) Correlation of pathologic findings with progression after radical retropubic prostatectomy. Cancer 71: 3586
42. Perez CA, Hanks GE, Leibel SA et al (1993) Localized carcinoma of the prostate (stages T1, T2 and T3). Cancer 72:3156–3173
43. Chybowski FM, Keller JL, Bergstrahl EJ, Oesterling JE (1991) Predicting radionuclide bone scan finding in patients with newly diagnosed untreated prostate cancer. J Urol 145:313–318
44. Andriole GL, Kavoussi LR, Torrence JR (1988) Transrectal ultrasonography in the diagnosis and staging of the carcinoma of the prostate. J Urol 140:758–760
45. Noldus J, Stamey TA (1996) Limitations of serum PSA in predicting peripheral and transition zone cancer volumes as measured by correlation coefficients. J Urol 155:232–237
46. Kelsey JL, Gammon MD (1995) The epidemiology of breast cancer. Cancer 41:146–165
47. Berg JW, Hutter RV (1995) Breast cancer. Cancer 75:257–269
48. Sondik EJ (1994) Breast cancer trends. Incidence, mortality and survival. Cancer 74:995–999
49. Possinger K, Große Y (2000) Mammakarzinome und gynäkologische Tumoren. In: Wilmanns W, Huhn D, Wilms K (eds) Internistische Onkologie. Thieme, Stuttgart
50. Spratt JS, Donegan WL (1979) Cancer of the breast. Saunders, Philadelphia
51. Tabar l, Grad A, Holmberg LH et al (1985) Reduction in mortality from breast cancer after mass screening with mammography. Lancet 1:829
52. Boag JW, Jaybittle JL, Fowler JR (1971) The number of patinets required in a clinical trial. Br J Radiol 44:122
53. Smart CR, Myers MH, Gloeckler LA (1978) Implications from SEER data on breast cancer management. Cancer 41:787
54. Koscielny SM, Tubiana M, Le MG et al (1984) Breast cancer. Relationship between the size of the primary tumor and the probability of metastatic dissemination. Br J Cancer 49:709
55. Donegan WL (1979) Epidemiology. In: Donegan WL, Spratt JS (eds) Cancer of the breast. Saunders, Philadelphia
56. Foster RS Jr, Lang SP, Constanza MC et al (1978) Breast self-examination practices and breast cancer stage. N Engl J Med 299: 265
57. Andersson I (1988) Mammographic screening and mortality from breast cancer: Malmö mammographic screening trial. Br J Med 297:943–948
58. Frisell J, Eklund G, Hellström L et al (1991) Randomized study of mammography screening – preliminary report on mortality in the Stockholm trial. Breast Cancer Res Treatment 18:49–56
59. Miller AB, Baines CJ, To T et al (1992) Canada national breast screening study. Can Med Assoc J 147:1459–1488
60. Meuret G (1995) Grundlagen des Mammakarzinoms. In: Meuret G (eds) Mammakarzinom. Thieme, Stuttgart
61. Clark GM, Sledge GW, Osborne CK, McGuire WL (1987) Survival from first recurrence: relative importance of prognostic factors in 1015 breast cancer patients. J Clin Oncol 5:55–61
62. Come SE, Schnipper LE (1991) Myelophtisisanemia and other aspects of bone marrow involvement. In: Harris JR, Hellman S, Henderson IC, Kinne DW (eds) Breast diseases. Lippincott, Philadelphia, pp 761–766
63. Perez DJ, Powles TJ, Milan J et al (1983) Detection of breast carcinoma metastases in bone: relative merits of x-rays and skeletal scintigraphy. Lancet 2:613–616
64. Rossing N, Munck O, Nielsen SP et al (1982) What do early bone scans tell about breast cancer patients? Eur J Cancer Clin Oncol 18:629–636
65. Kamby C, Bruun Rasmussen B, Kristensen B (1991) Prognostic indicators of metastatic bone disease in human breast cancer. Cancer 68:2045–2050
66. Muss HB (1992) Endocrine therapy for advanced breast cancer: a review. Breast Cancer Res Treat 21:15–26
67. Diel IJ, Solomayer EF, Costa SD et al (1998) Reduction in new metastases in breast cancer with adjuvant clodronate treatment. N Engl J Med 339:357–363
68. Conte N, Giannessi PG, Latreille J et al (1994) Delayed progression of bone metastaseswithb pamidronate therapy in breast cancer patients: a randomized, multicenter phase III trial. Br J Cancer 70:554–558
69. Van Holten-Verzantvoort ATM, Hermans J et al (1996) Does supportive pamodronate treatment prevent or delay the first manifestation of bone metastases in breast cancer patients. Eur J Cancer 32:450–454
70. Aberzik WJ, Silver B, Henderson IC et al (1986) The use of radiotherapy for treatment of isolated locoregional recurrence of breast carcinoma after mastectomy. Cancer 58:1214
71. Janjan NA, McNeese MD, Buzdar AU et al (1986) Management of locoregional recurrent breast cancer. Cancer 58:1552
72. Noguchi S, Miyauchi K, Nishizawa Y et al (1987) Results of surgical treatment for sternal metastases in breast cancer. Cancer 60:2524–2531
73. Schirrmeister H et al (1999) Early detection and accurate description of extent of metastatic bone disease in breast cancer with fluoride ion and positron emission tomography. J Clin Oncol 17:2381
74. Gambhir SS, Czernin J, Schwimmer J et al (2001) A tabulated summary of the FDG-PET literature. J Nucl Med 42:1S–93S
75. Blau M, Nagler W, Bender MA (1962) A new isotope for bone scanning. J Nucl Med 3:332–334
76. Cook G, Fogelman I (2001) The role of positron emission tomography in skeletal disease. Semin Nucl Med 1:50–61
77. Hawkins RA, Choi Y, Huang SC et al (1992) Evaluation of the skeletal kinetics of fluorine-18-fluoride ion with PET. J Nucl Med 33:633–642
78. Hoh CK, Hawkins RA, Dahlbom M et al (1993) Whole body skeletal imaging with F-18 fluoride ion and PET. J Comput Assist Tomogr 17:34–41
79. McNeil BJ et al (1973) Fluroine-18 bone scintigraphy in children with osteosarcoma or Ewing's sarcoma. Radiology 109:627–631
80. Buck AC et al (1975) Serial Fluorine-18 bone scans in the follow-up of carcinoma of the prostate. Br J Urol 47:287–294
81. Rosenfield N, Treves S (1974 Osseous and extraosseousuptake of fluorine-18 and techentium-99m polyphosphate in children with neuroblastoma. Radiology 111:127–133
82. Schirrmeister H, Rentschler M, Kotzerke J et al (1998) Skeletal imaging with F-18 NaF PET and comparison with planar scintigraphy. Fortschr Röntgenstr 168:451–456
83. Schirrmeister H, Guhlmann CA, Diederichs CG, Träger H, Reske SN (1999) Planar bone imaging vs. F-18 PET in patients with cancer of the prostate, thyroid and lung. J Nucl Med 40:1623–1629
84. Schirrmeister H, Glatting G, Hetzel J, Nussle K, Arslandemir C, Buck AK, Dziuk K, Gabelmann A, Reske SN, Hetzel M (2001) Prospective evaluation of the clinical value of planar bone scans, SPECT, and (18)F-labeled NaF PET in newly diagnosed lung cancer. J Nucl Med 42:1800–1804
85. Palmedo H, Schaible R, Textor J, Ko Y, Grohé C, von Mallek D, Ezziddin S, Reinhardt MJ, Biersack HJ (2002) PET with 18F Fluoride compared to bone scintigraphy in the diagnosis of bone metastases: results of a prospective study. J Nucl Med [Suppl] June, abstract 1150

CHAPTER 29

PET in Surgery

S. Yasuda · K. Nakai · M. Ide
S. Kawada · A. Shohtsu

29.1 Introduction

PET is not yet fully utilized in surgical-decision making. Surgeons are not well acquainted with the basics of PET and the interpretations of images. Their knowledge may be limited to "malignant lesions being visualized as hot spots." This simplistic view is not enough to convince surgeons of the value of PET. It is our responsibility as nuclear medicine physicians and radiologists engaged in PET oncology to inform surgeons of not only the advantages of PET, but also its limitations so that the capabilities of PET can be fully exploited in the surgical treatment of tumors, both malignant and benign.

29.2 Advantages of FDG-PET

The attractiveness of FDG PET imaging lies in its ability to detect lesions that are undetectable by conventional imaging modalities. Indeed, PET can non-invasively survey the entire body in a single examination and detect changes in local glucose metabolism.

29.3 Limitations of FDG-PET

FDG-PET was originally developed for in vivo measurement of local glucose metabolism. More studies remain to be done to exploit PET for this purpose in the field of oncology. What PET has been widely used for is tumor imaging. This has been since the development of whole-body scanning in 1990. FDG-PET has obvious limitations for tumor imaging, at present, however. These limitations pertain to three factors: tumor size, histology, and inflammation.

29.3.1 Tumor Size

With PET, we discovered a 6-mm breast cancer and a 6-mm thyroid cancer in asymptomatic screenees [80]. PET has the potential to detect small lesions. However, with current PET machines, the degree of FDG accumulation is underestimated for lesions less than twice the spatial resolution (e.g. 6–8 mm). Thus, PET is unable to detect small lesions (e.g. <1.5 cm). This size limitation is mentioned in reports repeatedly.

29.3.2 Histology

Even if tumor size is no problem, high FDG uptake is not observed in some types of tumor. For example, most lung carcinomas are FDG-avid, whereas bronchioloalveolar carcinoma is not [30]. Most colorectal carcinomas are FDG-avid, whereas high FDG uptake is not observed in mucinous adenocarcinoma of the colon and rectum probably because of the paucity of tumor cells [6]. The degree of FDG accumulation is lower in lobular carcinoma than in invasive ductal carcinoma of the breast [69]. The degree of FDG uptake differs depending not only on the organ involved, but also on the histopathologic type of tumor. When interpreting FDG-PET images, particular details concerning FDG uptake in individual tumor types must be kept in mind.

29.3.3 Inflammation

FDG accumulation in inflammatory lesions is a serious problem and an important factor diminishing the specificity of PET imaging. It is sometimes impossible with PET images alone to discriminate between lung carcinoma and granulomatous inflammation, pancreatic carcinoma and tumor-forming pancreatitis, colonic carcinoma and diverticulitis, and lymph node metastasis and lymphadenitis.

Alternatively, FDG-PET helps greatly in patients with tumors larger than 1.5 cm, with tumors of FDG-avid histopathology, and in tumors without inflammation. In this chapter, we discuss effective applications of PET in surgery for colorectal cancer, esophageal cancer, pancreatic cancer, lung cancer, and breast cancer.

29.4 Applications of FDG-PET in Surgery

29.4.1 Colorectal Cancer

29.4.1.1 *Evaluation of Primary Tumors*

FDG-PET can detect primary colorectal carcinomas. Abdel-Nabi et al. (1998) [1] reported the largest series of patients in which PET was used to detect primary tumor. High FDG uptake was observed in all 39 adenocarcinomas of 37 patients. This included the smallest rectal carcinoma, measuring 1.4 cm. PET results are likely to be positive in advanced colorectal carcinomas, although physiological bowel FDG uptake may hamper detection [78]. However, barium study and colonoscopy are excellent in the diagnosis of primary colorectal carcinoma. Therefore, PET has limited value in diagnosing primary lesions. In both barium study and colonoscopy, unpleasant cleansing of the bowel is essential, whereas PET does not require bowel preparation. PET can be applied in the differentiation between benign and malignant tumors, in observation of the oral side of colonic stricture, and in high-risk patients.

Histopathologically, all colorectal carcinomas in the above-mentioned reports were moderately differentiated adenocarcinomas. Generally, mucinous carcinomas account for approximately 3% of colorectal carcinomas, and signet-ring cell carcinoma account for 0.3% [36]. FDG uptake is not high in mucinous adenocarcinomas [6]. We have encountered a patient with a 2-cm signet-ring cell carcinoma and a false-negative PET scan. In our experience thus far, FDG uptake was not observed in advanced signet-ring cell carcinomas of the stomach. Although high FDG uptake may not be observed in these two types of colorectal carcinoma, approximately 95% of colorectal carcinomas are well, moderately, or poorly differentiated adenocarcinomas, and they are FDG-avid.

Among benign colorectal polyps, adenomatous polyps and hyperplastic polyps are the most prevalent. The adenomatous polyp has the potential for malignant transformation and is thought to be a premalignant lesion, whereas the hyperplastic polyp does not have this potential. High FDG uptake is observed in the adenomatous polyp [81] but not the hyperplastic polyp [1]. It is beneficial that the adenomatous polyp can be found with PET. It is important to recognize that adenomatous polyps or carcinoma can be found incidentally during FDG-PET studies. In cancer screenings with FDG-PET, potentially curable colonic adenomas and carcinomas have been found in asymptomatic screenees [80].

29.4.1.2 *Evaluation of Lymph Node Metastasis*

For preoperative study of advanced colorectal carcinoma, ultrasonography (US), computed tomography (CT), and occasionally magnetic resonance imaging (MRI) are used to evaluate local tumor extension, lymph node metastasis, and distant metastasis. Because of its poorer spatial resolution, PET cannot be used to determine the extent to which tumor involves adjacent organs. In this respect, CT is superior to PET.

PET is unable to discriminate lesions close to one another and thus to distinguish paracolic or pararectal lymph node metastases. This may partly explain the reported low sensitivity (29%) of PET [1] in detecting lymph node metastases; sensitivity is close to that of CT. However, in cases of advanced colorectal carcinoma, paracolic and pararectal lymph nodes are resected en block with the primary tumor. They are not left behind. Whether lymph node dissection is indicated depends on determining the presence or absence of metastasis in distal lymph nodes, that is, inferior mesenteric artery nodes, para-aortic nodes, and iliac nodes. PET seems to be superior to CT in this regard, although this has not been confirmed. Further studies are warranted.

29.4.1.3 *Evaluation of Distant Metastasis*

In cases of colorectal carcinoma, liver metastasis occurs at high rates. A solitary metastasis or a few metastatic lesions can be resected with a curative intent. In cases of unresectable metastasis, hepatic arterial infusion chemotherapy, systemic chemotherapy, or no treatment is chosen. During the initial surgery for primary colorectal cancer, as many as 15%–25% of patients show liver metastasis. Moreover, the most frequent site of recurrence is the liver [42, 64]. US and CT are currently used to detect liver metastasis, but with limited success. Colorectal surgeons are desirous of modalities that can detect smaller liver metastases sooner.

PET results for the detection of liver metastasis are shown in the Table 1. PET sometimes reveals liver metastasis that is undetectable with US or CT [1, 38]. PET would have high clinical impact if it could detect US- or CT-negative subclinical liver metastasis that is missed at the time of surgery. Some authors have reported high sensitivity for PET in detecting liver metastasis. On the resected liver, however, macroscopic metastases vary in size and there are not a few lesions less than 1 cm. Current PET scanners have obvious limitations in detecting carcinomas less than 1 cm. Actually, an increase in false-negative PET results has been reported for liver metastases less than 1 cm [13, 24, 38, 75, 87]. Therefore, we agree with the low sensitivity (71%) of PET in comparison to surgically resected liver [24]. If small metastases are in-

Table 1.
Detection of liver metastases from colorectal cancer

Reference	Number	PET Sensitivity (%)	Specificity (%)	CT Sensitivity (%)	Specificity (%)
[45]	34 Patients	93	57	100%	14%
[13]	127 Lesions	91	98	81%	60%
[56]	58 Patients	95	100	74%	85%
[83]	115 Patients	95	100	84%	95%
[21]	103 Patients	98	100	–	–
[24]	53 Lesions	71	–	–	–

cluded in the study, the sensitivity decreases even more. The important thing is whether PET can detect liver metastases that are undetectable with US, CT, and MRI.

Prior to liver resection for metastatic colorectal cancer, it is essential to confirm that there are no lesions in the residual liver or extrahepatic sites. If patients are screened by FDG-PET before liver resection, survival may be prolonged [75]. Candidates for liver resection with a curative intent deserve PET study.

CT and MRI have progressed steadily. Multidetector CT with contrast-enhancement (arterial phase) seems to be superior to conventional CT in the detection of small metastases. MRI with contrast-enhancement is capable of detecting small lesions. CT and MRI are formidable competitors to PET. PET will be expected to be more accurate than CT and MRI.

Lung metastases of no less than 6–7 mm are detectable with PET. Background FDG activity is lower in the lung than in the liver. Consequently, tumors of the same degree of FDG uptake are more easily visualized in the lung than in the liver. Nevertheless, CT is superior to PET in detecting lung metastases. Ordinarily, CT can identify 3- to 4-mm metastases; thus, sensitivity is high for detection of lung metastases. However, PET is more sensitive than CT in detecting mediastinal and chest wall metastases.

PET is also more sensitive than CT in detecting peritoneal metastases. The ability to detect peritoneal metastases is one of the advantages of PET, although false-negative results can be obtained for lesions less than 1 cm [38]. PET seems to be sensitive in detecting bone metastases, although there is not sufficient data on this subject.

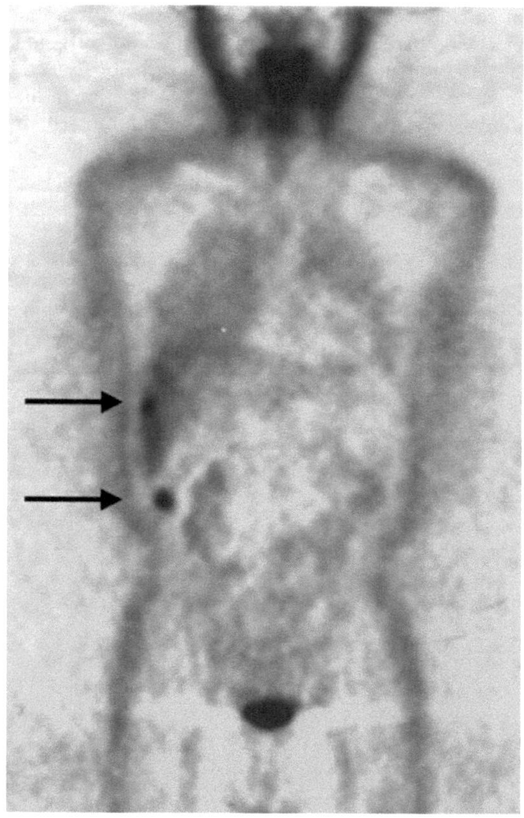

Fig. 1. An FDG-PET image showing liver and peritoneal metastases in a patient with recurrent colon cancer. The peritoneal metastasis was not detected with CT

29.4.1.4
Diagnosis of Recurrence

Carcinoembryonic antigen (CEA) is usually used in the post-surgery follow-up of patients with colorectal cancer. The American Society of Clinical Oncology guidelines suggest that repeating CEA measurement every 2–3 months after resection may be useful [15]. PET can disclose sites of recurrence in colorectal carcinoma patients with CEA elevation after surgery and negative results from conventional imaging studies [23]. CEA elevation with an unknown recurrence site is a good indication for PET. The current recommendations are as follows: patients with increasing serum CEA levels should undergo conventional studies. If the results are negative, the patient should undergo FDG-PET scanning. If the FDG-PET scan does not show any evidence of recurrent disease, serial CEA studies and selective repeat imaging at 3- to 6-month intervals should be undertaken. For patients who are found to have a single site of otherwise resectable disease on conventional images, an FDG-PET scan should be obtained to rule out additional disease sites [47].

Arulampalam et al. (2001) [3] showed in their excellent review that PET has clinical importance in the management of recurrent colorectal cancer. In one prospective study, PET directly influenced management decisions in 59 % of patients [38]. Unnecessary surgery can be avoided (Fig. 1). It is important to add PET study routinely in the follow-up of patients after surgery [73].

PET can be used to predict the effectiveness of chemotherapy and radiotherapy in patients with colorectal carcinoma. Patients with good tumor response after chemotherapy show decreased uptake of FDG [20, 52]. After radiation therapy for rectal carcinomas, FDG uptake decreases significantly due to a reduction in the number of viable tumor cells related to tumor necrosis [58, 67]. Quantification of glucose metabolism by PET should be exploited more in the treatment of colorectal cancer.

29.4.2 Esophageal Cancer

In comparison to colorectal cancer, esophageal cancer is uncommon but more aggressive; patients with esophageal cancer have a poorer prognosis. PET has not been fully utilized in the management of patients with esophageal cancer.

29.4.2.1 *Evaluation of Primary Tumors*

Contrast radiography and endoscopy are excellent for identifying the primary tumor in patients with esophageal cancer. Chromoendoscopy (endoscopy and iodine staining) can even detect superficial lesions that might be missed by conventional endoscopy [50]. Histopathologically, most esophageal carcinomas are squamous cell carcinomas or adenocarcinomas. Although both types are FDG-avid, a certain tumor volume is required for PET visualization. Superficial carcinomas are undetectable with PET. PET imaging can depict primary lesions invading the submucosal layer (pT1b or greater), but carcinomas confined to the mucosal layer (Tis or T1a) are undetectable [22, 31]. PET can be used to detect primary tumors (pT1b or greater) and extraluminal lesions that cannot be observed endoscopically (Fig. 2).

29.4.2.2 *Evaluation of Lymph Node Metastasis*

Lymph node metastasis is frequent in cases of esophageal cancer, and it is an important prognostic factor.

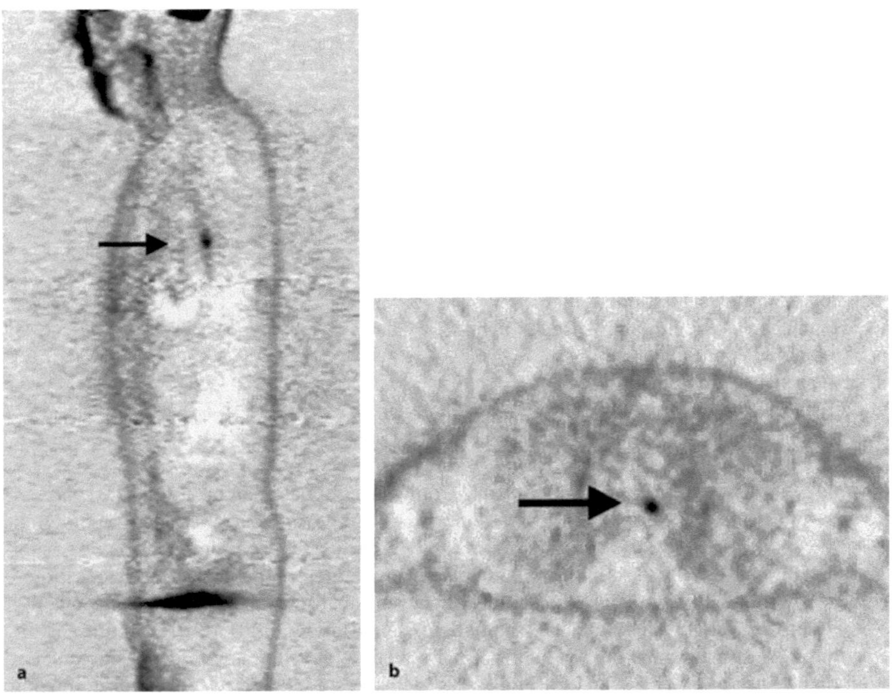

Fig. 2a, b. Small esophageal cancer detected incidentally during preoperative PET study for lung cancer (lung cancer is not shown on this image)

Even at the superficial cancer stage, the rate of nodal metastasis increases according to the depth of invasion [43]. Superficial cancer without nodal metastasis can be treated by endoscopic mucosal resection. In cases of nodal metastasis, lymph node dissection is carried out. This is most impressively illustrated by the three-field lymphadenectomy [61]. In this highly invasive operation, lymph nodes are dissected extensively through cervical, thoracic, and abdominal skin incisions. The invasiveness of treatment differs according to nodal status. In the diagnosis of lymph node metastasis.

CT and endoscopic ultrasonography (EUS) are of limited value. Correct identification of nodal status before or during surgery is very important.

A prospective study for nodal staging (i.e. N0, N1, N2) showed that for local (N1) and regional (N2) lymph nodes, the sensitivity of PET (22 %) is lower than that of the combined use of CT+EUS (83 %), but the specificity is higher at 91 % for PET versus 45 % for CT+EUS. For distant nodal metastasis, sensitivity and specificity are higher for PET (77 %) than for CT+EUS (46 %). The important finding is the significantly higher overall specificity of PET (90 %) versus that of CT+EUS (69 %) [46].

Choi et al. (2000) [11] studied the correlation between individual nodal groups and histologic nodal status in patients who underwent extensive lymph node dissection. The sensitivity, specificity, and accuracy were 57 %, 97 %, and 86 %, respectively, for PET and 18 %, 97 %, and 86 %, respectively, for CT. Another study showed sensitivity, specificity, and accuracy to be 42 %, 100 %, and 92 %, respectively, for PET and 38 %, 96 %, and 88 %, respectively, for CT [31].

The sensitivity of PET for detecting lymph node metastasis is low when the histologic findings obtained from extensive lymph node dissection are used as the gold standard. False-negative PET lesions are found in lymph nodes with only partial or microscopic tumor invasion or necrosis. Furthermore, micrometastases can be disclosed by immunohistochemistry [35]. Negative PET scans can not rule out the presence of lymph node metastasis.

29.4.2.3
Evaluation of Distant Metastasis

There are not many reports on PET detection of distant metastasis from esophageal cancer. Lung, liver, adrenal gland, and bone metastases have been detected with PET [7, 49]. One study demonstrated detection of distant metastases in 7 of 35 patients with negative findings on conventional images [49]. In a group of 58 patients with esophageal cancer, sensitivity for detecting distant metastasis was 100 % for PET and 29 % for CT [7].

The use of PET to supplement CT in patients with potentially resectable esophageal cancer improves our ability to classify patients as having either resectable or unresectable disease [7, 49]. PET should be exploited more in the evaluation of distant metastases.

29.4.2.4
Evaluation of Preoperative Chemotherapy

Preoperative chemotherapy is used in some patients with advanced esophageal carcinoma [41]. FDG-PET can be used to evaluate tumor response in the early phase. It is hypothesized that biochemical changes in tumor tissue induced by therapy precede changes in tumor size [62]. Studies have shown that metabolic measurements by FDG-PET provide for early differentiation of responding and non-responding tumors during preoperative chemotherapy of adenocarcinoma and squamous cell carcinoma of the esophagus [8, 89]. The decrease in tumor FDG uptake correlates well with the histopathologic response findings.

The FDG-PET findings do not only correlate well with subsequent response; they are also of prognostic relevance [89]. Measurement of tumor glucose metabolism was shown to be useful for predicting outcome; patients with high FDG uptake had a significantly worse outcome [27]. Thus, pre-treatment evaluation with PET seems to be beneficial in selected patients.

29.4.3
Pancreatic Cancer

At present, not many surgeons have acknowledged that FDG-PET study helps in decision-making for pancreatic cancer. For pancreatic surgery, differentiation between benign and malignant tumors and resectability are important issues.

29.4.3.1
Evaluation of Primary Tumors

It is sometimes impossible to differentiate between benign and malignant pancreatic masses by conventional imaging modalities (US, CT, MRI, ERCP, EUS). Histology of the resected specimen is still the most accurate means of diagnosing suspicious pancreatic masses. However, this is associated with invasive procedures. Nowadays, it is impossible even for the experienced surgeon to avoid over-surgery in some cases of benign pancreatic mass. There is a need for noninvasive identification of pancreatic cancer. Pancreatic surgeons desire modalities that can identify pancreatic carcinomas precisely.

Recent results of PET for the differentiation of pancreatic masses are shown in Table 2. The reported sensitivities are 71 %–92 % and specificities are 64 %–90 %. In many cases, PET can correctly differentiate between pancreatic cancer and chronic pancreatitis [33, 40, 60, 74]. However, there are not a few false-negative or false-

Table 2. Differentiation of pancreatic masses

Reference	Number	Sensitivity (%)	Specificity (%)	Accuracy (%)
[92]	106	85	84	85
[14]	65	92	85	91
[32]	48	96	90	94
[71]	42	71	64	69
[39]	103	84	66	85
[44]	86	82	81	81

positive results. The three factors limiting PET are particularly evident in this respect. First of all, small tumors can yield false-negative results [33]. There is a high rate of false-negative results in stage I (≥2 cm) cancers [25, 74], whereas three 1.5-cm pancreatic cancers were correctly diagnosed [71], and a CT-negative 1.2-cm pancreatic cancer was detected with PET [37]. Histopathology influences FDG uptake. Most frequent histopathologic type of pancreatic carcinomas is ductal adenocarcinoma. Other types include acinar cell adenocarcinoma, mucinous adenocarcinoma, cystadenocarcinoma, and malignant islet cell tumor (or pancreatic endocrine tumor including insulinoma, glucagonoma, and gastrinoma). The degree of FDG uptake relates to the histopathology. Mucinous adenocarcinoma, a low cellularity tumor, is subject to being false-negative [40, 71]. FDG accumulation was reported in islet cell tumors [33], a malignant insulinoma [2], and glucagonomas [19, 40, 53, 77], although the number of reports is still few. High FDG uptake is observed in some benign cystadenomas [33, 44]. Inflammation also influence FDG uptake. Chronic pancreatitis can be false-positive [14, 25, 40, 44, 74]. Inflammation can give rise to focal FDG uptake even when WBC, amylase, and lipase are normal [72]. In such false-positive cases, acute pancreatitis [32, 44, 72] or marked lymphocyte accumulation [40] is recognized histologically. It must be understood that an active inflammatory process at the histological level can lead to FDG accumulation [72].

29.4.3.2
Evaluation of Resectability

With regard to resectability, PET cannot be used to evaluate local tumor extension and the relation of the tumor to surrounding vessels. CT is, of course, more accurate in predicting resectability because of its anatomical delineation around the pancreas and its ability to detect vascular involvement [37].

PET has potential for detecting CT-negative liver metastasis from pancreatic adenocarcinoma [63]. However, the sensitivity decreases for small metastases ≤1 cm [26]. False-positive results are observed in patients with marked intrahepatic cholestasis that may accompany inflammatory reactions or abscesses in the bile duct system [26]. PET is capable of detecting peritoneal metastases that are undetectable with CT and MRI [70], although subcentimeter peritoneal implants are below the detection sensitivity of PET [63].

Some surgeons argue strongly that PET does not alter management of patients with pancreatic or periampullary cancer [37, 39]. Those who have used conventional modalities in surgical decision-making for a long time may not easily accept new approaches.

Taking into account the limited spatial resolution of PET, we had better deal with pancreatic masses larger than 1.5 cm. For these lesions, if the PET scan is entirely normal, the chance of malignancy may be negligible. PET is applicable for the detection of recurrent disease. However, there are no effective therapies or experimental protocols for recurrent disease [37].

Serum glucose levels should be checked in hyperglycemic patients. Patients with pancreatic cancer sometimes have diabetes mellitus. Markedly elevated plasma glucose levels greatly impair the detection of pancreatic malignancies [16, 71, 92]. Delbeke et al. (1999) [14] report measuring serum glucose in patients just before the administration of FDG, and regular insulin is administered to reduce the serum glucose level to below 150 mg/100 ml.

A study showed that FDG-PET has the potential to detect tumor response to neoadjuvant therapy in patients with pancreatic adenocarcinoma [63]. Application of FDG-PET for this purpose needs further study.

29.4.4
Lung Cancer

In surgery for lung carcinoma, it is crucial to characterize the solitary pulmonary nodule (SPN) and estimate resectability of the tumor.

29.4.4.1
Evaluation of Lung Tumors

FDG-PET is reliable in differentiating between benign and malignant SPNs. In a prospective multicenter trial with 89 patients having indeterminate SPN, PET showed an overall sensitivity and specificity of 92% and 90%, respectively [48].

Lung carcinomas tend to be visualized with high contrast owing to the low background FDG activity. However, small-sized carcinomas can yield false-negative results due to the limited resolution of the PET scanner. In the above-mentioned study [48], nodules less than 7 mm were excluded. A decrease in sensitivity from 92% to 80% was seen when the nodules were ≤1.5 cm. In most cases, CT is more sensitive than PET in detecting nodules less than 1 cm. However, CT has limited value in patients who have abnormal lung shadows secondary to thoracic surgery, atelectasis, emphysema, or fibrosis. In these situations, PET is superior to CT. We discovered a 1.0-cm lung carcinoma in a patient with emphysema [80]. CT was incapable of differentiating the carcinoma from fibrosis.

The histopathology of primary lung carcinoma includes adenocarcinoma (including bronchioloalveolar carcinoma), squamous cell carcinoma, small cell carcinoma, large cell carcinoma, and others. Primary lung carcinomas, with the exception of small cell carcinoma, can be candidates for surgery and are called non-small cell lung cancer (NSCLC). Small cell carcinoma is highly malignant and FDG-avid [91]. Among the NSCLCs, bronchioloalveolar carcinoma is not aggressive [55] and not so FDG-avid [30].

FDG accumulates in the presence of inflammation, and so in pneumonia. Benign lung nodules that can be false-positive with PET are granulomas with active inflammation such as tuberculoma [28], histoplasmosis, aspergillosis, coccidiomycosis, blastomycosis, fungal granuloma, necrotizing granuloma, and sarcoidosis [48, 76]. To confirm the histopathology in such cases, video assisted thoracoscopic surgery is one option that is less invasive than conventional thoracotomy [34]. Some granulomatous inflammations like tuberculoma sometimes require drug treatment based on histopathology.

29.4.4.2
Lymph Node Staging

Nodal metastasis is classified as N0 (no lymph node metastasis), N1 (metastasis to intrapulmonary or hilar lymph nodes), N2 (metastasis to ipsilateral mediastinal lymph nodes), and N3 (metastasis to contralateral mediastinal or supraclavicular lymph nodes). N3 lung cancer is contraindicated for surgery. Treatments for N2 lung cancer differ from country to country. Surgeons in Japan usually perform ipsilateral mediastinal lymph node dissection with a curative intent.

For detecting mediastinal lymph node metastasis from NSCLC, PET is superior to CT. Dwamena et al. (1999) [17] reviewed the published studies in the 1990s and reported that sensitivity and specificity were 60% and 77%, respectively, for CT and 79% and 91%, respectively, for PET. PET was significantly more accurate than CT for characterization of mediastinal lymph nodes. In a prospective study conducted by Pieterman et al. (2000) [65] sensitivity and specificity were 75% and 66%, respectively, for CT and 91% and 86%, respectively, for PET. PET was significantly superior to CT. PET+CT is significantly more accurate than CT alone in lymph node staging of NSCLC [85].

It should be noted, however, that in these studies PET results were not given for individual nodes. Lymph nodes were grouped by stations or compartments, and a positive PET scan was one that had at least one hot spot [65, 85]. Strictly speaking, for precise determination of nodal status, surgeons have to perform extensive lymph node dissection, not only of enlarged nodes but also of normal appearing nodes. Furthermore, conventional histopathologic examination is insufficient. Immunohistochemical staining or RT-PCR techniques are necessary to reveal micrometastases. When such histopathologic results are used as the gold standard, the sensitivity of PET is lowered. PET is incapable of detecting minimal disease in lymph nodes. The important thing is that PET can increase diagnostic accuracy for mediastinal lymph node metastasis by combined use with CT.

29.4.4.3
Evaluation of Distant Metastasis

One of the benefits of using PET is that it can disclose unsuspected lesions. Unsuspected extrathoracic metastasis were detected in 14% of patients with stage IIIa or less NSCLC [90]. The metastatic sites were bone, liver, and adrenal glands [10, 18, 90]. FDG-PET detected unsuspected lesions in as many as 24.6% of cases that would not have been discovered by conventional staging [86]. A prospective randomized study showed that PET can reduce the number of futile thoracotomies [84]. The value of PET is thus substantial for patients with lung carcinoma (Fig. 3).

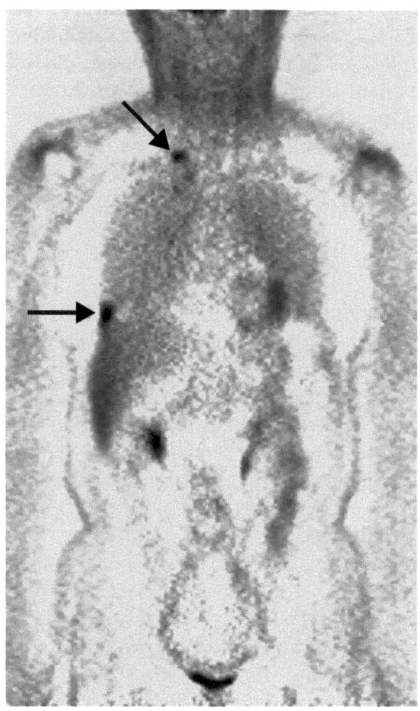

Fig. 3. Recurrent lung cancer at the upper mediastinum and chest wall. CT failed to detect the lesions

29.4.5 Breast Cancer

29.4.5.1 *Evaluation of Primary Tumors*

Recent studies of FDG-PET for differentiation between benign and malignant tumors of the breast showed 80%–93% sensitivity and 75%–76% specificity [5, 69]. Small carcinomas tend to yield false-negative findings. Avril et al. 2000 [5] showed the sensitivity of PET to be 48%–68% in pT1 tumors (≤2 cm), 81%–91% in pT2 tumors (>2 to 5 cm), and 79%–100% in pT3 tumors (>5 cm). We discovered a small breast carcinoma by PET in an asymptomatic screenee [79]. The surgical specimen was 6 mm, and the pathological specimen was 3 mm. Although this patient had undergone a PET study 9 months earlier, abnormal FDG uptake was not observed at that time even on retrospective analysis. This indicates a size limitation for detecting small breast cancer with PET.

Histopathologically, high FDG uptake is observed in ductal carcinoma. Lobular carcinomas comprise 7%–10% of invasive breast carcinomas, and tubular carcinoma 1%–2%, and both can yield false-negative findings [69]. High FDG uptake is reported in some fibroadenomas [69], whereas high FDG uptake is not observed in fibrocystic disease. The sensitivity of detecting breast carcinoma by FDG-PET seems to be dependent not only on tumor size but also on the histopathologic subtype [69].

Positive PET scans provide a high positive-predictive value (96.6%) for breast carcinoma [5]. However, distinguishing malignant from benign disease seems better addressed by aspiration cytology or breast biopsy. Therefore, PET is not recommended for routine use in the characterization of breast tumor.

29.4.5.2 *Axillary Staging*

In cases of axillary lymph node metastasis, FDG-PET showed 50%–79% sensitivity and 92%–100% specificity [4, 69, 82]. We obtained 70% sensitivity and 100% specificity [57]. Identification of nodal metastasis with PET is highly dependent on the tumor volume in the lymph nodes. The detection of small axillary lymph node metastasis is limited by the currently achievable spatial resolution of PET imaging. Of course, PET cannot detect micrometastases (≤2 mm) [29].

For axillary staging, sentinel lymph node biopsy (SLNB) has the ability to detect micrometastasis [54]. SLNB is indicated in patients with N0 breast cancer. For determination of N0 status, PET seems to be superior to physical examination and US. Patients with PET-negative findings for axillary nodes are indications for SLNB [69]. Patients with positive PET findings should undergo definitive surgery with full axillary dissection [88].

29.4.5.3 *Evaluation of Distant Metastasis*

With respect to bone metastasis, FDG-PET can detect more bone lesions than can be detected by 99mTc-MDP bone scintigraphy (bone scintigraphy). PET and bone scintigraphy exploit different mechanisms to detect tumor involvement. Bone scintigraphy relies on the osteoblastic bone response to tumor, whereas FDG-PET measures glucose uptake of the tumor cells. The radiographic appearance of bone metastases can be classified as osteolytic or osteoblastic (sclerotic). Higher standardized uptake values have been observed for osteolytic rather than osteoblastic disease (mean, 6.77 and 0.95, respectively; $p < 0.01$) [12]. Thus, PET is more sensitive than bone scintigraphy for lytic lesions. For sclerotic lesions, bone scintigraphy depicts more abnormalities than are depicted by PET. Sclerotic metastases are relatively acellular, and as such the lower volume of viable tumor tissue within individual lesions may influence the degree of FDG uptake. Patients with lytic bone metastasis have a poorer prognosis than that of patients with sclerotic bone metastasis. High sensitivity has been shown with F-18 PET in comparison to bone scintigraphy, although this method is not widely used at present [68].

We had a patient who had lung metastasis disclosed with PET just before surgery for the primary tumor. Chest radiography findings were negative. In another patient with right breast carcinoma and right axillary nodal metastases, PET disclosed left axillary nodal metastases. Surgery was canceled and chemotherapy was started. There is no evidence of disease in this patient, now 8 years after the start of chemotherapy. In the detection of recurrent or metastatic breast carcinoma, sensitivity and specificity of PET were 93% and 79%, respectively [51]. PET can help to detect more lesions than can be detected by MMG, US, chest radiography, and bone scintigraphy. For the assessment of systemic metastatic disease, however, some caution is in order: small lesions, sclerotic bone metastases, and brain metastases [88]. FDG-PET cannot be recommended for routine evaluation of the breast cancer, and it is best applied to resolve difficult imaging questions in specific patients [88].

29.4.5.4 *Quantification of Glucose Metabolism*

FDG-PET is used to assess glucose metabolism of breast carcinoma. Patients with a primary tumor of high FDG uptake have a poorer prognosis than those with primary tumor of low FDG uptake [59]. Among patients with advanced breast carcinoma undergoing primary chemotherapy, FDG-PET differentiates responders from nonresponders early in the course of therapy, providing an opportunity to offer nonresponders alternative therapies and thereby spare them from unwarranted toxicity [9, 66]. However, FDG-PET can not predict complete pathological response (no residual viable tumor) in patients achieving a good clinical response to neoadjuvant chemotherapy for primary breast cancer. Therefore, postoperative histological examination is required to confirm complete pathological response [9]. It appears reasonable to conclude that failure of a chemotherapy regimen to decrease FDG uptake promptly in a breast cancer portends a poor prognosis [88].

29.5 Summary

The attractiveness of PET imaging lies in its ability to detect lesions that are undetectable by conventional imaging modalities. Future PET scanners with a higher resolution could increase the potential to detect smaller lesions, improving the clinical benefits of PET. However, all imaging studies have an unavoidable limitation; they cannot detect microscopic lesions. For the small cancerous lesion, a positive PET image can indicate the abnormality, whereas a negative PET image cannot rule out the presence of a lesion. In some malignant tumors, FDG uptake is low, whereas in some benign tumors, FDG uptake is high. The degree of FDG uptake depends on the histopathologic tumor types. Finally, the presence of inflammation at the histological level can give rise to focal FDG uptake. If these are recognized, the results of FDG-PET studies will help in surgical decision-making.

References

1. Abdel-Nabi H, Doerr RJ, Lamonica DM et al (1998) Staging of primary colorectal carcinomas with fluorine-18 fluorodeoxyglucose whole-body PET: correlation with histopathologic and CT findings. Radiology 206:755–760
2. Adams S, Baum R, Rink T et al (1998) Limited value of fluorine-18 fluorodeoxyglucose positron emission tomography for the imaging of neuroendocrine tumors. Eur J Nucl Med 25:79–83
3. Arulampalam THA, Costa DC, Loizidou M et al (2001) Positron emission tomography and colorectal cancer. Br J Surg 88:176–189
4. Avril N, Schelling M, Dose J et al (1999) Utility of PET in breast cancer. Clin Pos Imag 2:261–271
5. Avril N, Rose CA, Schelling M et al (2000) Breast imaging with positron emission tomography and fluorine-18 fluorodeoxyglucose: use and limitations. J Clin Oncol 18:3495–3502
6. Berger KL, Nicholson SA, Dehdashti F et al (2000) FDG-PET evaluation of mucinous neoplasms: correlation of FDG uptake with histopathologic features. Am J Roentgenol 174:1005–1008
7. Block MI, Patterson GA, Sundaresan RS et al (1997) Improvement in staging of esophageal cancer with the addition of positron emission tomography. Ann Thorac Surg 64:770–777
8. Brücher BLDM, Weber W, Bauer M et al (2001) Neoajuvant therapy of esophageal squamous cell carcinoma: response evaluation by positron emission tomography. Ann Surg 233:300–309
9. Burcombe RJ, Makris A, Pittam M et al (2002) Evaluation of good clinical response to neoadjuvant chemotherapy in primary breast cancer using [18F]-fluorodeoxyglucose positron emission tomography. Eur J Cancer 38:375–379
10. Bury T, Barreto A, Daenen F et al (1998) Fluorine-18 deoxyglucose positron emission tomography for the detection of bone metastases in patients with non-small cell lung cancer. Eur J Nucl Med 25:1244–1247
11. Choi JY, Lee KH, Shim YM et al (2000) Improved detection of individual nodal involvement in squamous cell carcinoma of the esophagus by FDG PET. J Nucl Med 41:808–815
12. Cook GJ, Houston S, Rubens R et al (1998) Detection of bone metastases in breast cancer by 18FDG PET: differing metabolic activity in osteoblastic and osteolytic lesions. J Clin Oncol 16:3375–3379
13. Delbeke D, Vitola JV, Sandler MP et al (1997) Staging recurrent metastatic colorectal carcinoma with PET. J Nucl Med 38:1196–1201
14. Delbeke D, Rose DM, Chapman WC et al (1999) Optimal interpretation of FDG PET in the diagnosis, staging and management of pancreatic carcinoma. J Nucl Med 40:1784–1791
15. Desch CE, Benson AB, Smith TJ et al (1999) Recommended colorectal cancer surveillance guidelines by the American Society of Clinical Oncology. J Clin Oncol 17:1312
16. Diederichs CG, Staib L, Glatting G et al (1998) FDG PET: elevated plasma glucose reduced both uptake and detection rate of pancreatic malignancies. J Nucl Med 39:1030–1033
17. Dwamena BA, Sonnad SS, Angobaldo JO et al (1999) Metastases from non-small cell lung cancer: mediastinal staging in the 1990 s – meta-analytic comparison of PET and CT. Radiology 213:530–536
18. Erasmus JJ, Patz EF, McAdams HP et al (1997) Evaluation of adrenal masses in patients with bronchogenic carcinoma using 18F-fluorodeoxyglucose positron emission tomography. AJR 168:1357–1360
19. Femandez-Represa JA, Rodriguez DF, Contin MJP et al (2000) Pancreatic glucagonoma: detection by positron emission tomography. Eur J Surg 166:175–176
20. Findlay M, Young H, Cunningham D et al (1996) Noninvasive monitoring of tumor metabolism using fluorodeoxyglucose and positron emission tomography in colorectal cancer liver metastases: correlation with tumor response to fluorouracil. J Clin Oncol 14:700–708
21. Flamen P, Stroobants S, van Custem E et al (1999) Additional value of whole-body positron emission tomography with fluorine-18-2-fluoro-2-deoxy-D-glucose in recurrent colorectal cancer. J Clin Oncol 17:894–901
22. Flamen P, Lerut A, Cutsem EV et al (2000) Utility of positron emission tomography for the staging of patients with potentially operable esophageal carcinoma. J Clin Oncol 18:3202–3210
23. Flamen P, Hoekstra OS, Homans F et al (2001) Unexplained rising carcinoembryonic antigen (CEA) in the postoperative surveillance of colorectal cancer: the utility of positron emission tomography (PET). Eur J Cancer 37:862–869
24. Fong Y, Saldinger PF, Akhurst T et al (1999) Utility of 18F-FDG positron emission tomography scanning on selection of patients for resection of hepatic colorectal metastases. Am J Surg 178:282–287
25. Friess H, Langhans J, Ebert M et al (1995) Diagnosis of pancreatic cancer by 2[18F]-fluoro-2-deoxy-D-glucose positron emission tomography. Gut 36:771–777
26. Fröhlich A. Diederichs CG, Staib L et al (1999) Detection of liver metastases from pancreatic cancer. using FDG PET. J Nucl Med 40:250–255
27. Fukunaga T, Okazumi S, Koide S et al (1998) Evaluation of esophageal cancers using fluroine-18-fluorodeoxyglucose PET. J Nucl Med 39:1002–1007
28. Goo JM, Im JG, Do KH et al (2000) Pulmonary tuberculoma evaluated by means of FDG PET: findings in 10 cases. Radiology 216:117–121
29. Guller U, Nitzsche EU, Schirp U et al (2002) Selective axillary surgery in breast cancer patients based on positron emission tomography with 18F-fluoro-2-deoxy-D-glucose: not yet! Breast Cancer Res Treat 71:171–173
30. Higashi K, Ueda Y, Seki H et al (1998) Fluorine-18-FDG imaging is negative in bronchioloalveolar lung carcinoma. J Nucl Med 39:1016–1020

31. Himeno S, Yasuda S, Shimada H et al (2002) Evaluation of esophageal cancer by positron emission tomography. Jpn J Clin Oncol 32:340–346
32. Imdahl A, Nitzsche E, Krautmann F et al (1999) Evaluation of positron emission tomography with 2-[18F]fluoro-2-deoxy-D-glucose for the differentiation of chronic pancreatitis and pancreatic cancer. Br J Surg 86:194–199
33. Inokuma T, Tamaki N, Torizuka T et al (1995) Evaluation of pancreatic tumors with positron emission tomography and F-18 fluorodeoxyglucose: comparison with CT and US. Radiology 195:345–352
34. Iwasaki M, Nishiumi N, Maitani F et al (1996) Thoracoscopic surgery for lung cancer using the two small skin incision method. Two window method. J Cardiovasc Surg 37:79–81
35. Izbicki JR, Hosch SB, Pichlmeier U et al (1997) Prognostic value of immunohistochemically identifiable tumor cells in lymph nodes of patients with completely resected esophageal cancer. N Engl J Med 337:1188–1194
36. Japanese Society for Cancer of the Colon and Rectum (2002) Multi-institutional registry of large bowel cancer in Japan, vol 22, Tokyo
37. Kalady MF, Clary BM, Clark LA et al (2002) Clinical utility of positron emission tomography in the diagnosis and management of periampullary neoplasms. Ann Surg Oncol 9:799–806
38. Kalff V, Hicks RJ, Ware RE et al (2002) The clinical impact of 18F-FDG PET in patients with suspected or confirmed recurrence of colorectal cancer: a prospective study. J Nucl Med 43: 492–499
39. Kasperk RK, Riesener KP, Wilms K et al (2001) Limited value of positron emission tomography in treatment of pancreatic cancer: surgeon's view. World J Surg 25:1134–1139
40. Kato T, Fukatsu H, Ito K et al (1995) Fluorodeoxyglucose positron emission tomography in pancreatic cancer: an unsolved problem. Eur J Nucl Med 22:32–39
41. Kelsen DP, Ginsberg R, Pajak TF et al (1998) Chemotherapy followed by surgery compared with surgery alone for localized esophageal cancer. N Engl J Med 339:1979–1984
42. Kemeny N, Huang Y, Cohen AM et al (1999) Hepatic arterial infusion of chemotherapy after resection of hepatic metastases from colorectal cancer. N Engl J Med 341:2039–2048
43. Kodama M, Kakegawa T (1998) Treatment of superficial cancer of the esophagus: a summary of responses to a questionnaire on superficial cancer of the esophagus in Japan. Surgery 123: 432–439
44. Koyama K, Okamura T, Kawabe J et al (2001) Diagnostic usefulness of FDG PET for pancreatic mass lesions. Ann Nucl Med 15: 217–224
45. Lai DT, Fulham M, Stephen MS et al (1996) The role of whole-body positron emission tomography with [18F]fluorodeoxyglucose in identifying operable colorectal cancer metastases to the liver. Arch Surg 131:703–707
46. Lerut T, Flamen P, Ectors N et al (2000) Histopathologic validation of lymph node staging with FDG-PET scan in cancer of the esophagus and gastroesophageal junction. Ann Surg 232: 743–752
47. Libutti SK, Alexander HR Jr, Choyke P et al (2001) A prospective study of 2-[18F]fluoro-2-deoxy-D-glucose/positron emission tomography scan, 99mTc-labeled arcitumomab (CEA-scan), and blind second-look laparotomy for detecting colon cancer recurrence in patients with increasing carcinoembryonic antigen levels. Ann Surg Oncol 8:779–786
48. Lowe VJ, Fletcher JW, Gobar L et al (1998) Prospective investigation of positron emission tomography in lung nodules. J Clin Oncol 16:1075–1084
49. Luketich JD, Friedman DM, Weigel TL et al (1999) Evaluation of distant metastases in esophageal cancer: 100 consecutive positron emission tomography scans. Ann Thorac Surg 68:1133–1137
50. Makuuchi H (1996) Endoscopic mucosal resection for early esophageal cancer – indication and technique. Dig Endosc 8: 175–179
51. Moon DH, Maddahi J, Silverman DHS et al (1998) Accuracy of whole-body fluorine-18-FDG PET for the detection of recurrent or metastatic breast carcinoma. J Nucl Med 39:431–435
52. Nagata Y, Yamamoto K, Hiraoka M et al (1990) Monitoring liver tumor therapy with [18F]FDG positron emission tomography. J Comput Assist Tomogr 14:370–374
53. Nishiguchi S, Shiomi S, Ishizu H et al (2001) A case of glucagonoma with high uptake on F-18 fluorodeoxyglucose positron emission tomography. Ann Nucl Med 15:259–262
54. Noguchi M (2002) Sentinel lymph node biopsy and breast cancer. Br J Surg 89:21–34
55. Noguchi M, Morikawa A, Kawasaki M et al (1995) Small adenocarcinoma of the lung. Cancer 75:2844–2852
56. Ogunbiyi OA, Flanagan FL, Dehashi F et al (1997) Detection of recurrent and metastatic colorectal cancer: comparison of positron emission tomography and computed tomography. Ann Surg Oncol 4:613–620
57. Ohta M, Tokuda Y, Saitoh Y et al (2000) Comparative efficacy of positron emission tomography and ultrasonography in preoperative evaluation of axillary lymph node metastases in breast cancer. Breast Cancer 7:99–103
58. Oku S, Nakagawa K, Momose T et al (2002) FDG-PET after radiotherapy is a good prognostic indicator of rectal cancer. Ann Nucl Med 16:409–416
59. Oshida M, Uno K, Suzuki M et al (1998) Predicting the prognosis of breast carcinoma patients with positron emission tomography using 2-deoxy-2-fluoro[18F]-D-glucose. Cancer 82: 2227–2234
60. Rajput A, Stellato TA, Faulhaber PF et al (1998) The role of fluorodeoxyglucose and positron emission tomography in the evaluation of pancreatic disease. Surgery 124:793–798
61. Rice TW (1999) Superficial oesophageal carcinoma: is there a need for three-field lymphadenectomy? Lancet 354:792–794
62. Romer W, Hanauske AR, Ziegler S et al (1998) Positron emission tomography in non-Hodgkin's lymphoma: assessment of chemotherapy with fluorodeoxyglucose. Blood 91:4464–4471
63. Rose DM, Delbeke D, Beauchamp RD et al (1998) 18Fluorodeoxyglucose-positron emission tomography in the management of patients with suspected pancreatic cancer. Ann Surg 229:729–738
64. Ruers T, Bleichrodt RP (2002) Treatment of liver metastases, an update on the possibilities and results. Eur J Cancer 38:1023–1033
65. Pieterman RM, Van Putten JWG, Meuzelaar JJ et al (2000) Preoperative staging of non-small-cell lung cancer with positron-emission tomography. N Engl J Med 343:254–261
66. Schelling M, Avril N, Nahrig J et al (2000) Positron emission tomography using [(18)F]fluorodeoxyglucose for monitoring primary chemotherapy in breast cancer. J Clin Oncol 18:1689–1695
67. Schiepers C, Haustermans K, Geboes K et al (1999) The effect of preoperative radiation therapy on glucoses utilization and cell kinetics in patients with primary rectal carcinoma. Cancer 85: 803–811
68. Schirrmeister H, Guhlmann A, Kotzerke J et al (1999) Early detection and accurate description of extent of metastatic bone disease in breast cancer with fluoride ion and positron emission tomography. J Clin Oncol 17:2381–2389
69. Schirrmeister H, Kuhn T, Guhlmann A et al (2001) Fluorine-18 2-deoxy-2-fluoro-D-glucose PET in the preoperative staging of breast cancer: comparison with the standard staging procedure. Eur J Nucl Med 28:351–358
70. Schwart M, Pauls S, Sokiranski R et al (2001) Is a preoperative multidiagnostic approach to predict surgical resectability of periampullary tumors still effective ? Am J Surg 182:243–249
71. Sendler A, Avril N, Helmberger H et al (2000) Preoperative evaluation of pancreatic masses with positron emission tomography using 18F-fluorodeoxyglucose: diagnostic limitations. World J Surg 24:1121–1129
72. Shreve PD (1998) Focal fluorine-18 fluorodeoxyglucose accumulation in inflammatory pancreatic disease. Eur J Nucl Med 25:259–264
73. Staib L, Schirrmeister H, Reske SN et al (2000) Is 18F-fluorodeoxyglucose positron emission tomography in recurrent colorectal cancer a contribution to surgical decision making? Am J Surg 180:1–5
74. Stollfuss JC, Glatting G, Friess H et al (1995) 2-[fluorine-18]-flu-

oro-2-deoxy-D-glucose PET in detection of pancreatic cancer: value of quantitative image interpretation. Radiology 195:339–344, World J Surg 24:1121–1129
75. Strasberg SM, Dehdashti F, Siegel BA et al (2001) Survival of patients evaluated by FDG-PET before hepatic resection for metastatic colorectal carcinoma: a prospective database study. Ann Surg 233:293–299
76. Yasuda S, Shohtsu A, Ide M et al (1996) High fluorine-18 labeled deoxyglucose uptake in sarcoidosis. Clin Nucl Med 21:983–984
77. Yasuda S, Shohtsu A, Tomioka K (1998) F-18 fluorodeoxyglucose positron emission tomography imaging in ectopic nonfunctioning glucagonoma. Clin Nucl Med 23:474–475
78. Yasuda S, Takahashi W, Takagi S et al (1998) Factors influencing physiological FDG uptake in the intestine. Tokai J Exp Clin Med 23:241–244
79. Yasuda S, Kubota M, Tajima T et al (1999) A small breast cancer detected by PET. Jpn J Clin Oncol 29:387–389
80. Yasuda S, Ide M, Fujii H et al (2000) Application of positron emission tomography imaging to cancer screening. Br J Cancer 83:1607–1611
81. Yasuda S, Fujii H, Nakahara T et al (2001) 18F-FDG PET detection of colonic adenomas. J Nucl Med 42:989–992
82. Yutani K, Shiba E, Kusuoka H et al (2000) Comparison of FDG-PET with MIBI-SPECT in the detection of breast cancer and axillary lymph node metastasis. J Comput Assist Tomogr 24: 274–280
83. Valk PE, Abella Columna E, Haseman MK et al (1999) Whole-body PET imaging with [18F]fluorodeoxyglucose in management of recurrent colorectal cancer. Arch Surg 134:503–511
84. Van Tinteren H, Hoekstra OS, Smit EF et al (2002) Effectiveness of positron emission tomograph in the preoperative assessment of patients with suspected non-small-cell lung cancer: the PLUS multicentre randomised trial. Lancet 359:1388–1392
85. Vansteenkiste JF, Stroobants SG, de Leyn PR et al (1998) Lymph node staging in non-small-cell lung cancer with FDG-PET scan: a prospective study on 690 lymph node stations from 68 patients. J Clin Oncol 16:2142–2149
86. Vesselle H, Pugsley JM, Vallieres E et al (2002) The impact of fluorodeoxyglucose F 18 positron-emission tomography on the surgical staging of non-small cell lung cancer. J Thorac Cardiovasc Surg 124:511–519
87. Vitola JV, Delbeke D, Sandler MP et al (1996) Positron emission tomography to stage suspected metastatic colorectal carcinoma to the liver. Am J Surg 171:21–26
88. Wahl RL (2001) Current status of PET in breast cancer imaging, staging, and therapy. Semin Roentgenol 36:250–260
89. Weber WA, Ott K, Becker K et al (2001) Prediction of response to preoperative chemotherapy in adenocarcinomas of the esophagogastric junction by metabolic imaging. J Clin Oncol 19:3058–3065
90. Weder W, Schmid RA, Bruchhaus H et al (1998) Detection of extrathoracic metastases by positron emission tomography in lung cancer. Ann Thorac Surg 66:886–893
91. Zhao DS, Valdivia AY, Blaufox LY (2002) 18Fofluorodeoxyglucose positron emission tomography in small-cell lung cancer. Semin Nucl Med 32:272–275
92. Zimny M, Bares R, Fass J, et al (1997) Fluorine-18 fluorodeoxyglucose positron emission tomography in the differential diagnosis of pancreatic carcinoma: a report of 106 cases. Eur J Nucl Med 24:678–682

CHAPTER 30

PET and Radiotherapy

V.J. Lowe

30.1 Background

In the late 1800s radioactivity and X-rays were discovered. The uses of radioactive treatment developed over subsequent years and in the early 1900s some of the standard radiotherapy principles were devised. Experimentation led to the law of Bergonie and Tribondeau which states that radiosensitivity is highest in tissues with a high mitotic index. Other scientists from this time described the dependence of radiation response to oxygen. Further advancement in radiation production equipment and computer assisted treatment planning then occurred. This brought us the radiotherapy practice of today that is able to generate controlled radiation doses and deliver radiation to precise tissue areas, thus optimizing desired radiation dosage.

Radiotherapy induction of cellular toxicity results from a combination of direct and indirect action. Radiotherapy can directly ionize the DNA molecule and lead to DNA strand breaks which, when multiple, can result in cell death. Radiation also has an indirect effect by creating free radicals of which the most important is likely the hydroxyl radical. Free radicals may then damage DNA or other important targets of cellular reproduction. Experts believe that roughly two thirds of total radiotherapy toxicity can be attributed to the actions of free radicals [1].

Assessing the effects of radiation therapy can be a difficult endeavor. Some aspects of radiotherapeutic assessment have been very difficult to determine in humans prior to the advent of PET. The following sections will deal with the use of PET in aiding the planning and assessment of radiation therapy.

30.2 PET Before Radiation Therapy

PET scans before, during and after treatment may each provide information that is useful for managing patients undergoing radiation therapy. In patients with locally advanced cancer, FDG-PET imaging performed before radiation therapy can be a valuable tool. It can assist in radiation therapy planning by helping to focus radiation ports to precise areas of tumor activity.

One group has described an evaluation of the possible effect of PET in altering radiation treatment plans. This group performed a retrospective assessment of whether PET would have changed treatment regions. A qualitative assessment was performed to determine whether abnormal thoracic PET activity was present in areas regarded as normal by diagnostic imaging. Additionally, adequacy of coverage of each patient's abnormal PET activity by the actual radiation field was assessed. Of 15 patients analyzed, 26.7% (four patients) would have had their radiotherapy volume influenced by PET findings [2].

Hughes and coworkers used PET in the dosing design for stereotactic implantation of iodine-125 seeds for the palliative treatment of recurrent malignant gliomas [3]. This group describes using three-dimensional (3D) models of PET and anatomic imaging to aid in dosage design.

Treatment planning with PET will likely require substantial image manipulation and compatibility with existing 3D planning computers. Treatment planning in a pilot group was evaluated by Erdi and coworkers [4]. They found that there was a change in treatment planning volumes when PET was used that improved definition of the primary tumor and lymph nodes involved. Malyapa and authors looked at 3D brachytherapy treatment planning for cervical cancer using PET and found that PET gave a reliable estimate of the tumor volume and improved isodose tumor coverage[5]. Although no studies presently demonstrate improved outcome from using PET in treatment planning, these data are promising and hopefully will improve the likelihood of achieving local disease control.

30.3 PET During Radiation Therapy

Further work needs to be done to evaluate the use of PET during radiation therapy as data is very sparse. Some data suggests that radiotherapy may induce early acute inflammatory hypermetabolism that can be confused with tumor hypermetabolism. In addition, some investigators have concluded that an early decrease in FDG uptake did not necessarily indicate a good prognosis.

Hautzel showed in a single patient that after only 6 Gy the metabolic level in cancer can increase and then subsequently decrease [6]. This highlights the need for detailed time course and treatment response parameter evaluations in this setting as uptake may be influenced by a variety of metabolic changes that may be unrelated to tumor response.

In sarcomas treated with combined radiotherapy and hyperthermia, well-defined central regions of absent uptake, with reduction of peripheral uptake, developed on FDG-PET 1–3 weeks after initiating therapy [7]. Immediately after completion of radiation therapy, PET demonstrated continued uptake, albeit less in some cases than in the pretreatment tumor, in the periphery of the tumor. This FDG accumulation was found to correlate pathologically with the formation of a fibrous pseudocapsule rather than residual disease [7]. In cases where tumor kill was over 90 %, such residual hypermetabolism was seen but was usually at some reduced level from the pretreatment PET. Brun and coworkers looked at the implications of PET in the early weeks of therapy. They concluded that a rapid reduction from a high metabolic level may imply a higher likelihood of response [8].

30.4 Deoxygenation and PET

Reoxygenation is the process by which tumor cells that were once hypoxic, regain access to oxygen due to shrinkage of tumor secondary to therapy. Animal models have demonstrated that reoxygenation occurs at different rates with different tumors. Because oxygen is needed for the production of free radicals, reoxygenation is an essential factor for optimal tumor kill [1]. Fractionated radiation therapy takes advantage of reoxygenation for more complete tumor kill. An initial dose will sterilize only the oxygenated cells, but, with a subsequent dose, cells that were once hypoxic that have become reoxygenated will be susceptible. There are no radiation therapy studies of this effect in humans but PET can offer a method to evaluate tumor hypoxia and reoxygenation in humans.

PET imaging of [F-18]fluoromisonidazole (FMISO) uptake allows noninvasive assessment of tumor hypoxia. Increased uptake is seen where cell hypoxia is present due to bioreduction and deposition of the agent, but FMISO is rapidly removed from well-oxygenated areas. Koh and colleagues used FMISO to assess tumors undergoing fractionated therapy and concluded that although there is a general tendency toward improved oxygenation in human tumors during fractionated radiotherapy, these changes were unpredictable and insufficient to overcome the negative effects of existing pretreatment hypoxia [9]. They suggested that trials including pretreatment hypoxia assessments with PET would be recommended for further test fractionated therapy protocols.

Minn and coworkers have also described the visualization of hypoxia with the metabolic tracers 2-[5,6-3H]fluoro-2-deoxy-D-glucose ([3H]FDG), L-[methyl-3H] methionine ([3H]MET), and L-[1-3H]leucine ([3H]LEU) [10]. This group showed that [3H]FDG accumulation is increased in hypoxic squamous cell cancer. They saw a decrease in acid-precipitable [3H]LEU uptake in hypoxia that may indicate a decline in protein synthesis, while unchanged [3H]MET uptake may reflect unaffected amino acid transport.

Further study of this type of assessment by PET may lead to improved radiation therapy planning. Fractionated radiation regimens would be more effective on tumors that are able to reoxygenate more quickly and can demonstrate reductions in tumor hypoxic fractions as radiation therapy is ongoing.

30.5 PET Imaging After Completion of Radiation Therapy

Radiotherapy response has traditionally been associated with reduction in tumor size. Complete response is generally felt to be the only standard for indicating tumor control. A partial response is considered to be a radiotherapeutic failure in most cases. The definition of complete response can be problematic as complete disappearance of the tumor may only occur rarely and more commonly residual tissue, whether it be scar or residual tumor, can remain.

PET has been used to assess the therapeutic response to radiation therapy. FDG-PET can identify changes in glucose uptake after treatment and may prove to be a better indicator of a favorable response to therapy. However, it may be important to differentiate between a decrease in FDG uptake and the complete absence of FDG uptake. Some investigators have concluded that a simple decrease in FDG uptake does not necessarily indicate a good prognosis [11]. Rather, it has been suggested that a decrease in FDG uptake may only indicate a partial response due to destruction of cells sensitive to the therapy while other resistant cells continue to be metabolically active. This is consistent with current thinking by radiotherapists of a partial response.

Post-treatment normalization of FDG uptake, on the other hand, appears to be a good prognostic sign. One study by Hebert and coworkers has demonstrated that negative PET findings after radiation therapy, even in the presence of non-specific radiographic changes, are an indicator of a good response [12]. Hebert noted that all of their patients with negative PET findings were alive at 2 years after treatment, whereas 50 % of patients with residual hypermetabolism, albeit reduced, had expired within that same 2-year period. Other investigators have used this logic to justify further treatment of

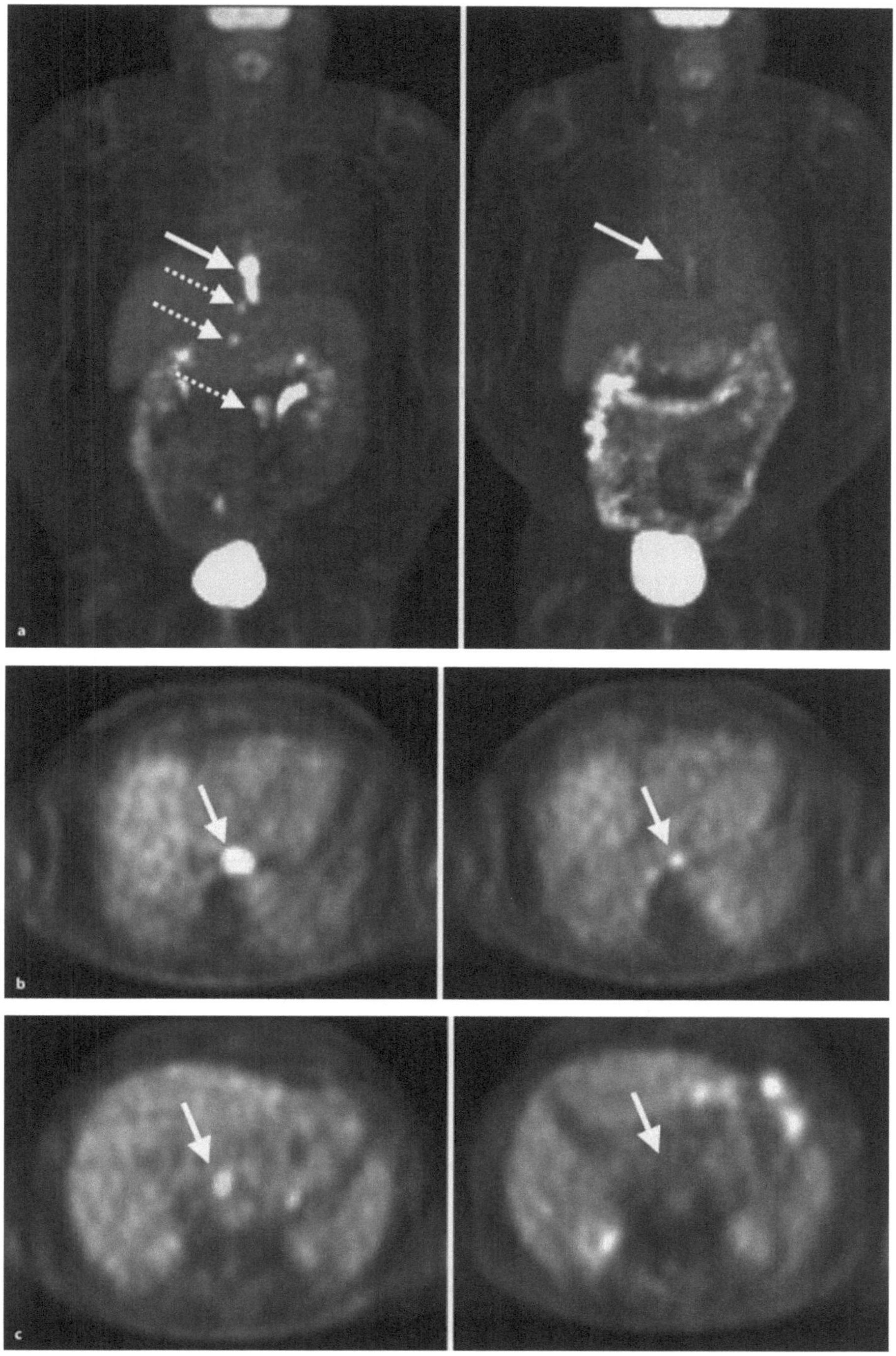

Fig. 1. a Coronal PET images pre- and post-neoadjuvant chemoradiotherapy for esophageal cancer. The esophageal tumor (*arrow*) largely resolves and the nodal disease (*dashed arrows*) completely resolves. **b, c** Axial views pre- and post-therapy of the primary tumor (*arrows*) (**b**) and a common hepatic lymph node (*arrows*) (**c**). Surgical pathology showed residual lymph node disease and microscopic residual esophageal tumor with post-treatment inflammation. The good PET response seen is predictive of good outcome even in the face of some minimal residual disease that was resected. The patient had no evidence of disease at 18 months after treatment

asymptomatic individuals whose PET scans demonstrate residual hypermetabolism after an initial course of therapy. Frank and colleagues treated five such asymptomatic patients in their study based solely on residual hypermetabolism and all were alive at 3 years [13].

Head and neck cancer reports have resulted in similar findings. Lindholm and others described C^{11} methionine PET imaging as it relates to treatment response [14]. They showed that reduced methionine uptake after therapy was more likely to indicate response. Minn and coworkers described the reduction in FDG uptake in patients imaged after radiation therapy and prior to surgery. A complete histological response was verified in none of nine cases with a post-irradiation SUV larger than 3.1, whereas 7 of the 10 cases with a SUV of 3.1 or smaller had complete response. This was a statistically significant finding ($p = 0.003$) [15].

Data has also shown that esophageal cancer neoadjuvant therapy can be assessed using PET. Combined radiochemotherapy has been looked at in a few studies in this regard [16, 17]. In one study by Flamen and coworkers [17], a group of 36 patients with locally advanced esophageal cancer (clinical T4 stage) without organ metastases, underwent FDG-PET before and 1 month after CRT. Resolution of tumor and all lymph node FDG uptake was considered to be indicative of a major response. They found that PET was 67% (4/6) sensitive and 50% (4/8) specific for a pathologic complete response and therefore was not a good predictor of pathologic response. This was due to microscopic residual disease and inflammatory hypermetabolism, respectively. However, the data was very promising in that a PET tumor complete response was still predictive of improved survival. The median survival was 16.3 months in PET responders and 6.4 months in non-responders. Given this data, patients would still need surgical removal of minimal residual tumor in PET "responders" but these patients will survive longer (Fig. 1).

30.6 Diagnosing Recurrent Disease with PET

Diagnosis of recurrent cancer is another potential use of FDG-PET after radiation therapy. Radiologic changes such as scarring and necrosis which occur after radiotherapy may obscure the identification of recurrent tumor unless significant volume changes occur over time. The interpretation of recurrence is often not made until the disease progresses to the point of marked enlargement of questionable abnormalities. Unfortunately, a tissue biopsy that is negative for tumor in such situations is suspect due to the inherent difficulty in identifying and accurately sampling the areas of viable tumor in the midst of scar. A PET evaluation of tumor recurrence can potentially assist in this determination.

For example, patients who have chest radiographic findings suspicious for tumor recurrence can be accurately characterized by FDG-PET. Benign, nonspecific pleural thickening is another example of post-treatment changes which may be difficult to differentiate from recurrent disease. Pleural biopsy itself may be relatively unreliable when performed percutaneously. PET imaging can differentiate recurrent tumor from radiation inducing benign pleural thickening [18]. Patz and coworkers [19] demonstrated a very high accuracy of PET in distinguishing recurrent disease from benign treatment effects when patients were scanned after therapy. The report of Inoue and coworkers [20] yielded similar results. Greven, in a nonblinded, prospective, single institution study, assessed 18 patients after radiation therapy and found a 100% sensitivity and a 92% specificity for detection of residual or recurrent head and neck cancer [21].

30.7 Timing of PET After Radiation Therapy

Normal tissues can manifest radiotherapy toxicity to different degrees. Some tissue will demonstrate toxicity in a few days. These tissues are bone marrow, gonads, lymph nodes, salivary glands, gastrointestinal tract, larynx, and skin. Other tissues demonstrate radiation damage in weeks to months and some examples are lung, liver, kidney, spinal cord and brain. Because of these effects, significantly increased FDG uptake can be seen in selected soft tissue regions that are irradiated. Data suggests that radiotherapy may induce early acute inflammatory hypermetabolism on PET that is likely related to healing of tissues damaged by radiation. This effect will likely depend on the radiosensitivity of the normal tissues being irradiated.

In chest radiotherapy, increased FDG uptake in the chest wall correlates with clinical evidence of radiation damage. Increased FDG accumulation in normal chest wall tissue can be statistically significant at least 12–16 months after treatment. The standardized uptake ratio (SUR) of this radiation related uptake is generally less than what is found in recurrent tumor (SUR<2.5) [22]. Nevertheless, FDG uptake from radiation effects can in a few cases be in a range that is worrisome for malignancy. This study showed that normal tissue activity inflammatory responses are maximum at about 6 months but can be seen for at least 1 year. (Fig. 2)

The study by Jones et al. suggests that immediately following radiation, a hypermetabolic pseudocapsule can be seen that may appear to falsely represent tumor [7]. And still, Greven and coworkers showed that within 1 month of radiation it is slightly more likely to see negative PET scans in people with some minimal residual disease. They also found that a 4-month PET assessment did not demonstrate any false negatives [21]. (Figs. 3, 4)

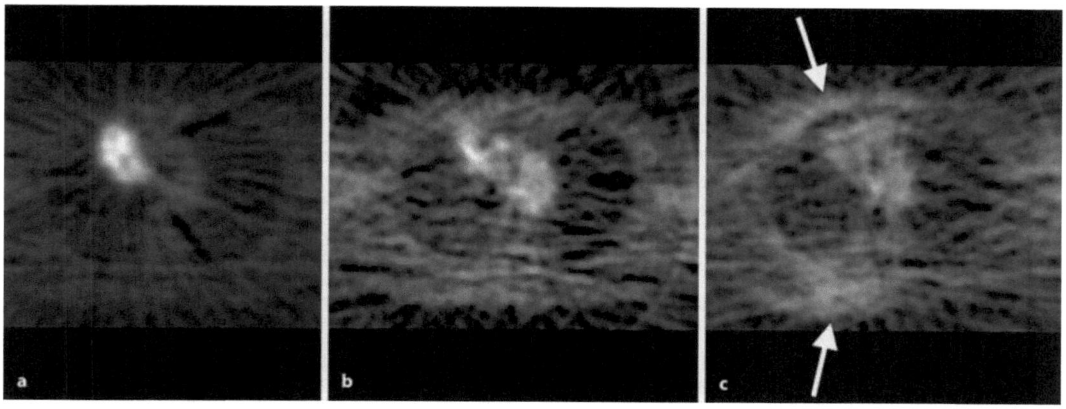

Fig. 2a–c. Axial FDG-PET images of a patient with right lung cancer before (**a**), 1 month after (**b**) and 6 months after (**c**) radiation therapy with 73.6 Gy. Mild chest wall inflammatory hypermetabolism is seen on the 6-month scan in radiation port locations (*arrows*). The tumor activity continues to decrease over the period but is only less intense than blood pool activity (negative for disease) at 6 months. The patient was free of disease 1 year later

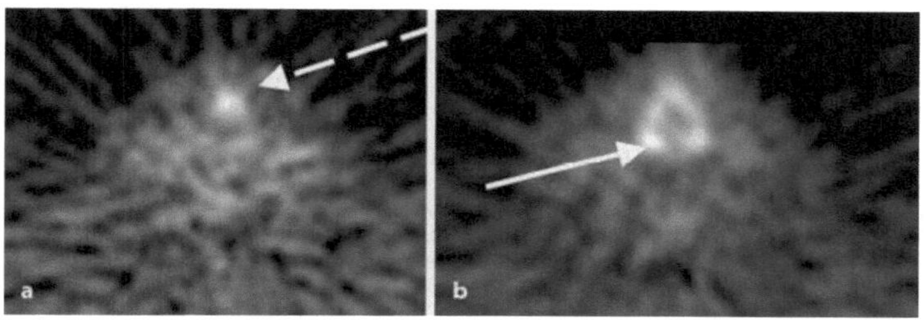

Fig. 3a,b. Axial FDG-PET images of a patient with T1 larynx cancer (*broken arrow*) before (**a**) and 1 month after (**b**) radiation therapy with 68 Gy. Hypermetabolism in the arytenoid cartilage regions is intense on the post-therapy scan because they are very radiation sensitive (*solid arrow*). Additional uptake more anteriorly in the vocal cords due to inflammation or muscle activity makes interpretation difficult in this 1 month post-therapy scan. The patient was disease-free 2 years later

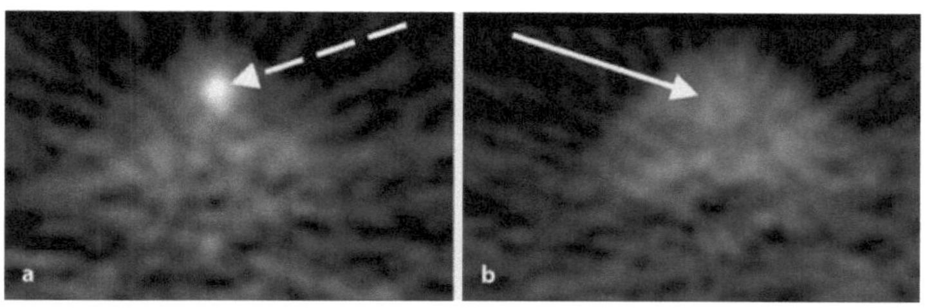

Fig. 4a,b. Axial FDG-PET images of a patient with T2 larynx cancer (*broken arrow*) before (**a**) and 4 months after (**b**) radiation therapy with 70 Gy. No intense post-therapy uptake is seen although mild uptake is present in the vocal cord region (*arrow*). This post-therapy scan is confidently negative. The patient was disease-free 2 years later

A fair compromise may be to recommend PET imaging 4–6 months after completion of radiation if possible. This would allow for assessment of early recurrence and probably give high accuracy of treatment assessment. If inflammatory hypermetabolism is confusing, a follow-up scan may be required to see if the activity diminishes over time. If one is forced to image earlier due to clinical necessity, particular attention should be paid to the patterns of any hypermetabolism present in the hope of distinguishing inflammation from residual disease. As in the esophageal cancer data, some loss in accuracy relative to pathologic response can be expected when imaging is performed early, but the predictive nature of a marked reduction in FDG for improved survival appears to be maintained and appears to be superior to any other imaging metric.

30.8 Summary

PET imaging can aid in radiation therapy planning and in the assessment of residual or recurrent disease. Areas of ongoing research that hold promise for additional uses of PET include early assessment of radiation effects and assessment of tumor hypoxia.

References

1. Hall EJ, Cox JD (1994) Physical and biologic basis of radiation therapy. In: Cox JD (ed) Moss' radiation oncology. Mosby-Year Book, St Louis, pp 3–66
2. Kiffer JD et al (1998) The contribution of 18F-fluoro-2-deoxyglucose positron emission tomographic imaging to radiotherapy planning in lung cancer. Lung Cancer 19:167–177
3. Hughes SW et al (1995) Computer planning of stereotactic iodine-125 seed brachytherapy for recurrent malignant gliomas. Br J Radiol 68:175–181
4. Erdi YE et al (2002) Radiotherapy treatment planning for patients with non-small cell lung cancer using positron emission tomography (PET). Radiother Oncol 62:51–60
5. Malyapa RS et al (2002) Physiologic FDG-PET three-dimensional brachytherapy treatment planning for cervical cancer. Int J Radiat Oncol Biol Phys 54:1140–1146
6. Hautzel H, Muller GH (1997) Early changes in fluorine-18-FDG uptake during radiotherapy. J Nucl Med 38:1384–1386
7. Jones DN et al (1996) Monitoring of neoadjuvant therapy response of soft-tissue and musculoskeletal sarcoma using fluorine-18-FDG PET. J Nucl Med 37:1438–1444
8. Brun E et al (1997) Early prediction of treatment outcome in head and neck cancer with 2–18FDG PET. Acta Oncologica 36: 741–747
9. Koh WJ et al (1995) Evaluation of oxygenation status during fractionated radiotherapy in human nonsmall cell lung cancers using [F-18]fluoromisonidazole positron emission tomography. Int J Radiat Oncol Biol Phys 33:391–398
10. Minn H, Clavo AC, Wahl RL (1996) Influence of hypoxia on tracer accumulation in squamous-cell carcinoma: in vitro evaluation for PET imaging. Nucl Med Biol 23:941–946
11. Ichiya Y et al (1991) Assessment of response to cancer therapy using fluorine-18-fluorodeoxyglucose and positron emission tomography. J Nucl Med 32:1655–1660
12. Hebert ME et al (1996) Positron emission tomography in the pretreatment evaluation and follow-up of non-small cell lung cancer patients treated with radiotherapy: preliminary findings. Am J Clin Oncol 19:416–421
13. Frank A et al (1995) Decision logic for retreatment of asymptomatic lung cancer recurrence based on positron emission tomography findings. Int J Radiat Oncol Biol Phys 32:1495–512
14. Lindholm P et al (1995) Evaluation of response to radiotherapy in head and neck cancer by positron emission tomography and [11C]methionine. Int J Radiat Oncol Biol Phys 32:787–794
15. Minn H et al (1997) Prediction of survival with fluorine-18-fluoro-deoxyglucose and PET in head and neck cancer. J Nucl Med 38:1907–1911
16. Brucher BL et al (2001) Neoadjuvant therapy of esophageal squamous cell carcinoma: response evaluation by positron emission tomography. Ann Surg 233:300–309
17. Flamen P et al ((2002) Positron emission tomography for assessment of the response to induction radiochemotherapy in locally advanced oesophageal cancer. Ann Oncol 13:361–368
18. Lowe VJ et al (1994) FDG-PET evaluation of pleural abnormalities. J Nucl Med 35:229P
19. Patz EJ et al (1994) Persistent or recurrent bronchogenic carcinoma: detection with PET and 2-[F-18]-2-deoxy-D-glucose. Radiol 191:379–382
20. Inoue T et al (1995) Detecting recurrent or residual lung cancer with FDG-PET. J Nucl Med 36:788–793
21. Greven KM et al (1994) Positron emission tomography of patients with head and neck carcinoma before and after high dose irradiation (see comments). Cancer 74:1355–1359
22. Lowe VJ, Naunheim KS (1998) Positron emission tomography in lung cancer. Ann Thorac Surg 65:1821–1829

CHAPTER 31

Cancer Screening with 18F FDG-PET

K. Nakai · S. Yasuda · M. Ide
S. Kawada · A. Shohtsu

Whole-body positron emission tomography (PET) with ^{18}F-fluorodeoxyglucose (FDG) is frequently used for tissue characterization, staging and therapy control images (Conti et al. 1996; Sven and Jorg 2001). We examined the potential application of ^{18}F FDG-PET for cancer screening in a large number of asymptomatic individuals (Yasuda and Shohtsu 1997; Ide and Suzuki 1996). A wide variety of cancers have been detected at potentially curable stages in asymptomatic individuals. However, FDG-PET study has obvious limitations in the detection of urological cancers, cancers of low cell density, small cancers and hypometabolic or FDG-negative cancers. Thus conventional examinations are also needed for cancer screening in conjunction with FDG-PET and understanding the images obtained in such cases helps in preventing misinterpretation of PET images (Yasuda et al. 2000). In the following section we report on our 7-year experience with whole-body PET for cancer screening in asymptomatic individuals.

31.1 Background

We evaluated the PET images using a simple visual analysis without transmission scanning to save time. Lesions (98.1%) were recognizable on uncorrected images as well as corrected images in an earlier study of patients with various cancers (Yasuda et al. 1996a).

In a simple visual analysis without attenuation correction, the boundary between the lung and the liver was not distinct. Furthermore intensity was enhanced in directions tangential to the body surface in lesions located near the body surface and the anteroposterior dimension appears longer on uncorrected images because of the elliptical cross section of the body. Though these image distortions were observed, lesion contrast was not diminished.

31.2 Subjects and Methods

Our institution is a medical health club located in Yamanashi, Japan. Our cancer screening program includes whole-body PET in conjunction with conventional screening modalities including physical examination, laboratory study, ultrasonography (upper abdomen, thyroid gland and breast), spiral CT (chest) and MRI (lower abdomen). Under our current protocol, all subjects fast for at least 6 hours before FDG injection. Water intake is encouraged to dilute the urinary concentration of FDG. Coffee intake is also allowed to reduce myocardial FDG uptake, although the effect is not evident. We use a dose of 260 MBq FDG. Resting is encouraged during the uptake period to prevent FDG uptake in the muscles, especially the skeletal, oculomotor, and laryngeal muscles. After an uptake period of 45–60 min, the subjects are encouraged to void. To minimize bladder activity, emission scanning (3 min for each bed position) starts from the pelvis and moves upward to the maxilla. Gray-scale hard copy images of transaxial slices are printed out and interpreted visually; images of coronal and sagittal slices are also made available.

31.3 Results

Between October 1994 and April 2002, 6147 asymptomatic club members participated in 13,243 screening sessions (3824 men and 2323 women, mean age was 52.2 ± 10.4 yeas). Malignant tumors were discovered in 129 of the 6147 participants (2.1%) and 13,243 screening sessions (0.97%) (Table 1).

FDG-PET findings were true-positive in 69 of the 129 cancers (53%) (Table 2). These 69 cases include 19 lung, 18 thyroid, ten colon, nine breast, three stomach cancers and one case each of pancreas, esophagus, kidney, liver, and ovary cancer. In particular, the cases of pancreas, esophageal and ovarian cancer could not be detected without FDG-PET examination. Microscopic metastatic foci were observed in a dissected lymph node in one patient with breast cancer, but lymph node metastasis was not observed in any other patient. All lung cancers were pathological Stage I. Most of the 69 patients underwent potentially curative surgery with the exception of one lymphoma patient, thus a wide variety of cancers were detected by FDG-PET (Figs. 1–10).

FDG-PET findings were false-negative in 60 of the 129 patients (47%). Of these 60, 30 (50%) were of uro-

Table 1. Cancers detected at the HIMEDIC Imaging Center (13,243 studies/6147 subjects) between October 1994 and April 2002

Cancer	Cases (*n*)	PET (+)	PET(−)	Other methods of detection
Lung	28	19	9	CT
Thyroid	26	18	8	US
Prostatic	17	0	17	DRE, PSA
Breast	12	9	3	US
Colorectal	10	10	0	-
Renal	7	1	6	US, CT
Hepatoma	7	1	6	US
Gastric	6	3	3	US
Bladder	5	0	5	US, MRI
Metastatic liver	2	2	0	US
Pancreas	2	1	1	US, CT
Uterine	2	0	2	MRI
Esophageal	1	1	0	-
Malignant lymphoma	1	1	0	-
Ovarian	1	1	0	-
Parapharyngeal	1	1	0	-
Chronic myelogenous leukemia	1	1	0	-
Total	129	69	60	-

Table 2. FDG-PET positive studies (13,243 studies/6147 subjects) obtained between October 1994 and April 2002

Cancer	Cases (*n*)	Size
Lung	19	1.0–3.6 cm
Thyroid	18	0.6–3.0 cm
Colorectal	10	3.5–6.0 cm
Breast	9	0.6–2.4 cm
Gastric	3	3.5 cm
Metastatic liver	2	0.6–2.4 cm
Hepatoma	1	
Pancreas	1	2.0 cm
Esophageal	1	2.0 cm
Renal	1	4.0 cm
Malignant lymphoma	1	-
Ovarian	1	-
Parapharyngeal	1	4.0 cm
Chronic myelogenous leukemia	1	-
Total	69	-

Table 3. FDG-PET negative studies (13,243 studies/6147 subjects) obtained between October 1994 and April 2002

Cancer	Cases (*n*)	Size
Prostatic	17	A2–D2
Lung	9	0.8–2.0 cm
Thyroid	8	1.0–2.0 cm
Renal	6	1.5–6.0 cm
Hepatoma	6	1.5–3.0 cm
Bladder	5	1.0–2.0 cm
Breast	3	0.5 cm
Gastric	3	1.5 cm
Uterine	2	4.0 cm
Pancreas	1	-
Total	60	-

genital origin (Table 3). There were nine false-negative lung cancers including an 8-mm tubular adenocarcinoma, a 1.2-cm bronchoalveolar adenocarcinoma, and a 1.5-cm bronchoalveolar adenocarcinoma. These were also negative with chest radiography. Five hepatomas were negative with PET and positive with ultrasonography. And there were three false-negative breast cancers including a scirrhous-type breast cancer (1.5-cm), which were negative with PET and positive with ultrasonography.

A substantial number of benign lesions were detected with PET. Unnecessary surgery was performed in one case of chronic thyroiditis encountered early in our study (Yasuda et al. 1997a). The result of ultrasonographic diagnosis in this case was thyroid tumor. Three subjects with benign pulmonary lesions (one 1-cm tuberculoma and two 1-cm organized pneumonias), for whom PET and CT scans were inconclusive, had to undergo surgery before definite diagnoses could be obtained. High FDG uptake was noted in other benign lesions such as colonic adenoma (Yasuda et al. 1998a), Warthin's tumor (Horiuchi et al. 1998), thyroid adenoma, sarcoidosis (Yasuda et al. 1996b), chronic maxillary sinusitis, and lymphadenitis.

31.4 Cancer Screening

Positron emission tomography (PET) with ^{18}F-fluorodeoxy-glucose (FDG) has been developed to quantitatively assess local glucose metabolism. Because malignant tumors exhibit increase of glucose metabolism, quantification of FDG uptake by PET helps to differentiate between benign and malignant tumors (Rigo et al. 1996), to determine the degree of malignancy (Adler et al. 1991), to evaluate the effectiveness of chemotherapy or radiotherapy (Price and Jones 1995), and to predict prognosis (Okada et al. 1994; Nakata et al. 1997; Oshida et al. 1998). Since the invention of the whole-body imaging technique (Guerrero et al. 1990), PET has also been used to depict hypermetabolic cancers. PET imaging has been shown to be sensitive enough to detect various cancers including lung, breast, colorectal, pancreatic and head and neck cancer, and malignant lymphoma

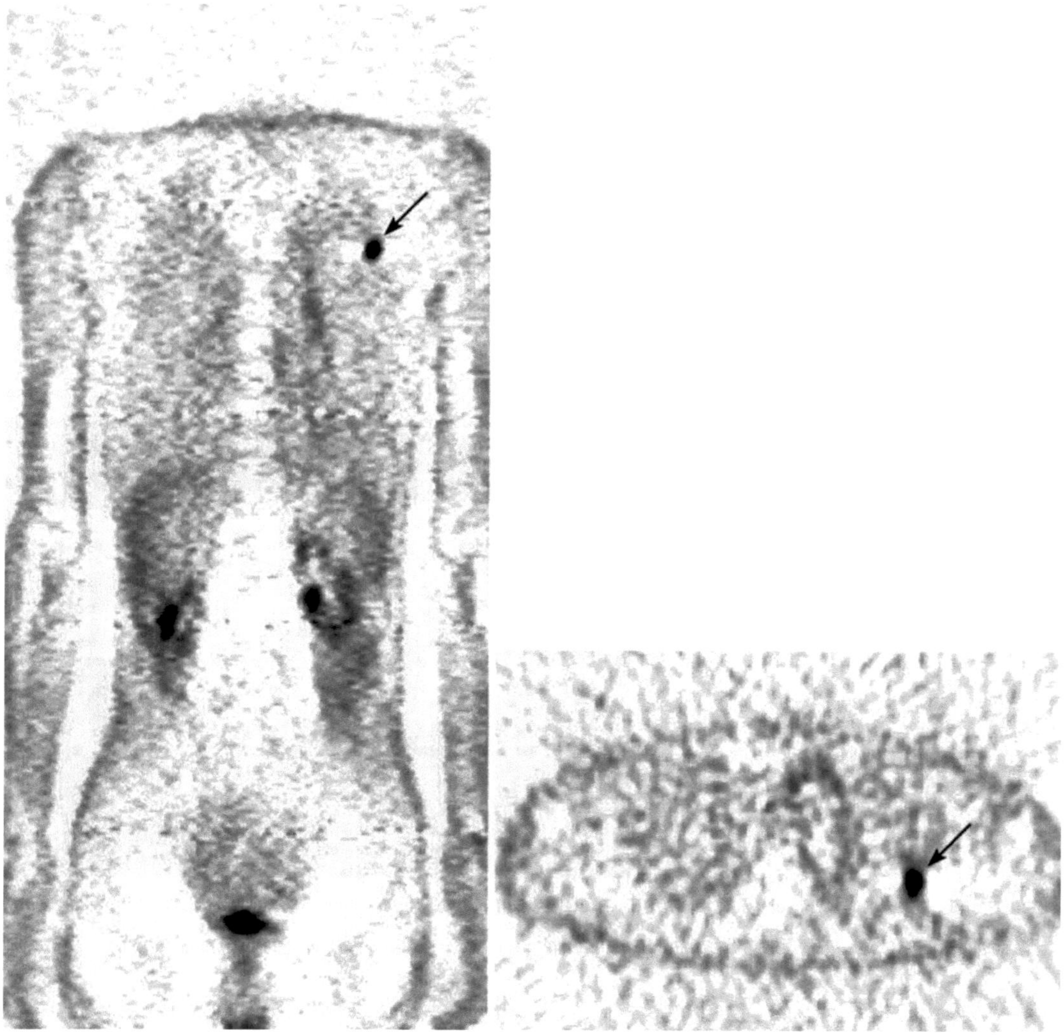

Fig. 1. Lung cancer in a 66-year-old man. On coronal and axial tomographic PET images, high FDG uptake was observed in the left upper lobe of the lung (*arrow*). CR and CT were inconclusive. Surgery was performed. Histopathologically, the lesion was a 1.0-cm papillary adenocarcinoma. Lymph node metastasis was not observed

and melanoma (Conti et al. 1996; Rigo et al. 1996; Delbeke 1999). It can also be used successfully in patients with unknown primary tumor (Lassen et al. 1999). Thus PET imaging has the potential to detect cancers of many types at early stages with a single study.

Cancer screening is a major healthcare issue because cancer is still a major cause of death. Screening modalities are constantly changing due to improvements in technology. The efficacy of cancer screening to date has been confirmed by the fecal occult blood test for colorectal cancer (Hardcastle et al. 1996), by low-dose computed tomography (CT) for lung (Kaneko et al. 1996; Henschke et al. 1999), and by mammography for breast cancer in women in their fifth decade (Taubes 1997). In addition, several studies are underway to determine the efficacy of screening for prostate cancer and ovarian cancer (Kramer et al. 1994). Current screening methods target single organs or a few organs independently. Furthermore, these mass screening programs do not target low-prevalence cancers, primarily because of cost–benefit considerations.

Whole-body PET can be used to survey the entire body seamlessly; the targets are not confined to single organs in cancer screening. Ovarian cancer, pancreatic cancer, and lymphoma can be targeted, although there is still no evidence that PET can be used to detect these cancers in resectable stages in asymptomatic individuals. However, when cancer detection by a single exami-

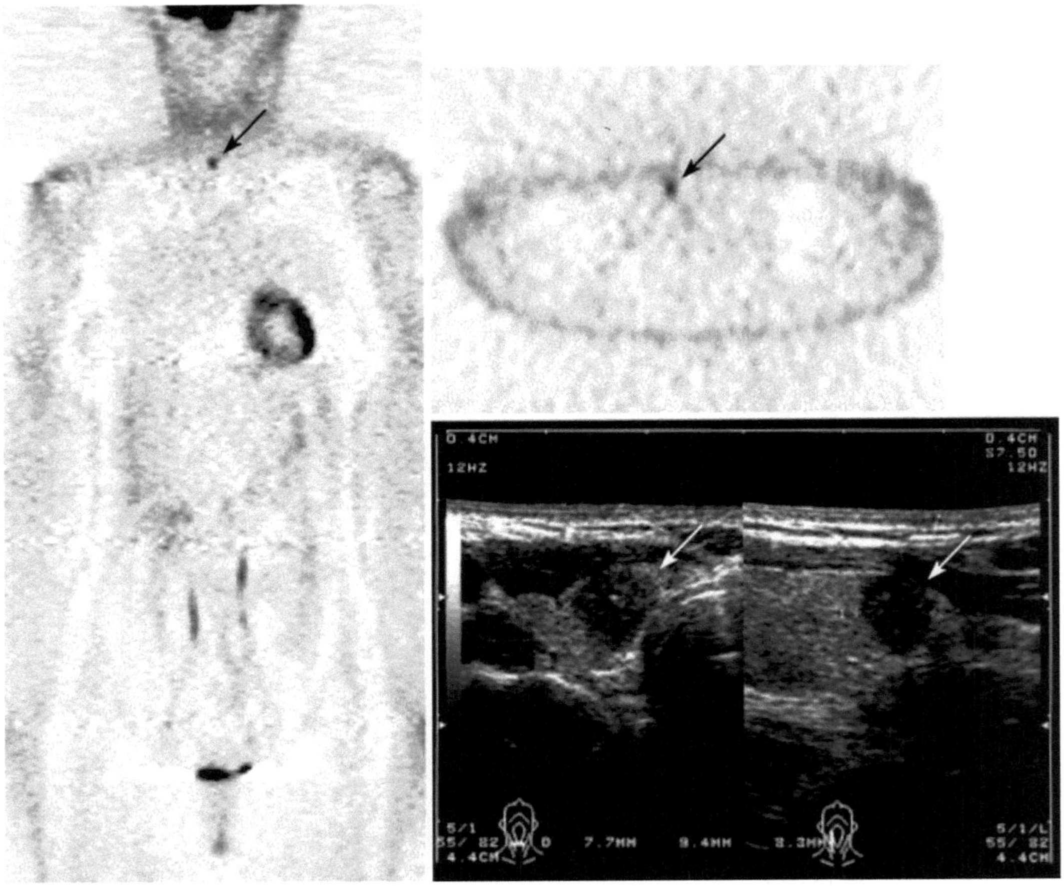

Fig. 2. Thyroid cancer in a 39-year-old woman. High FDG uptake was noticed in the thyroid gland (*arrow*). An ultrasound examination showed a nodule with intense FDG uptake in the right lobe. Ultrasound-guided biopsy was performed, and histological diagnosis was papillary adenocarcinoma. A right hemithyroidectomy was performed and the lesion was 0.6 cm in diameter

nation is considered, PET proves to be superior to other screening methods in hypermetabolic cancers. Cancers of many types can be detected in resectable stages.

Cancer screening raises issues of cost and risk. PET examination does entail a substantial cost. At our center the members themselves pay the cost of the examination. In order to win widespread acceptance, screening methods must be not only of high quality but also inexpensive. Because of the short half-life of FDG, the radiation dose to the individual is low. It can be further reduced if the patient voids at the proper times (Mejia et al. 1991). To date, PET imaging is not suited to screening tests for the general population because PET examination involves substantial cost.

31.4.1 PET-Negative Cancers

PET-negative cancers were identified in our series of studies and were tentatively categorized as belonging to one of four groups on the basis of our observations:

1. Urologic cancers, and adjacent area
2. Cancers of low cell density
3. Small-sized cancers
4. Hypometabolic cancers

All 17 prostate cancers were PET-negative in our PET screening, and they were all detected by measurement of prostate-specific antigen levels in serum. Although urinary excretion of FDG may hamper the detection of urologic cancers, there may be another reasons for the false-negative results in the case of urologic cancers. For example, the positive rate was less than 50 % in our study of

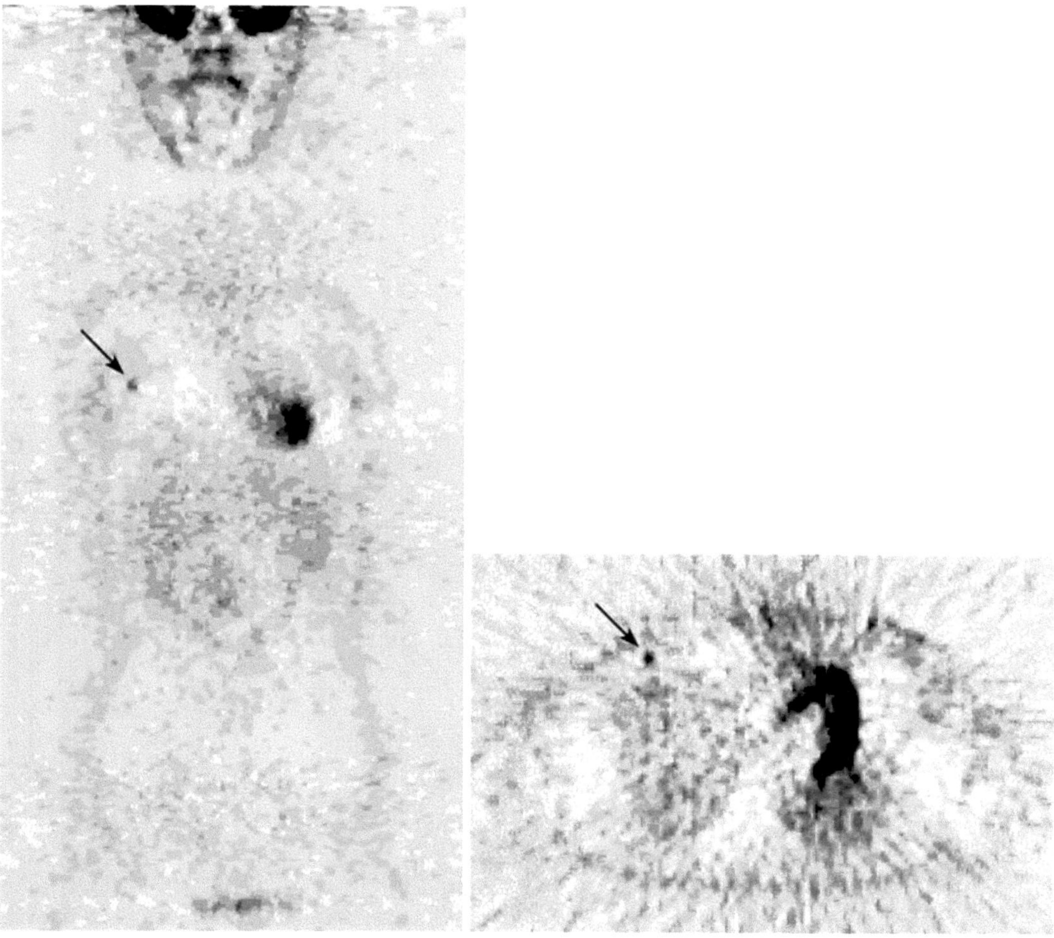

Fig. 3. Breast cancer in a 43-year-old woman. A small high FDG uptake was noted in the right breast on coronal and transaxial PET images (*arrow*). An ultrasonographic image obtained after the PET study displays a low echoic area measuring 4 mm in diameter. No positive findings were seen on the mammogram and MR image in other institute. Breast-conserving therapy was performed. According to the cut surface of the resected specimen, the tumor was 6 mm in diameter

19 patients with renal cancer (unpublished results). Low tumor cellularity, such as in signet-ring cell cancers or mucinous cancers, may result in low FDG accumulation. The spatial resolution of our PET scanner is approximately 6 mm, and partial-volume effects decrease the sensitivity in tumors smaller than twice that resolution.

In our study, there were a few cases of gastric cancer, one of the most prevalent cancers in Japan where gastric cancer screening is common. Many of our subjects had undergone stomach examinations at other institutions. In any event, endoscopy is superior to PET for detecting superficial lesions, especially in the stomach.

Furthermore, hypometabolic cancers exist. A 1.5-cm bronchoalveolar carcinoma of the lung was PET-negative in our study. Bronchoalveolar cancers of certain histologic types show the most favorable prognosis (Noguchi et al. 1995). How glucose metabolism relates to biological malignancy is not well known. Furthermore, in spite of a high avidity for FDG of cervical cancers (Rose et al. 1999), the artifact of urinary bladder disturbed the detection of cervical cancers without continuous bladder irrigation in our study of asymptomatic individuals. These limitations must be recognized in PET screening. Therefore, conventional examinations are also needed for cancer screening in conjunction with FDG-PET.

31.4.2 Benign Lesions with High FDG Uptake

It has been thought that FDG-PET is not suitable for unselected screening because of the likelihood of false positives (Rigo et al. 1996). Our study is the first to deal

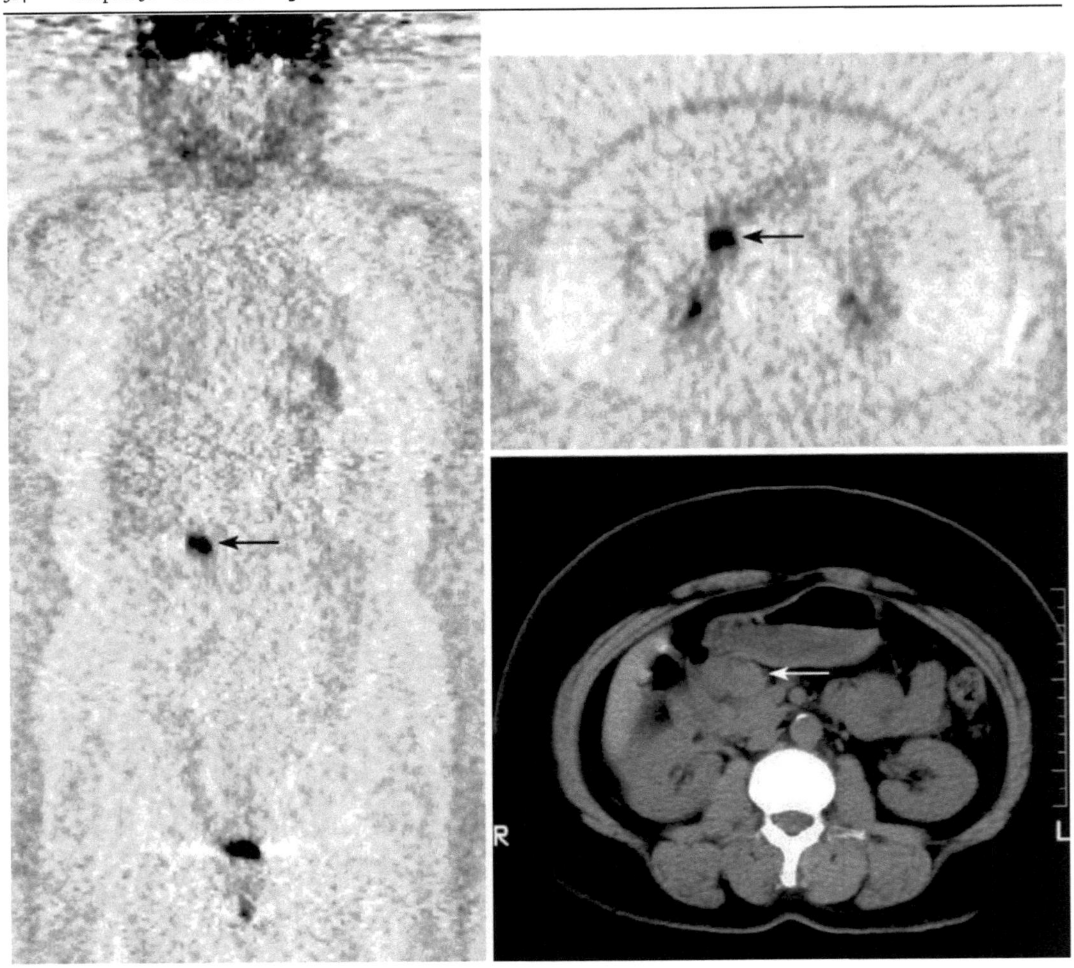

Fig. 4. Pancreatic cancer in a 47-year-old woman. A high FDG uptake was noted in the right upper abdomen on coronal and transaxial PET images (*arrow*). Plain CT was inconclusive. Surgery was performed. Histopathologically, the lesion was 3×2 cm in diameter. Lymph node metastasis was not observed. The patient was still alive 12 months after surgery without recurrence

with a large number of asymptomatic persons. Although false-positive lesions were occasionally discovered, these subclinical lesions were thought to warrant further clinical examination or follow-up. Early in our study we found that diffuse thyroidal FDG uptake was not uncommon in otherwise healthy women and that it was a sign of subclinical chronic thyroiditis or Hashimoto's thyroiditis (Yasuda et al. 1997a).

Other benign lesions with High FDG uptake are as follows:

- Gingivitis: It is not uncommon to see focal FDG accumulation in the gingiva. Granulomas may accumulate a high level of FDG in this region.
- Maxillary sinusitis: Unilateral maxillary FDG accumulation is not rare. FDG tends to accumulate along the sinus wall.
- Periarthritis of the shoulder: arch-shaped FDG accumulation along the shoulder joints is strongly suggestive of periarthritis of the shoulder. There may be a correlation between the intensity of FDG uptake and clinical symptoms (pain and restriction of movement). FDG accumulation in this area is not uncommon in PET screening.
- Contusion of the chest: Faint FDG accumulation was observed at the chest wall on PET images.
- Bronchopneumonia: High FDG uptake is occasionally observed in pneumonia in PET screening. In such cases it is necessary to perform a spiral CT scan of the chest simultaneously.
- Sarcoidosis: Multiple FDG accumulation is occasionally observed in lymph nodes of the lung hilum in healthy subjects. The etiology is unknown.

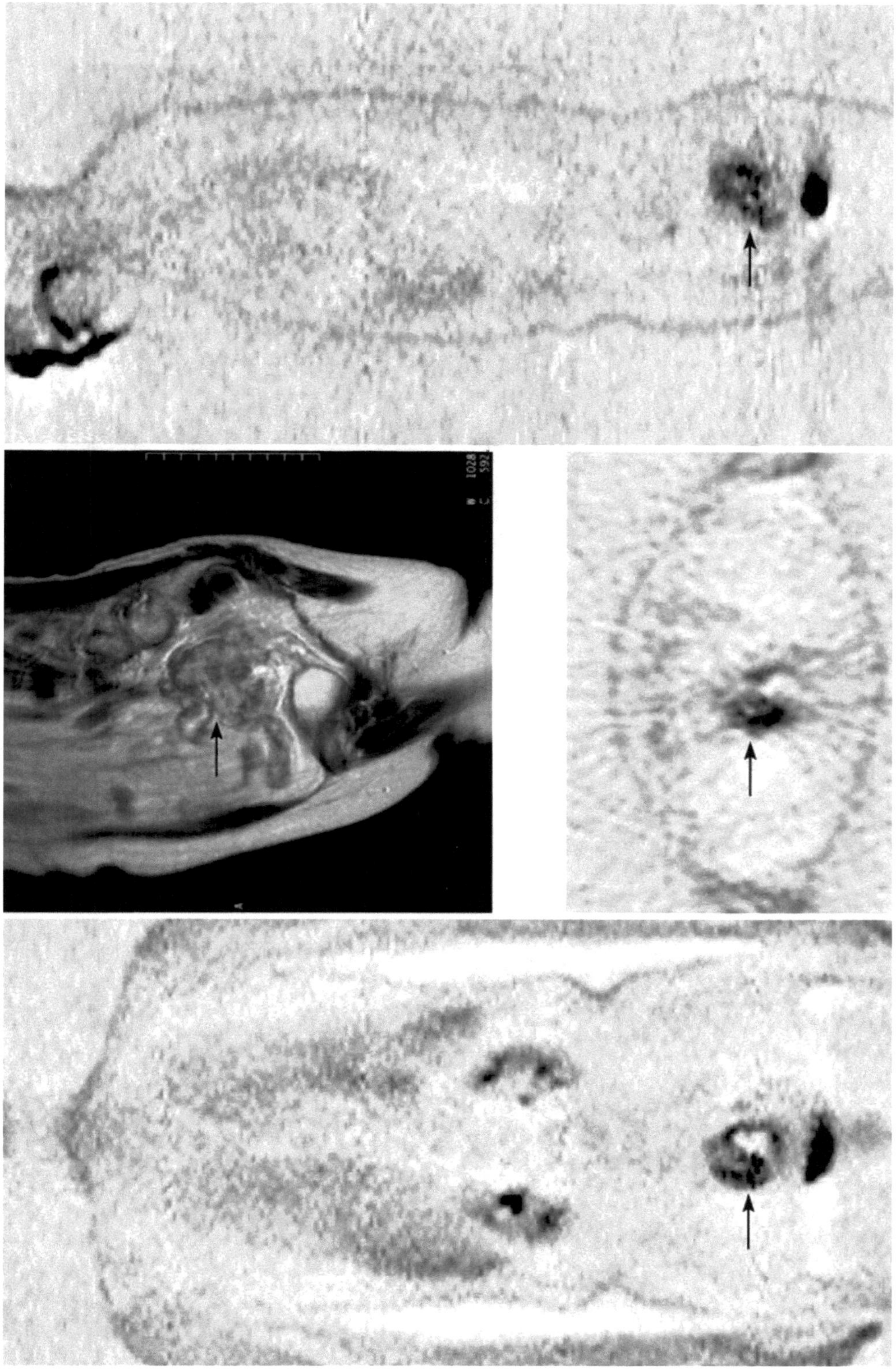

Fig. 5. Ovarian cancer in a 71-year-old woman. A spotty FDG uptake was noted in the pelvis on coronal, transaxial and sagittal PET images (*arrow*) and she visited a gynecologist on our advice. However, because MRI and other conventional examinations were inconclusive, she was not treated for 18 months. Finally, pelvic exenteration was performed after her symptoms were apparent. It is important to understand useful indications for a PET in oncology generally

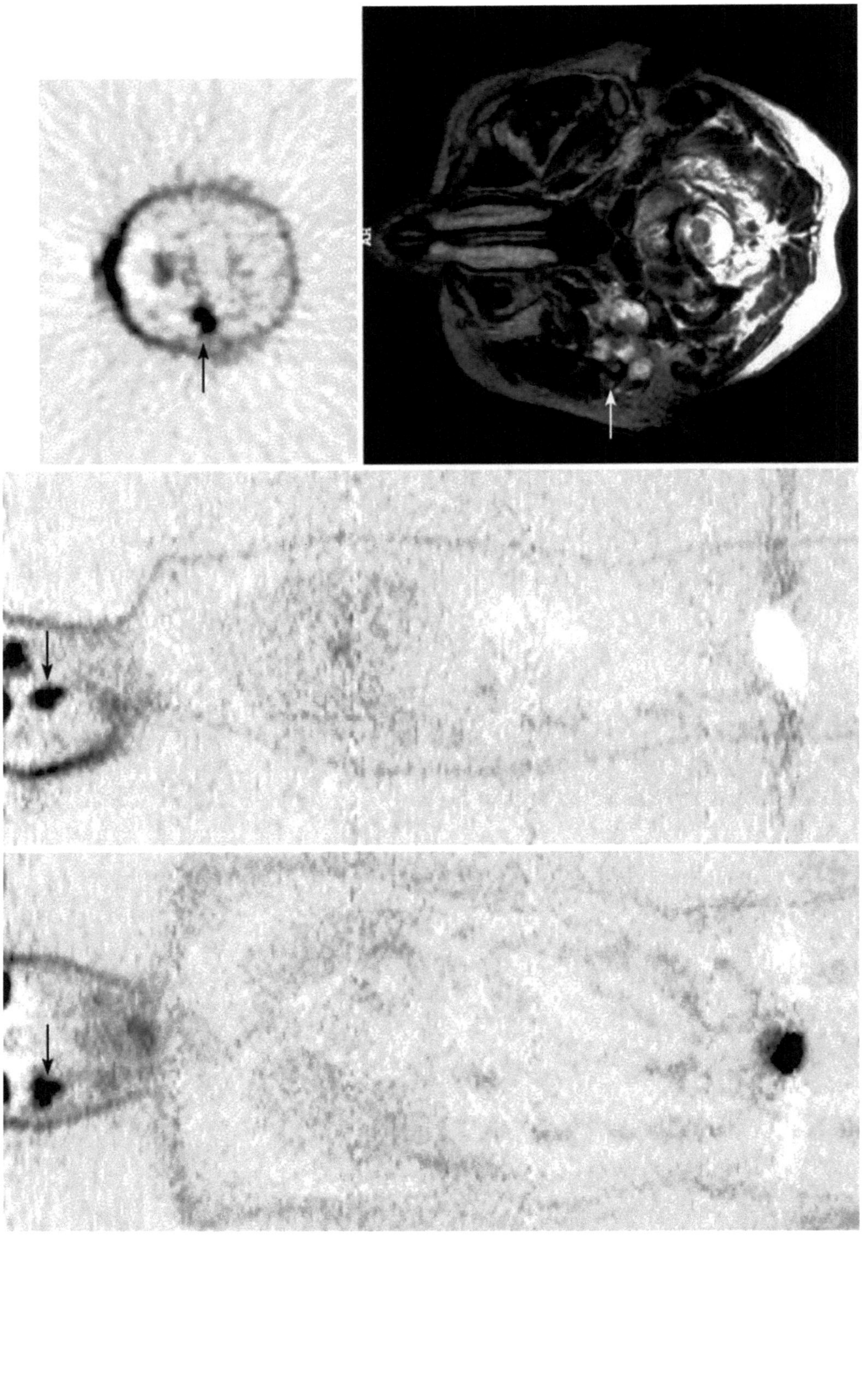

Fig. 6. Adenoid cystic carcinoma in a 64-year-old man. High FDG uptake was noticed in the right side of the parapharyngeal space asymmetrically on coronal, transaxial and sagital PET images (*arrow*). Surgery was performed and histological diagnosis was adenoid cystic carcinoma

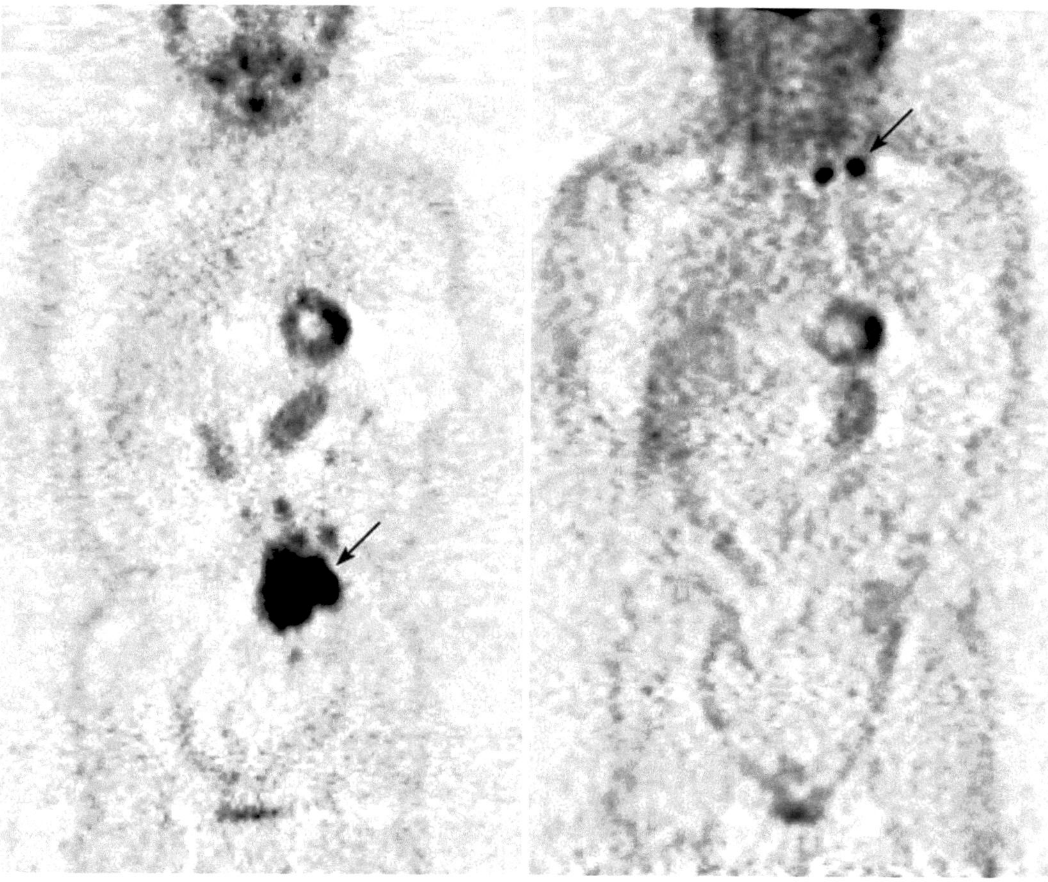

Fig. 7. Non-Hodgkin's lymphoma in a 59-year-old woman. High FDG uptake was noticed in the mesenteric and para-aortic nodes on left coronal PET image (*arrow*). She was diagnosed with non-Hodgkin's lymphoma, Stage II, in November 2000, and treated with chemotherapy and radiotherapy. These primary lesions were found incidentally. Despite this, high FDG uptake was observed in the left supraclavicular region on right coronal PET image in June 2002 (*arrow*), at which point she was treated again

- Colonic adenoma: High FDG uptake is observed in an adenoma of the colon (Yasuda et al. 2001).

However, PET is sensitive for detecting hypermetabolic sites. As regards cancer detection by means of a single examination, PET is superior to other methods in hypermetabolic cancers. Although benign lesions exhibiting hypermetabolism were detected, they were worthy of clinical attention. False-positive interpretations can be avoided by recognizing potential sites and characteristics of benign lesions.

31.4.3 Physiological FDG Accumulation

Physiologically increased FDG uptake is occasionally noted in PET screening. FDG accumulation can be observed in the uterus during menstruation (Yasuda et al. 1997b). High FDG uptake can be observed in lactating mammary glands (Binns and Hicks 1997). Increased FDG uptake may be observed in skeletal muscles after exercise (Yasuda et al. 1998b). FDG appears to accumulate in laryngeal muscles in proportion to contractile activity during speech (Kostakoglu et al. 1996). Although patients' eyes are closed during the period of FDG uptake, this does not prevent FDG accumulation in the oculomotor muscles.

Intense FDG uptake was observed occasionally in the myocardium. Image artifacts caused by intense myocardial FDG accumulations result in incomplete examinations of the neighboring organs such as lungs, mediastinum, and esophagus. We tried administering Intralipid (10 %, 100 ml) intravenously in ten patients to increase serum FFA levels (Nuutila et al. 1992). However, we did not observe significant reduction of myocardial FDG uptake as compared with a control group. Intense FDG

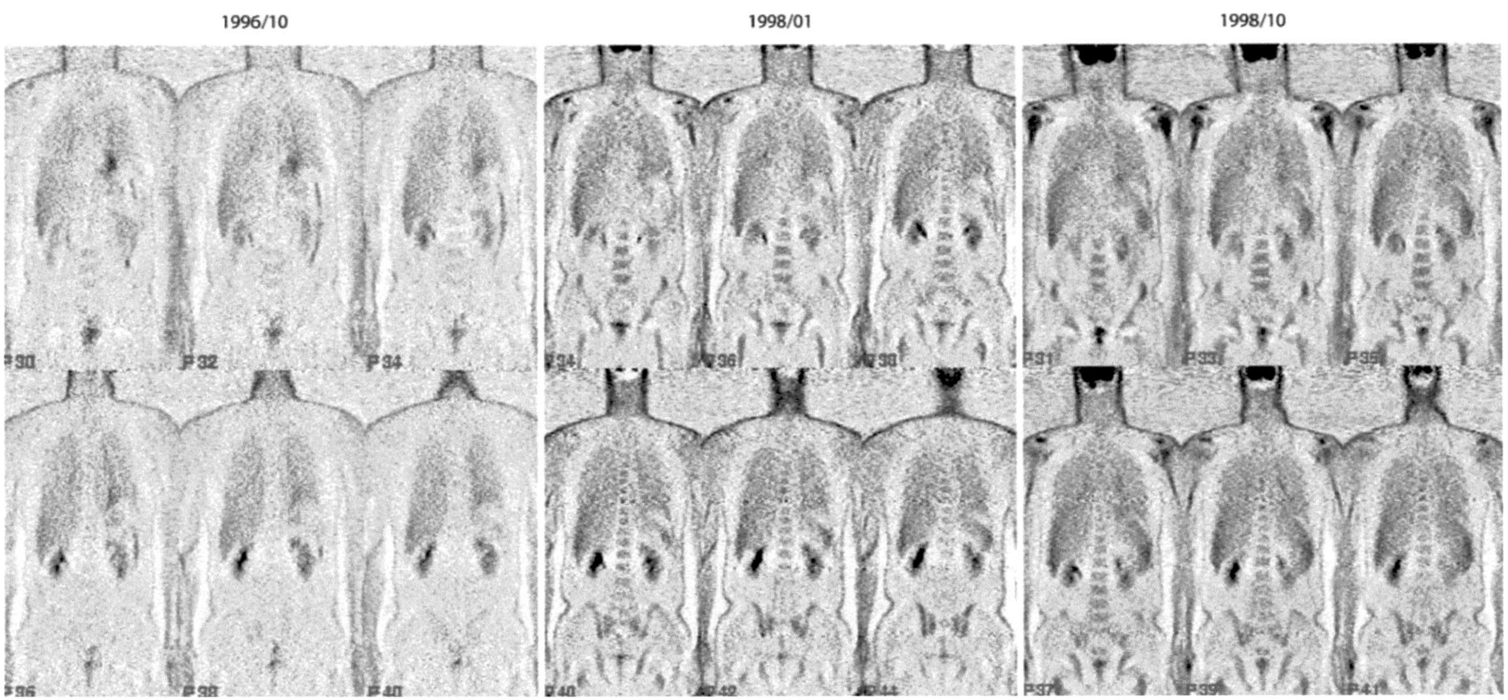

Fig. 8. Chronic myeloid leukemia in a 70-year-old man. On the *left* consecutive six coronal PET images obtained in October 1996, the bone marrow uptake of FDG was not observed and a white blood cell count was 8400/μl. In January 1998, mild bone marrow uptake of FDG was observed on the *middle* consecutive six coronal PET images. However, the white blood cell count was 23,900/μl and no abnormal cells were observed in peripheral blood. Bone marrow aspiration showed no abnormal findings. On the *right* consecutive six coronal PET images obtained in October 1998, diffusely increased marrow uptake, intense focal uptake within the humeri and splenomegaly were observed. The white blood cell count was 41,500/μl and the patient was diagnosed as having chronic myelomonocytic leukemia

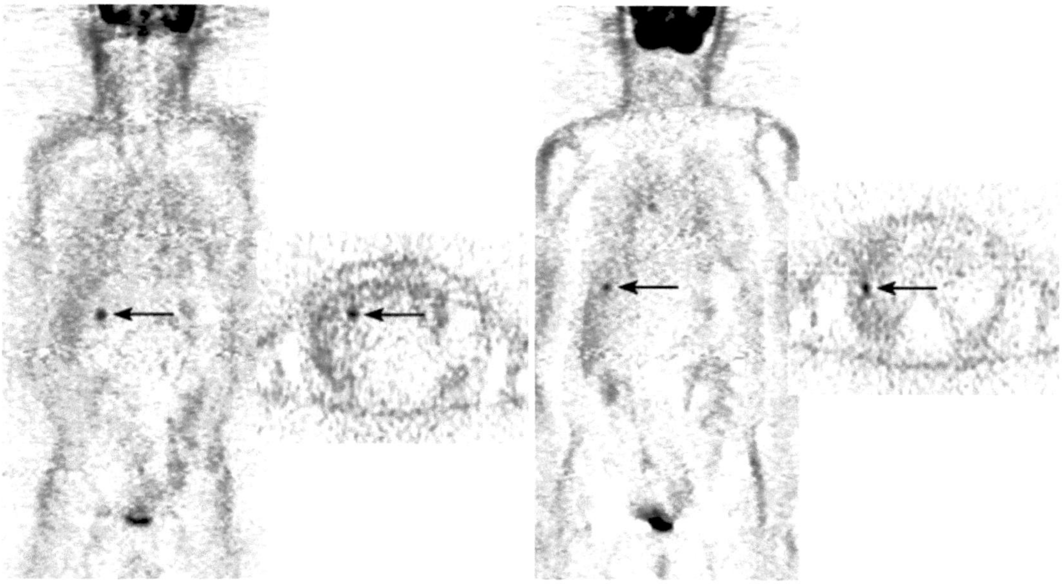

Fig. 9. Metastatic liver cancer in a 61-year-old man. Two high FDG uptakes were noted in the liver on coronal and transaxial PET images (*arrow*). The lesions were 1 cm and 1.5 cm in diameter

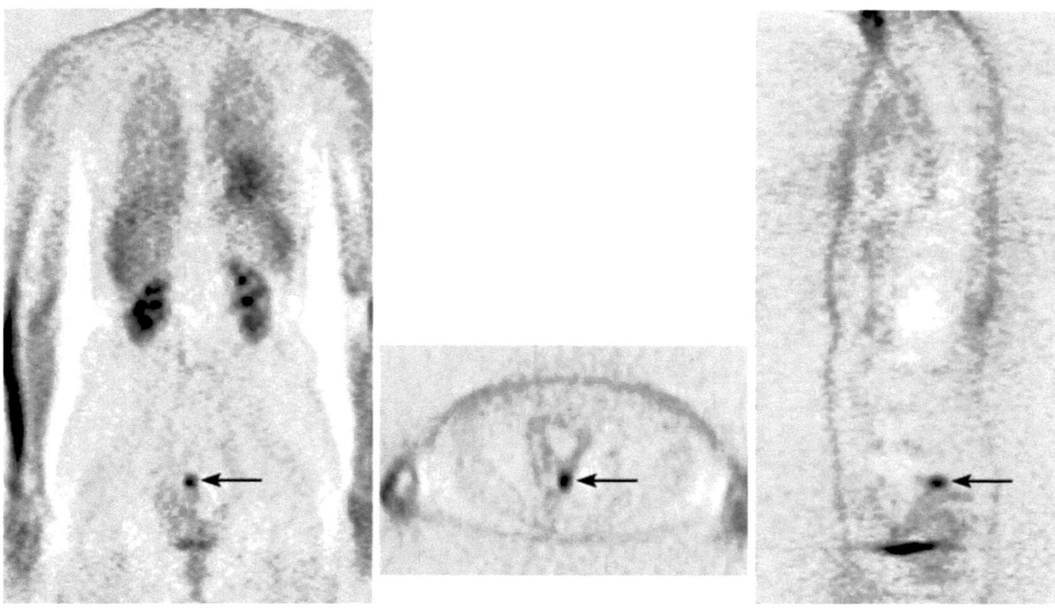

Fig. 10. Early colonic cancer in a 56-year-old woman). High FDG uptake was noticed in the lower abdomen on coronal and transaxial PET images (*arrow*). After PET study, she underwent colonoscopy, which revealed sessile polyp in the sigmoid colon. Polypectomy was performed, and histopathologic study showed 23-mm adenocarcinoma with submucosal invasion

uptake was observed in the myocardium in the case of serum FFA levels below than 0.3 mEq/ml. And FDG uptake was not observed in the myocardium in the case of serum blood sugar levels above 220 mg/dl.

Similarly, intense FDG accumulations in the bowel result in incomplete bowel examinations. We also tried administering scopolamine butylbromide (Buscopan) intravenously in ten patients in order to reduce bowel peristalsis. But in this case as well, we did not observe any significant reduction in bowel FDG uptake when compared with a control group. Further studies are required in order to find a way to reduce FDG uptake in the myocardium and bowel.

31.5. Conclusions

FDG-PET imaging has the potential to detect a wide variety of cancers at potentially curable stages in asymptomatic individuals. But PET cannot be used as an alternative to all other conventional methods because any FDG-PET study has obvious limitations in the detection of urological cancers, cancers of low cell density, small cancers and hypometabolic or FDG-negative cancers. Therefore, conventional examinations are also needed for cancer screening in conjunction with FDG-PET. Our experience over 7 years showed that PET can be used to detect a wide variety of cancers at resectable stages in asymptomatic individuals. However, PET imaging is not suited to screening tests for the general population because PET examination still involves substantial cost, but further technological advances will likely increase the usefulness and significance of PET for cancer screening.

References

Binns D, Hicks RJ (1997) Pattern of F-18 FDG uptake and excretion in the lactating breast. 9th ICP Conference. Poster abstract p3 Eur I Nucl Med 23:1677–1679

Conti PS, Lilien DL, Hawley K et al (1996) PET and [18F]-FDG in oncology: a clinical update. Nucl Med Biol 23:717–35

Hardcastle JD, Chamberlain JO, Robinson MHE et al (1996) Randomised controlled trial of faecal-occult-blood screening for colorectal cancer. Lancet 348:1472–1477

Horiuchi M, Yasuda S, Shohtsu A et al (1998) Four cases of Warthin's tumor of the parotid gland detected with FDG PET. Ann Nucl Med 12:47–50

Ide M, Suzuki Y (1996) A window on Japan: medical health club with clinical PET

Kostakoglu L, Wong JCH, Barrington SF et al (1996) Speech-related visualization of laryngeal muscles with fluorine-18-FDG. J Nucl Med 37:1771–1773

Kramer BS, Gohagan I, Prorok PC (1994) NIH consensus 1994: screening. Gynecol Oncol 55:20–21

Mejia AA, Nakamura T, Itoh M et al (1991) Estimation of absorbed dose in humans due to intravenous administration of fluorine-18-fluorodeoxyglucose in PET studies. J Nucl Med 32:699–706

Noguchi M, Morikawa A, Kawasaki M et al (1995) Small adenocarcinoma of the lung. Histologic characteristics and prognosis. Cancer 75:2844–2852

Nuutila P, Koivisto A, Knuuti J et al (1992) Glucose-free fatty acid cycle operates in human heart and skeletal muscle in vivo. J Clin Invest 89:1767–1774

Rigo P, Paulus P, Kaschten BJ et al (1996) Oncological application of positron emission tomography with fluorine-18 fluorodeoxyglucose. Eur J Nucl Med 23:1641–1674

Rose PG, Adler LP, Rodriguez M et al (1999) Positron emission tomography for evaluating para-aortic nodal metastasis in locally advanced cervical cancer before surgical staging: a surgicopathologic study. J Clin Oncol 17:41–45

Sven NR, Jorg K (2001) FDG-PET for clinical use. Eur J Nucl Med 28:1707–1723

Taubes G (1997) The breast-screening brawl. Science 275:1056–1059

Yasuda S, Shohtsu A (1997) Cancer screening with whole-body 18F-fluorodeoxyglucose positron-emission tomography. Lancet 359:1819

Yasuda S, Ide M, Takagi S et al (1996a) Cancer detection with whole-body FDG PET images without attenuation correction. Jpn J Nucl Med 33:367–373

Yasuda S, Shohtsu A, Ide M et al (1996b) High fluorine-18 deoxyglucose uptake in sarcoidosis. Clin Nucl Med 21:983–984

Yasuda S, Shohtsu A, Ide M et al (1997a) Diffuse F-18 FDG uptake in chronic thyroiditis. Clin Nucl Med 22:341

Yasuda S, Ide M, Takagi S et al (1997b) Intrauterine accumulation of F-18 FDG during menstruation. Clin Nucl Med 22:793–794

Yasuda S, Ide M, Takagi S et al (1998a) F-18 FDG uptake in colonic adenoma. Clin Nucl Med 23:99–100

Yasuda S, Ide M, Takagi S et al (1998b) High fluorine-18 fluorodeoxyglucose uptake in skeletal muscle. Clin Nucl Med 23:111–112

Yasuda S, Ide M, Fujii H et al (2000) Application of positron emission tomography imaging to cancer screening. Br J Cancer 83: 1607–1611

Yasuda S, Fujii H, Nakahara T et al (2001) 18F-FDG PET detection of colonic adenomas. J Nucl Med 42:989–992

CHAPTER 32

Cost-Effectiveness Studies of PET in Oncology

K.A. Miles · L.B. Connelly

32.1 Introduction

The ever-increasing need to rigorously demonstrate the cost-effectiveness of PET and other new diagnostic imaging modalities has emerged in the current context of evidence-based medicine. Governments and other purchasers of health care have a responsibility to ensure that there is good evidence that the procedures purchased on behalf of patients are both safe and effective. For example, since 1998, the Australian government has adopted mechanisms to ensure that new and existing medical procedures attracting government benefits are supported by scientific evidence of cost effectiveness [1]. The inevitable constraints of fixed budgets for health care results in a need to compare the value for money obtained by one procedure in comparison to another. Hence the beneficial health effects produced by a particular health intervention need to be balanced against the cost of producing this effect, a process known as cost-effectiveness or cost-benefit analysis. This chapter reviews the available methods for assessing the cost-effectiveness of diagnostic imaging modalities and reviews the results of studies assessing the cost-effectiveness of various clinical applications of PET imaging. The difficulties in translating cost-effectiveness studies from one country to another will also be addressed.

32.1.1 The Role of Evaluation

PET imaging specialists are likely to see the role of cost-effectiveness studies as a means to promoting acceptance of PET techniques into medical practice and to support funding of PET by governments and other health purchasers. Yet, different parties or ‚stakeholders' may perceive such evaluations as serving different purposes and may well have different views about which costs and consequences matter for a given diagnostic procedure. Thus, economists use the terms ‚economic evaluation' and ‚financial evaluation' to distinguish between differences in focus or „perspective". Economic evaluation refers to those assessments that take account of **all** of the costs and benefits of the alternatives considered, regardless of which parties incur the costs and receive the benefits, corresponding to a ‚social perspective'. Financial evaluations, on the other hand, employ a more exclusive conception of the costs and consequences and typically they are concerned only with the subset of costs and consequences that affect the party that has commissioned the evaluation. Thus, the term financial evaluation can be employed when a perspective is taken that excludes the consideration of some affected constituent of society. Hence, the evaluation techniques discussed in this chapter can be useful for organisations with quite different goals.

32.2 Definitions

32.2.1 Cost

Regardless of whether cost-effectiveness analysis (CoEA) or cost-benefit analysis (CoBA) is employed (see 2.3 below), the costs of alternative investments are expressed as money values. Measuring the costs of the alternatives may not be straightforward, especially when the more inclusive, economic, definition of costs is employed. Hence measuring costs is generally less time-consuming for a financial evaluation than for a full economic evaluation. In economics, the concept of ‚opportunity cost' is employed. The opportunity cost of any activity is measured as the benefit that is foregone to undertake it. This is not a simple concept to understand, but it is one of the central and distinguishing features of *economic*, as opposed to *financial*, analysis.

Initially, for simplification, we illustrate the concept of opportunity costs with a non-medical example. Suppose you own the title to a holiday home at a popular beach and, of the infinite possible uses of your home when you are unable to occupy it, you have narrowed the choice down to two options. Option 1 is to allow your friends and family to use the property, free of charge. Option 2 is to rent your property, at market rates, to other holiday makers. How would you quantify the opportunity cost of pursuing Option 1 or 2? If Option 1 is your choice, the opportunity cost can be measured as the return you have foregone by not letting your property for that period. This might be easy to calculate, because the rental on your property as well as the costs incurred as a result of rental may be quite clear. Importantly, though, the fact that you own the property does not render the opportunity cost of letting it to friends and relatives, zero (and, hopefully, your lucky tenants will appreciate this)! What would the opportunity cost be if you chose Option 2? Once again, it isn't zero. Conceptually, the opportunity cost of renting your holiday home to holiday-makers is the benefit that you would have received by choosing Option 1 (i.e., letting the home to your friends and relatives free of charge). Measuring that opportunity cost as a dollar value may be somewhat more difficult. However, since you chose Option 2, the satisfaction it provides to you presumably exceeds that provided by Option 1. In turn, it might at least be deduced that the opportunity cost of Option 2, is **no greater** than the net money benefit produced by Option 2, itself.

The preceding example illustrates that sometimes the costs and benefits of activities are not easily identifiable in terms of prices, or cost and revenue streams. When confronted with choices about how to allocate finite resources to produce the greatest net benefit, economists emphasise that the absence of a money price should not be assumed to indicate a zero economic value for the purposes of economic (or ‚social') decision-making. When evaluating diagnostic modalities such as PET, it is also important to bear in mind that the opportunities forgone may be non-diagnostic. In fixed-budget settings, an increase in expenditure on diagnosis may dictate reduced expenditure on another activity, such as treatment.

Financial cost data for existing diagnostic and therapeutic procedures are increasingly available from governments and other third party payers such as health insurance companies. Institutional costs have often been used in published cost-effectiveness analyses but it is frequently difficult to extrapolate the results of such studies to other institutions. The evaluation of PET, the cost of PET is a major determinant of the resulting cost-effectiveness. However, PET costs may also vary considerably depending on the model of delivery of PET services adopted. The use of partial ring detectors or hybrid coincidence gamma cameras as an alternative to dedicated full-ring PET systems has the potential to save costs but it is essential that such service delivery models be supported by appropriate evidence of diagnostic performance for that particular technology.

32.2.2 Effectiveness and the Measurement of Outcomes

The effectiveness of a diagnostic test can be considered at a number of different levels representing a hierarchy through which imaging modalities frequently pass during their development and subsequent clinical evaluation (Fig. 1) [2].

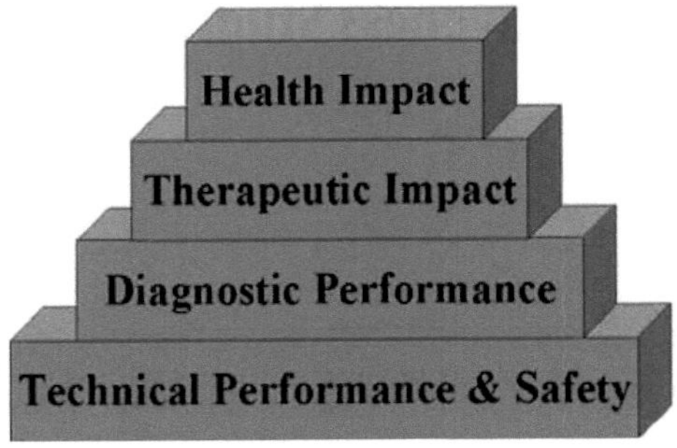

Fig. 1. Evaluation hierarchy for the effectiveness of diagnostic tests

Safety and technical performance comprises the most basic level of assessment. In the case of FDG-PET, this would include evidence that administration of FDG is without significant complication and that the imaging process truly reflects the glucose metabolism within tumour and other tissues.

Diagnostic performance is most commonly expressed as diagnostic accuracy, reported as sensitivity, specificity, positive predictive value and negative predictive value (Table 1). Receiver operating characteristic (ROC) analysis is a more sophisticated method that assesses diagnostic performance over a range of conditions for diagnosis. For example, with FDG-PET, sensitivity and specificity values might be determined for each of a range of threshold values for the specific uptake value (SUV) that indicates malignancy in a lung nodule.

Generally, diagnostic accuracy data can be obtained from searches of the medical literature. However, it is important that studies identified by such a search are assessed for quality and for the presence of bias in particular. Detailed descriptions of such evaluation methods are available elsewhere [3], but ideally studies will have undertaken an independent, masked comparison of the new test (e.g. PET) against a reference standard within an appropriate population of consecutive patients.

Table 1. Definitions for common measures of diagnostic performance

Accuracy	The proportion of all tests giving the correct result
Sensitivity	The proportion of patients with the disease that are correctly identified by the test
Specificity	The proportion of patients without the disease that are correctly identified by the test
Positive predictive value	The proportion of positive tests that correctly identify patients with the disease
Negative predictive value	The proportion of negative tests that correctly identify patients without the disease

Therapeutic impact assessments aim to determine the extent to which, having made the diagnosis, the new test alters the clinical management of the patient. In general, such evaluations would determine whether the treatment has changed, for instance the frequency with which FDG-PET changes management from surgical intervention to conservative therapy.

Health Impact assessments provide the highest-level assessment of effectiveness. These assessments aim to determine the effect that management changes induced by the new diagnostic test alter ultimate health outcomes such as mortality, quality of life and quality adjusted survival, measured in quality-adjusted life years (QALYs) for example. Clearly, little benefit is gained if a new diagnostic test directs patients to a treatment that is ineffective. However, ultimate outcomes are primarily a function of the effectiveness of treatment rather than the effectiveness of diagnosis. It can therefore be argued that measuring ultimate outcomes generally should not be a priority in the evaluation of diagnostic technology for symptomatic patients (as opposed to screening) [4]. As many steps in the care process intervene between diagnostic imaging and ultimate outcome, the statistical variance that arises at each of these steps obscures the effects of imaging, making the effect of imaging on the ultimate outcome difficult or even impossible to observe. Thus, when subsequent treatments have already been shown to be effective, it is usually appropriate for technology assessment in diagnostic imaging to use more proximal (or intermediate) outcomes, such as change in management [4].

Outcome measures such as median survival times with or without therapy (e.g. surgery versus no treatment for particular stages of cancer) can be obtained from a literature search. However, it should be borne in mind that these treatment outcomes would have been measured using populations selected for treatment on the basis of previous diagnostic methods. (It may be possible to correct for this problem with appropriate modelling.) Quality of life measures are less commonly available from the literature. If no quality of life studies are available, an estimate of quality of life can be made using a time-trade off method. For instance, a cost-effectiveness study of FDG-PET in head and neck cancer surveyed head and neck surgery residents to assess how much healthy life they would be willing to trade to avoid the morbidity of a range of treatment options [5].

32.2.3 Cost-Benefit and Cost-Effectiveness

Once the outcomes of the alternative diagnostic tests have been quantified, there are two general approaches that can be applied to evaluate the alternatives.

Cost-benefit analysis (CoBA) is one possible approach. In CoBA, not only the costs but also the consequences of the alternatives are measured in monetary units, e.g. dollars. An advantage of CoBA is that, by measuring costs and consequences in comparable units, one can answer the question ‚Do the benefits outweigh the costs' for any one of the evaluated tests, on its own. Furthermore, comparing the net benefits of each (calculated by subtracting the cost of each diagnostic approach from its benefits) allows one to identify the test that creates the greatest net benefit and to choose between the alternatives, if they are mutually exclusive. However, in the context of health sector decisions, it is often difficult task to assign monetary values to the benefits of health sector activities.

Cost-effectiveness analysis (CEfA) is an alternative to CBA and is more commonly used in the health sector because it removes the need to assign monetary values to health benefits. In CEfA, the consequences of alternative investments are compared in physical units, rather than in dollar terms. Thus, CEfA cannot be used to answer the question ‚Do the benefits [of some intervention] outweigh the costs?' because the costs and consequences are measured in different units, e.g. dollars, and life-years saved. Furthermore, conventional CEfA cannot be used to compare production processes (e.g., diagnostic tests) that produce qualitatively different outputs. The need to standardise endpoints of effectiveness has already been identified within the nuclear medicine literature [6] but the ability to standardise measurements of health outcomes has been enhanced by the work of health economists to produce measures of the qualitatively-different health outcomes of different health sector activities. These outcomes can now be approached using a range of concepts such as QALYs, disability-adjusted life-years (DALYs) and health year equivalents (HYEs). CEfAs that invoke these measures are sometimes referred to as ‚cost-utility analyses'.

32.2.4 Marginal Analysis and the Incremental Cost-Effectiveness Ratio (ICER)

Marginal analysis refers to the practice of analysing the costs and benefits that occur with small changes in investments, or programs of a given kind. In economic evaluations, rather than calculating the total or average costs and benefits of various alternatives, an ‚incremental' approach is often taken. The incremental approach involves calculating the *additional* costs and benefits associated with a change of some kind. For example, the cost and effectiveness of a new imaging strategy are commonly compared to an existing management strategy by using the incremental cost-effectiveness ratio (ICER), defined as:

$$\text{ICER} = \frac{\text{Cost}_{\text{new strategy}} - \text{Cost}_{\text{current strategy}}}{\text{Effectiveness}_{\text{new strategy}} - \text{Effectiveness}_{\text{current strategy}}} \quad (1)$$

Note that if the new strategy has a greater effectiveness for a lower cost, the ICER is negative and the new strategy is said to „dominate". The ICER will also be negative if the new strategy has greater cost for lower effectiveness but in these circumstances the current strategy is „dominant". If the new strategy has improved effectiveness but with greater cost, the ICER will be positive and a judgement has to be made as to whether the additional benefit is worth the additional cost. There is no generally accepted ICER value beyond which health sector interventions are considered ‚acceptable' and such judgements may vary considerably between different countries and health care systems. A $50,000 per life year or QALY threshold value for ICER is frequently applied in the PET literature from the USA but readers should be aware that economists have questioned the appropriateness of using such cost-per-QALY benchmarks as guidelines for health policy formulation [7].

32.3 Techniques for Assessing Cost-Effectiveness

The techniques most commonly employed for cost-effectiveness analysis of diagnostic imaging tests can be broadly classified as a) case-tracking methods, or b) modelling approaches. Clinical consensus offers a lower level of evidence, but has been used widely to establish guidelines for the effective use of diagnostic imaging in several countries. Often a combined approached is most expedient in which the results of case-tracking studies can be used to confirm the validity of particular models [8] with clinical consensus used to fill in the gaps where these higher levels of evidence are absent.

32.3.1 Case-Tracking Methods

Case-tracking studies centre on a series of patients who undergo the new diagnostic test and individual patients are tracked to determine the costs and benefits that accrue from the application of the new technology. Ideally, such studies would have a randomised-controlled design with patients assigned either to the current diagnostic strategy or to the new strategy. However, randomised controlled trials (RCT), although well established in the assessment of therapeutic manoeuvres, present distinct difficulties when applied to diagnostic imaging technologies.

RCTs are likely to be expensive, being in the order of US$ 1–2 million per study, and often take a long time to accomplish, some protocols requiring in excess of four years to complete [4]. As diagnostic imaging technologies are evolving very rapidly and unpredictably, such prolonged studies are at risk of being out-dated by their time of completion. RCTs can also be associated with ethical difficulties that result from the requirement to randomise patients to a study arm comprising a diagnostic imaging method already shown to be less accurate than the new technology under evaluation. This is likely to be a particular problem when the new imaging technology has already become widely accepted in other countries.

A self-controlled study design offers an alternative that avoids some of the difficulties associated with the application of RCTs to diagnostic imaging. In a prospective study, the clinician is asked to record, at the time of referral, the clinical management intended had the new imaging modality not been available. Case tracking is then used to determine the actual clinical management that occurred following receipt of the imaging results with the actual clinical management compared to the originally intended plan. Any changes in management can be observed and their costs and benefits assessed.

32.3.2 Modelling Approaches

Approaches that model the decision-making processes involved in health care have emerged as a rapid and relatively low-cost method for assessing the cost effectiveness of diagnostic imaging strategies. Such techniques are commonly referred to as „decision tree analysis", for each management strategy is represented by a horizontal flow chart with branching points at which a decision is made, resulting in a range of possible outcomes. Figure 2 provides an illustrative decision tree in which the current CT only strategy is compared to a new strategy in which patients with a negative CT result undergo PET imaging. Detection of the disease, in this case disseminated metastases, indicates that patients are unsuitable for surgery and therefore undergo follow-up only.

Once the decision trees are defined, the next stage is to input a range of assumptions about the patient population, the diagnostic and therapeutic procedures and the possible outcomes. The prevalence (or prior probability) of the disease within the population and diagnostic performance (sensitivity and specificity) of each diagnostic test are estimated along with cost of each diagnostic and therapeutic procedure. To assess the effectiveness of each strategy, a value is assigned for each outcome. This value may reflect an ultimate outcome such as life expectancy or quality adjusted life-years. Alternatively, an intermediate outcome can be assessed by assigning a value of 1 to desired outcomes and 0 to unfavourable outcomes. For example, in Fig. 3, assigning a value of 1 to the terminal nodes representing outcomes in which patients with disseminated metastases are treated non-surgically will enable the number of unnecessary surgical procedures avoided to be quantified for each strategy. The likelihood, cost and value of each outcome associated with both strategies is determined and the average cost and outcome per patient is calcu-

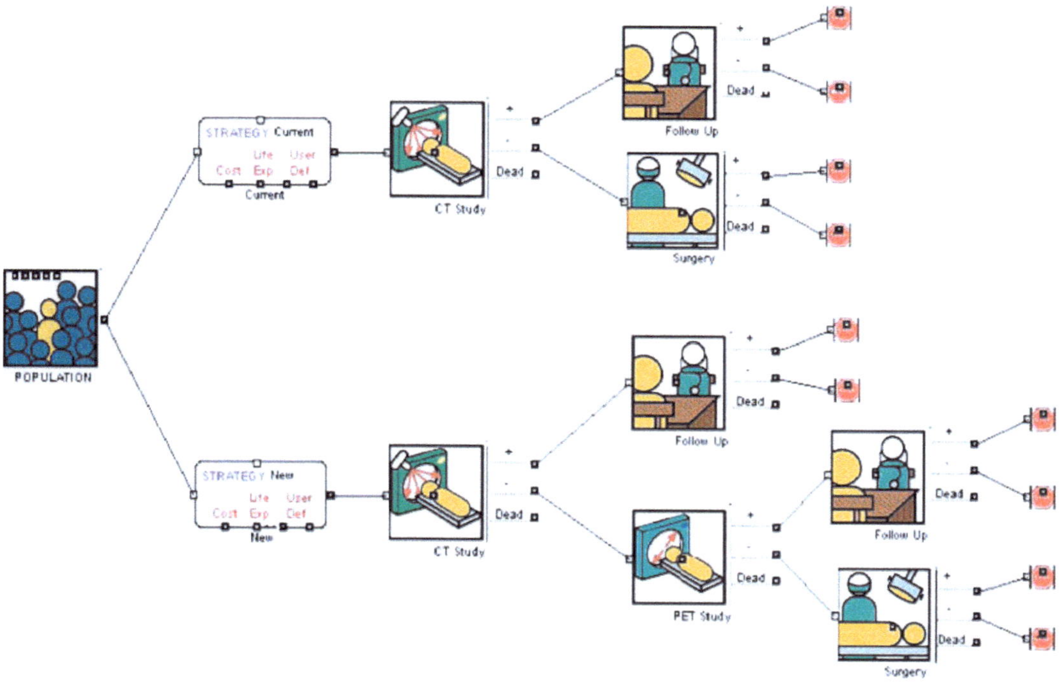

Fig. 2. Illustrative decision tree comparing a new PET-based strategy to a current CT only strategy. [Produced using Extend_ software (Imagine That, Inc. San Jose, USA) with medical imaging blocks from the Crump Institute, UCLA.]

lated (e.g., in QALYs), thereby enabling a comparison of the cost-effectiveness of the two strategies.

The decision tree methodology can be extended by performing ‚sensitivity analysis' to determine the conditions under which the new test remains cost-effective. This achieved by entering into the model different values for the cost and the diagnostic performance (sensitivity and specificity) of procedures and the prevalence of the disease, thereby determining the effect that variations in these parameters will have upon the cost-effectiveness of one or the other strategy. A "one-way" sensitivity analysis entails variation of only one variable (e.g. disease prevalence, Fig. 3), whereas a „two-way" analysis involves simultaneous variation of two input variables (e.g. disease prevalence and cost of PET). Two-way sensitivity analyses can also be displayed graphically where two selected parameters are represented on the graph axes (Fig. 4). The graph is divided into two areas by a line that indicates equivalent cost-effectiveness for the two strategies. The most cost-effective strategy can be determined for given values of the plotted parameters by comparing the relative position of any point to the plotted line.

Sensitivity analysis is a useful technique because it can allow for any uncertainty about the input assumptions and can also be used to model the effects that any potential differences between populations from differ-

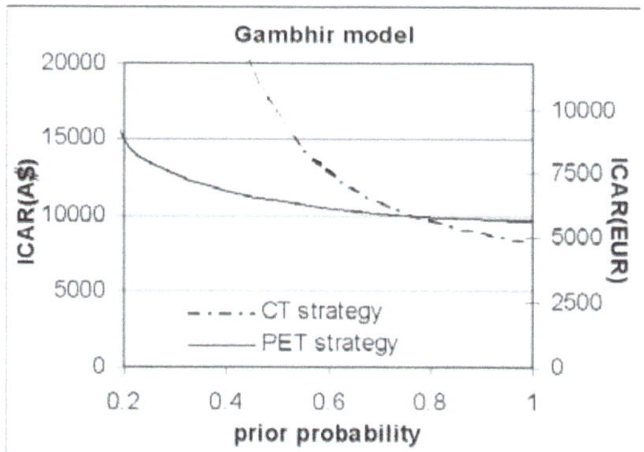

Fig. 3. One-way sensitivity analyses demonstrating the effect of prior probability of malignancy on cost-effectiveness (expressed as the incremental cost-accuracy ratio, ICAR) for CT-based (dotted line) and PET-based (solid line) strategies for the investigation of solitary pulmonary nodules. The decision tree model described by Gambhir et al. [10] has been studied using Australian data. The PET strategy is more cost-effective at low and medium levels of prior probability. The CT strategy becomes more cost-effective at high levels of prior probability (Reproduced with permission from figure 3 in Keith CJ, Miles KA, Pitman A, Hicks RJ. Solitary pulmonary nodules: Accuracy and cost-effectiveness of sodium iodide FDG-PET using Australian data. Eur J Nucl Med 2002; 29: 1016–1023, © Springer [11])

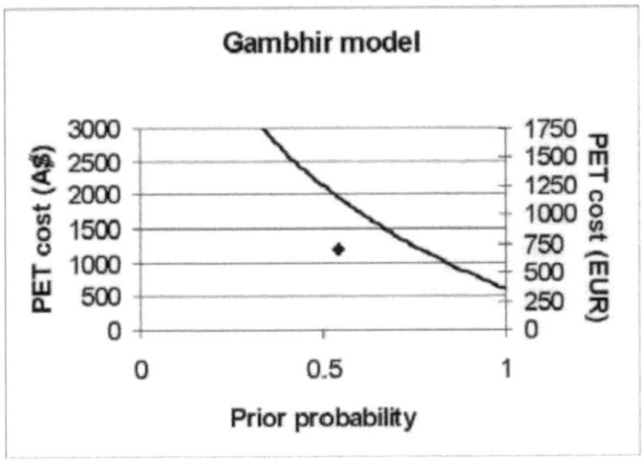

Fig. 4. Two-way sensitivity analysis demonstrating the simultaneous effects of prior probability of malignancy and cost of PET on cost-effectiveness (expressed as the incremental cost-accuracy ratio, ICAR) for the CT-based and PET-based strategies in Fig. 3. Paired values of prior probability and PET cost falling to the left of the solid line are associated with greater cost-effectiveness. The points indicated are values derived using Australian data. (Reproduced with permission from figure 4 in Keith CJ, Miles KA, Pitman A, Hicks RJ. Solitary pulmonary nodules: Accuracy and cost-effectiveness of sodium iodide FDG-PET using Australian data. Eur J Nucl Med 2002; 29: 1016–1023, © Springer [11])

ent countries might have upon the cost-effectiveness of the new imaging modality (see section 4 below). Performance of decision tree sensitivity analysis is aided by the availability of commercial software designed for the task.

Finally, if the costs and consequences of the interventions analysed occur over a period of more than one year, variations to the so-called ‚discount rate' - the rate at which future benefits and costs are adjusted to ‚present values' - constitute another important type of sensitivity analysis. An introductory discussion of the rationale for discounting, and its application in the context of sensitivity analysis may be found in [9].

32.4 Cost-Effectiveness Studies of PET in Oncology

Although limited in size, the body of literature assessing the cost-effectiveness of PET in oncology is generally larger than that found for other imaging techniques such as CT. To some extent, this situation has resulted from the pressure placed upon PET protagonists to demonstrate cost-effectiveness for PET in the face of the widespread perception that PET is a highly expensive technique. The perception of high expense is, to some degree, justified when one considers that PET developed primarily as a research tool often associated with relatively high overheads. However, recent years have seen the emergence of less expensive models for PET focusing on clinical service delivery. The cost-effectiveness literature for PET in oncology is also limited to the application of FDG. As yet, other radiotracers have not shown sufficient clinical impact.

32.4.1 The Investigation of the Solitary Pulmonary Nodule (SPN)

The investigation of SPNs has been one of the first PET applications analysed for cost-effectiveness and has now been assessed in several countries around the world. The potential for PET to be cost-effective in this clinical situation arises because its superior diagnostic accuracy over CT may enable the cost and morbidity associated with needle biopsy or excision surgery to be avoided for those patients in whom the PET scan implies benign disease.

In a USA case-tracking study in 1996, Valk et al. reported that the use of PET for characterisation of SPNs would have produced savings of approximately $2200 per patient by avoiding the costs associated with thoracotomy and/or fine needle biopsy [12]. In the same year, Gambhir et al described a US-based decision tree sensitivity analysis for the investigation for SPNs [10]. Measuring incremental cost per life year gained compared to a „watch and wait" baseline strategy, a strategy combining CT and PET was more cost-effective than CT alone over a wide range of pre-test likelihood for malignancy within the nodules (0.12 to 0.69), with potential savings of $91 to $2,200 per patient.

Miles [8] re-worked these and other studies using Australian costs and demonstrated cost-savings of between AUS$505 and AUS$935 per patient. A later Australian decision tree analysis using local data for PET diagnostic performance and pre-test likelihood of malignancy, determined savings of AUS$774 per patient when using the CT and PET strategy in preference to CT alone [11]. Sensitivity analysis showed that the cost-effectiveness, expressed as incremental cost per additional correctly managed patient, was greatest for the CT and PET strategy over wide ranges of prior probability of malignancy and PET cost (Figs. 3, 4). In Japan, Kosuda et al. [13] determined an ICER of Y218,000 ($1557) per life-year gained for a CT and PET strategy versus CT alone. In Germany, Dietlein et al. [14] have shown similar results with a lower ICER for a PET-based investigation algorithm (EUR 3218 per life year gained) than alternative strategies. For both these studies, the authors considered the cost per life year gained acceptable.

Thus, PET has proved to be cost-effective for the investigation of SPNs for a range of countries with differing health care cost structures and prevalence of malignancy within nodules. Studies have shown that PET-based strategies either dominate or produce life-expectancy gains at modest cost. CT-based strategies are only likely to be cost-effective for patients with a high pre-test probability of malignancy, for example a 75 year old male smoker (1.5 packs/day) with a 2 cm nodule (probability of malignancy 0.8 [10]). The cost-effectiveness advantages of PET for this indication may be further advanced by the fact that whole-body PET imaging may often detect incidental but significant findings, such as other malignancies, producing changes in clinical management with additional cost savings [15].

32.4.2 PET in Pre-Operative Staging of Non-small Cell Lung Cancer (NSCLC)

PET has the potential to be cost-effective in the pre-operative staging of NSCLC through identification of otherwise unsuspected tumour sites outside of the proposed operative field, either mediastinal nodal disease (stages N2 or N3) or distant metastases (stage M1). Surgery would then become inappropriate for such patients thereby saving the associated morbidity, mortality and cost.

To date, cost-effectiveness studies in this area have produced variable results, making it difficult to draw any definite conclusions about the cost-effectiveness of PET in the staging of NSCLC. The variability in results is largely due to differences in the ratio of PET costs to surgical costs and to whether PET is used for all patients or reserved to those without nodal enlargement on CT.

An early US study by Gambhir et al using decision tree analysis, found that a staging strategy in which all patients underwent PET, dominated the CT-based strategy, saving $1154 per patient with a small life-expectancy gain of 2.96 days [16]. However, in a subsequent decision tree analysis from the USA, Scott et al reported that the only PET strategy to be considered cost-effective was one in which the utilisation of PET was restricted to those patients without enlarged mediastinal nodes on CT [17]. This PET strategy did not dominate but produced a life expectancy gain at an average cost of $25,286 per year of life, hence falling below the $50,000/life-year threshold commonly quoted as an indication of cost-effectiveness in the USA (see section 2.4). Furthermore, Scott et al used Medicare reimbursement rates whereas Gambhir used institutional costs, resulting in a significantly lower ratio of PET to surgical costs in the Scott study. Nevertheless, US Medicare reimbursement rates were used in the case-tracking study Valk et al [12] which showed that PET would have produced cost-savings of approximately $1200 per patient.

Studies of the cost-effectiveness of PET in staging NSCLC in other countries include an Australian re-working of the studies of Gambhir and Valk showing more modest cost-savings of between AUS$35 and AUS$360 per patient [8]. Cost-savings remained if the prevalence of non-resectable disease was above 0.3. In Japan, a decision tree sensitivity analysis by Kosuda et al. [18] considered the whole management of NSCLC, including diagnosis of the SPN and staging of those patients with malignancy. A strategy that reserved PET for patients without enlarged mediastinal lymph nodes or distant metastases on CT, dominated the conventional imaging strategy with cost savings of between US$951 and US$1,493 and a modest gain in life-expectancy of 0.0136 and 0.0246 years. The cost-savings remained over a wide-range of values for pre-test probability of malignancy within a SPN and prevalence of non-resectable disease. A Swiss case-tracking study by Von Schultess et al. [19] demonstrated cost-savings of 1616 Sfr per patient studied by PET and CT in preference to CT with bone scintigraphy. On the other hand, a German decision tree analysis showed that use of PET for patients without mediastinal nodal enlargement on CT was more costly but produced a gain in life-expectancy with an ICER of EUR 143/life-year [20]. A similar PET strategy in a decision tree analysis undertaken by the Scottish Health Technology Board (HTB) also increased costs but with slight improvement in average life-expectancy [21]. The ICER compared to a theoretical strategy comprising surgery in all patients was $48,000/QALY but only $18,250 when compared to current management practices.

32.4.3 The Cost-Effectiveness of PET for Patients with Recurrent Colorectal Cancer

PET is potentially cost-effective in the assessment of patients with known or suspected recurrent colorectal cancer due to the technique's ability to depict small but significant tumour foci undetected by CT or other appropriate diagnostic modalities. The impact is likely to be greatest for patients under consideration of surgery for an apparently isolated metastasis, particularly isolated hepatic metastases, for which hepatic resection has been shown to result in improved life-expectancy. However, there is also the potential for improved survival for patients with raised tumour markers, such as carcinoembryonic antigen (CEA), with normal conventional imaging. Although not yet confirmed in practice, detection and early resection of an isolated metastasis in a patient with a raised CEA would be expected to have a survival benefit.

In a US case-tracking study comprising patients under consideration of surgical resection of metastatic lesions as well as patients with elevated CEA, Valk et al. [12] reported that PET contraindicated surgery in 25% of patients, representing a cost-saving of $2618 per patient. Using Australian costs, Miles [8] calculated the cost-savings produced by the management changes reported in three studies [12, 22, 23] to be lower at AUS$ 249. However, restricting the calculations to a single Australian series of patients under consideration for hepatic resection [22] produced greater cost-savings of AUS$1723 per patient. In contrast, a more recent decision tree sensitivity analysis from the Crump Institute, USA, found a CT + PET strategy was higher in mean cost by $429 per patient but resulted in an increase in average life-expectancy of 9.527 [24]. The authors concluded that PET was cost-effective as the ICER of $16,437/life-year was less than the US $50,000/life-year threshold.

32.4.4 The Cost-Effectiveness of PET for Patients with Head and Neck Cancer

PET has been reported to be cost-effective in the assessment of patients with head and neck cancer in US two studies, one using a case-tracking approach, the other decision tree analysis. Valk et al. [12] considered patients under consideration for major surgery for either primary tumours or recurrent disease. By demonstrating unsuspected distant metastases that contraindicated surgery, the use of PET produced cost-savings of $500 per patient. Hollenbeak et al. [5] used decision tree sensitivity analysis to evaluate the cost-effectiveness of PET more specifically in a group of patients with head and neck squamous cell carcinoma with no evidence of lymph node metastases on clinical examination or CT (stage N0). The potential for cost-effectiveness of PET in this group of patients arose from the ability of PET to demonstrate nodal disease not found by CT. By avoiding the morbidity, poorer survival and quality of life, and in some cases greater costs, associated with delayed treatment, the PET strategy led to improved outcomes with gains in average life expectancy and quality adjusted life-years of 0.13 years and 0.44 QALY respectively. The additional cost incurred by the PET strategy was $1107 giving ICERs of $8718/life-year and $2505/QALY. Sensitivity analysis showed that the cost per QALY remained below the $50,000 threshold if the prevalence of unsuspected nodal disease was between 16% and 36%.

32.4.5 The Cost-Effectiveness of PET in Staging Patients with Lymphoma

There have been two case-tracking studies reporting a cost-effective role for PET in the staging of lymphoma, one from the USA, the other from Germany. Both studies considered the relative costs and staging accuracy of a PET based staging compared to a conventional staging approach. The costs of subsequent management were not included in either case. The US study by Hoh et al. [25] comprised 18 patients who underwent conventional staging followed by PET. By using PET as the primary staging investigation, the accuracy of staging improved from 83% to 94% whilst the average cost of staging fell by $1685 per patient. The German study by Klose et al. [26] reported a similar increase in staging accuracy (82% to 100%) but found PET based staging to be more costly. The cost per correctly staged patient were EUR 478 for CT and EUR 3133 for PET, which would give an ICER for PET over CT of EUR 15,065 per additional correctly staged patient. The judgement as to whether PET for lymphoma staging represents value for money in the German context would require an evaluation of the financial benefits of more accurate staging.

32.4.6 Cost-Effectiveness Studies for the Utilisation of PET in Other Tumours

Evidence offered for the cost-effectiveness of PET in the assessment of other tumours includes a US case-tracking study by Valk et al. [12] comprising 45 patients with metastatic or recurrent melanoma, including 29 patients being evaluated for resectability of an apparently isolated lesion. PET contraindicated surgery in 12 (27%) patients, either by demonstrating the putative lesion to be benign or by revealing disseminated disease, representing a saving of $2175 per patient. The cost-effectiveness of PET in axillary staging of breast cancer has been evaluated in the US by Adler et al. [27] and in Australia by Miles [8]. The US study identified cost savings of $2,300 per patient compared to up to AUS$550 in Australia. However, following the advent of sentinel node detection, the role of PET in detection of axillary metastases is unclear, and to date, no study has compared the cost-effectiveness of the two techniques.

32.5 Translating the Results of Cost-Effectiveness Studies to Other Countries

The overview of the cost-effectiveness studies described above illustrates the enormous variability of results from one country to the next. Cost-effectiveness of a PET application in one country cannot be assumed to apply elsewhere. The costs of PET procedures in different countries are often compared. Yet, rather than the absolute cost, it is the cost of PET relative to any therapeutic procedures avoided by its use, especially major surgery, that largely accounts for differences in the results of cost-effectiveness studies. This ratio is particularly likely to vary between countries (Table 2) because of differences in (i) the relative prices of PET and therapeutic procedures in various countries, (ii) the approaches taken by researchers to the measurement of costs and outcomes, and (iii) variations that are due to changes to price relativities over time (e.g. the relative fall in the prices of some technologies as they diffuse). PET is more likely to prove cost-effective for a broader range of indications in those countries where this ratio is lowest. This fact provides a challenge for PET providers in those countries where surgical costs are low, to find equally cost-ef-

Table 2. Estimated ratios of PET costs to surgical costs in different countries

Country	Ratio of PET costs to surgical costs	References
USA	4%–13%	[5, 10, 16, 17]
Switzerland	6%	[19]
Japan	6%–13%	[13, 18]
Germany	11%	[20]
Australia	13–16%	[8, 11]
United Kingdom	30%	[21]

fective solutions for the provision of clinical PET services that will convince governments and health purchasers to fund this technically effective technology.

Although the costs and prices of medical inputs used in a study from one country can be substituted with costs and prices from another, the applicability of the result will remain in question due to other potential differences between populations. The prior probability or prevalence of the disease to be detected can vary considerably between populations. Yet disease prevalence can have a significant impact on cost-effectiveness (see Figs. 3, 4). The diagnostic performance of PET may also vary between countries. Assuming comparable equipment, techniques and reporting skills, the ability to detect the disease, i.e. the sensitivity, should be similar between countries. However, the specificity may vary due to differences in the prevalence of a second disease that produces false positive PET results. One example would be the variable prevalence of granulomatous disease of the lung, a recognised cause for false positive FDG uptake in a SPN, found between different areas of the USA and elsewhere resulting in varying reports of specificity of PET in SPN characterisation [10]. The effect these parameters can have on cost-effectiveness is illustrated by two decision tree analyses assessing PET in the characterisation of SPNs as described above, both using local input data. The Australian study by Keith et al. [11] produced one of the most PET cost-effective results whilst describing a disease prevalence of 0.54 and PET specificity of 0.95. The Japanese study by Kosuda et al. [13] was amongst the least favourable for PET and assumed a higher disease prevalence at 0.71 and a lower specificity value for PET of 0.79.

Case-tracking cost-effectiveness studies are only applicable to populations with a similar disease prevalence and PET diagnostic performance. Hence, the results of such studies cannot be readily transferred between one country and another. However, the sensitivity analyses incorporated into decision tree methodologies can be used to model the effects that any population differences may have upon cost-effectiveness. Ideally, local data for disease prevalence and PET diagnostic performance should be used where possible. Nevertheless, even if the precise nature of any population differences is unknown, sensitivity analysis can define the conditions under which PET is likely to be cost-effective and so provide a level of confidence that population differences could exist without eliminating cost-effectiveness. A two-way sensitivity analysis that evaluates the effects on cost-effectiveness not only of disease prevalence but also of PET costs relative to surgical costs is likely to be particularly helpful. However, decision tree analyses are only useful when the model closely approximates actual clinical practice. Demonstrating that the results of case-tracking studies are consistent with the findings of decision tree analysis can usefully validate the model employed.

32.6 Summary

Techniques for demonstrating the cost-effectiveness of PET and other imaging modalities are being used with ever-increasing frequency and now appear regularly in the medical imaging literature. It therefore behoves PET imaging specialists to become familiar with the techniques employed, along with their advantages and limitations. Decision tree analysis has emerged as a particularly powerful tool and the models employed are becoming increasingly complex to more accurately reflect actual clinical practice. To date, the available data support the cost-effectiveness of PET for a variety of applications across a range of countries despite differences in medical costs and population characteristics and is perhaps strongest for the role of PET in characterising solitary pulmonary nodules. However, much more work is required to develop the evidence base of cost-effectiveness for other PET applications. In general, the difficulty in transferring the results of cost-effectiveness studies from one country to another will mean that individual studies need to be repeated for the population of interest. Reimbursement for PET is now available in several countries around the world (see chapter 33) and it is likely that the techniques and studies reviewed in this chapter contributed to those determinations. Yet, in the final analysis, it should be remembered that the decision to fund a particular health intervention often rests on factors other than simple financial considerations.

References

1. Medicare Services Advisory Committee. Background to establishment of MSAC (updated 22/06/2001). Available at http://www.health.gov.au/msac/bckgrd.htm
2. Mackenzie R, Dixon AK (1995) Measuring the effects of imaging: an evaluative framework. Clin Radiol 50:513–518
3. Cochrane Methods Group on Systemic Review of Screening and Diagnostic Tests: Recommended Methods (updated 6 June 1996). Available at http://www.cochrane.org/cochrane/satdoc1.htm

4. Sunshine JH, McNeil BJ (1997) Rapid method for rigorous assessment of radiologic imaging technologies. Radiology 202: 549–557
5. Hollenbeak CS, Lowe VJ, Stack BC Jr (2001) The cost-effectiveness of fluorodeoxyglucose 18-F positron emission tomography in the N0 neck. Cancer 92:2341–2348
6. Dietlein M, Knapp WH, Lauterbach KW, Schicha H (1999) Economic evaluation studies in nuclear medicine: the need for standardization. Eur J Nucl Med 26:663–680
7. Birch S, Gafni A (1992) Cost effectiveness/utility analyses: do current decision rules lead us to where we want to be? J Health Econ 11:279–296
8. Miles KA (2001) An approach to demonstrating cost-effectiveness of diagnostic imaging modalities in Australia illustrated by Positron Emission Tomography. Austr Radiol 45:9–18
9. Drummond MF, O'Brien B, Stoddart GL, Torrance GW (1997) Methods for the economic evaluation of health care programmes, 2nd edn. Oxford University Press, Oxford
10. Gambhir SS, Shepherd JE, Shah BD, Hart E, Hoh CK, Valk PE, Emi T, Phelps ME (1998) Analytical decision model for the cost-effective management of solitary pulmonary nodules. J Clin Oncol 16:2113–2125
11. Keith CJ, Miles KA, Griffiths MR, Wong D, Pitman AG, Hicks RJ (2002) Solitary pulmonary nodules: accuracy and cost-effectiveness of sodium iodide FDG-PET using Australian data. Eur J Nucl Med Mol Imag 29:1016–1023
12. Valk PE, Pounds TR, Tesar RD et al (1996) Cost-effectiveness of PET imaging in clinical oncology. Nucl Med Biol 23:737–743
13. Kosuda S, Ichihara K, Watanabe M, Kobayashi H, Kusano S (2000) Decision-tree sensitivity analysis for cost-effectiveness of chest 2-fluoro-2-D-[(18)F]fluorodeoxyglucose positron emission tomography in patients with pulmonary nodules (non-small cell lung carcinoma) in Japan. Chest 117:346–353
14. Dietlein M, Weber K, Gandjour A, Moka D, Theissen P, Lauterbach KW, Schicha H (2000) Cost-effectiveness of FDG-PET for the management of solitary pulmonary nodules: a decision analysis based on cost reimbursement in Germany. Eur J Nucl Med 27:1441–1456
15. Zhuang HM, Duarte P, Pourdehnad M, Yamamoto AJ, Loman JC, Sinha P, Alavi A (2000) Incidental findings should be included in the analysis of cost-effectiveness for evaluation of pulmonary nodules by FDG-PET. Clin Positron Imag 3:180
16. Gambhir SS, Hoh CK, Phelps ME, Madar I, Maddahi J (1996) Decision tree sensitivity analysis for cost-effectiveness of FDG-PET in the staging and management of non-small-cell lung carcinoma. J Nucl Med 37:1428–1436
17. Scott WJ, Shepherd J, Gambhir SS (1998) Cost-effectiveness of FDG-PET for staging non-small cell lung cancer: a decision analysis. Ann Thorac Surg 66:1876–1883
18. Kosuda S, Ichihara K, Watanabe M, Kobayashi H, Kusano S (2002) Decision-tree sensitivity analysis for cost-effectiveness of whole-body FDG PET in the management of patients with non-small-cell lung carcinoma in Japan. Ann Nucl Med 16:263–271
19. Von Schulthess GK, Steinert HC, Dummer R, Weder W (1998) Cost-effectiveness of whole-body PET imaging in non-small cell lung cancer and malignant melanoma. Acad Radiol 5 [Suppl 2]:S300–S302
20. Dietlein M, Weber K, Gandjour A, Moka D, Theissen P, Lauterbach KW, Schicha H (2000) Cost-effectiveness of FDG-PET for the management of potentially operable non-small cell lung cancer: priority for a PET-based strategy after nodal-negative CT results. Eur J Nucl Med 27:1598–1609
21. Bradbury I, Boynton J, Facey K, Iqbal K, McDonald C, Parpia T, Sharp P, Walker A (2002) Health technology assessment of positron emission tomography (PET) imaging in cancer management: staging non-small cell lung cancer (NSCLC). Consultation Assessment Report Health Technology Board for Scotland. Glasgow, HTBS
22. Lai DTM, Fulham M, Stephen MS et al (1996) The role of whole-body positron emission tomography with [18F] fluorodeoxyglucose in identifying operable colorectal cancer metastases to the liver. Arch Surg 131:703–707
23. Delbeke D, Vitola JV, Sandler MP et al (1997) Staging recurrent metastatic colorectal cancer with PET. J Nucl Med 38:1196–1201
24. Park KC, Schwimmer J, Shepherd JE, Phelps ME, Czernin JR, Schiepers C, Gambhir SS (2001) Decision analysis for the cost-effective management of recurrent colorectal cancer. Ann Surg 233:310–319
25. Hoh CK, Glapsy J, Rosen P, Dahlbom M, Lee SJ et al (1997) Whole-body FDG-PET imaging for staging of Hodgkin's disease and lymphoma. J Nucl Med 38:343–348
26. Klose T, Leidl R, Buchmann I, Brambs HJ, Reske SN (2000) Primary staging of lymphomas: cost-effectiveness of FDG-PET versus computed tomography. Eur J Nucl Med 27:1457–1464
27. Adler LP, Faulhaber PF, Schnur KC et al (1997) Axillary lymph node metastases: screening with [F-18] 2-deoxy-2-fluoro-D-glucose (FDG) PET. Radiology 203:323–327

PET Reimbursement: Europe

M. Dietlein

Reimbursement of the "dedicated" PET with a full-ring detector system and of the coincidence gamma-camera differs both among European countries and between regions within countries. In most European countries the regulations of reimbursement are under discussion. However, there is an increasing tendency for national or social insurances to cover the well-documented PET indications in oncology.

The following data is based on a questionnaire sent in January 2003 to those PET institutions which published clinical PET studies in international journals between 1998 and 2002. Data have been gathered from Belgium, the Netherlands, France, the United Kingdom, Italy, Spain, Finland, Switzerland, Austria and Germany. The references to the personal communication were given with consent in the questionnaires. The other answers of the PET centres were not cited but evaluated. If the information received from the same country was divergent in the questionnaires the data were re-evaluated by the authors (Dietlein and Schicha 2003). Therefore the data of each country were not always identical to the regulations described in the references.

Table 1. The number of PET institutions in European countries in January 2003 (modified from Dietlein and Schicha 2003)

Country	Number of PET institutions
Germany	>60 in university hospitals, in private institutions and non-university hospitals
Austria	Eight dedicated PET units 12 coincidence cameras
Belgium	13 recognized PET institutions (six university hospitals, six private institutions) Five PET institutions without official authorization
Italy	18
Spain	15
France	11 An increase to 20 PET institutions by the end of 2003 and to 60 PET institutions (relation PET to inhabitants 1:1,000,000) in the next 4 years was predicted by the experts
Switzerland	7
United Kingdom	6[a]
Netherlands	Four dedicated PET unit One mobile PET unit One coincidence camera
Finland	One dedicated PET unit Six coincidence cameras

[a] A total of 14 PET institutions was reported by the German Wissenschaftsrat in 2000

33.1.1 Relation of PET Institutions to Inhabitants

The relation of PET institutions to inhabitants ranged from 1:500,000 (*Belgium*) and 1:1,000,000 (*Germany, Austria, Switzerland*) to 1:4,000,000 (*Italy, Spain, France, the Netherlands*). Details are reported in Table 1. At the beginning of 2003 the relation in *France* was only 1:5,000,000, but a rapid increase of PET institutions to the relation of 1:1,000,000 was predicted by experts. The relation of approximately 1:1,000,000 was already reached in *Germany, Austria* and *Switzerland*. In Germany and Austria there was no regular financing by the national insurance and it seemed that the high capacity of the already installed PET machines rendered the regulations of reimbursement more difficult.

33.1.2 Procedure of Reimbursement

The procedures of refinancing varied from country to country. In *France* a sum of 450,000 EUR per year was granted to the public hospitals. Therefore, the cancer patients are covered up to 100 % by the public social security. In France, two PET machines were used in private practices. These practices were able to reach an agreement with the social insurance. In *Belgium* the reimbursement was two-fold, differentiating between recognized and not recognized PET centres, as well as to listed and other not listed indications. Each recognized PET centre received a direct financial contribution from the Belgian state of approximately 446,000 EUR per year. This amount had been calculated on a basis of 1000 patients scanned per year. Each procedure within the listed indications was additionally reimbursed by 150 EUR plus 173 EUR for the tracer FDG. Thus, the reimbursement was 446 EUR + 150 EUR + 173 EUR = 769 EUR per procedure with regard to the recognized indications.

For all other indications the recognized PET centres received 250 EUR plus 29 EUR per procedure. The PET centres which were not recognized were allowed to charge 250 EUR plus 29 EUR per examination, regardless of indication.

In *Italy*, *Switzerland* and the *Netherlands* the fee for a PET examination performed in an in-patient setting was included either in the DRG rate („diagnosis related groups") or in the general hospital flat fee. A separate reimbursement was paid on an out-patient basis in these countries. In *Germany* and *Austria* PET was generally not covered if the patient was insured by the national health insurance, whereas reimbursement was unproblematic in private care. In view of the "federalism" in Germany there were some exceptions: PET would be covered in some out-patients (1225 EUR) if the examination was recommended to an individual patient by the experts of the national insurance service, but their interpretation of the evidence of the published PET studies was heterogeneous and less than 20% of the indications proposed were accepted. Another exception was that a fixed sum of about 320 EUR would be paid if PET was performed in out-patients within an interval between 5 days prior to hospitalisation and 14 days after discharge from hospital. But this special regulation will be stopped as soon as the DRG system is implemented in Germany in 2003/2004. In some regions of Germany, university hospitals or non-university hospitals received a fixed annual financial contribution for an annually calculated number of patients. But the majority of the PET examinations in university hospitals were covered by the medical faculties. In Germany the reimbursement of PET would be rejected by the national insurance if patients were included in clinical trials.

33.1.3 Accepted Indications for FDG-PET

The indications mainly used or reimbursed are shown in Table 2. In *Belgium* a lower fee for the PET examination was covered if the not listed indication gave rise to the PET examination. In *France*, *Italy*, *the Netherlands* and *the United Kingdom* reimbursement of PET in cancer patients was not restricted to official indications, but in France priority was given to lung cancer, head and neck cancer, lymphoma, colorectal cancer and melanoma. In *the Netherlands* the efficacy of PET (outcome-measurement) was evaluated for the indications: lung cancer, colorectal cancer, head and neck cancer, lymphoma, oesophageal cancer and breast cancer. The PLUS multicentre randomised trial in the Netherlands has shown that the addition of PET to conventional workup prevented unnecessary surgery in one out of five patients with suspected non-small cell lung cancer (NSCLC) (van Tinteren et al. 2002). As a consequence PET has become a standard procedure for the staging of NSCLC in the Netherlands. In *Italy* PET indications

Table 2. PET in oncology: indications reimbursed in European countries in January 2003 (modified from Dietlein and Schicha 2003)

Indication	Belgium[b]	Netherlands[a]	France[a]	United Kingdom[a]	Italy[a]	Finland	Switzerland[c]	Spain	Austria	Germany
NSCLC	+	+[e]	+[d]	+	+	+	+	+		
Colorectal cancer	+	+[d]	+[d]	+	+	+	+	+		
Head and neck cancer	+	+[d]	+[d]	+	+	+		+		
Lymphoma	+	+[d]	+[d]	+	+	+	+	+		
Melanoma	+	+	+[d]	+	+	+	+	+		
Oesophageal cancer	+	+[d]	+	+	+	+		+		
Pancreatic carcinoma	+	+	+	+	+	+				
Ovary cancer	+	+	+	+	+					
Breast cancer		+[d]	+	+	+	(+)	+	+		
Testicular cancer		+	+	+	+		+			
Thyroid cancer		+	+	+	+	(+)				
Brain tumour	+	+	+	+	+	+	+			
Others, CUP		+	+	+	+	+		+		

+, Indication accepted; (+), indication accepted but not commonly asked.
[a] No officially limited indications.
[b] In Belgium: NSCLC (diagnosis benign or malignant, D; pretherapeutic staging, St; detection and/or restaging of recurrence, Re), colorectal cancer (Re), head and neck cancer (Re), lymphoma (St, Re), melanoma (St, Re), oesophageal cancer (St), pancreatic carcinoma (D, St; Re), ovary cancer (Re), brain tumour (Re).
[c] In Switzerland: colorectal cancer (Re).
[d] Priority given to the evaluation of efficacy.
[e] PET as a standard modality.
CUP, carcinoma of unknown primary; NSCLC, non-small cell lung cancer.

Table 3. The level of reimbursement in European countries in January 2003 (modified from Dietlein and Schicha 2003)

Country	Level of reimbursement	Commentary
Belgium	769 EUR	446,000 EUR annually granted to public hospitals
Switzerland	1000–2000 EUR	Re: out-patients and private care; in-patients covered by the hospital flat rate
United Kingdom	1600 EUR	
Netherlands	1150 EUR	Separate fee interfered with the budget system in hospitals
Italy	1190 EUR	Re: out-patients; in-patients covered by the DRG system
Finland	1400 EUR	
Spain	900–1200 EUR	
Austria	1055 EUR	Re: private care
Germany	1225 EUR (exception) 1500–1900 EUR	Only if the national insurance service consented, <20 % Re: private care

were limited to those patients in whom there is diagnostic doubt regarding the presence of cancer lesions not solved by a previous morphologic imaging modality.

33.1.4 "Dedicated" PET and Dual-Head Coincidence System

What were the differences in reimbursement between a full-ring detector machine and dual-head coincidence systems? In *Finland* and *Germany* the centres using dual-head coincidence systems for FDG-imaging received charges as for SPECT.

The respondents in *France, the United Kingdom* and *Italy* were not aware of different fees for the two different techniques.

In the *Netherlands* the coincidence-imaging was only reimbursed for myocardial viability on the level of SPECT. In *Belgium* the law stated that a full-ring machine had to be used. The few centres using dual-head systems for FDG imaging received charges as for scintigraphy. In *Switzerland* and *Spain* coincidence-conventional imaging was in principle not reimbursed.

33.1.5 Level of Reimbursement

What was the level of reimbursement for a whole-body scan using FDG and a full-ring machine? The levels given in Table 3 were not directly comparable to each other because reimbursement differed between in-patients and out-patients, a separate fee interfered with the DRG system or an annual sum was granted to the recognized institutions in *France* and *Belgium*. The average reimbursed fee was approximately 1200 EUR.

References

Carrio I (2003) Personal communication
Comans EFI (2003) Personal communication
Corstens F (2003) Personal communication
Dietlein M, Schicha H (2003) Reimbursement of the PET in oncology in Europe: a questionnaire based survey. Nuklearmedizin 42:80–85
Knuuti J (2003) Personal communication
Lind P (2003) Personal communication
Lonneux M, Pauwels S (2003) Personal communication
Ribeiro MJ (2003) Personal communication
Von Schulthess G (2003) Personal communication
Talbot JN (2003) Personal communication
Van Tinteren H, Hoekstra OS, Smit EF, van den Bergh JHAM, Schreurs AJM, Stallaert RALM, van Velthoven PCM, Comans EFI, Diepenhorst FW, Verboom P, van Mourik JC, Postmus PE, Boers M, Teule GJJ, and the PLUS study group (2002) Effectiveness of positron emission tomography in the preoperative assessment of patients with suspected non-small-cell lung cancer: the PLUS multicentre randomised trial. Lancet 359:1388–1392
Wissenschaftsrat (2001) Stellungnahme zur Positronen-Emissions-Tomographie (PET) in Hochschulkliniken und außeruniversitären Forschungseinrichtungen, 13.7.2001, Greifswald

PET Reimbursement: United States

R.E. Coleman · R.D. Tesar

The utilization of positron emission tomography (PET) is increasing and its major impact at this time is on the management of oncology patients. The utilization of PET scans in oncologic patients is benefiting only a small percentage of patients who could benefit from having a PET scan. Since the initial coverage of lung cancer indications by Medicare in January 1998, several cancers are now covered by Medicare and other third-party payers. The delay in utilization relates to several factors: lack of knowledge about PET by referring physicians; lack of knowledge about PET by patients; limited number of PET scanners available; and limited number of physicians trained to read PET scans. With the recent introduction of combined PET and computed tomography (CT) devices, additional complexity in performing and interpreting PET scans is introduced. Now we have the decision to make concerning the technologist who performs the study, i.e., is it a radiologic technologist, a nuclear medicine technologist, or both, and the physician interpreting the study, i.e., is it a diagnostic radiologist alone or a nuclear medicine physician interpreting the PET scan and a diagnostic radiologist interpreting the CT scan?

In this section of the chapter, we will provide a background on the payment for PET in the United States covering the regulatory and reimbursement issues, an overview of the PET market, the costs of doing PET, and a summary of the current status of coverage.

33.2.1 Background

The first PET scans were performed in the United States in the early 1970s, soon after the introduction of CT for brain imaging. The first report of PET scans and magnetic resonance imaging (MRI) scans occurred at about the same time. MRI developed into a clinical imaging modality much more rapidly than did PET imaging. PET imaging remained as an expensive, difficulty research imaging modality at a few academic medical centers. PET was used to provide elegant in vivo studies of blood flow, metabolism, receptor density, etc. With the development of 2-F-18-2-fluorodeoxyglucose (FDG) in the late 1970s, the potential clinical applications of PET became apparent in the 1980s. The initial studies demonstrated clinical utility in the evaluation of disorders of the brain and heart. The role of PET in brain tumors was demonstrated to be the grading of the degree of malignancy and the differentiation of recurrent tumor from necrosis after therapy. The role in refractory seizure disorders was also well documented, and the potential role in evaluation dementia was demonstrated. FDG-PET myocardial viability studies were demonstrated to be very accurate for determining the patients that would benefit from revascularization procedures.

In the 1990s, the whole-body techniques for evaluating cancer patients became widely utilized and the results were very good. At that time, much concern and criticism were occurring related to the rapid increase in utilization of CT and MRI. Health care costs were increasing at an alarming rate, and the new imaging modalities were seen as a major cause in the increasing cost of medical care. Several studies and reports were published during the 1990s that were critical of the approval process for coverage of CT and MRI, and suggested that there was marked over utilization of these imaging modalities. Thus, as PET was starting to be reviewed as a clinical imaging modality, it came under heightened scrutiny compared to CT and MRI.

An issue for PET imaging was obtaining a New Drug Application (NDA) for FDG. When reimbursement was sought from the Health Care Financing Administration (HCFA), now Centers for Medicare and Medicaid Services (CMS), which administers Medicare, and other third-party payers, the status of approval of FDG by the FDA was raised. Because there were essentially no policies for reimbursement at that time, there was no commercial entity interested in producing FDG. The Institute of Clinical PET (ICP) was formed in the early 1990s to work on getting appropriate regulatory approval and reimbursement. Medicare and other third-party payers were not going to provide coverage without an NDA for FDG.

The ICP worked with the FDA in trying to develop a mechanism for approval of FDG. The FDA knew how to regulate large pharmaceutical companies, but they were unable to develop a mechanism for regulating FDG that was produced and used on a local or regional basis. In 1997, Congress changed the regulation of PET radiopharmaceuticals when it passed the Food and Drug Modernization Act (FDAMA). In that law, PET radiopharmaceuticals that were included in the United States Pharmacopoeia were given the equivalence of FDA approval. The law stated that for the next two years, the FDA must work with the PET community to develop a mechanism for regulating PET radiopharmaceuticals and that the PET community would have two years to come into compliance. The PET community is continuing to work with the FDA to develop appropriate regulatory guidelines. Thus, the process is many years behind the schedule outlined in the FDAMA.

During 1996 and 1997, representatives of ICP were interacting with representatives of HCFA concerning reimbursement. Medicare provides coverage for persons age 65 and older. Most third party payers have policies to cover at least what Medicare covers. The reimbursement by the other third party payers is determined by a variety of methods including fee for service, discounted rates and captivation. Payment for PET by Medicare was placed under a "National Coverage Determination" that made it unique from CT and MRI because PET would only be covered as a result of a formalized coverage process. There is a statement of "non-coverage" meaning that PET scans would not be paid by Medicare even if local carriers determined that the indication met medical necessity requirements unless there was a national coverage policy. PET and other medical procedures are paid by the Medicare System by several methods. If the patient is an outpatient seen in the hospital, the payment is made by a special outpatient rate through the Hospital Outpatient Prospective Payment System (HOPPS) under the Ambulatory Payment Classification (APC) at the current rate of $1768. If the patient is an outpatient seen in an imaging center independent from the hospital, the reimbursement rate is determined by the local carrier and is generally greater than the HOPPS rate – now is approximately $2100. If the patient is an inpatient, procedures performed while in the hospital are paid under one payment for the entire hospitalization under the diagnostic related groups (DRGS). The hospital determines how the reimbursement is divided amongst the departments caring for the patients under each DRG. Americans who meet financial need requirements with incomes below the poverty levels are covered under Medicaid, which is administered by the CMS.

After FDG received approval by the FDAMA, HCFA announced that it would cover FDG-PET scans for two indications starting January 1, 1998: evaluation of the indeterminate solitary pulmonary nodule and the initial staging of lung cancer. This coverage decision had a major impact on the development of PET in the United States. Indications for coverage developed by Medicare are generally covered by other third-party payers. Several of the large third-party payers have their own technology assessment panels and do their own evaluations. However, most third-party payers cover at least what Medicare does, and many cover indications not approved by Medicare.

The announcement of coverage of PET scans starting in 1998 resulted in an industry developing around the production of FDG and PET scanners. Before that time, a limited number of PET scanners were being sold. With the start of reimbursement, more scanners were sold and more money went into research and development of new scanners. Furthermore, FDG was available commercially at only a very few number of sites in the United States in 1997, and the reimbursement policies resulted in an expansion of the number of commercial entities distributing FDG and the number of sites producing FDG.

33.2.2 PET Market

Because of the reimbursement and the rapid expansion of clinical indications, the PET market grew rapidly. The number of clinical PET scans performed in 1998 was estimated at 150,000, and the number in 2002 was estimated at 650,000. The number of FDG distribution sites in the United States in 1998 was estimated at 10, and the number in 2002 was estimated at 70. Most metropolitan areas have ready access to FDG, and back-up production sites are generally available to provide FDG if a primary site has a problem.

According to National Equipment Manufacturer Association (NEMA) reports, 100 new scanners were sold in 2000, 200 in 2001 and 327 in 2002. It is estimated that PET will be a billion-dollar market in 2003. At this time, approximately 60% of all PET scanners are sold as combined PET/CT devices.

The reasons that PET only systems are being bought are the following: software image fusion can provide registration of the PET with CT or MRI images; CT adds from $600,000 to $1,000,000 to the cost of the device; and PET alone is exempt from the Stark law; thus permitting partnerships with oncology, radiation oncology and surgery groups. The reasons that combined PET/CT devices are being bought are the following: noise free attenuation correction; short duration transmission scans; shorter duration scans and faster patient throughput; anatomic lesion localization; potential added revenue from CT; competition factor (having the newest and best); adjunct to already established CT service (additional CT access); and improved registration, not only for diagnostic purposes but also for use with radiation oncology for radiation therapy planning and intensity modulated radiation therapy.

33.2.3 Costs of PET

The costs for doing PET are the capital costs for the scanner, the space for housing the scanner, waiting room, injection room, etc; staff; ancillary items, such as FDG, contrast, injectors; additional software such as for calcium scoring, lung nodule volume measurement, etc; and interpretation fees.

The following scenario is developed for leasing a PET scan that has an initial acquisition cost of $1,200, 000 and a PET/CT scan that has an initial acquisition cost of $1,900,000. The cost of FDG is $400 per dose. The total expenses for the first year for a PET/CT scanner is $1,775,011. In 2003, Medicare reimbursed $2137 for a PET scan performed in a freestanding center and $1768 for a PET scan performed in a hospital outpatient center and reimbursed under the Ambulatory Payment Classification (APC) system. The APC payment amount for a CT scan of the chest, abdomen and pelvis is approximately $280 for each body area scanned. If the scanner does 4 patients on the PET scanner per day, the revenue is $2,222,480. If 8 patients per day have a PET scan, the revenue is $4,264,000. If a CT scan is performed and billed in 30% of patients having a PET scan, the annual revenue would be $360,360 for 4 PET patients per day and $1,096,640 if 8 patients have PET scans per day.

If a center has a PET scanner without CT capability, the breakeven point is 2.23 patients per day or 580 patients per year. For a center with a combined PET/CT scanner that does not bill for the CT scan, the breakeven point is 2.92 patients per day or 760 patients per year. For a PET/CT scanner that bills for 30% of the CT scans, the breakeven point is 2.52 patients per day or 656 patients per year.

Thus, at reimbursement rates prevalent today in the United States, between 2 and 3 patients per day are needed to break even on purchasing a PET (closer to 2) or PET/CT (closer to 3) scanner. In 2001, the average number of patient studies performed on a PET scanner was 2.1. As more patient studies are performed on a scanner each day, the costs per patient decrease. It is likely that reimbursement rates for PET will decrease in the coming years.

33.2.4 Current Status of Coverage

After the initial Medicare coverage for evaluation of solitary pulmonary nodules and initial staging of lung cancer become effective in January 1998, the types of cancer and indications have increased. Starting in 1999, Medicare added colorectal cancer with rising CEA, initial staging and restaging of Hodgkin and non-Hodgkin lymphoma and initial staging and restaging of melanoma. In 2000, Medicare provided coverage for the diagnosis, staging and restaging of the following malignancies: lung cancer, colorectal cancer, head and neck cancer, esophageal cancer, melanoma, and Hodgkin and non-Hodgkin lymphoma. Brain tumors and thyroid cancer were specifically excluded from coverage in the head and neck cancer category.

In October 2002, Medicare started covering breast cancer for staging, restaging, and monitoring of therapy. This monitoring of therapy for breast cancer was the first time that this indication was approved.

A thyroid cancer indication has been approved and coverage will begin October 2003. Many other indications for FDG have been submitted including small cell lung cancer, cervical cancer, brain tumor, pancreatic cancer, ovarian cancer, multiple myeloma, gastrointestinal stromal tumors, recurrent prostate cancer, testicular cancer, and pediatric cancers. It is anticipated that these reviews will be completed in 2003, and new policies for reimbursement will occur in 2004. In addition to the petition to increase the number of cancers covered for imaging with FDG, a request for coverage of F-18 fluoride for assessing altered mineral metabolism such as occurs in metastatic disease has been submitted.

Subject Index

N

O

T

U

MIX
Papier aus verantwortungsvollen Quellen
Paper from responsible sources
FSC® C105338

If you have any concerns about our products,
you can contact us on
ProductSafety@springernature.com

In case Publisher is established outside the EU,
the EU authorized representative is:
Springer Nature Customer Service Center GmbH
Europaplatz 3, 69115 Heidelberg, Germany

Printed by Libri Plureos GmbH
in Hamburg, Germany